Advances in Anticancer Agents in Medicinal Chemistry

Volume 2

Edited By:

Michelle Prudhomme

Institut de Chimie de Clermont-Ferrand ICCF
CNRS UMR 6296 24 Avenue des Landais 63177 Aubiere Cedex
France

Bentham Science Publishers
Executive Suite Y - 2
PO Box 7917, Saif Zone
Sharjah, U.A.E.
subscriptions@benthamscience.org

Bentham Science Publishers
P.O. Box 446
Oak Park, IL 60301-0446
USA
subscriptions@benthamscience.org

Bentham Science Publishers
P.O. Box 294
1400 AG Bussum
THE NETHERLANDS
subscriptions@benthamscience.org

CONTENTS

Contd.....

FOREWORD

This eBook in the Advances in *Anticancer Agents in Medicinal Chemistry* series continues the concept put together so well in the first volume of the series. By drawing on original articles published during 2008-2010 in *Anticancer Agents in Medicinal Chemistry*, and having them updated, the volume provides up-to-date reviews on a wide range of drug classes, including marine macrolides, metal-based complexes and glycoconjugate-based vaccines. Also discussed are biological targets through which to control leukemia stem cells, mitosis, metastasis, DNA repair and estrogen receptor modulation. Michelle Prudhomme, Editor-in-Chief of *Anticancer Agents in Medicinal Chemistry*, is to be commended for this new series, and for the selection of such a wide-ranging set of interesting reviews in Volume 2.

William A. Denny
Auckland Cancer Society Research Centre
University of Auckland
New Zealand

PREFACE

In Volume 2 of the eBook series *Advances in Anticancer Agents in Medicinal Chemistry* are gathered chapters on several classes of molecules exhibiting anticancer potentialities as well as some important targets for the development of novel anticancer drugs.

Marine macrolides are fascinating molecules with a large number of chiral centers. In the first chapter of Volume 2, Antonio H. Daranas, José J. Fernández and colleagues discuss the potential of marine macrolides in cancer therapy. Various families of marine macrolides and their biological targets are presented.

Since the discovery of cisplatin, a huge interest has been paid to metal-based complexes as anticancer drugs. The second chapter by Chang-He Zhou *et al.* reviews the recent research and development of organometallic supramolecular complexes as anticancer agents. Whereas in the third chapter, Dolores Fregona and colleagues develop the potential of gold-based anticancer agents, in particular gold(III)-dithiocarbamato complexes which, due to their lower toxicity compared to the platinum drugs, could provide an interesting alternative.

In the search for anticancer vaccines, recent synthetic strategies towards glycoconjugates have been developed. These strategies and the development of glyconanoparticles are reviewed by Laura Cipolla and co-workers.

Isatin is an oxidised derivative of indole. Various substituted isatins exhibiting anticancer properties have been identified in plants and microorganisms. Isatin is a simple and excellent scaffold for the construction of new compounds of biological interest. Kara L. Vine, Lidia Matesic and colleagues summarize the recent structure-activity relationship studies on isatin-based compounds as anticancer agents.

The tripentone family represents a promising class of compounds, some of them exhibiting a potent cytotoxicity towards cancer cells. In their chapter, Patrick Dallemagne and collaborators review the different synthetic routes to tripentones and the emergence of the highly cytotoxic MR22388.

Endocrine therapy targeting to estrogen receptors (ER) and especially ER alpha has been very successful in the treatment and prevention of breast cancer. Virgil C. Jordan and co-workers provide an excellent update on the potential of selective estrogen receptor modulators.

Leukemia stem cells (LSCs) are defined as a small cell population required for the initiation and maintenance of leukemia. The chapter by Shaoguang Li and collaborators gives an overview on the development of new therapeutic strategies and drugs targeting LSCs.

Glioblastoma (GBM) is an aggressive disease associated with a poor prognostic due to a rapid migration of the GBM cells. In this review, Cory Adamson and colleagues describe various potential targets that may be exploited to inhibit the migration GBM cells.

The last chapter by Yves Pommier *et al.* is devoted to a DNA repair protein Tyrosyl-DNA phosphodiesterase 1 (Tdp1), an enzyme implicated in the repair of irreversible Top1-DNA covalent complexes. Rationale for the development of Tdp1 inhibitors for cancer therapy is discussed.

Michelle Prudhomme
Institut de Chimie de Clermont-Ferrand ICCF
CNRS UMR 6296 24 Avenue des Landais 63177 Aubiere Cedex
France

LIST OF CONTRIBUTORS

José G. Napolitano
Instituto Universitario de Bioorgánica "Antonio González", Astrofísico Fco. Sánchez 2, Universidad de La Laguna, La Laguna 38206, Canary Islands, Spain

Antonio H. Daranas
Departamento de Ingeniería Química y Tecnología Farmacéutica, Astrofísico Fco. Sánchez 2, Universidad de La Laguna, La Laguna 38071, Canary Islands, Spain

Manuel Norte
Instituto Universitario de Bioorgánica "Antonio González", Astrofísico Fco. Sánchez 2, Universidad de La Laguna, La Laguna 38206, Canary Islands, Spain

José J. Fernández
Instituto Universitario de Bioorgánica "Antonio González", Astrofísico Fco. Sánchez 2, Universidad de La Laguna, La Laguna 38206, Canary Islands, Spain

Cheng-He Zhou
Laboratory of Bioorganic & Medicinal Chemistry, School of Chemistry and Chemical Engineering, Southwest University, Chongqing 400715, P.R. China

Hui-Zhen Zhang
Laboratory of Bioorganic & Medicinal Chemistry, School of Chemistry and Chemical Engineering, Southwest University, Chongqing 400715, P.R. China

Sheng-Feng Cui
Laboratory of Bioorganic & Medicinal Chemistry, School of Chemistry and Chemical Engineering, Southwest University, Chongqing 400715, P.R. China

Jing-Song Lv
Laboratory of Bioorganic & Medicinal Chemistry, School of Chemistry and Chemical Engineering, Southwest University, Chongqing 400715, P.R. China

Cong-Yan Yan
Laboratory of Bioorganic & Medicinal Chemistry, School of Chemistry and Chemical Engineering, Southwest University, Chongqing 400715, P.R. China

Kun Wan
Laboratory of Bioorganic & Medicinal Chemistry, School of Chemistry and Chemical Engineering, Southwest University, Chongqing 400715, P.R. China

Yi-Yi Zhang
Laboratory of Bioorganic & Medicinal Chemistry, School of Chemistry and Chemical Engineering, Southwest University, Chongqing 400715, P.R. China

Shao-Lin Zhang
Laboratory of Bioorganic & Medicinal Chemistry, School of Chemistry and Chemical Engineering, Southwest University, Chongqing 400715, P.R. China

Gui-Xin Cai
Laboratory of Bioorganic & Medicinal Chemistry, School of Chemistry and Chemical Engineering, Southwest University, Chongqing 400715, P.R. China

Rong-Xia Geng
Laboratory of Bioorganic & Medicinal Chemistry, School of Chemistry and Chemical Engineering, Southwest University, Chongqing 400715, P.R. China

Guri L.V. Damu
Laboratory of Bioorganic & Medicinal Chemistry, School of Chemistry and Chemical Engineering, Southwest University, Chongqing 400715, P.R. China

Luca Ronconi
The Biomedicinal Chemistry Research Group, Department of Chemical Sciences, University of Padova, Padova, Italy

Chiara Nardon
The Biomedicinal Chemistry Research Group, Department of Chemical Sciences, University of Padova, Padova, Italy

Giulia Boscutti
The Biomedicinal Chemistry Research Group, Department of Chemical Sciences, University of Padova, Padova, Italy

Dolores Fregona
The Biomedicinal Chemistry Research Group, Department of Chemical Sciences, University of Padova, Padova, Italy

Luca Gabrielli
Department of Biotechnology and Biosciences, University of Milano-Bicocca, P.za della Scienza 2, 20126 Milano, Italy

Alice Capitoli
Department of Biotechnology and Biosciences, University of Milano-Bicocca, P.za della Scienza 2, 20126 Milano, Italy

Laura Russo
Department of Biotechnology and Biosciences, University of Milano-Bicocca, P.za della Scienza 2, 20126 Milano, Italy

David Bini
Department of Biotechnology and Biosciences, University of Milano-Bicocca, P.za della Scienza 2, 20126 Milano, Italy

Francesca Taraballi
Department of Biotechnology and Biosciences, University of Milano-Bicocca, P.za della Scienza 2, 20126 Milano, Italy

Cristina Lupo
Department of Biotechnology and Biosciences, University of Milano-Bicocca, P.za della Scienza 2, 20126 Milano, Italy

Laura Cipolla
Department of Biotechnology and Biosciences, University of Milano-Bicocca, P.za della Scienza 2, 20126 Milano, Italy

Kara L. Vine
School of Biological Sciences, University of Wollongong, Wollongong, NSW, 2522, Australia

Lidia Matesic
Life Sciences Division, Australian Nuclear Science and Technology Organisation, Lucas Heights, NSW, 2234, Australia

Julie M. Lock
Intelligent Polymer Research Institute, University of Wollongong, Wollongong, NSW, 2522, Australia

Danielle Skropeta
Centre for Medicinal Chemistry, University of Wollongong, Wollongong, NSW, 2522, Australia

Christophe Rochais
Université de Caen Basse-Normandie, CERMN EA 4258 – FR CNRS 3038 INC3M – SF 4206 ICORE, Bd Becquerel 14032 Caen Cedex, France

Sylvain Rault
Université de Caen Basse-Normandie, CERMN EA 4258 – FR CNRS 3038 INC3M – SF 4206 ICORE, Bd Becquerel 14032 Caen Cedex, France

Patrick Dallemagne
Université de Caen Basse-Normandie, CERMN EA 4258 – FR CNRS 3038 INC3M – SF 4206 ICORE, Bd Becquerel 14032 Caen Cedex, France

Surojeet Sengupta
Department of Oncology, Lombardi Cancer Center, Georgetown University Medical Center, Washington, DC 20057, USA

Jing Peng
Fox Chase Cancer Center, Philadelphia, PA 19111-2497, USA

Virgil C. Jordan
Department of Oncology, Lombardi Cancer Center, Georgetown University Medical Center, Washington, DC 20057, USA

Yaoyu Chen
Division of Hematology/Oncology, Department of Medicine, University of Massachusetts Medical School, 364 Plantation Street, Worcester, MA 01605, USA

Cong Peng
Division of Hematology/Oncology, Department of Medicine, University of Massachusetts Medical School, 364 Plantation Street, Worcester, MA 01605, USA

Dongguang Li
Division of Hematology/Oncology, Department of Medicine, University of Massachusetts Medical School, 364 Plantation Street, Worcester, MA 01605, USA

Shaoguang Li
Division of Hematology/Oncology, Department of Medicine, University of Massachusetts Medical School, 364 Plantation Street, Worcester, MA 01605, USA

Ranjith Babu
Preston Robert Tisch Brain Tumor Center, Departments of Surgery (Neurosurgery) and Neurobiology, Duke University; Neurosurgery Section, Durham VA Medical Center, NC 27710, USA

Chunhui Di
Preston Robert Tisch Brain Tumor Center, Departments of Surgery (Neurosurgery) and Neurobiology, Duke University; Neurosurgery Section, Durham VA Medical Center, NC 27710, USA

Austin K. Mattox
Preston Robert Tisch Brain Tumor Center, Departments of Surgery (Neurosurgery) and Neurobiology, Duke University; Neurosurgery Section, Durham VA Medical Center, NC 27710, USA

Steve Harward
Preston Robert Tisch Brain Tumor Center, Departments of Surgery (Neurosurgery) and Neurobiology, Duke University; Neurosurgery Section, Durham VA Medical Center, NC 27710, USA

Cory Adamson
Preston Robert Tisch Brain Tumor Center, Departments of Surgery (Neurosurgery) and Neurobiology, Duke University; Neurosurgery Section, Durham VA Medical Center, NC 27710, USA

Thomas S. Dexheimer
NIH Chemical Genomics Center, National Center for Advancing Translational Sciences, National Institutes of Health, 9800 Medical Center Dr., Rockville, MD 20850, USA

Yves Pommier
Laboratory of Molecular Pharmacology, Center for Cancer Research, National Cancer Institute, National Institutes of Health, 37 Convent Dr., Building 37, Room 5068, Bethesda, Maryland, MD 20892-4255, USA

Shar-yin N. Huang
Laboratory of Molecular Pharmacology, Center for Cancer Research, National Cancer Institute, National Institutes of Health, 37 Convent Dr., Building 37, Room 5068, Bethesda, Maryland, MD 20892-4255, USA

Smitha Antony
Laboratory of Molecular Pharmacology, Center for Cancer Research, National Cancer Institute, National Institutes of Health, 37 Convent Dr., Building 37, Room 5068, Bethesda, Maryland, MD 20892-4255, USA

Christophe Marchand
Laboratory of Molecular Pharmacology, Center for Cancer Research, National Cancer Institute, National Institutes of Health, 37 Convent Dr., Building 37, Room 5068, Bethesda, Maryland, MD 20892-4255, USA

Advances in Anticancer Agents in Medicinal Chemistry, 2013, Vol. 2, 3-45 3

CHAPTER 1

Marine Macrolides: Blue Biotechnology Against Cancer

José G. Napolitano[1], Antonio H. Daranas[*,1,2], Manuel Norte[1] and José J. Fernández[*,1]

[1]Instituto Universitario de Bioorgánica "Antonio González", Astrofísico Fco. Sánchez 2, Universidad de La Laguna, La Laguna 38206, Canary Islands, Spain; [2]Departamento de Ingeniería Química y Tecnología Farmacéutica, Astrofísico Fco. Sánchez 2, Universidad de La Laguna, La Laguna 38071, Canary Islands, Spain

Abstract: Chemical study of marine organisms has revealed them as a rich source of natural products with unique structural characteristics and outstanding biological activities. Marine macrolides are a unique group of natural products that frequently include a highly oxygenated polyene backbone and a macrocyclic lactone as a conformational constraint. Many of them have shown unparalleled cell growth antiproliferative properties, making them valuable molecular probes for the discovery of new biochemical pathways or as promising lead compounds in the development route to new antitumor chemotherapeutic agents. This bibliographic review has been focussed on marine macrolides with strong cytotoxic activity and potential in cancer research and therapy, as well as those macrolides either in the market or currently in clinical trials and/or preclinical development.

Keywords: Marine macrolides, antitumor agents, blue biotechnology, natural products, cytotoxicity, cancer.

1. INTRODUCTION

Oceans cover more than 70% of the earth's surface and approximately 90% of the total global species live in the marine habitat [1]. The immense biodiversity of marine biosphere has proved to be an extraordinary source of new metabolites isolated from numerous organisms, including algae, sponges, molluscs, tunicates and phytoplankton [2]. Therefore, a wide range of novel natural products had been isolated during the systematic investigation of marine environments as a source of new therapeutic agents. Many of these marine metabolites not only

***Address correspondence to Antonio H. Daranas and José J. Fernández:** Instituto Universitario de Bioorgánica "Antonio González", Astrofísico Fco. Sánchez 2, Universidad de La Laguna, La Laguna 38206, Canary Islands, Spain; Tel: +34922318586; Fax: +34922318571; E-mail: adaranas@ull.es; jjfercas@ull.es

Michelle Prudhomme (Ed)

possess unique molecular architectures, but also exhibit an unparalleled range of biological activities [2,3]. Over the last forty years, pharmaceutical industry have made a continued effort aimed at the discovery of novel and clinically useful antitumor agents, many times derived from marine organisms. This task has been mainly achieved through a preclinical research focused on studies with novel agents discovered to be active against specific cancer-related targets, followed by clinical studies with the most promising compounds. In fact, most currently known antitumor natural products were initially discovered because they exhibited potent *in vitro* cytotoxicity against murine or human cancer cell lines, and it was only later that their mechanisms of action were established [3].

One of the most interesting groups of marine natural products is formed by macrolides, macrocyclic lactones which typically possess a pattern of oxygenation, alkylation and dehydration along the primary aliphatic chain that is indicative of a polyketide biosynthetic origin [4]. Marine macrolides possess some of the most intricate structures of any compounds used in medicinal chemistry research. Their structural elucidation frequently includes a challenging assignment, and determination of the stereochemistry of each individual domain embedded into the macrocyclic frame of these natural products is the main objective of several research groups. Marine macrolides have also contributed to the growth of synthetic organic chemistry, since the successful synthesis of these and related compounds commonly involve the development of new synthetic methodology [5]. Moreover, because the majority of marine macrolides exhibit potent biological activities, an important area of research in pharmacology is therefore to determine the modes of action of these compounds.

Bryostatins are definitely the best example of the importance of marine macrolides from a therapeutic viewpoint [6]. These macrocylic lactones are known to bind to C1 domain of protein kinase C (PKC) and to regulate its activity. Currently there are more than twenty bryostatins isolated from the bryozoan *Bugula neritina*, although the bacterial origin of these complex polyketides was recently established with the identification of the putative biosynthetic genes in uncultured symbiotic bacterium "*Candidatus* Endobugula sertula" [7]. The best studied and most abundant compound, bryostatin 1 (**1**), has a wide range of biological activities including immune stimulation, growth inhibition and induction of differentiation [8]. Consequently, several studies on the molecular and cellular level have been carried out involving this compound. Furthermore, in various studies bryostatin 1 has been shown to reverse multidrug resistance, restore apoptotic function, and act synergistically with other cytotoxic compounds, with motivating benefits such as an improvement in the outcome of treatment and a lowering of dosage of cytotoxic compounds, thus avoiding possible side effects [6,9]. The exceptional activity, potency, and selectivity of bryostatin 1 against several cancer cell lines make it a potentially powerful agent for cancer therapy, and therefore it is currently being evaluated alone and in combination with other chemotherapeutic agents in a number of phase II/III clinical trials.

In recent years many remarkable aspects of the chemistry and pharmacology of marine macrolides have been comprehensively studied and competently reviewed in numerous articles [3,5] and books chapters [10]. Herein, we intended to present an overview of the most representative marine macrolides currently in clinical trials and preclinical development, accompanied by several examples of macrolides with potent cytotoxic activity that could be used as lead compounds in antitumor drug design or as molecular probes on physiological studies. In this review the identified cellular and molecular targets are used to subdivide and categorise the marine macrolides according to their specific mechanisms of action. It is necessary to point out that amphidinolides, an important family of cytotoxic macrolides isolated from dinoflagellates of the genus *Amphidimiun*, have been extensively reviewed in recent years [11], and thus they have been excluded from the present review. Cryptophycins and scytophycins are also out of the scope of this review, since these macrolides were originally isolated from terrestrial cyanophyte.

2. MACROLIDES TARGETING CYTOSKELETON

The cytoskeleton is an intricate network of protein filaments that provides structure and organization to the cytoplasm and determines the shape of eukaryotic cells. Small molecules able to act on the cytoskeleton alter the abnormal growth properties of tumor cells, their ability to adhere to tissue, and their increased ability to metastasize. Therefore, proteins involved in intracellular trafficking, intracellular organization and cell division represent attractive targets for development of new chemotherapeutic agents. The main mechanisms of action for the majority of marine macrolides consist on interfering with the polymerization dynamics of two major components of the cytoskeleton: actin and tubulin subunits, which polymerize into microfilaments and microtubules, respectively.

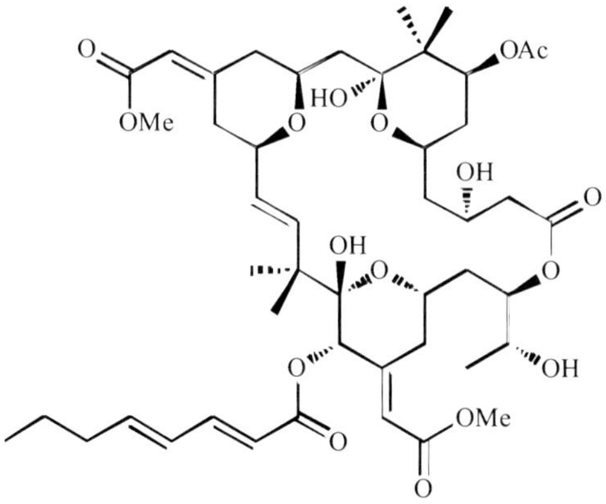

1

2.1. Macrolides Targeting Actin

Actin is the most abundant intracellular protein in eukaryotic cells. Actin filaments (F-actin), in the form of a right handed double-stranded helix, are formed by assembly of globular (G-actin) monomer subunits in a head-to-tail orientation. The actin cytoskeleton plays a critical role in many pathogenic cellular processes such as angiogenesis, cell adhesion, intracellular transportation, cytokinesis and metastasis. For this reason, actin cytoskeleton represents a key target in anticancer drug development.

Latrunculins A and B (**2-3**) were the first marine macrolides identified as actin-binding agents. These 2-thiazolidinone-containing 16-membered macrocyclic lactones, isolated from the Red Sea sponge *Latrunculia magnifica* [12], were found to cause major alterations in specific cytoskeletal proteins, inducing changes in morphology of NI1-115 neuroblastoma and 3T3 mouse fibroblast cells at submicromolar concentrations [13]. The relative configuration of latrunculins was extrapolated from that of latrunculin A methyl acetal derivative, while the absolute stereochemistry was secured by X-ray diffraction [13,14]. Later it was shown that latrunculin A affects the polymerization of actin *in vitro* forming a 1:1 molar complex with G-actin, thereby disrupting microfilament organization [15,16]. An interesting model of binding of these macrolides to actin was soon constructed using the crystal structure of actin in complex with gelsolin binding protein. This model suggested that latrunculin A binds in the interface between subdomains 2 and 4 and clamps the ATP binding site [17]. Further studies confirmed this assumption through the determination of the first X-ray crystallographic structure of actin in the absence of other actin-binding proteins. The actin-latrunculin A complex represents the first example of successful use of a marine natural product inhibitor of actin polymerization to stabilize actin for purposes of crystallization [18]. It is noteworthy that many of the studies that have identified roles of the actin cytoskeleton in different biological systems have made use of latrunculins as molecular probes. For example, latrunculin B was used in the work that established the critical and previously unknown role of the actin cytoskeleton in spindle orientation [19].

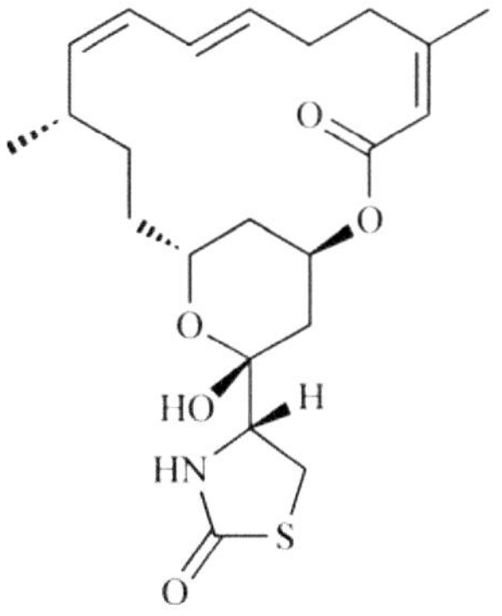

2

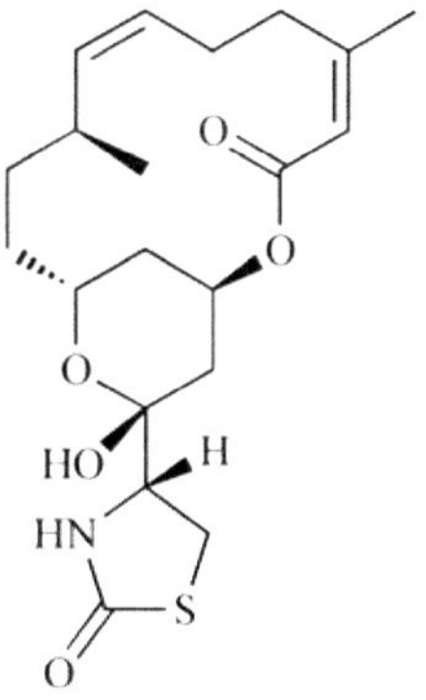

3

Trisoxazole-containing macrolides are among the better-characterized specific inhibitors of actin filaments network. This family of marine toxins comprises more than thirty 28-membered macrocyclic lactones bearing an unusual trisoxazole moiety and an aliphatic side chain with an *N*-methylformyl terminus. Some of the most representative members of this family of compounds are ulapualides and kabiramides, isolated from egg masses of the nudibranch *Hexabranchus sanguineus* [20,21], mycalolides obtained from the Japanese sponge *Mycale sp.* and the stony coral *Tubastrea faulkneri* [22], halichondramides and halishigamides purified from sponges of the genus *Halichondria* [23,24] and jaspisamides, from the Okinawan sponge *Jaspis sp.* [25]. The relative and absolute stereochemistry of these potent cytotoxic and antifungal macrolides were determined *via* the total synthesis of a diastereomer of ulapualide A (**4**) [26], followed by the asymmetric synthesis of some degradation products of the mycalolides [27]. Further synthetic efforts concluded with the first total synthesis of mycalolide A (**5**), which confirmed the stereochemical assignment of this natural product [28].

Mycalolide B (**6**) was the first trisoxazole-containing macrolide reported to interfere with normal actin filament dynamics and regulation, suppressing actin-activated myosin Mg^{2+}-ATPase activity [29]. Later it was shown that this compound binds to G-actin with a 1:1 molecular ratio, inhibiting its polymerization. Moreover, kinetics studies of depolymerization, in combination with viscometry and electron microscopy observation, suggested that mycalolide B severs F-actin [30]. Recent X-ray crystallographic structures of actin in complex with kabiramide C (**7**) and jaspisamide A (**8**) not only established the absolute stereochemistry of these toxins, but also revealed the main interactions between actin and the entire family of trisoxazole-containing macrolides: the three contiguous oxazole rings interacts with actin subdomain 1, while the aliphatic side chain is inserted into the hydrophobic cavity between subdomains 1 and 3, the same binding site occupied by actin-capping domain of the gelsolin superfamily of proteins [31]. Furthermore, competition-binding studies showed that kabiramide C binds to the same site on G-actin as gelsolin domain 1, suggesting that these small molecules might mimic an entire class of actin-binding proteins [32]. The recent publication of the high-resolution crystal structure of ulapualide A in a complex with G-actin has also revealed the absolute configuration of this compound [33].

Swinholide A (**9**) is a potent actin-binding macrolactone isolated from the sponge *Theonella swinhoei*. This potent cytotoxic and antifungal compound was originally formulated as a 22-membered macrolide [34], although its structure was later revised to a 44-membered dimeric dilactone [35]. The absolute stereochemistry of swinholide A was determined by the X-ray crystal analysis of its di-*p*-bromobenzylated diketone derivative, providing also some conformational characteristics of this family of C_2 symmetric macrodiolides [36]. The first total synthesis of swinholide A was achieved using a macrocyclization to generate the 44-membered ring, and was accompanied by the synthesis of the erroneous monomeric structure initially proposed, designated hemiswinholide A [37].

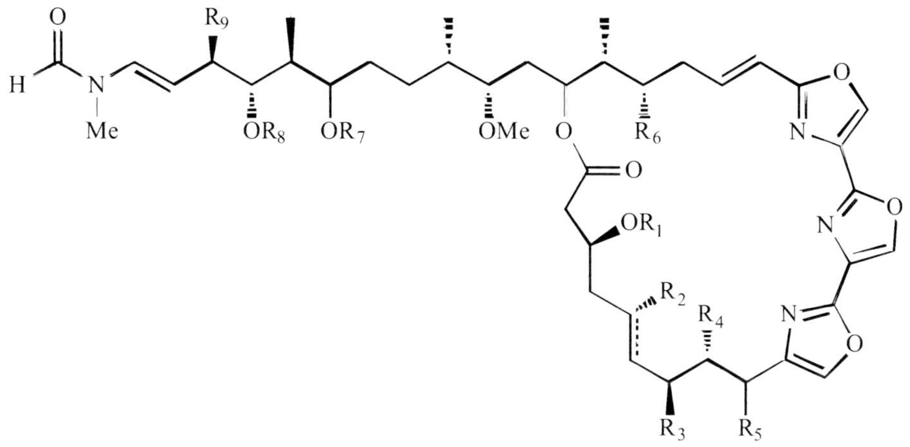

Compound	R_1	R_2	R_3	R_4	R_5	R_6	R_7	R_8	R_9	$\Delta_{5,6}$
Ulapualide A (**4**)	H	H	O	H	α-Me	OMe	O	Ac	Me	
Mycalolide A (**5**)	H	H	O	Me	β-OMe	OMe	O	Ac	Me	x
Mycalolide B (**6**)	H	H	O	Me	β-OMe	OMe	2,3-dimethoxypropanoyl	Me	Me	x
Kabiramide C (**7**)	$CONH_2$	Me	OH	Me	α-OMe	OMe	O	Me	Me	
Jaspisamide A (**8**)	H	OH	O	Me	β-OMe	H	O	Me	H	

Further studies revealed that swinholide A disrupts the actin cytoskeleton *in vivo*, inhibits the polymerization by sequestering G-actin (with one macrolide molecule binding with two actin monomers), and catalyzes depolymerization of actin filaments *in vitro* [38]. Misakinolide A (**10**, also known as bistheonellide A) is a 40-membered macrodiolide structurally similar to swinholide A, lacking only the C2-C3 and C2'-C3' double bonds [39]. Like swinholide A, misakinolide A is a readily cell permeable compound, it has a high specificity for G-actin and forms 1:2 complex with actin monomers, suggesting that the modification in the ring size does not change the actin-binding site. However, this compound does not sever F-actin [40,41]. Recently, taking advantage of the fact that actin complexed with swinholide A does not polymerize, the structure of the actin-swinholide A complex was determined by X-ray diffraction (Fig. **1**), revealing that swinholide A binds to actin monomers at the same region as trisoxazole-containing toxins, and thus highlighting the importance of exposed subdomains 1 and 3 in actin polymerization [42].

9, n = 1
10, n = 2

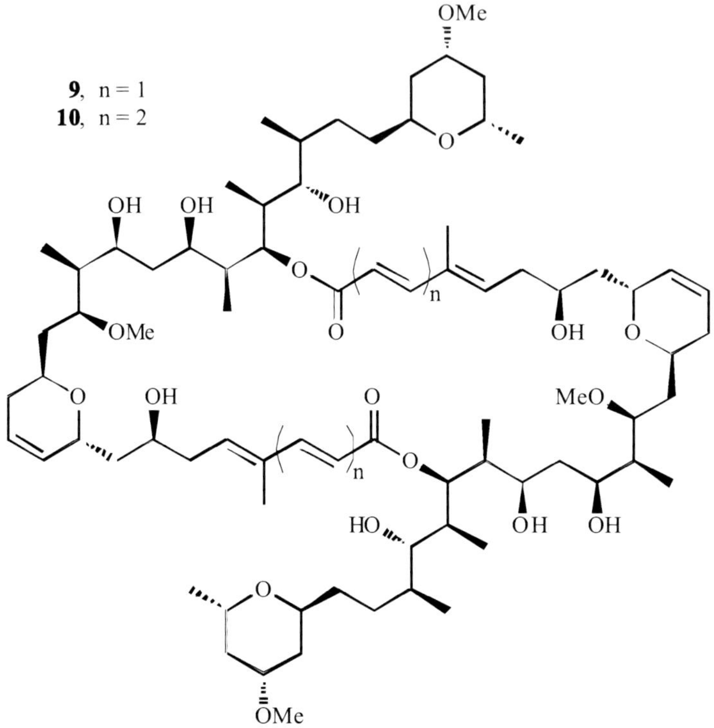

Sphinxolides (**11-13**), isolated from an unidentified nudibranch and from New Caledonian sponge *Neosiphonia superstes* [43], and reidispongiolides (**14-16**), obtained from New Caledonian sponge *Reidispongia coerulea* [44], are potent cytotoxins with several structural similarities to the macrocyclic frame of swinholide A (**9**), while their side chain holds an *N*-methylformyl moiety like trisoxazole macrolides. The relative configuration of these metabolites, often obtained in minute quantities from their natural sources, was proposed on the basis of a combination of NMR spectroscopy and computational methods [45]. This approach relying in quantum mechanics calculations and spin-spin coupling constants measurement has become an important tool for assignment of the relative configuration of flexible systems, being especially suitable for carbon frameworks containing several adjacent stereogenic centres [46].

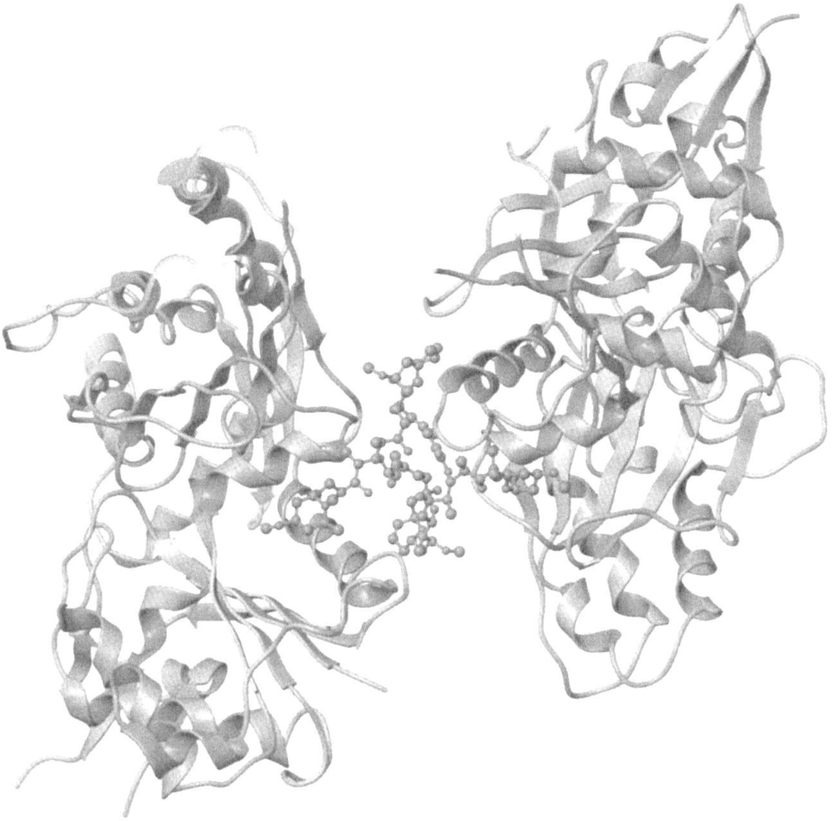

Fig. (1). X-ray structure of actin-swinholide A complex.

Pharmacological studies have shown that the cytotoxic activity of these 26-membered macrolides is associated with cell cycle arrest in G_2/M phase and induction of apoptosis. In addition, sphinxolides circumvented multidrug resistance and caused rapid loss of microfilaments in culture cells without affecting microtubule organization [47], demonstrating that these natural occurring compounds are potent and specific actin-binding agents that could be useful in the treatment of drug-resistant tumors. The recent determination of the actin-bound X-ray structure of reidispongiolides A and C (**14-16**) and sphinxolide B (**12**) has allowed not only the unequivocal assignment of the absolute configuration for each compound, but also the identification of their actin-binding site, located in the same region occupied by trisoxazole macrolides and swinholide A [48]. Recently, the first total synthesis of reidispongiolide A has been reported [49]. This achievement is an important step to assure the supply of material to support further pharmacological studies on reidispongiolide/ sphinxolide family of marine toxins, as well as a promising starting point in the design of novel analogues for structure-activity relationship studies.

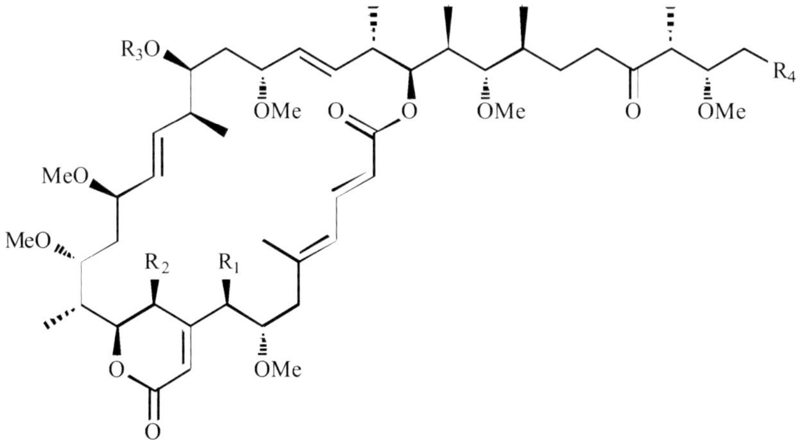

Compound	**R1**	**R2**	**R3**	**R4**
Sphinxolide A (**11**)	Me	OH	Me	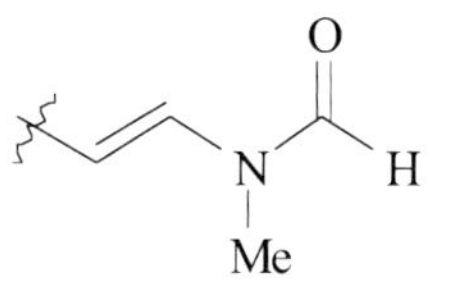
Sphinxolide B (**12**)	H	OH	H	
Sphinxolide C (**13**)	OMe	OH	Me	
Reidispongiolide A (**14**)	H	Me	Me	
Reidispongiolide B (**15**)	H	H	H	
Reidispongiolide C (**16**)	H	H	Me	CH_2COOH

Aplyronines (**17-24**) were initially purified from the Japanese sea hare *Aplysia kurodia* using a bioguided methodology. The major component, aplyronine A (**17**), exhibited strong *in vitro* cytotoxicity against HeLa-S_3 cells (IC_{50} 0.039 ng/mL) and exceedingly potent antitumor activity *in vivo* against P388 murine leukemia (T/C value of 545% at a dose of 0.08 mg/kg), Lewis lung carcinoma (T/C = 556%, 0.04 mg/kg), Ehrlich carcinoma (T/C = 398%, 0.04 mg/kg), colon 26 carcinoma (T/C = 255%, 0.08 mg/kg) and B16 melanoma (T/C = 201%, 0.04 mg/kg) [50]. Soon after the absolute stereochemistry of aplyronine A was

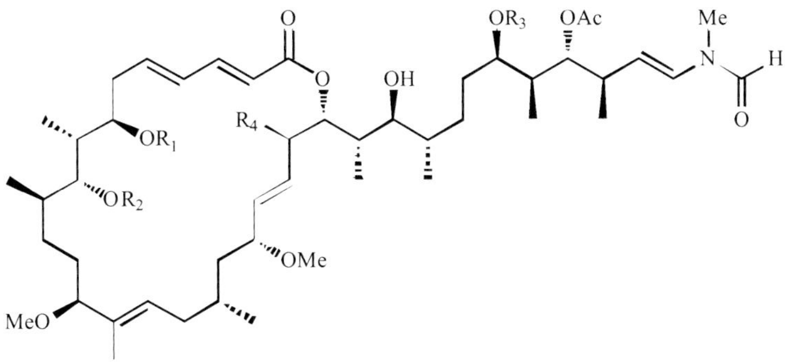

Compound	**R$_1$**	**R$_2$**	**R$_3$**	**R$_4$**
Aplyronine A (**17**)	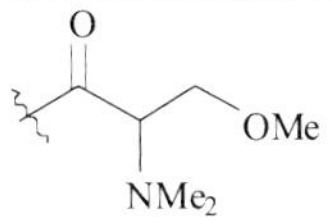	H	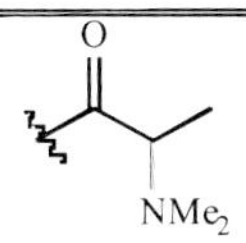	H
Aplyronine B (**18**)	H	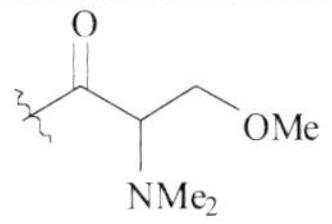	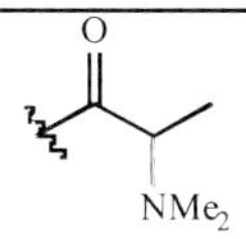	H
Aplyronine C (**19**)	H	H	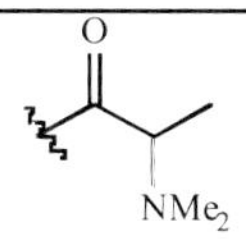	H
Aplyronine D (**20**)	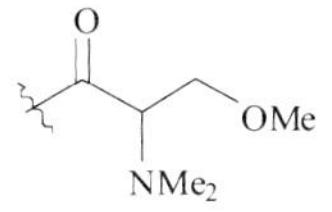	H	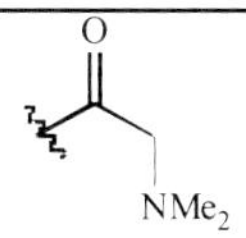	H
Aplyronine E (**21**)	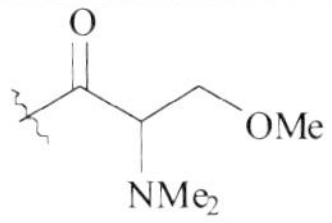	H	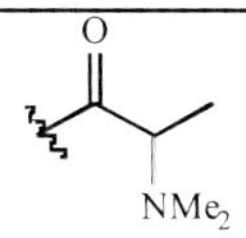	Me
Aplyronine F (**22**)	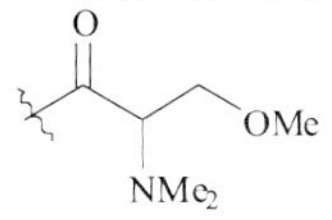	H	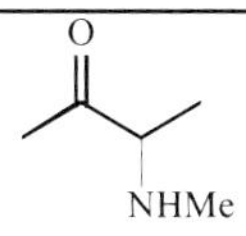	H
Aplyronine G (**23**)	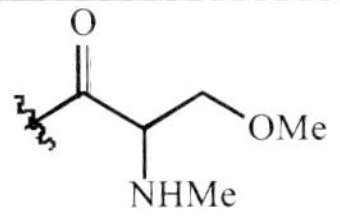	H	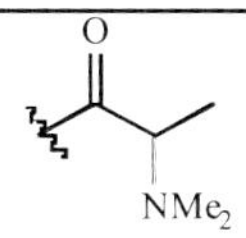	H
Aplyronine H (**24**)	H	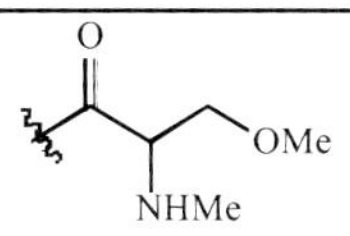	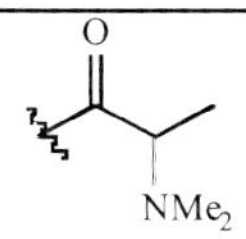	H

assigned on the basis of spectroscopic analysis and the enantioselective synthesis of degradation products [51], and the total synthesis of this 24-membered macrolide was immediately achieved by the same research group [52], followed by stereochemical assignment and the total syntheses of the minor constituents, aplyronines B-C (**18-19**) [53]. Recently, five new minoritary congeners, aplyronines D-H, were isolated. Among them, aplyronine D showed the strongest cytotoxicity (sixfold greater than aplyronine A) [54]. Additional synthetic efforts included initial structure-activity relationship studies, revealing the essential role of the side chain and the trimethylserine moiety in the potent cytotoxicity shown by aplyrorine A. Moreover, biological studies showed that this macrolide do not interact with DNA, tubulins, or cell cycle-regulating enzymes, but inhibited polymerization of G-actin to F-actin and depolymerized F-actin to G-actin [55].

Due to its strong actin-depolymerizing activity, the side chain portion of aplyronine A was later exploited as a ligand in the design of molecular probes, and further photoaffinity labelling experiments demonstrated that actin directly interacts with this structural feature of aplyronine A [56]. Recently, the structure of the actin-aplyronine A complex was determined by X-ray crystallographic analysis, revealing that aplyronine A binds to actin at the same location occupied by trisoxazole macrolides, intercalating its side chain portion into the actin molecule (Fig. **2**) [57]. Aplyronine A derivatives possessing a biotin moiety have been synthesised in order to investigate their target proteins in tumor cells. As a result, two actin-related proteins (Arp 2 and Arp 3) were found as targets of this molecule [58].

2.2. Macrolides Targeting Microtubules

Microtubules are polymers formed by tubulin subunits (a heterodimer of α- and β-tubulin) which are integral components of the mitotic spindle. Assembly and disassembly of tubulin subunits to form microtubules are processes in dynamic equilibrium. Therefore, small molecules that disturb this equilibrium can block mitosis and lead to cell death. Tubulin subunits are a familiar target in medicinal chemistry research due to the success of paclitaxel in cancer treatment. However, the development of new tubulin-binding agents is essential not only to improve the understanding of interactions between small molecules and tubulin, but also to overcome the clinical multidrug resistance phenomena.

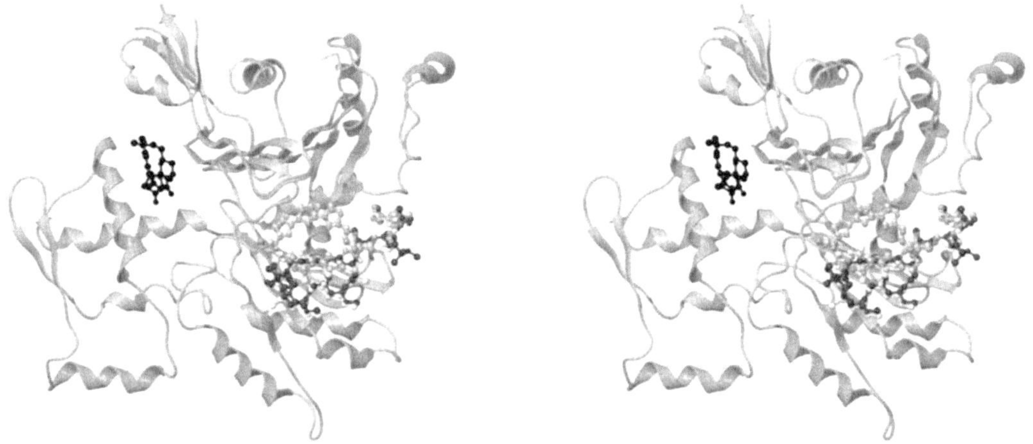

Fig. (2). Stereo view of the superimposed X-ray structures of actin in complex with latrunculin A, kabiramide C, jaspisamide A, reidispongiolide A and aplyronine A.

Halichondrins were the first marine macrolides established as powerful antimitotic agents. Originally isolated from the Japanese sponge *Halichondria okadai* [59], several members of this family of polyether macrolides have been obtained from sponges of the genera *Theonella*, *Lissodendoryx*, *Axinella* and *Phakellia* [60-65]. The complex structure of these polyketide-derived compounds was determined by X-ray crystallographic analysis [60]. Halichondrin B (**25**) was shown to be the most potent of the halichondrins, exhibiting subnanomolar growth inhibitory activities *in vitro* against numerous tumor cell lines and inhibiting proliferation of P388 leukemia, B16 melanoma, and L1210 leukemia cells *in vivo* [59]. Further studies revealed that halichondrins arrested cells in the G_2/M phase of the cell cycle and caused disruption of mitotic spindles, consistent with the antimitotic mechanism of several known tubulin-binding agents [66]. However, halichondrins are noncompetitive inhibitors of dolastatin 10 and vinca alkaloids, suggesting that these potent antimitotic agents bind to β-tubulin in a different binding site [67]. Because of their exceedingly potent biological activities, alongside with the serious obstacle of material supply, halichondrins rapidly became targets for chemical synthesis. Several approaches to their total syntheses have been reported [68], and the incessant design of structurally simplified halichondrin analogues eventually led to the discovery of the clinical candidate E7389 also known as eribulin (**32**), a potent antitumor macrocyclic ketone that inhibits vinblastine binding to tubulin in a competitive manner, in contrast to the noncompetitive inhibition seen with halichondrin B [69]. Recently, the United States Food and Drug Administration approved eribulin mesylate (Halaven ^{TM}) as a treatment for locally advanced and metastatic breast cancer [70,71]. In addition, several second-generation analogs with better bioavailability and efficacy against multidrug resistant tumors have been prepared by substitution of the 1,2-amino alcohol side chain with lipophilic fragments [72].

Spongipyrans (spongistatins, cinachyrolide and altohyrtins) were isolated by three independent research groups from sponges of genera *Spongia*, *Spirastrella*, *Cinachyra* and *Hyrtio*s using a bioassay-guided methodology [73-77]. These 42-membered macrolides possess two spiroketals systems and one bis(tetrahydropyran) fragment as prominent structural features. Their relative and absolute configurations were confirmed through the total syntheses of altohyrtins A and C (**33-35**) [78,79], followed by numerous synthetic approaches to other member of this family [80]. Spongipyrans are among the most powerful cytostatic agents tested to date in the NCI's panel of 60 human carcinoma cell lines. The most potent member, spongistatin 1 (altohyrtin A, **33**), was particularly effective against solid tumour cell lines derived from patients with melanoma, lung cancer, colon cancer and brain tumours (GI_{50} 0.02 – 0.4 nM), retaining its potency against a subset of highly chemoresistant tumours types (GI_{50} 0.03 nM) [81,82]. Spongistatin 1 also exhibited an exceedingly potent cytotoxic activity against L1210 murine leukemia cells (IC_{50} 0.02 nM) [73]. Later it was shown that spongistatin 1 inhibited glutamate-induced polymerization of purified tubulin at low micromolar concentrations [83]. Further studies revealed that spongipyrans, like halichondrins, are noncompetitive inhibitors of dolastatin 10 and vinca alkaloids [84].

Dictyostatin (**36**), a 22-membered macrolide which has some of the structural features of discodermolides, was originally isolated from the Maldivian sponge *Spongia sp.* and later from the Jamaican deep-water sponge *Corallistidae sp.* [85,86]. This compound exhibits potent cytotoxic activity toward several human

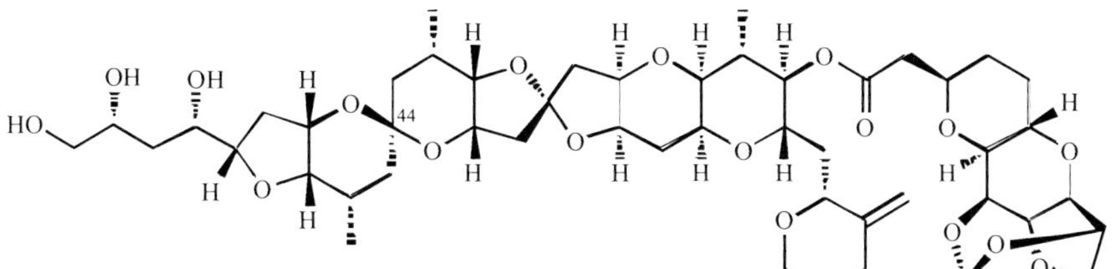
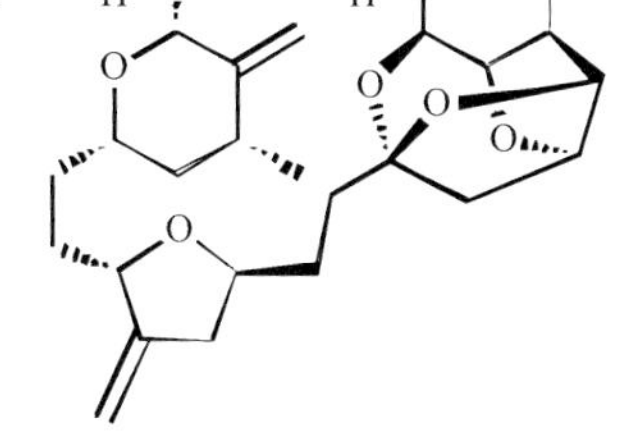

25

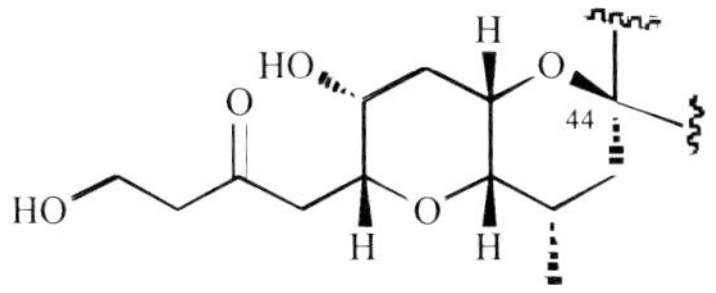

26

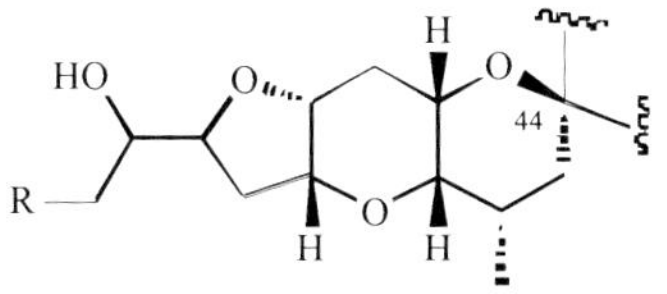

27, R = OH
28, R = Cl

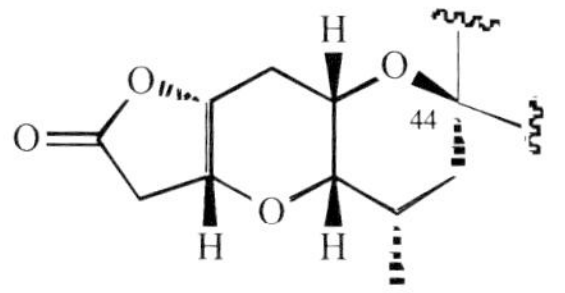

29

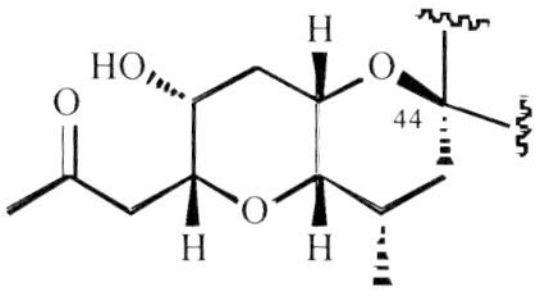

30

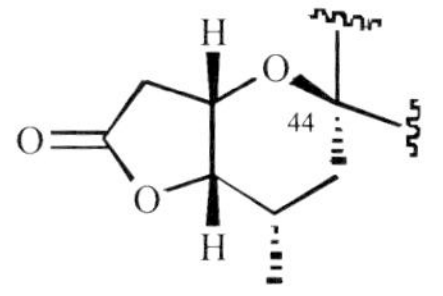

31

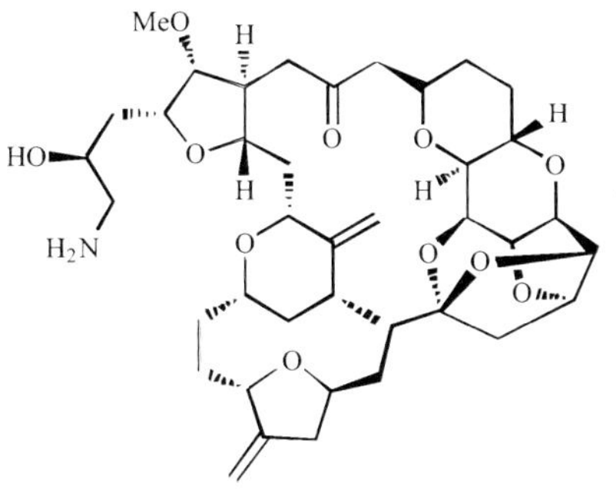

32

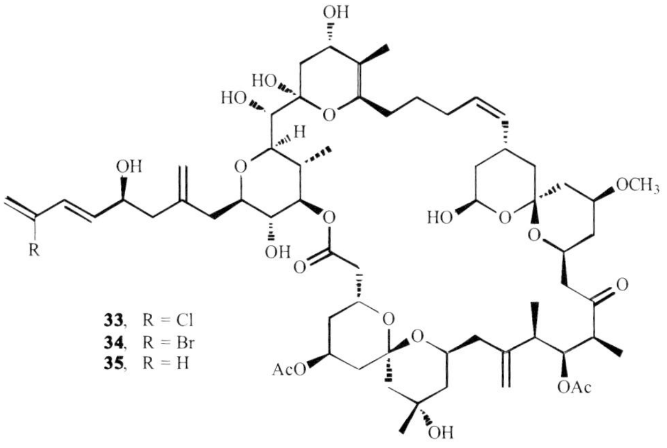

33, R = Cl
34, R = Br
35, R = H

cancer cell lines at low nanomolar concentrations, including those with multidrug-resistant phenotype. The relative stereochemistry of dictyostatin was assigned based on a combination of extensive high field NMR studies and molecular modeling [87], and soon the total synthesis of this paclitaxel-like antimitotic agent was accomplished by two different research groups [88]. Dictyostatin arrests human lung adenocarcinoma cells in the G_2/M phase of the cell cycle at concentrations as low as 10 nM, and also induces a rapid polymerization of purified bovine brain tubulin *in vitro* [89]. Further studies revealed that dictyostatin shares the same microtubule-stabilizing mechanism as paclitaxel and discodermolide, binding at β-tubulin with higher affinity than paclitaxel. These results are consistent with the idea that the macrocyclic structure of dictyostatin represents the template for the bioactive conformation of discodermolide [90]. Recent biochemical structure-activity studies with several dictyostatin analogues demonstrated that dictyostatin, discodermolide, epothilone B and paclitaxel have favourable interactions with Phe270 within the taxoid binding site on β-tubulin. Additionally, this analysis revealed that 7-*epi*- and 6-*epi*-dictyostatin are also potent microtubule-stabilizing agents, indicating that a change to the configuration of these stereocenters is well tolerated [90].

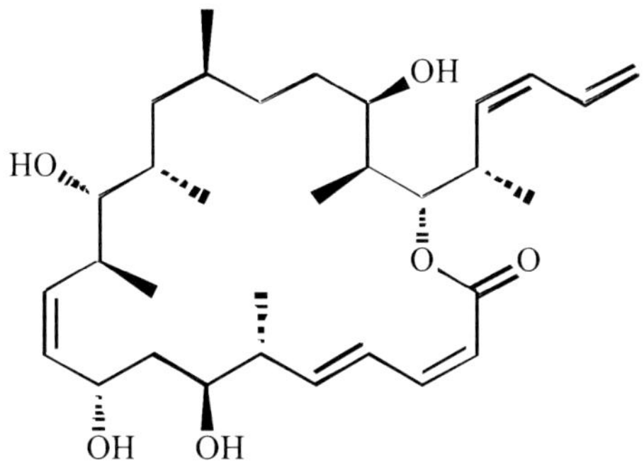

36

Laulimalide (**37**) and isolaulimalide (**38**), two 20-membered cytotoxic macrolides bearing two dihydropyran rings in their structure, were originally isolated from the Vanuatu sponge *Cacospongia mycofijiensis* [91], and later obtained from other sponges of the genera *Hyatella*, *Fasciospongia* and *Dactylospongia* [92,93]. The relative stereochemistry of laulimalides was assigned based on the analysis of spectroscopic data, and their absolute configurations were unequivocally determined *via* X-ray diffraction. The crystallographic structure also permitted a resolution of the contradictory conformational assignment made by NMR spectroscopy and revealed the conformational preferences operating in the solid state [14]. The unusual structure and interesting biological activities of laulimalide led to its total synthesis by several groups using diverse approaches [94].

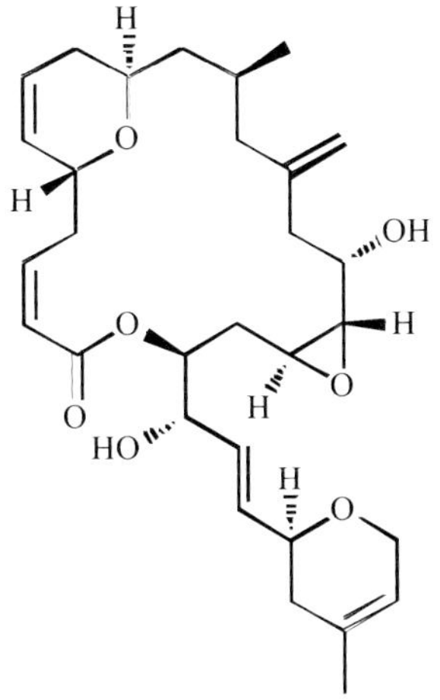

37

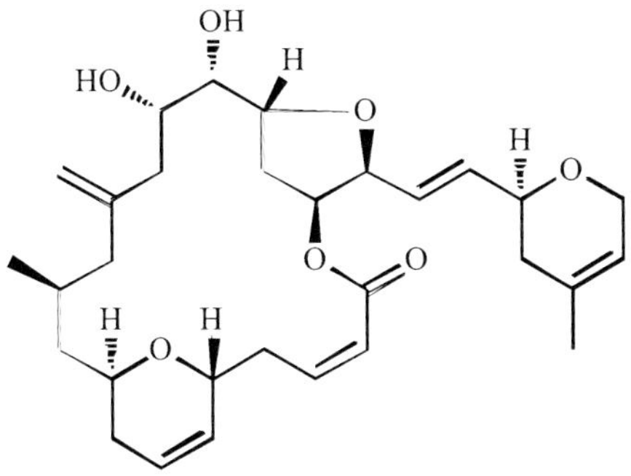

38

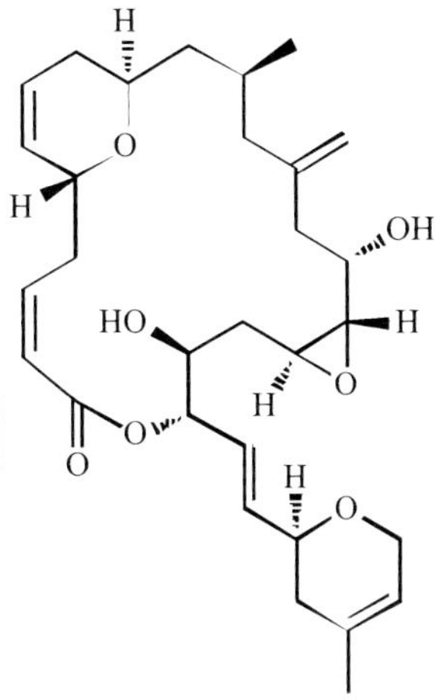

39

Laulimalide exhibit potent antiproliferative activity against several human carcinoma cell lines with IC_{50} values in the low nanomolar range, whereas isolaulimalide, a rearrangement of laulimalide formed through the acid-catalyzed attack of the side chain hydroxyl group on the *trans*-substituted epoxide moiety, is much less potent with IC_{50} values in the low micromolar range. In addition, laulimalide possess the ability to stimulate tubulin polymerization in a fashion that resembles paclitaxel [95]. Further studies revealed that laulimalide was unable to inhibit the binding of a fluorescent paclitaxel derivative to tubulin, indicating that this macrolide targets tubulin in a different location from that occupied by the taxoids. Moreover, laulimalides inhibits the proliferation of paclitaxel-resistant cell lines and has a synergistic effect on microtubule polymerization when combined with paclitaxel [96]. In recent years several laulimalide analogues as neolaulimide (**39**) had been prepared and evaluated against drug-sensitive cell lines, allowing the generation of preliminary structure-activity relationship data [97, 98]. Significantly, although these derivatives had lower potency than laulimalide, paclitaxel and epothilone-resistant cell lines were less resistant to some of these laulimalide analogues [99]. These results provide crucial information on the structural basis of laulimalide's mode of action and form the basis for the design of new analogues that could be advanced toward therapeutic applications.

Peloruside A (**40**), a 16-membered macrolide with structural similarity to epothilone, was isolated from the New Zealand sponge *Mycale hentscheli* [100]. The relative stereochemistry of peloruside A was assigned on the basis of extensive data gathered from a variety of high-field NMR experiments, while the absolute stereochemistry was established with the total synthesis of the natural product [101]. A natural congener, Peluroside B (**41**) was isolated in sub-milligram quantities from the same source and showed a comparable bioactivity [102]. Although peluroside A presents some structural similarities to the protein kinase C (PKC) binding pharmacophore of bryostatin, further studies revealed that peluroside A possesses a mode of action independent of PKC [103]. Like paclitaxel, peluroside A arrests cells in the G_2/M phase of the cell cycle and induces apoptosis. Additionally, peluroside A exhibits extremely potent cytotoxicity against several tumor cell lines and retains potency against cells lines expressing the P-glycoprotein efflux pump [104]. *In vitro* studies with purified tubulin indicate that peloruside A directly induces tubulin polymerization in the absence of microtubule-associated proteins, competing with laulimalide for the same or overlapping binding sites [105].

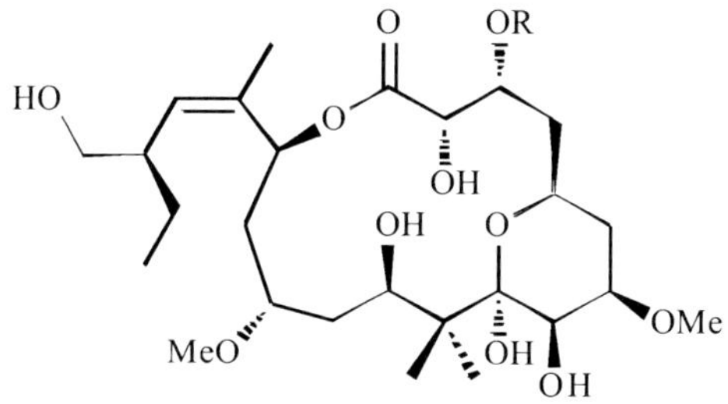

40, R = Me
41, R = H

Even though the location of the binding site(s) for laulimalides and peloruside A to tubulin is still undefined, several interesting computational approaches have been reported. Initial comparisons with tubulin-interacting drugs using docking and QSAR approaches point to a new binding site at the α subunit of tubulin [106]. Afterwards, the main conformations of peluroside A in water solution were deduced from NMR data, and a binding model between the bioactive conformation of peloruside A and the α-tubulin subunit was also proposed on the basis of molecular mechanics calculations and docking [107]. However, a new structural model of the peloruside-binding site located on the exterior of β-tubulin was recently suggested using a strategy involving comparative hydrogen-deuterium exchange mass spectrometry of different microtubule-stabilizing agents and data-directed docking [108]. Peloruside A represents a new class of antitumor agents with significant clinical potential, and thus new synthetic strategies to obtain this microtubule stabilizer have been reported [109].

2.3. Macrolides Targeting Intermediate Filaments

The cytoskeleton of cells is rich in intermediate filaments. These filaments are formed by staggered head-to-tail and side-by-side association of pairs of intermediate filament proteins such as keratins, lamins, vimentin and desmin, followed by further association to form two stranded α-helical coiled coils with globular domains at the ends. Intermediate filaments extend throughout the cytoplasm providing a mechanical support to the nuclear membrane and playing an important role in cell division, cell-cell adhesion and cell-matrix adhesion. Agents that interact with this structural framework affect morphology of invasive cancer cells and increase the risk of cell rupture. Therefore, intermediate filaments have become potentially interesting target for small molecule modulation.

Phorboxazoles A and B (**42-43**), two 26-membered macrolides with extraordinary cytostatic activity, were isolated from the methanol extract of the Indian Ocean sponge *Phorbas sp.* [110]. Both compounds inhibited the growth of most of the 60 cell lines used in NCI's assays at low nanomolar concentrations (GI_{50} 1.6 nM), and showed selectivity against solid tumor cells such as colon HCT 116 (IC_{50} 0.25 nM) [110,111]. These highly functionalized compounds possess three tetrahydropyran rings and one 2,4-substituted oxazole ring in their macrocyclic frame, with two additional cycles (one tetrahydropyran and one oxazole ring) in their side chain. The absolute configuration of phorboxazoles was determined by a combination of chemical degradation, synthesis of model compounds for NMR spectroscopic comparison, MTPA derivatization and CD measurements [111,112]. Although substantial efforts have yielded several total syntheses [113], the mechanism of action of phorboxazoles remained undefined until recent studies using fluorescent labeled derivatives, which elucidate the cellular uptake, localization and biomolecular association of these natural products. Phorboxazoles generated cell cycle arrest at S phase in HeLa cells at nanomolar concentrations, and produced a dramatic restructuring of intermediate filaments to form a large aggregate adjacent to the nucleus. Analysis of cytosolic partitions of HeLa cells treated with fluorescent phorboxazole analogues revealed that these macrolides target human cytokeratins and induce the association of these proteins with the cyclin-dependent kinase 4 (cdk4), an essential component of G_1/S phase cell cycle progression and a validated anticancer drug target [114]. Initial structure-activity relationship studies with phorboxazole analogues have shown that the entire macrocyclic core is indispensable for activity, whereas the side chain terminus can be modified without an important loss of potency [115]. The latter assumption recently led to the synthesis of an interesting phorboxazole congener with enhanced activity, chlorophorboxazole A (**44**), a potent cytostatic agent capable to inhibit several human solid tumor cancer cell lines at picomolar concentrations [116].

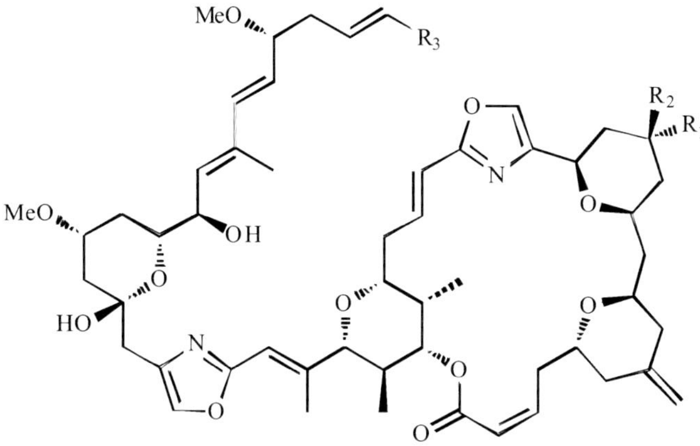

Compound	R1	R2	R3
Phorboxazole A (**42**)	H	OH	Br
Phorboxazole B (**43**)	OH	H	Br
Chlorophorboxazole (**44**)	OH	H	Cl

3. MACROLIDES TARGETING VACUOLAR TYPE (H^+)-ATPases

Vacuolar type (H^+)-ATPases (V-ATPases) are heteromultimeric, proton-translocating proteins which are located on membranes of vacuoles, endosomes, lysosomes, and other cellular organelles, as well as on the plasma membranes of certain cells, such as osteoclasts for bone degradation and macrophages for control of cytoplasmic pH [117]. These ATP-driven ion pumps are responsible for energize many different transport processes across eukaryotic membranes. Since V-ATPases appear to be involved in angiogenesis, cellular proliferation, tumor metastasis, apoptosis and programmed cell death, this enzyme system represent a plausible target from the perspective of medicinal chemistry and drug research [118,119].

Macrocyclic benzolactone enamides were the first *in vitro* V-ATPase inhibitors obtained from marine organisms. Salicylihalamides A and B (**45**, **46**), two 12-membered macrocyclic salicylates bearing a highly unsaturated enamide substituent, were originally purified from the organic extract of an unidentified sponge of genus *Haliclona* [120]. The differential cytotoxicity pattern of salicylhalamide A against NCI's 60-cell line human tumor panel did not match those of any known antitumor compounds. Following the isolation of salicylihalamides, six new macrolides, called lobatamides, were obtained from collections of the Australian tunicates *Aplidium lobatum*, *Aplidium sp.* and an unidentified Philippine ascidian [121]. Later it was shown that both salicylihalamides and lobatamides showed strong correlations with the differential

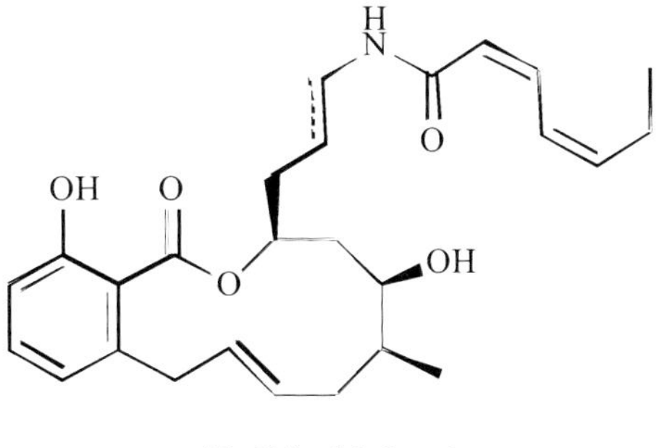

45, *E*-double bond
46, *Z*-double bond

cytotoxicity profiles of bafilomycins and concanamycins, the first known *in vitro* V-ATPase inhibitors. However, the new benzolactone enamide inhibitors showed an unprecedented selectivity for mammalian V-ATPase, with calculated IC_{50} values of 0.40 – 0.62 nM for salicylihalamide A and 0.68 – 14 nM for lobatamides A-F [122]. It is noteworthy that, despite binding to the same V_o sector, salicylihalamide A does not compete with bafilomycins and concanamycins for binding to V-ATPase [123].

The absolute stereochemistry of salicylihalamide A (**45**) was corrected following the total synthesis of this natural product [124], and confirmed after other synthetic efforts [125]. Initial structure-function studies of salicylihalamides revealed that the side chain and the salicylate moiety are indispensable for activity [126]. On the basis of these results, a series of simplified salicylihalamide analogues that retain the ability to inhibit V-ATPase were synthesized [127]. Salicylihalamides have received considerable attention as antitumor agents, and several efficient total syntheses have been presented as a critical source for obtaining enough material for preclinical development [128]. In the case of lobatamides, the total synthesis of lobatamide C (**47**) has been accomplished, thus determining its absolute stereochemistry [129]. Additionally, some acyclic lobatamide analogues have been synthesized and evaluated against bovine V-ATPase, confirming the importance of the salicylate ring and the enamide group for activity [130].

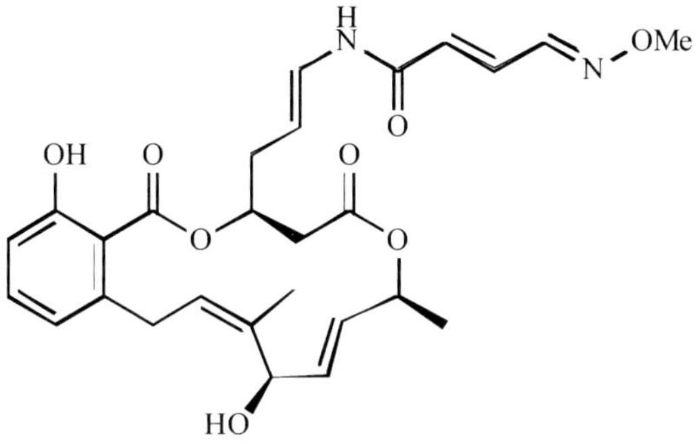

47

Chondropsins A and B (**48**, **49**), two polyketide-derived macrolide lactams isolated from the aqueous extract of an Australian collection of the sponge *Chondropsissp.* [131], along with other structurally related compounds isolated in minute quantities from sponges of the genera *Ircinia*, *Psammoclemma*, *Poecillastra*, *Jaspis* and *Siliquariaspongia* [132], comprise a new class of V-ATPase modulators. Although chondropsins are less potent than other inhibitors, they possess a unique specificity, inhibiting fungal V-ATPase (IC_{50} 0.04 – 0.7 μM) better than mammalian V-ATPase (IC_{50} 0.4 to > 10 μM). Chondropsins produced the same pattern of selective cytotoxicity in the NCI's 60-cell panel that is characteristic of other known *in vitro* V-ATPase inhibitors [133]. With ring sizes ranging from 33 to 37-membered ring systems, chondropsins are among the largest macrolides that could be used as structural lead to drug development, although notable efforts in organic synthesis would be necessary to obtain structurally simplified analogues and perform a precise stereochemical assignment.

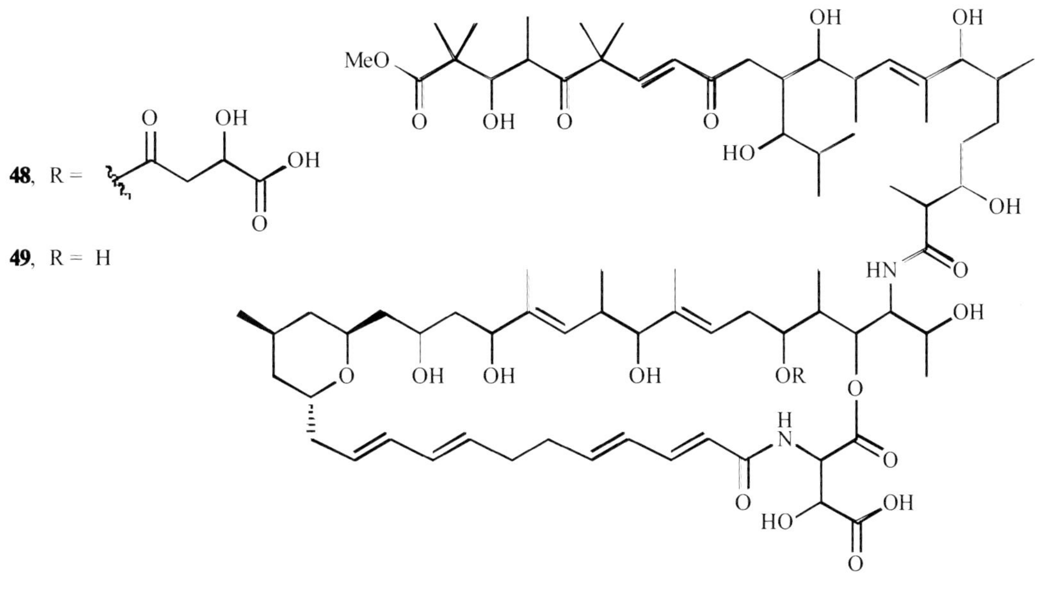

48, R =

49, R = H

Iejimalides A and B (**50**, **51**), the first macrocyclic lactones isolated from the tunicate *Eudistoma cf. rigida*, were recently identified as vacuolar ATPase inhibitors [134]. The stereochemistry of these 24-membered macrolides remained unsolved until the isolation of a relatively large amount of iejimalides from the Okinawan tunicate *Cystodytes sp.* [135]. The configuration of the serine residue adjacent to the *N*-formyl terminus was determined to be L-form by chiral HPLC analysis, and the stereochemistry of five stereocenters was assigned on the basis of detailed analysis of NMR data, along with CD measurements, chemical derivatization and distance geometry calculations [136]. The total synthesis of iejimalides by two different groups confirmed the proposed stereochemistry [137,138]. The IC_{50} values against partially purified *Saccharomyces cerevisiae* V-ATPase were calculated to be 71.1 and 95.0 nM, respectively. Furthermore, the nearly 4-fold decrease in the inhibitory activity of iejimalides against a bafilomycin-resistant mutant ATPase suggests that the binding site of iejimalides could be overlapping the bafilomycins/concanamycins-binding site [139].

Interestingly, a recent report revealed that iejimalides also induce severe changes in the actin cytoskeleton of 3T3 fibroblasts, exhibiting a potent actin-depolymerizing capacity comparable with the activity of latrunculins (**2**, **3**), while no significant effect on the tubulin cytoskeleton was observed [138]. Further studies with iejimalides carbamate derivatives confirmed that these natural products do not produce disruption of microtubules [140].

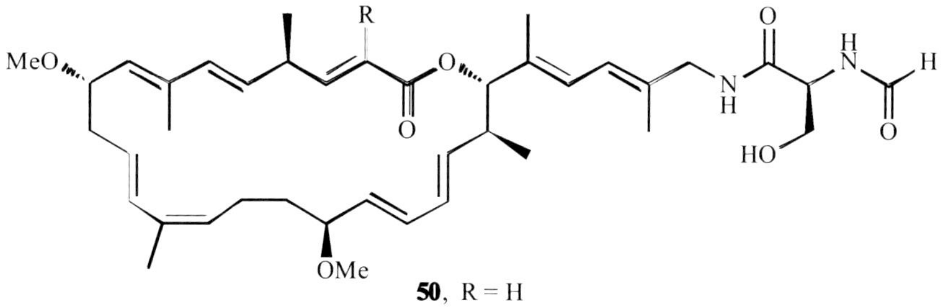

50, R = H
51, R = Me

Palmerolide A (**52**), an enamide-bearing macrolide isolated from the Antarctic tunicate *Synoicum adareanum*, inhibits vacuolar ATPase at nanomolar concentrations (IC_{50} 2 nM). Palmerolide A showed potent cytotoxicity against UACC-62 melanoma cells (LC_{50} 18 nM), but only modest activity against other cell lines such as HCC-2998 colon cancer cells (LC_{50} 6.5 μM) and RXF-393 renal cancer cells (LC_{50} 6.5 μM) [141]. Further degradative studies of palmerolide A to confirm the relative configuration have concluded with the reassignment of three stereocenters [142], and the absolute configuration of this 20-membered macrolide was recently determined with the total syntheses of the natural product and some stereoisomers [143]. Initial structure-activity relationship studies of palmerolide A have been reported, obtaining a 10-fold increase in potency against several tumor cell lines when the isopentenoyl group in the side chain of the natural product is replaced by a nonpolar aromatic system [144], a path pointing result for future design and synthesis of new palmerolide A analogues.

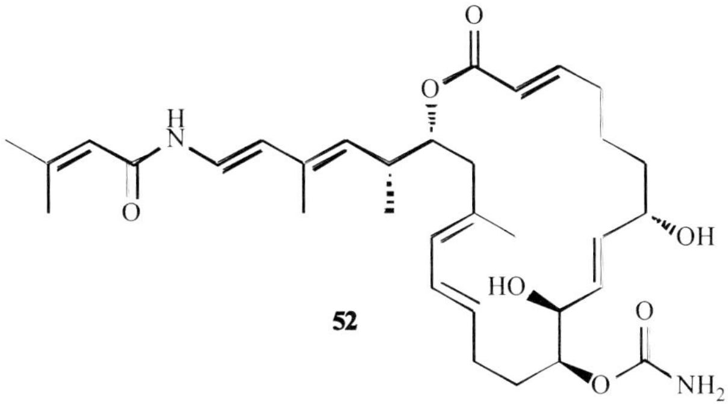

52

4. MACROLIDES TARGETING RIBOSOMES

Protein synthesis in living systems takes place on the ribosome, a complex macromolecular assembly responsible for the translation of genetic code in the mRNA into the correct amino acid sequence for each of the thousands of proteins present in the cell. The process of eukaryotic protein biosynthesis contains many potential targets for cancer therapy, such as the interaction of small molecules with ribosomal subunits or proteins involved in different steps of the complex translation process (initiation, elongation and termination). Although many structurally diverse natural products have been reported to inhibit protein synthesis, only a small number of marine macrolides can be considered as inhibitors of ribosomal function.

Pateamine A (**53**) is an immunosuppressive agent isolated from different species of sponges of the genus *Mycale* [145]. The bis-lactone core in pateamine A accommodate four asymmetric centres together with a thiazole ring and a *E,Z*-1,3-diene unit, and is substituted by an unusual all-*E* trienamine residue. Total syntheses of pateamine A led to the structural verification of all the four stereocenters, and initial structure-activity relationship studies indicated that both the macrocycle and the trienamine side chain are important to retain immunosuppressive activity [146]. Further studies demonstrated that the C1-C5 sector of the molecule (including the C3 amino group) serves as a scaffold for the remaining conformationally rigid sector of the molecule, and thus it could be exploited as a site of attachment for hybrid molecules useful for target identification and/or isolation of the cellular receptor [147].

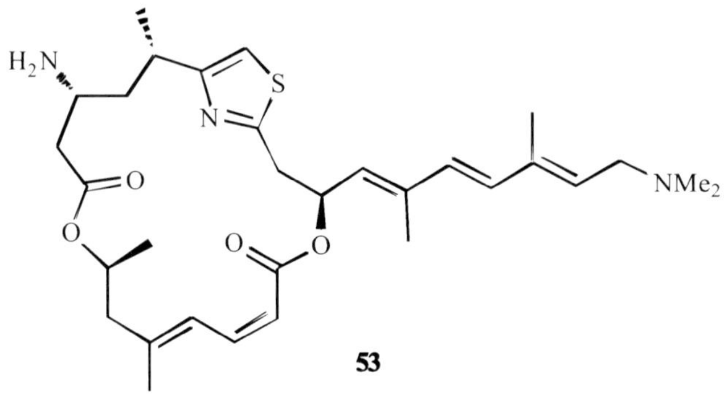

53

Later it was shown that pateamine A is a selective inhibitor of cap-dependent translation initiation that binds to eukaryotic initiation factor 4A (eIF4A), disturbing its protein-protein interactions and enhancing its RNA-dependent ATPase and ATP-stimulated RNA binding activities [148]. Further studies on the mechanism of action of pateamine A revealed that this natural product is a chemical inducer of dimerization that forces an engagement between eIF4A and RNA and prevents eIF4A from participating in the ribosome-recruitment step of translation initiation [149]. The specific binding of pateamine A to eIF4A, a member of DEAD/H box RNA helicases family, demonstrates the viability of selective targeting of highly conserved enzymes with small molecules. Recent studies indicate that pateamine A could be used as a valuable pharmacological and biochemical tool to study the molecular mechanism of eukaryotic translation initiation, and also as a promising lead compound for the development of anticancer agents [150].

13-Deoxytedanolide (**54**) is the only marine macrolide reported to inhibit eukaryotic protein synthesis specifically. This macrolide, originally isolated from the lipophilic extract of the sponge *Mycale adhaerens*, shows potent *in vitro* cytotoxicity against P388 murine leukemia cells (IC_{50} 0.094 ng/mL) and decreases the growth rate of P388 tumors implanted in mice with a T/C value of 189% at a dose of 0.125 mg/kg [151]. Further studies revealed that 13-deoxytedanolide strongly binds to the 60S large ribosomal subunit, causing *in vitro* inhibition of polypeptide elongation in *Saccharomyces cerevisiae.* Interestingly, 13-

deoxytedanolide does not inhibit the polypeptide synthesis in *Escherichia coli*, even at micromolar concentrations [152]. A recent X-ray crystallographic structure of 13-deoxytedanolide bound to the 50S ribosomal subunit from *Haloarcula marismortui* has shown that 13-deoxytedanolide binds to the E site of the 50S subunit at the same location as the CCA of tRNA, and thus appears to act as a competitive inhibitor of tRNA interaction with the E site. The specificity of 13-deoxytedanolide for eukaryotic ribosomes is explained by its interactions with protein L44e, which is an E site component of eukaryotic ribosomes, but not of eubacterial ribosomes [153].

13-Deoxytedanolide is the most potent compound of the tedanolide family of macrocyclic polyketides, which includes five 18-membered macrolides with potent cytotoxic activity [154,155]. The parent compound, tedanolide (**55**), was isolated from the Caribbean sponge *Tedania Ignis* and its structure as well as the absolute configuration were unambiguously determined by X-ray crystallographic analysis [154]. The stereochemistry of 13-deoxytedanolide was proposed to be the same of tedanolide, since ^{1}H and ^{13}C chemical shifts are very similar in both compounds [155]. In the past five years, several total syntheses of 13-deoxytedanolide and tedanolide had been reported [156]. Moreover, structure-activity relationship studies using a total of ten 13-deoxytedanolide analogues have shown that the southern hemisphere of the molecule and the epoxide-bearing side chain are critical to retain the cytotoxic activity against P388 murine leukemia cells and the inhibitory activity of polypeptide elongation in yeast cell lysate, while the northern hemisphere appears to play a essential role to maintain the conformation of the molecule in a suitable form to bind to its cellular target [157].

5. PERSPECTIVES

Marine organisms have become an area of major attention due to the broad structural diversity and the immense pharmacological potential presented by metabolites isolated from these organisms. Marine macrolides are among the most stunning natural products isolated ever, and some of these compounds could play a fundamental role as potential lead compounds for drug development or as useful tools in biomedical research. However, their complexity and low natural abundance make them inaccessible in sufficient amounts and therefore preclude an easy access to derivatives that could contribute to our understanding of their mode of action. Advances in biotechnological sciences are of paramount importance to achieve a continuous source of producing organisms. Alternatively, multigram total chemical synthesis is the other alternative route to provide larger quantities of these fascinating substances. However, in most cases these approaches have been very difficult to achieve. Recent identification of the biosynthetic gene cluster of bryostatins from a bacterial symbiont opens a new way to produce some of these bioactive compounds through the heterologous expression of biosynthetic genes in a suitable host.

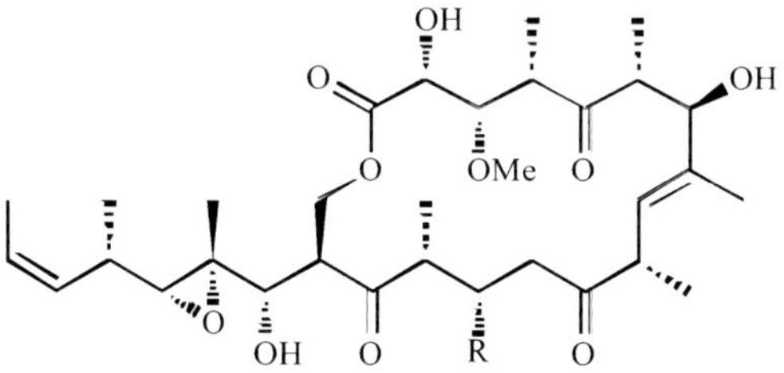

54, R = H
55, R = OH

In addition to the previously clustered structures, a number of very interesting new macrolides with unknown and potentially novel modes of action have been discovered in recent times. Among them, leiodermatolide (**56**) formed by an unprecedented 16-membered macrolide skeleton attached to an unsaturated side chain that includes a δ-lactone, exhibited potent antimitotic activity (IC_{50}< 10 nM) against a panel of cancer cell lines and belizeanolide (**57**) a 54-membered lactone attached to an acyclic portion that contains an unprecedented diene unit [158]. Interestingly the opened form of **57**, belizeanolic acid (**58**), showed a ten fold better cytotoxic activity against a variety of human solid tumor cells [159]. Finally, it is worth mentioning that even though a significant number of marine macrolides have been summarized in this review, bryostatin 1 and halichondrin B are the only metabolites currently involved in clinical trials, whereas laulimalide, salicylihalamides, peluroside A, and aplyronine A are presently in preclinical development. Therefore, solving the supply problem will be essential in order to gain more insight into the true clinical potential of these promising compounds.

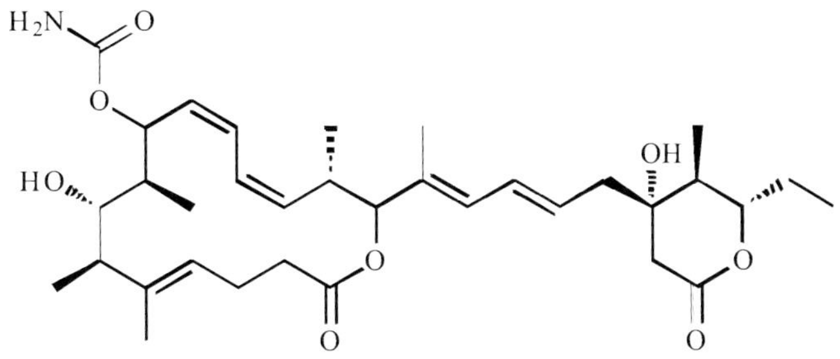

56

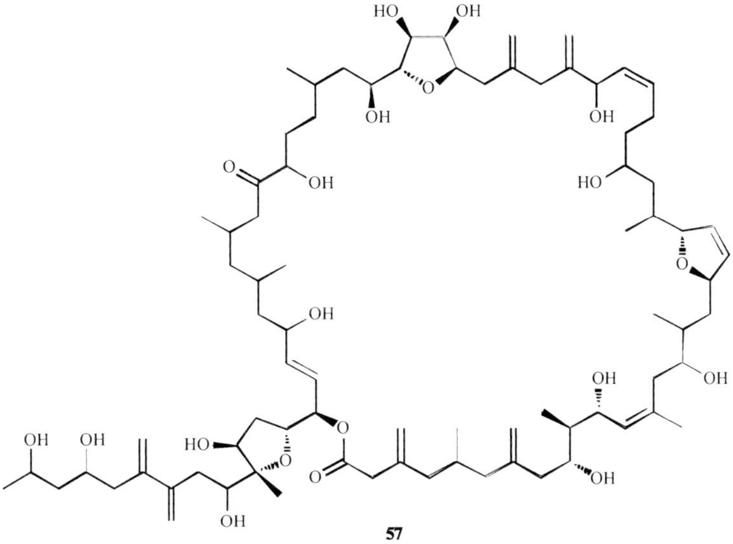

57

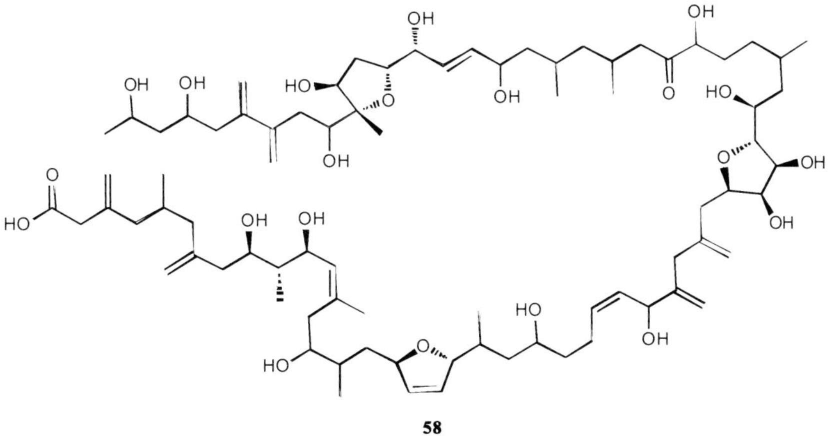

58

CONFLICT OF INTEREST

The authors declare that there is no conflict of interest.

ACKNOWLEDGEMENTS

This work was supported by Spanish Ministerio de Economía y Competitividad (SAF2011-28883-C03-01).

DISCLOSURE

This e-Book chapter is an updated version of the article entitled "Marine Macrolides, a Promising Source of Antitumor Compounds" published in *Anti-Cancer Agents in Medicinal Chemistry*, **2009**, *9*(2), 122-137.

REFERENCES

[1] Harvey, A. Strategies for discovering drugs for previously unexplored natural products. *Drug Discovery Today*, **2000**, *5*, 294.

[2] For recent reviews on marine natural products, see: Blunt, J.W.; Copp, B.R.; Hu, W.-P.; Munro, M.H.G.; Northcote, P.T.; Prinsep, M.R. Marine natural products. *Nat. Prod. Rep.*, **2012**, *29*, 144. Blunt, J.W.; Copp, B.R.; Hu, W.-P.; Munro, M.H.G.; Northcote, P.T.; Prinsep, M.R. Marine natural products. *Nat. Prod. Rep.*, **2011**, *28*, 196. Blunt, J.W.; Copp, B.R.; Hu, W.-P.; Munro, M.H.G.; Northcote, P.T.; Prinsep, M.R. Marine natural products. *Nat. Prod. Rep.*, **2010**, *27*, 165. Blunt, J.W.; Copp, B.R.; Hu, W.-P.; Munro, M.H.G.; Northcote, P.T.; Prinsep, M.R. Marine natural products. *Nat. Prod. Rep.*, **2009**, *26*, 170. Blunt, J.W.; Copp, B.R.; Hu, W.-P.; Munro, M.H.G.; Northcote, P.T.; Prinsep, M.R. Marine natural products. *Nat. Prod. Rep.*, **2008**, *25*, 35. Blunt, J.W.; Copp, B.R.; Hu, W.-P.; Munro, M.H.G.; Northcote, P.T.; Prinsep, M.R. Marine natural products. *Nat. Prod. Rep.*, **2007**, *24*, 31. Blunt, J.W.; Copp, B.R.; Munro, M.H.G.; Northcote, P.T.; Prinsep, M.R. Marine natural products. *Nat. Prod. Rep.*, **2006**, *23*, 26. Blunt, J.W.; Copp, B.R.; Munro, M.H.G.; Northcote, P.T.; Prinsep, M.R. Marine natural products. *Nat. Prod. Rep.*, **2005**, *22*, 15. Blunt, J.W.; Copp, B.R.; Munro, M.H.G.; Northcote, P.T.; Prinsep, M.R. Marine natural products. *Nat. Prod. Rep.*, **2004**, *21*, 1. Newman, D.J.; Cragg, G.M.; Snader, K.M. Natural products as sources of new drugs over the period 1981-2002. *J. Nat. Prod.*, **2003**, *66*, 1022. For reviews on synthesis of marine natural products, see: Morris, J.C.; Phillips, A.J. Marine natural products: synthetic aspects. *Nat. Prod. Rep.*, **2008**, *25*, 95. Morris, J.C.; Nicholas, G.M.; Phillips, A.J. Marine natural products: synthetic aspects. *Nat. Prod. Rep.*, **2007**, *24*, 87.

[3] For recent reviews on pharmacological aspects of marine natural products, see: Fusetani, N. Biotechnological potential of marine natural products. Pure Appl Chem., **2010**, *8*, 17. Banerjee, S.; Wang, Z.; Mohammad, M.; Sarkar, F.H.; Mohammad, R.M. Efficacy of selected natural products as therapeutic agents against cancer. *J. Nat. Prod.*, **2008**, *71*, 492. Nakao, Y.; Fusetani, N. Enzyme inhibitors from marine invertebrates. *J. Nat. Prod.*, **2007**, *70*, 689. Newman, D.J.; Cragg, G.M. Natural products as sources of new drugs over the last 25 years. *J. Nat. Prod.*, **2007**, *70*, 461. Dixon, N.; Wong, L.S.; Geerlings, T.H.; Micklefield, J. Cellular targets of natural products. *Nat. Prod. Rep.*, **2007**, *24*, 1288. Baker, D.D.; Chu,

M.; Oza, U.; Rajgarhia, V. The value of natural products to future pharmaceutical discovery. *Nat. Prod. Rep.*, **2007**, *24*, 1225. Mayer, A.M.S.; Gustafson, K.R. Marine pharmacology in 2003–2004: anti-tumourand cytotoxic compounds. *Eur. J. Cancer*, **2006**, *42*, 2241. Drahl, C.; Cravatt, B.F; Sorensen, E.J. Protein-reactive natural products. *Angew. Chem. Int. Ed.*, **2005**, *44*, 5788. Butler, M.S. The role of natural product chemistry in drug discovery. *J. Nat. Prod.*, **2004**, *67*, 2141. Newman, D.J.; Cragg, G.M. Marine natural products and related compounds in clinical and advancedpreclinical trials. *J. Nat. Prod.*, **2004**, *67*, 1216. Cragg, G.M.; Newman, D.J. A tale of two tumor targets: topoisomerase I and tubulin. The Wall and Wani contribution to cancer chemotherapy. *J. Nat. Prod.*, **2004**, *67*, 232. Mayer, A.M.S.; Gustafson, K.R. Marine pharmacology in 2001–2: antitumour andcytotoxic compounds. *Eur. J. Cancer*, **2004**, *40*, 2676.

[4] Rawlings, B.J. Biosynthesis of polyketides (other than actinomycetemacrolides). *Nat. Prod. Rep.*, **1999**, *16*, 425.

[5] For recent reviews on synthesis of macrolides, see: Florence, G.J.; Gardner, N.M.; Paterson, I. Development of practical syntheses of the marine anticancer agentsdiscodermolide and dictyostatin. *Nat. Prod. Rep.*, **2008**, *25*, 342. Yeung, K.-S.; Paterson, I. Advances in the total synthesis of biologically important marine macrolides. *Chem. Rev.*, **2005**, *105*, 4237. Yeung, K.-S.; Paterson, I. Actin-binding marine macrolides : total synthesis and biological importance. *Angew. Chem. Int. Ed.*, **2002**, *41*, 4632.

[6] Mutter, R.; Wills, M. Chemistry and clinical biology of the bryostatins. *Bioorg. Med. Chem.*, **2000**, *8*, 1841.

[7] Sudek, S.; Lopanik, N.B.; Waggoner, L.E.; Hildebrand, M.; Anderson, C.; Liu, H.; Patel, A.; Sherman, D.H.; Haygood, M.G. Identification of the putative bryostatin polyketide synthase gene cluster from "*Candidatus*endobugula sertula", the uncultivated microbial symbiont of the marine bryozoan*Bugula neritina*. *J. Nat. Prod.*, **2007**, *70*, 67.

[8] Kortmansky, J.; Schwartz, G.K. Bryostatin-1: a novel PKC inhibitor in clinical development. *Cancer Investigation*, **2003**, *21*, 924.

[9] Mohammad, R.M.; al-Katib, A.; Pettit, G.R.; Sensenbrenner, L.L. Successful treatment of human Waldenstrom's macroglobulinemia with combination biological and chemotherapy agents. *Cancer Res.*, **1994**, *54*, 165. Mohammad, R.M.; Varterasian, M.L.; Almatchy, V.P.; Hannoudi, G.N.; Pettit, G.R.; al-Katib, A. Successful treatment of human chronic lymphocytic leukemia xenografts with combination biological agents auristatin PE and bryostatin 1. *Clin. Cancer Res.*, **1998**, *4*, 1337. Mohammad, R.M.; Wall, N.R.; Dutcher, J.A.; al-Katib, A. The addition of bryostatin 1 to cyclophosphamide, doxorubicin, vincristine, and prednisone (CHOP) chemotherapy improves response in a CHOP-resistant human diffuse large cell lymphoma xenograft model. *Clin. Cancer Res.*, **2000**, *6*, 4950.

[10] Newman, D.J.; Cragg, G.M. In *Natural Products: Drug Discovery and Therapeutic Medicine*; Zhang, Demain, Eds.; Humana Press Inc.: Totowa, **2005**; pp. 129-168. Ishibashi, M. In *Macrolide Antibiotics: Chemistry, Biology and Practice*, Second Edition; Omura, Ed.; Elsevier Science Inc.: San Diego, **2002**; pp. 57-98.

[11] Kobayashi, J.; Kubota, T. Bioactive macrolides and polyketides from marine dinoflagellates of the genus*Amphidinium*. *J. Nat. Prod.*, **2007**, *70*, 451. Kobayashi, J.; Tsuda, M. Amphidinolides, bioactive macrolides from symbiotic marinedinoflagellates. *Nat. Prod. Rep.*, **2004**, *21*, 77. Kobayashi, J.; Shimbo, K.; Kubota, T.; Tsuda, M. Bioactive macrolides and polyketides frommarine dinoflagellates. *Pure Appl. Chem.*, **2003**, *75*, 337.

[12] Kashman, Y.; Groweiss, A.; Shmueli, U. Latrunculin, a new 2-thiazolidinone macrolide from the marine sponge *Latrunculia magnifica*. *Tetrahedron Lett.*, **1980**, *21*, 3629.

[13] Groweiss, A.; Shmueli, U.; Kashman, Y. Marine toxins of *Latrunculia magnifica*. *J. Org. Chem.*, **1983**, *48*, 3512.

[14] Jefford, C.W.; Bernardelli, G.; Tanaka, J.; Higa, T. Structures and absolute configurations of the marine toxins, latrunculin A and laulimalide. *Tetrahedron Lett.*, **1996**, *37*, 159.

[15] Spector, I.; Shochet, N.R.; Kashman, Y.; Groweiss, A. Latrunculins: novel marine toxins that disrupt microfilament organization in cultured cells. *Science.*, **1983**, *219*, 493.

[16] Coue, M.; Brenner, S.L.; Spector, I.; Korn, E.D. Inhibition of actin polymerization by latrunculin A. *FEBS Lett.*, **1987**, *213*, 316.

[17] Morton, W.M.; Ayscough, K.R.; McLaughlin, P.J. Latrunculin alters the actin-monomer subunit interface to prevent polymerization. *Nature Cell Biol.*, **2000**, *2*, 376.

[18] Yarmola, E.G.; Somasundaram, T.; Boring, T.A.; Spector, I.; Bubb, M.R. Actin-latrunculin A structure and function. *J. Biol. Chem.*, **2000**, *275*, 28120.

[19] Gachet, Y.; Tournier, S.; Millar, J.B.A.; Hyams, J.S. A MAP kinase-dependent actin checkpoint ensures proper spindle orientation in fission yeast. *Nature*, **2001**, 41*2*, 352.

[20] Roesener, J.A.; Scheuer, P.J. Ulapualide A and B, extraordinary antitumor macrolides from nudibranch eggmasses. *J. Am. Chem. Soc.*, **1986**, *108*, 846.

[21] Matsunaga, S.; Fusetani, N.; Hashimoto, K. Kabiramide C, a novel antifungal macrolide from nudibranch eggmasses. *J. Am. Chem. Soc.*, **1986**, *108*, 847. Matsunaga, S.; Fusetani, N.; Hashimoto, K.; Koseki, K.; Noma, M.; Noguchi, H.; Sankawa, U. Further kabiramides and halichondramides, cytotoxic macrolides embracing trisoxazole, from the *Hexabranch*us egg masses. *J. Org. Chem.*, **1989**, *54*, 1360.

[22] Fusetani, N.; Yasumuro, K.; Matsunaga, S.; Hashimoto, K. Mycalolides A-C, hybrid macrolides of ulapualides and halichondramide, from a sponge of the genus *Mycale*. *Tetrahedron Lett.*, **1989**, *30*, 2809. Rashid, M.A.; Gustafson, K.R.; Cardellina, II, J.H.; Boyd, M.R. Mycalolides D andE, new cytotoxic macrolides from a collection of the stony coral *Tubastrea faulkneri*. *J. Nat. Prod.*, **1996**, *58*, 1120.

[23] Kernan, M.R.; Faulkner, D.J. Halichondramide, an antifungal macrolide from the sponge *Halichondria* sp. *Tetrahedron Lett.*, **1987**, *28*, 2809. Kernan, M.R.; Molinski, T.F.; Faulkner, D.J. Macrocyclic antifungal metabolites from the spanish dancer nudibranch *Hexabranchus sanguineus* and sponges of the genus *Halichondria*. *J. Org. Chem.*, **1988**, *53*, 5014.

[24] Kobayashi, J.; Tsuda, M.; Fuse, H.; Sasaki, T.; Mikami, Y. Halishigamides A-D, new cytotoxic oxazole-containing metabolites fromOkinawan spongeHalichondriasp. *J. Nat. Prod.*, **1997**, *60*, 150.

[25] Kobayashi, J.; Murata, O.; Shigemori, H. Jaspisamides A-C, new cytotoxic macrolides from the Okinawan sponge *Jaspis* sp. *J. Nat. Prod.*, **1993**, *56*, 787.

[26] Chattopadhyay, S.K.; Pattenden, G. Total synthesis of Ulapualide A, a novel *tris-oxazole* containing macrolide from the marine nudibranch *Hexabranchus sanguineus*. *Tetrahedron Lett.*, **1998**, *39*, 6095. Chattopadhyay, S.K.; Pattenden, G. A total synthesis of the unique tris-oxazole macrolide ulapualide Aproduced by the marine nudibranch *Hexabranchus sanguineus*. *J. Chem. Soc., Perkin Trans. 1*, **2000**, 2429.

[27] Matsunaga, S.; Liu, P.; Celatka, C.A.; Panek, J.S.; Fusetani, N. Relative and absolute stereochemistry ofmycalolides, bioactive macrolides from the marinesponge*Mycale magellanica*. *J. Am. Chem. Soc.*, **1999**, *121*, 5605.

[28] Liu, P.; Panek, J.S. Total synthesis of (-)-Mycalolide A. *J. Am. Chem. Soc.*, **2000**, *122*, 1235. Liu, P.; Panek, J.S. Total synthesis of the actin-depolymerizing agent (-)-mycalolide A: application of chiral silane-based bond construction methodology. *J. Am. Chem. Soc.*, **2000**, *122*, 11090.

[29] Hori, M.; Saito, S.; Shin, Y.; Ozaki, H.; Fusetani, N.; Karaki, H. Mycalolide-B, a novel and specific inhibitor of actomyosin ATPase isolated from marine sponge. *FEBS Lett.*, **1993**, *322*, 151.

[30] Saito, S.; Watabe, S.; Ozaki, H.; Fusetani, N.; Karaki, H. Mycalolide B, a novel actin depolymerizing agent. *J. Biol. Chem.*, **1994**, *269*, 29710.

[31] Klenchin, V.A.; Allingham, J.S.; King, R.; Tanaka, J.; Marriott, G.; Rayment, I. Trisoxazole macrolide toxins mimic the binding of actin-capping proteins to actin. *Nature Structural Biol.*, **2003**, *10*, 1058.

[32] Tanaka, J.; Yan, Y.; Choi, J.; Bai, J.; Klenchin, V.A.; Rayment, I.; Marriott, G. Biomolecular mimicry in the actin cytoskeleton: mechanisms underlying the cytotoxicity of kabiramide C and related macrolides. *Proc. Natl. Acad. Sci. USA.*, **2003**, *100*, 13851.

[33] Allingham, J.S.; Tanaka, J.; Marriott, G.; Rayment, I. Absolute stereochemistry ofulapualide A. *Org. Lett.*, **2004**, *6*, 597.

[34] Carmely, S.; Kashman, Y. Structure of swinholide A, a new macrolide from the marine sponge *Theonella swinhoei. Tetrahedron Lett.*, **1985**, *26*, 511.

[35] Kobayashi, M.; Tanaka, J.; Katori, T.; Matsuura, M.; Kitagawa, I. Structure of swinholide A, a potente cytotoxic macrolide from the Okinawan marine sponge *Theonella swinhoei. Tetrahedron Lett.*, **1989**, *30*, 2963.

[36] Kitagawa, I.; Kobayashi, M.; Katori, T.; Yamashita, M. Absolute stereostructure of swinholide A, a potent cytotoxic macrolide from the okinawan marine sponge *Theonella swinhoei. J. Am. Chem. Soc.*, **1990**, *112*, 3710. Doi, M.; Ishida, T.; Kobayashi, M.; Kitagawa, I. Molecular conformation of swinholide A, a potent cytotoxic dimeric macrolide from the Okinawan marine sponge *Theonella swinhoei:* X-ray crystal structure of its diketone derivative. *J. Org. Chem.*, **1991**, *56*, 3629.

[37] Paterson, I.; Yeung, K.-S.; Ward, R.A.; Cumming, J.G.; Smith, J.D. Total synthesis of swinholide A and hemiswinholide A. *J. Am. Chem. Soc.*, **1994**, *116*, 9391.

[38] Bubb, M.R.; Spector, I.; Bershadsky, A.D.; Korn, E.D. Swinholide A is a microfilament disrupting marine toxin that stabilizes actin dimers and severs actin filaments. *J. Biol. Chem.*, **1995**, *270*, 3463.

[39] Kato, Y.; Fusetani, N.; Matsunaga, S.; Hashimoto, K.; Sakai, R.; Higa, T.; Kashman, Y. Antitumor macrodiolides isolated from a marine sponge *Theonella* sp.: structure revision of misakinolide A. *Tetrahedron Lett.*, **1987**, *28*, 6225.

[40] Watabe, S.; Wada, S.; Saito, S.; Matsunaga, S.; Fusetani, N.; Ozaki, H.; Karaki, H. Cellularchangesofratembryonicfibroblastsbyanactin-polymerizationinhibitor, bistheonellideA, fromamarinesponge. *Cell Structure Function*, **1996**, *21*, 199.

[41] Terry, D.R.; Spector, I.; Higa, T.; Bubb, M.R. Misakinolide A is a marine macrolide that caps but does notsever filamentous actin. *J. Biol. Chem.*, **1997**, *272*, 7841.

[42] Klenchin, V.A.; King, R.; Tanaka, J.; Marriott, G.; Rayment, I. Structural basis ofswinholide A binding to actin. *Chem. Biol.*, **2005**, *12*, 287.

[43] Guella, G.; Manzini, I.; Chiasera, G.; Pietra, F. Sphinxolide, a 26-membered antitumoral macrolide isolated from an unidentified Pacific nudibranch. *Helv. Chim. Acta.*, **1989**, *72*, 237. D'Auria, M.V.; Gomez-Paloma, L.; Minale, L.; Zampella, A.; Verbist, J.-F.;

Roussakis, C.; Debitus, C. Three new potent cytotoxic macrolides closely related to sphinxolide from the New Caledonian sponge *Neosiphonia superstes*. *Tetrahedron.*, **1993**, *49*, 8657.

[44] D'Auria, M.V.; Gomez-Paloma, L.; Minale, L.; Zampella, A.; Verbist, J.-F.; Roussakis, C.; Debitus, C.; Patissou, J. Reidispongiolide A and B, two new potent cytotoxic macrolides from the New Caledonian sponge *Reidispongia coerulea*. *Tetrahedron,* **1994**, *50*, 4829. Carbonelli, S.; Zampella, A.; Randazzo, A.; Debitus, C.; Gomez-Paloma, L. Sphinxolides E-G and reidispongiolide C: four new cytotoxic macrolides from the New Caledonian lithistida sponges *N. superstes* and *R. coerulea*. *Tetrahedron.*, **1999**, *55*, 14665.

[45] Bassarello, C.; Bifulco, G.; Zampella, A.; D'Auria, M.V.; Riccio, R.; Gomez-Paloma, L. Stereochemical studies on sphinxolide: advances in theJ-Based NMR. Determination of the relative configuration of flexible systems. *Eur. J. Org. Chem.*, **2001**, 39.

[46] Riccio, R.; Bifulco, G.; Cimino, P.; Bassarello, C.; Gomez-Paloma, L. Stereochemical analysis of natural products. Approaches relying on the combination of NMRspectroscopy and computational methods. *Pure Appl. Chem.*, **2003**, *75*, 295. Bifulco, G.; Bassarello, C.; Riccio, R.; Gomez-Paloma, L. Quantum mechanical calculations ofNMR Jcoupling values in thedetermination of relative configurationin organic compounds. *Org. Lett.*, **2004**, *6*, 1025. Bifulco, G.; Dambrouso, P.; Gomez-Paloma, L.; Riccio, R. Determination of relative configuration in organic compounds by NMRspectroscopy and computational methods. *Chem. Rev.*, **2007**, *107*, 3744.

[47] Zhang, X.; Minale, L.; Zampella, A.; Smith, C.D. Microfilament depletion and circumvention of multiple drug resistance bys phinxolides. *Cancer Res.*, **1997**, *57*, 3751.

[48] Allingham, J.S.; Zampella, A.; D'Auria, M.V.; Rayment, I. Structures of microfilament destabilizing toxins bound to actin provide insight into toxin design and activity. *Proc. Natl. Acad. Sci. USA.*, **2005**, *102*, 14527.

[49] Paterson, I.; Ashton, K.; Britton, R.; Cecere, G.; Chouraqui, G.; Florence, G.J.; Stafford, J. Total synthesis of (-)-reidispongiolide A, an actin-targeting marinemacrolide. *Angew. Chem. Int. Ed.*, **2007**, *46*, 6167.

[50] Yamada, K.; Ojika, M.; Ishigaki, T.; Yoshida, Y.; Ekimoto, H.; Arakawa, M. Aplyronine A, a potent antitumor substance, and the congeners aplyronines B and C isolated from the sea hare *Aplysia kurodai*. *J. Am. Chem. Soc.*, **1993**, *115*, 11020.

[51] Ojika, M.; Kigoshi, H.; Ishigaki, T.; Tsukuda, I.; Tsuboi, T.; Ogawa, T.; Yamada, K. Absolute stereochemistry of aplyronine A, a potent antitumor substance of marine origin. *J. Am. Chem. Soc.*, **1994**, *116*, 7441.

[52] Kigoshi, H.; Ojika, M.; Ishigaki, T.; Suenaga, K.; Mutou, T.; Sakakura, A.; Ogawa, T.; Yamada, K. Total synthesis of aplyronine A, a potent antitumor substance of marine origin. *J. Am. Chem. Soc.*, **1994**, *116*, 7443.

[53] Suenaga, K.; Ishigaki, T.; Sakakura, A.; Kigoshi, H.; Yamada, K. Absolute stereochemistry and synthesis of aplyronines B and C, the congeners of aplyronine A, a potent antitumor substance of marine origin. *Tetrahedron Lett.*, **1995**, *36*, 5053.

[54] Ojika, M.; Kigoshi, H.; Suenaga, K.; Imamura, Y.; Yoshikawa, K.; Ishigaki, T.; Sakakura, T.; Sakakura, A.; Mutou, T.; Yamada, K. Aplyronines D-H from the sea hare *Aplysia kurodai*: isolation, structures, and cytotoxicity. *Tetrahedron*, **2012**, *68*, 982.

[55] Kigoshi, H.; Suenaga, K.; Mutou, T.; Ishigaki, T.; Atsumi, T.; Ishiwata, H.; Sakakura, A.; Ogawa, T.; Ojika, M.; Yamada, K. Aplyronine A, a potent antitumor substance of marine origin, aplyronines B and C, and artificial analogues: total synthesisand structure-

cytotoxicity relationships. *J. Org. Chem.*, **1996**, *61*, 5326. Kigoshi, H.; Suenaga, K.; Takagi, M.; Akao, A.; Kanematsu, K.; Kamei, N.; Yamada, K. Cytotoxicity and actin-depolymerizing activity of aplyronine A, a potent antitumor macrolide of marine origin, and its analogs. *Tetrahedron.*, **2002**, *58*, 1075.

[56] Kuroda, T.; Suenaga, K.; Sakakura, A.; Handa, T.; Okamoto, K.; Kigoshi, H. Study of the interaction between actin and antitumor substance aplyronine Awith a novel fluorescent photoaffinity probe. *Bioconjugate Chem.*, **2006**, *17*, 524.

[57] Hirata, K.; Muraoka, S.; Suenaga, K.; Kuroda, T.; Kato, K.; Tanaka, H.; Yamamoto, M.; Takata, M.; Yamada, K.; Kigoshi, H. Structure basis for antitumor effect of aplyronine A. *J. Mol. Biol.*, **2006**, *356*, 945.

[58] Kita, M.; Hirayama, Y.; Sugiyama, M.; Kigoshi, H. Development of highly cytotoxic and actin-depolymerizing biotin derivatives of aplyronine A. *Angew. Chem. Int. Ed.* **2011**, *50*, 9871.

[59] Hirata, Y.; Uemura, D. Halichondrins – antitumor polyethers macrolides from a marine sponge. *Pure Appl. Chem.*, **1986**, *58*, 701.

[60] Uemura, D.; Takahashi, K.; Yamamoto, T.; Katayama, C.; Tanaka, J.; Okumura, Y.; Hirata, Y. Norhalichondrin A: an antitumor polyether macrolide from a marine sponge. *J. Am. Chem. Soc.*, **1985**, *107*, 4796.

[61] Pettit, G.R.; Herald, C.L.; Boyd, M.R.; Leet, J.E.; Dufresne, C.; Doubek, D.L.; Schmidt, J.M.; Cerny, R.L.; Hooper, J.N.; Rutzler, K.C. Antineoplastic agents 219. Isolation and structure of the cell growth inhibitory constituents from the Western Pacific marine sponge *Axinella* sp. *J. Med. Chem.*, **1991**, *34*, 3339.

[62] Pettit, G.R.; Tan, R.; Williams, M.D.; Doubek, D.L.; Boyd, M.R.; Schmidt, J.M.; Chapuis, J.-C.; Hamel, E.; Bai, R.; Hooper, J.N.; Tackett, L.P. Isolation and structure of halistatin 1 from the eastern Indian ocean marine sponge *Phakellia carteri*. *J. Org. Chem.*, **1993**, *58*, 2538.

[63] Litaudon, M.; Hart, J.B.; Blunt, J.W.; Lake, R.J.; Munro, M.H.G. Isohomohalichondrin B, a new antitumor polyether macrolide from the New Zealand deep water sponge *Lissodendoryx* sp. *Tetrahedron Lett.*, **1994**, *35*, 9435.

[64] Pettit, G.R.; Ichihara, Y.; Wurzel, G.; Williams, M.D.; Schmidt, J.M.; Chapuis, J.-C. Isolation and structure of halistatin 3 from the western Pacific (Chuuk) marine sponge *Phakellia* sp. *J. Chem. Soc., Chem. Commun.*, **1995**, 383.

[65] Hickford, S. J. H.; Blunt, J. W.; Munro, H. G. Antitumour polyether macrolides: Four new halichondrins from the New Zealand deep-water marine sponge *Lissodendoryx sp. Bioorg. Med. Chem.*, **2009**, *17*, 2199.

[66] Luduena, R.F.; Roach, M.C.; Prasad, V.; Pettit, G.R. Interaction of halichondrin B and homohalichondrin B with bovine brain tubulin. *Biochem. Pharmacol.*, **1993**, *45*, 421.

[67] Bai, R.L.; Paull, K.D.; Herald, C.L.; Malspeis, L.; Pettit, G.R.; Hamel, E. Halichondrin B and homohalichondrin B, marine natural product binding in the vinca domain of tubulin. *J. Biol. Chem.*, **1991**, *266*, 15882.

[68] Cooper, A.; Salomon, R. Total synthesis of halichondrins: enantioselective construction of a homochiral pentacyclic C1-C15 intermediate from D-ribose. *Tetrahedron Lett.*, **1990**, *31*, 3813. Aicher, T.D.; Buszek, K.R.; Fang, F.G.; Forsyth, C.J.; Jung, S.H.; Kishi, Y.; Scola, P.M.; Spero, D.M.; Yoon, S.K. Total synthesis of halichondrin B and norhalichondrin B. *J. Am. Chem. Soc.*, **1992**, *114*, 3162.

[69] Stamos, D.P.; Chen, S.S.; Kishi, Y.; New synthetic route to the C14-C38 segment of halichondrins. *J. Org. Chem.,* **1997**, *62*, 7552. Wang, Y.; Habgood, G.; Christ, W.; Littlefield, B.Y.; Melvin, J. Structure-activity studies of halichondrin B analogues: modifications at C30-C38. *Bioorg. Med. Chem. Lett.,* **2000**, *10*, 1029. Towle, M.J.; Salvato, K.A.; Budrow, J. *In vitro* and *in vivo* anticancer activities of synthetic macrocyclic ketone analogues of halichondrin B. *Cancer Res.,* **2001**, *61*, 1013. Namba, K.; Jun, H.-S.; Kishi, Y.; A simple but remarkably effective device for forming C8-C14 polycyclic ring system of halichondrin B. *J. Am. Chem. Soc.,* **2004**, *126*, 7770.

[70] Twelves, C.; Cortes, J.; Vahdat, L.T.; Wanders, J.; Akerele, C.; Kaufman, P. A. Phase III trials of eribulin mesylate (E7389) in extensively pretreated patients with locally recurrent or metastatic breast cáncer. *Clin. Breast Cancer***2010**, 10, 160.

[71] Cortes, J.; Vahdat, L.; Blum, J.L.; Twelves, C.; Campone, M.; Roche, H.; Bachelot, T.; Awada, A.; Paridaens, R.; Goncalves, A.; Shuster, D.E.; Wanders, J.; Fang, F.; Gurnani, R.; Richmond, E.; Cole, P.E.; Ashworth, S.; Allison, M. A. Phase II study of the halichondrin B analog eribulin mesylate in patients with locally advanced or metastatic breast cancer previously treated with an anthracycline, a taxane, and capecitabine. *J. Clin. Oncol.* **2010**, 28, 3922.

[72] Narayan, S.; Carlson, E. M.; Chen, H.; Du, H.; Hu, Y.; Jiang, Y.; Lewis, B.M.; Seletsky, B.M.; Tendyke, K.; Zhang, H. ; Zheng, W.; Littlefield, B.A.; Tole, M.J.; Yu, M.J. Novel second generation analogs of eribulin. Part I: Compounds containing a lipophilic C32 side chain overcome P-glycoprotein susceptibility. *Biorg. Med. Chem. Letters*, **2011**, 21, 1630.

[73] Pettit, G.R.; Cichacz, Z.A.; Gao, F.; Herald, C.L.; Boyd, M.R.; Schmidt, J.M.; Hooper, J.N.A. Isolation and structure of spongistatin 1. *J. Org. Chem.,* **1993**, *58*, 1302.

[74] Fusetani, N.; Shinoda, K.; Matsunaga, S. Cinachyrolide A: a potent cytotoxic macrolide possessing two spiro ketals from marine sponge *Cinachyra* sp. *J. Am. Chem. Soc.,* **1993**, *115*, 3977.

[75] Kobayashi, M.; Aoki, S.; Sakai, H.; Kawazoe, K.; Kihara, N.; Sasaki, T.; Kitagawa, I. Altohyrtin A, a potent anti-tumor macrolide from the Okinawan marine sponge *Hyrtios altum*. *Tetrahedron Lett.,* **1993**, *34*, 2795.

[76] Kobayashi, M.; Aoki, S.; Sakai, H.; Kihara, N.; Sasaki, T.; Kitagawa, I. Altohyrtins B and C and 5-desacetylaltohyrtin A, potent cytotoxic macrolide congeners of altohyrtin A, from the Okinawan marine sponge *Hyrtios altum*. *Chem. Pharm. Bull.,* **1993**, *41*, 989.

[77] Kobayashi, M.; Aoki, S.; Gato, K.; Kitagawa, I. Marine natural products XXXVIII. Absolute stereostructures of altohyrtins A, B and C and 5-desacetylaltohyrtin A, potent cytotoxic macrolides, from the Okinawan marine sponge *Hyrtios altum*. *Chem. Pharm. Bull.,* **1996**, *44*, 2142.

[78] Evans, D.A.; Coleman, P.J.; Diaz, L.C. Enantioselective synthesis of altohyrtin C (spongistatin 2): synthesis of the AB- and CD-spiroketal subunits. *Angew. Chem. Int. Ed.,* **1997**, *36*, 2737.

[79] Guo, J.; Duffy, K.J.; Stevens, K.L.; Dalko, P.I.; Roth, R.M.; Wayward, M.M.; Kishi, Y. Total synthesis of altohyrtin A (spongistatin 1). *Angew. Chem. Int. Ed.,* **1998**, *37*, 187.

[80] Claffey, M.M.; Heathcock, C.H. A method for constructing the C2-C12 dispiroacetal moiety of altohyrtin A. *J. Org. Chem.,* **1996**, *61*, 7646. Paquette, L.A.; Zuey, D. A modular approach to marine macrolide construction 1. An enantiocontrolled route to the C1-C12 (AB) spiroacetal sector. *Tetrahedron Lett.,* **1997**, *38*, 5115. Paterson, I.; Oballa, R.M.; Norcross, R.D. Studies in marine macrolide synthesis. Stereocontrolled syntesis of the AB-

spiroacetal subunit of spongistatin 1 (altohyrtin A). *Tetrahedron Lett.,* **1996**, *37*, 8581. Smith, III, A.B.; Zhuang, L.; Brook, C.S.; Boldi, A.M.; McBriar, M.D.; Hoser, W.H.; Murase, N.; Nakayama, K.; Verhoest, P.R.; Lin, Q. Spongistatin synthetic studies. 1. Construction of a C(29-48) subtarget. *Tetrahedron Lett.,* **1997**, *38*, 8667. Pietruszka, J. Spongistatins, cynachyrolides, or altohyrtins marine macrolides in cancer therapy. *Angew. Chem. Int. Ed.,* **1998**, *37*, 2629.

[81] Pettit, G.R.; Cichacz, Z.A.; Gao, F.; Herald, C.L.; Boyd, M.R. Isolation and structure of the remarkable human cancer cell growth inhibitors spongistatins 2 and 3 from an eastern Indian ocean *Spongia* sp. *J. Chem. Soc., Chem. Comunn.,* **1993**, 1166.

[82] Pettit, R.K.; McAllister, S.C.; Pettit, G.R.; Herald, C.L.; Johnson, J.M.; Cichacz, Z.A. A broad spectrum antifungal from the marine sponge *Hyrtios erecta. Int. J. Antimicrob. Agents.,* **1998**, *9*, 147.

[83] Uckun, F.M.; Mao, C.; Jan, S.-T.; Huang, H.; Vassilev, A.O.; Navara, C.S.; Narla, R.K. Spongistatins as tubulin targeting agents. *Curr. Pharm. Des.,* **2001**, *7*, 1291.

[84] Bai, R.; Taylor, G.F.; Cichacz, Z.A.; Herald, C.L.; Kepler, J.A.; Pettit, G.R.; Hamel, E. The spongistatins, potently cytotoxic inhibitors of tubulin polymerization, bind in a distinct region of the vinca domain. *Biochemistry,* **1995**, *34*, 9714.

[85] Pettit, G.R.; Chicacz, Z.A.; Gao, F.; Boyd, M.R.; Schmidt, J.M. Isolation and structure of the cancer cell growth inhibitor dictyostatin 1. *J. Chem. Soc., Chem. Commun.*, **1994**, 1111.

[86] Isbruker, R.A.; Cummins, J.; Pomponi, S.A.; Longley, R.E.; Wright, A.E. Tubulin polymerizing activity of dictyostatin-1, a polyketide of marine sponge origin. *Biochem. Pharmacol.*, **2003**, *66*, 75.

[87] Paterson, I.; Britton, R.; Delgado, O.; Wright, A.E. Stereochemical determination of dictyostatin, a novelmicrotubule-stabilising macrolide from the marine sponge *Corallistidaesp. Chem. Commun.*, **2004**, 632.

[88] Paterson, I.; Britton, R.; Delgado, O.; Meyer, A.; Poullennec, K.G. Total synthesis and configurational assignmentof (-)-dictyostatin, a microtubule-stabilizingmacrolide of marine sponge origin. *Angew. Chem. Int. Ed.*, **2004**, *43*, 4629. Shin, Y.; Fournier, J.-H.; Fukui, Y.; Brückner, A.M.; Curran, D.P. Total synthesis of (-)-dictyostatin : confirmationof relative and absolute configurations. *Angew. Chem. Int. Ed.*, **2004**, *43*, 4634.

[89] Madiraju, C.; Edler, M.C.; Hamel, E.; Raccor, B.S.; Balachandran, R.; Zhu, G.; Giuliano, K.A.; Vogt, A.; Shin, Y.; Fournier, J.-H.; Fukui, Y.; Brückner, A.M.; Curran, D.P.; Day, B.W. Tubulin assembly, taxoid site binding, and cellular effects of themicrotubule-stabilizing agent dictyostatin. *Biochemistry*, **2005**, *44*, 15053.

[90] Raccor, B.S.; Vogt, A.; Sikorski, R.P.; Madiraju, C.; Balachandran, R.; Montgomery, K.; Shin, Y.; Fukui, Y.; Jung, W.-H.; Curran, D.P.; Day, B.W. Cell-based and biochemical structure-activity analyses of analogs of the microtubule stabilizer dictyostatin. *Mol. Pharmacol.*, **2008**, *73*, 718.

[91] Quiñoa, E.; Kakou, Y.; Crews, P. Fijianolides, polyketide heterocycles from a marine sponge. *J. Org. Chem.*, **1988**, *53*, 3642.

[92] Corley, D.G.; Herb, R.; Moore, R.E.; Scheuer, P.J.; Paul, V.J. Laulimalides: new potent cytotoxic macrolides from a marine sponge and a nudibranch predator. *J. Org. Chem.*, **1988**, *53*, 3644.

[93] Cutignano, A.; Bruno, I.; Bifulco, G.; Casapullo, A.; Debitus, C.; Gomez-Paloma, L.; Riccio, R. Dactylolide, a new cytotoxic macrolide from the Vanuatu sponge *Dactylospongia* sp. *Eur. J. Org. Chem.*, **2001**, *775*.

[94] For a recent review on synthesis of laulimalide and analogues, see: Mulzer, J.; Ohler, E. Microtubule-stabilizing marine metabolite laulimalide and its derivatives:synthetic approaches and antitumor activity. *Chem. Rev.* **2003**, *103*, 3753.

[95] Mooberry, S.L.; Tien, G.; Hernandez, A.H.; Plubrukarn, A.; Davidson, B.S. Laulimalide and isolaulimalide, new paclitaxel-like microtubule-stabilizing agents. *Cancer Res.*, **1999**, *59*, 653.

[96] Pryor, D.; O'Brate, A.; Bilcer, G.; Díaz, J.F.; Wang, Y.; Wang, Y.; Kabaki, M.; Jung, M.K.; Andreu, J.M., Ghosh, A.K.; Giannakakou, P.; Hamel, E. The microtubule stabilizing agent laulimalide does not bind in the taxoid site, kills cells resistant to paclitaxel and epothilones, and may not require itsepoxide moiety for activity. *Biochemistry*, **2002**, *41*, 9109. Gapud, E.J.; Ghosh, A.K.; Hamel, E. Laulimalide and paclitaxel: a comparison of their effect on tubulin assembly and their synergistic action when present simultaneously. *Mol. Pharmacol.*, **2004**, *66*, 113.

[97] Wender, P.A.; Hedge, S.G.; Hubbard, R.D.; Zhang, L.; Mooberry, S.L. Synthesis and biological evaluation of(−)-laulimalide analogues. *Org. Lett.*, **2003**, *5*, 3507.

[98] Gollner, A.; Altmann, K.; Gertsch, J.; Mulzer, J. The leulimalide family: total synthesis and biological evaluation of neolaulimalide, isolaulimalide, laulimalide and a non-natural analogue. *Chem. Eur. J.* **2009**, *15*, 5979.

[99] Mooberry, S.L.; Randall-Hlubek, D.A.; Leal, R.M.; Hedge, S.G.; Hubbard, R.D.; Zhang, L.; Wender, P.A. Microtubule-stabilizing agents based on designed laulimalide analogues. *Proc. Natl. Acad. Sci. USA*, **2004**, *101*, 8803.

[100] West, L.M.; Northcote, P.T.; Battershill, C.N. Peloruside A: a potent cytotoxic macrolide isolated from theNew Zealand marine sponge*Mycale*sp. *J. Org. Chem.*, **2000**, *65*, 445.

[101] Liao, X.; Wu, Y.; De Brabander, J.K. Total synthesis and absolute configuration of thenovel microtubule-stabilizing agentpeloruside A. *Angew. Chem. Int. Ed.*, **2003**, *42*, 1648.

[102] Singh, A.J.; Xu, C.; Xu, X.; West, L.M.; Wilmes, A.; Chan, A.; Hamel, E.; Milleer, J.H.; Northcote, P.T.; Ghosh, A.K. Peloruside B, a potent antitumor macrolide from the New Zealand marine sponge *Mycale hentscheli*: isolation, structure, total synthesis and bioactivity. *J. Org. Chem.* **2010**, 75, 2.

[103] Hood, K.A.; Bäckström, B.T.; West, L.M.; Northcote, P.T.; Berridge, M.V.; Miller, J.H. The novel cytotoxic sponge metabolite peloruside A, structurally similar to spongistatin 1, has unique bioactivity independent of protein kinase C. *Anticancer Drug Des.*, **2001**, *16*, 155.

[104] Hood, K.A.; West, L.M.; Rouwé, B.; Northcote, P.T.; Berridge, M.V.; Wakefield, S.J.; Miller, J.H. Peloruside A, a novel antimitotic agent with paclitaxel-like microtubule-stabilizing activity. *Cancer Res.*, **2002**, *62*, 3356.

[105] Gaitanos, T.N.; Buey, R.M.; Díaz, J.F.; Northcote, P.T.; Teesdale-Spittle, P.; Andreu, J.M.; Miller, J.H. Peloruside A does not bind to the taxoid site onβ-tubulin and retains itsactivity in multidrug-resistant cell lines. *Cancer Res.*, **2004**, *64*, 5063.

[106] Pineda, O.; Farràs, J.; Maccari, L.; Manetti, F.; Botta, M.; Vilarrasa, J. Computational comparison of microtubule-stabilising agentslaulimalide and peloruside with taxol and colchicine. *Bioorg. Med. Chem. Lett.*, **2004**, *14*, 4825.

[107] Jiménez-Barbero, J.; Canales, A.; Northcote, P.T.; Buey, R.M.; Andreu, J.M.; Díaz, J.F. NMR determination of the bioactive conformation ofpeloruside A bound to microtubules. *J. Am. Chem. Soc.*, **2006**, *128*, 8757.

[108] Huzil J.T.; Chik, J.K.; Slysz, G.W.; Freedman, H.; Tuszynski, J.; Taylor, R.E.; Sackett, D.L.; Schriemer, D.C. A unique mode of microtubule stabilization induced by peloruside A. *J. Mol. Biol.*, **2008**, *378*, 1016.

[109] Jin, M.; Taylor, R.E. Total synthesis of (+)-peloruside A. *Org. Lett.*, **2005**, *7*, 1303. Ghosh, A.K.; Xu, X.; Kim, J.-H.; Xu, C.-X. Enantioselective total synthesis ofpeloruside A: a potent microtubulestabilizer. *Org. Lett.*, **2008**, *10*, 1001.

[110] Searle, P.A.; Molinski, T.F. Phorboxazoles A and B: potent cytostatic macrolides from marine sponge *Phorbas* sp. *J. Am. Chem. Soc.*, **1995**, *117*, 8126.

[111] Molinski, T.F. Absolute configuration of phorboxazoles A and B from the marine sponge, *Phorbas* sp. 2.C43 and complete stereochemistry. *Tetrahedron Lett.*, **1996**, *37*, 7879.

[112] Searle, P.A.; Molinski, T.F. Absolute configuration of phorboxazoles A and Bfrom the marine sponge*Phorbas*sp. 1. Macrolideand hemiketal rings. *J. Am. Chem. Soc.*, **1996**, *118*, 9422.

[113] Forsyth, C.J.; Ahmed, F.; Cink, R.D.; Lee, C.S. Total synthesis of phorboxazole A. *J. Am. Chem. Soc.*, **1998**, *120*, 5597. Smith, III, A.B.; Verhoest, P.R.; Minbiole, K.P.; Schelhaas, M. Total synthesis of (+)-phorboxazole A. *J. Am. Chem. Soc.*, **2001**, *123*, 4834. Gonzalez, M.A.; Pattenden, G. A convergent total synthesis ofphorboxazole A. *Angew. Chem. Int. Ed.*, **2003**, *42*, 1255. Wang, B.; Forsyth, C.J. Stereoselective synthesis of thephorboxazole A macrolide byring-closing metathesis. *Org. Lett.*, **2006**, *8*, 5223. Li, D.-R.; Zhang, D.-H.; Sun, C.-Y.; Zhang, J.-W.; Yang, L.; Chen, J.; Liu, B.; Su, C.; Zhou, W.-S.; Lin, G.-Q. Total synthesis of phorboxazole B. *Chem. Eur. J.*, **2006**, *12*, 1185. Lucas, B.S.; Gopalsamuthiram, V.; Burke, S.D. Total synthesis of phorboxazole B. *Angew. Chem. Int. Ed.*, **2007**, *46*, 769. Smith, III, A.B.; Razler, T.M.; Ciavarri, J.P.; Hirose, T.; Ishikawa, T.; Meis, R.M. A second-generation total synthesis of (+)-phorboxazole A. *J. Org. Chem.*, **2008**, *73*, 1192.

[114] Forsyth, C.J.; Ying, L.; Chen, J.; La Clair, J.J. Phorboxazole analogues induce association of cdk4 with extranuclearcytokeratin intermediate filaments. *J. Am. Chem. Soc.*, **2006**, *128*, 3858.

[115] Uckun, F.M.; Forsyth, C.J. Anticancer activity of synthetic analogues of the phorboxazoles. *Bioorg. Med. Chem. Lett.*, **2001**, *11*, 1181.

[116] Smith, III, A.B.; Razler, T.M.; Meis, R.M.; Pettit, G.R. Synthesis and biological evaluation of phorboxazole congeners leading to the discovery and preparative-scale synthesis of(+)-chlorophorboxazole a possessing picomolar human solidtumor cell growth inhibitory activity. *J. Org. Chem.*, **2008**, *73*, 1201.

[117] Wieczorek, H.; Brown, D.; Grinstein, S.; Ehrenfeld, J.; Harvey, W.R. Animal plasma membrane energization by proton-motive V-ATPases. *Bioessays*, **1999**, *21*, 637.

[118] Torigoe, T.; Izumi, H.; Ishiguchi, H.; Uramoto, H.; Murakami, T.; Ise, O.; Yoshida, Y.; Tanabe, M.; Nomoto, M.; Itoh, H.; Kohno, K. Enhanced expression of the human vacuolar H+-ATPase c subunit gene (*ATP6L*) in response to anticancer agents. *J. Biol. Chem.*, **2002**, *277*, 36534. Lu, X.; Qin, W.; Li, J.; Tan, N.; Pan, D.; Zhang, H.; Xie, L.; Yao, G.; Shu, H.; Yao, M.; Wan, D.; Gu, J.; Yang, S. The growth and metastasis of human hepatocellular carcinoma xenografts are inhibited by small interfering RNA targeting to the subunit ATP6L of proton pump. *Cancer Res.*, **2005**, *65*, 6843.

[119] For recent reviews on vacuolar ATPase inhibitors, see: Beutler, J.A.; McKee, T.C. Novel marine and microbial natural product inhibitors of vacuolar ATPase. *Curr. Med. Chem.*,

2003, *10*, 787. Yet, L. Chemistry and biology of salicylihalamide A and related compounds. *Chem. Rev.*, **2003**, *103*, 4283.

[120] Erickson, K.L.; Beutler, J.A.; Cardellina II, J.H.; Boyd, M.R. Salicylihalamides A and B, novel cytotoxic macrolides from themarine sponge*Haliclona*sp. *J. Org. Chem.*, **1997**, *62*, 8188.

[121] Galinis, D.L.; McKee, T.C.; Pannell, L.K.; Cardellina II, J.H.; Boyd, M.R. Lobatamides A and B, novel cytotoxic macrolides from the tunicate*Aplidiumlobatum*. *J. Org. Chem.*, **1997**, *62*, 8968. McKee, T.C.; Galinis, D.L.; Pannell, L.K.; Cardellina II, J.H.; Laakso, J.; Ireland, C.M.; Murray, L.; Capon, R.J.; Boyd, M.R. The lobatamides, novel cytotoxic macrolides from southwesternpacific tunicates. *J. Org. Chem.*, **1998**, *63*, 7805.

[122] Boyd, M.R.; Farina C.; Belfiore, P.; Gagliardi, S.; Kim, J.-W.; Hayakawa, Y.; Beutler, J.A.; McKee, T.C.; Bowman, B.J.; Bowman, E.J. Discovery of a novel antitumor benzolactone enamide class that selectively inhibits mammalian vacuolar-type (H+)-ATPases. *J. Pharmacol. Exp. Ther.*, **2001**, *297*, 114.

[123] Huss, M.; Ingenhorst, G.; König, S.; Gaßel, M.; Dröse, S.; Zeeck, A.; Altendorf, K.; Wieczorek, H. Concanamycin A, the specific inhibitor of V-ATPases, binds to theVosubunit c. *J. Biol. Chem.*, **2002**, *277*, 40544. Xie, X.-S.; Padron, D.; Liao, X.; Wang, J.; Roth, M.G.; De Brabander, J.K. Salicylihalamide A inhibits the V0sector of the V-ATPase through amechanism distinct from bafilomycin A1. *J. Biol. Chem.*, **2004**, *279*, 19755.

[124] Wu, Y.; Esser, L.; De Brabander, J.K. Revision of the absolute configuration of salicylihalamide A through asymmetric total syntesis. *Angew. Chem. Int. Ed.*, **2000**, *39*, 4308.

[125] Snider, B.B.; Song, F. Total synthesis of (−)-salicylihalamide A. *Org. Lett.*, **2001**, *3*, 1817. Labrecque, D.; Charron, S.; Rej, R.; Blais, C.; Lamothe, S. Enantioselective total synthesis of salicylihalamides A and B. *Tetrahedron Lett.*, **2001**, *42*, 2645.

[126] Wu, Y.; Seguil, O.R.; De Brabander, J.K. Synthesis and initial structure–activityrelationships of modifiedsalicylihalamides. *Org. Lett.*, **2000**, *2*, 4241.

[127] Lebreton, S.; Xie, X.-S.; Ferguson, D.; De Brabander, J.K. Ring-closing metathesis: a powerful tool for the synthesis ofsimplified salicylihalamide-based V-ATPase inhibitors. *Tetrahedron,* **2004**, *60*, 9635.

[128] Herb, C.; Maier, M.E. A formal total synthesis of the salicylihalamides. *J. Org. Chem.*, **2003**, *68*, 8129. Herb, C.; Bayer, A.; Maier, M.E. Total synthesis of salicylihalamides A and B. *Chem. Eur. J.*, **2004**, *10*, 5649. Haack, T.; Haack, K.-L.; Diederich, W.E.; Blackman, B.; Roy, S.; Pusuluri, S.; Georg, G.I. Formal total syntheses of the (-)-salicylihalamides A and B fromD-glucose andL-rhamnose. *J. Org. Chem.*, **2005**, *70*, 7592.

[129] Shen, R.; Lin, C.T.; Porco, Jr., J.A. Total synthesis and stereochemical assignment of the salicylate antitumormacrolide lobatamide C. *J. Am. Chem. Soc.*, **2002**, *124*, 5650.

[130] Shen, R.; Lin, C.T.; Bowman, E.J.; Bowman, B.J.; Porco, Jr., J.A. Synthesis and V-ATPase inhibition ofsimplified lobatamide analogues. *Org. Lett.*, **2002**, *4*, 3103.

[131] Cantrell, C.L.; Gustafson, K.R.; Cecere, M.R.; Lewis, K.P.; Boyd, M.R. Chondropsins A and B: novel tumor cell growth-inhibitorymacrolide lactams from the marine sponge*Chondropsis*sp. *J. Am. Chem. Soc.*, **2000**, *122*, 8825.

[132] Rashid, M.A.; Gustafson, K.R.; Boyd, M.R. New chondropsin macrolide lactams from marine sponges in thegenus*Ircinia*. *Tetrahedron Lett.*, **2001**, *42*, 1623. Rashid, M.A.; Cantrell, C.L.; Gustafson, K.R.; Boyd, M.R. Chondropsin D, a new 37-membered-ring

macrolide lactam from the marinespongeChondropsisspecies. *J. Nat. Prod.,* **2001**, *64*, 1341. Rashid, M.A.; Gustafson, K.R.; Crouch, R.C.; Groweiss, A.; Pannell, L.K.; Van, Q.N.; Boyd, M.R. Application of high-field NMR andcryogenic probe technologies in thestructural elucidation of poecillastrin A, a new antitumor macrolide lactam fromthe sponge*Poecillastra*species. *Org. Lett.,* **2002**, *4*, 3293. Takemoto, D.; Takekawa, Y.; Van Soest, R.W.M.; Fusetani, N.; Matsunaga, S. Poecillastrin D: A new cytotoxin of the chondropsin classfrom marine sponge*Jaspis serpentina. Biosci. Biotechnol. Biochem.,* **2007**, *71*, 2697. Takada, K.; Choi, B.W.; Rashid, M.A.; Gamble, W.R.; Cardellina, II, J.H.; Van, Q.N.; Lloyd, J.R.; McMahon, J.B.; Gustafson, K.R. Structural assignment of poecillastrins B and C, macrolide lactams from the deep-waterCaribbean sponge*Poecillastra*species. *J. Nat. Prod.,* **2007**, *70*, 428. Plaza, A.; Baker, H.L.; Bewley, C.A. Mirabilin, an antitumor macrolide lactam from the marine sponge*Siliquariaspongiamirabilis*. *J. Nat. Prod.,* **2008**, *71*, 473.

[133] Bowman, E.J.; Gustafson, K.R.; Bowman, B.J.; Boyd, M.R. Identification of a new chondropsin class of antitumor compoundthat selectively inhibits V-ATPases. *J. Biol. Chem.,* **2003**, *278*, 44147.

[134] Kobayashi, J.; Cheng, J.; Ohta, T.; Nakamura, H.; Nozoe, S.; Hirata, Y.; Ohizumi, Y.; Sasaki, T. Iejimalides A and B, novel 24-membered macrolides with potent antileukemic activity from the Okinawan tunicate *Eudistoma* cf. *rigida. J. Org. Chem.,* **1988**, *53*, 6147.

[135] Shimbo, K.; Tsuda, M.; Fukushi, E.; Kawabata, J.; Kobayashi, J. Dytesinins A and B, new clerodane-type diterpenes with a cyclopropane ring from the tunicate *Cystodytes* sp. *Tetrahedron.,* **2000**, *56*, 7923.

[136] Tsuda, M.; Nozawa, K.; Shimbo, K.; Ishiyama, H.; Fukushi, E.; Kawabata, J.; Kobayashi, J. Stereochemistry of iejimalide B. *Tetrahedron Lett.,* **2003**, *44*, 1395. Nozawa, K.; Tsuda, M.; Ishiyama, H.; Sasaki, T.; Tsuruo, T.; Kobayashi, J. Absolute stereochemistry and antitumor activity of iejimalides. *Bioorg. Med. Chem.,* **2006**, *14*, 1063.

[137] Fürstner, A.; Nevado, C.; Tremblay, M.; Chevrier, C.; Teply, F.; Aïssa, C.; Waser, M. Total synthesis of iejimalide B. *Angew. Chem. Int. Ed.,* **2006**, *45*, 5837.

[138] Fürstner, A.; Nevado, C.; Waser, M.; Tremblay, M.; Chevrier, C.; Teply, F.; Aïssa, C.; Moulin, E.; Müller, O. Total synthesis of iejimalide A-D and assessment of theremarkable actin-depolymerizing capacity of these polyenemacrolides. *J. Am. Chem. Soc.,* **2007**, *129*, 9150.

[139] Kazami, S.; Muroi, M.; Kawatani, M.; Kubota, T.; Usui, T.; Kobayashi, J.; Osada, H. Iejimalides show anti-osteoclast activity *via* V-ATPase inhibition. *Biosci. Biotechnol. Biochem.,* **2006**, *70*, 1364.

[140] Schweitzer, D.; Zhu, J.; Jarori, G.; Tanaka, J.; Higa, T.; Davisson, V.J.; Helquist, P. Synthesis of carbamate derivatives of iejimalides. Retentionof normal antiproliferative activity and localization of bindingin cancer cells. *Bioorg. Med. Chem.,* **2007**, *15*, 3208.

[141] Diyabalange, T.; Amsler, C.D.; McClintock, J.B.; Baker, B.J. Palmerolide A, a cytotoxic macrolide from the antarctic tunicate*Synoicum adareanum. J. Am. Chem. Soc.,* **2006**, *128*, 5630.

[142] Lebar, M.D.; Baker, B.J. On the stereochemistry of palmerolide A. *Tetrahedron Lett.,* **2007**, *48*, 8009.

[143] Jiang, X.; Liu, B.; Lebreton, S.; De Brabander, J.K. Total synthesis and structure revision of the marine metabolitepalmerolide A. *J. Am. Chem. Soc.,* **2007**, *129*, 6386. Nicolaou, K.C.; Guduru, R.; Sun, Y.-P.; Banerji, B.; Chen, D.Y.-K. Total synthesis of the originally

proposed and revised structures ofpalmerolide A. *Angew. Chem. Int. Ed.*, **2007**, *46*, 5896. Nicolaou, K.C.; Sun, Y.-P.; Guduru, R.; Banerji, B.; Chen, D.Y.-K. Total synthesis of the originally proposed and revisedstructures of palmerolide A and isomers thereof. *J. Am. Chem. Soc.*, **2008**, *130*, 3633.

[144] Nicolaou, K.C.; Leung, G.Y.C.; Dethe, D.H.; Guduru, R.; Sun, Y.-P.; Lim, C.S.; Chen, D.Y.-K. Chemical synthesis and biological evaluation of palmerolide A analogues. *J. Am. Chem. Soc.*, **2008**, *130*, 10019.

[145] Northcote, P.T.; Blunt, J.W.; Munro, M.H.G. Pateamine: a potent cytotoxin from the New Zealand sponge, *Mycale* sp. *Tetrahedron Lett.*, **1991**, *32*, 6411. Hood, K.A.; West, L.M.; Northcote, P.T.; Berridge, M.V.; Miller, J.H. Induction of apoptosis by the marinesponge (Mycale) metabolites, mycalamide A and pateamine. *Apoptosis*, **2001**, *6*, 207.

[146] Rzasa, R.M.; Shea, H.A.; Romo, D. Total synthesis of the novel, immunosuppressiveagent (-)-pateamine A from*Mycale*sp. employing aβ-lactam-based macrocyclization. *J. Am. Chem. Soc.*, **1998**, *120*, 591. Romo, D.; Rzasa, R.M.; Shea, H.A.; Park, K.; Langenhan, J.M.; Sun, L.; Akhiezer, A.; Liu, J.O. Total synthesis and immunosuppressive activity of (-)-pateamine Aand related compounds: implementation of aβ-lactam-basedmacrocyclization. *J. Am. Chem. Soc.*, **1998**, *120*, 12237.

[147] Romo, D.; Choi, N.S.; Li, S.; Buchler, I.; Shi, Z.; Liu, J.O. Evidence for separate binding and scaffolding domains inthe immunosuppressive and antitumor marine naturalproduct, pateamine A: design, synthesis, and activitystudies leading to a potent simplified derivative. *J. Am. Chem. Soc.*, **2004**, *126*, 10582.

[148] Bordeleau, M.; Matthews, J.; Wojnar, J.M.; Lindqvist, L.; Novac, O.; Jankowsky, E.; Sonenberg, N.; Northcote, P.; Teesdale-Spittle, P.; Pelletier, J. Stimulation of mammalian translation initiation factor eIF4A activity by a small molecule inhibitor of eukaryotic translation. *Proc. Natl. Acad. Sci. USA.*, **2005**, *102*, 10460. Low, W.-K.; Dang, Y.; Schneider-Poetsch, T.; Shi, Z.; Choi, N.-S.; Merrick, W.C.; Romo, D.; Liu, J.O. Inhibition of eukaryotic translation initiation by the marine natural product pateamine A. *Mol Cell.*, **2005**, *20*, 709.

[149] Bordeleau, M.; Cencic, R.; Lindqvist, L.; Oberer, M.; Northcote, P.; Wagner, G.; Pelletier, J. RNA-mediated sequestration of the RNA helicase eIF4A by pateamine A inhibits translation initiation. *Chem. Biol.*, **2006**, *13*, 1287.

[150] Low, W.-K.; Dang, Y.; Schneider-Poetsch, T.; Shi, Z.; Choi, N.-S.; Rzasa, R.M.; Shea, H.A.; Li, S.; Park, K.; Ma, G.; Romo, D.; Liu, J.O. Isolation and identification of eukaryotic initiation factor 4A as a molecular target for the marine natural product pateamine A. *Methods Enzymol.*, **2007**, *431*, 303. Low, W.-K.; Dang, Y.; Bhat, S.; Romo, D.; Liu, J.O. Substrate-dependent targeting of eukaryotic translation initiation factor 4a by pateamine A: Negation of domain-linker regulation of activity. *Chem Biol.*, **2007**, *14*, 715.

[151] Fusetani, N.; Sugawara, T.; Matsunaga, S. Cytotoxic metabolites of the marine sponge *Mycale adhaerens* Lambe. *J. Org. Chem.*, **1991**, *56*, 4971.

[152] Nishimura, S.; Matsunaga, S.; Yoshida, S.; Nakao, Y.; Yokoyama, S.; Fusetani, N. 13-Deoxytedanolide, a marine sponge-derived antitumormacrolide, binds to the 60S large ribosomal subunit. *Bioorg. Med. Chem.*, **2005**, *13*, 449.

[153] Schroeder, S.J.; Blaha, G.; Tirado-Rives, J.; Steitz, T.; Moore, P.B. The structures of antibiotics bound to the E site region of the 50 S ribosomal bubunit of *Haloarcula marismortui*: 13-deoxytedanolide and girodazole. *J. Mol. Biol.*, **2007**, *367*, 1471.

[154] Schmitz, F.J.; Gunasekera, S.P.; Yalamanchili, G.; Hossain, M.B.; Van der Helm, D. Tedanolide: A potent cytotoxic macrolide from the Caribbean sponge *Tedania ignis*. *J. Am. Chem. Soc.*, **1984**, *106*, 7251.

[155] Chevallier, C.; Bugni, T.S.; Feng, X.; Harper, M.K.; Orendt, A.M.; Ireland, C.M. Tedanolide C: A potent new 18-membered-ringcytotoxic macrolide isolated from the PapuaNew Guinea marine sponge*Ircinia*sp. *J. Org. Chem.*, **2006**, *71*, 2510. Meragelman, T.L.; Willis, R.H.; Woldemichael, G.M.; Heaton, A.; Murphy, P.T.; Snader, K.M.; Newman, D.J.; Van Soest, R.; Boyd, M.R.; Cardellina, II, J.H.; McKee, T.C. Candidaspongiolides, distinctive analogues of tedanolide from sponges of the genus*Candidaspongia*. *J. Nat. Prod.*, **2007**, *70*, 1133.

[156] Smith, III, A.B.; Adams, C.M.; Lodise Barbosa, S.A.; Degnan, A.P. Total synthesis of (+)-13-deoxytedanolide. *J. Am. Chem. Soc.*, **2003**, *125*, 350. Julian, L.D.; Newcom, J.S.; Roush, W.R. Total synthesis of (+)-13-deoxytedanolide. *J. Am. Chem. Soc.*, **2005**, *127*, 6186. Ehrlich, G.; Hassfeld, J.; Eggert, U.; Kalesse, M. The total synthesis of (+)-tedanolide. *J. Am. Chem. Soc.*, **2006**, *128*, 14038. Smith, III, A.B.; Lee, D. Total synthesis of (+)-tedanolide. *J. Am. Chem. Soc.*, **2007**, *129*, 10957. Ehrlich, G.; Hassfeld, J.; Eggert, U.; Kalesse, M. The total synthesis of (+)-tedanolide—A macrocyclic polyketide frommarine sponge*Tedania ignis*. *Chem. Eur. J.*, **2008**, *14*, 2232.

[157] Nishimura, S.; Matsunaga, S.; Yoshida, S.; Nakao, Y.; Hirota, H.; Fusetani, N. Structure–activity relationship study on 13-deoxytedanolide, a highly antitumor macrolide from the marine sponge*Mycaleadhaerens*. *Bioorg. Med. Chem.*, **2005**, *13*, 455.

[158] Paterson, I.; Dalby, S.M.; Roberts, J.C.; Naylor, G.J.; Guzman, E.A.; Isbrucker, R.; Pittis, T.P.; Linley, P.; Divlianska, D.; Reed, J.K.; Wright, A.E. Leiodermatolide, a potent antimitotic macrolide from the marine sponge *Leiodermatum sp*. *Angew. Chem. Int. Ed.* **2011**, *50*, 3219.

[159] Napolitano, J.G.; Norte, M.; Padrón, J.M.; Fernández, J.J.; Daranas, A.H. Belizeanolide, ac cytotoxic macrolide from dinoflagellate *Prorocentrum belizeanum*. *Angew. Chem. Int. Ed.* **2009**, *48*, 796.

CHAPTER 2

Recent Developments in Organometallic Supramolecular Complexes as Anticancer Drugs

Cheng-He Zhou*, Hui-Zhen Zhang, Sheng-Feng Cui, Jing-Song Lv, Cong-Yan Yan, Kun Wan, Yi-Yi Zhang, Shao-Lin Zhang, Gui-Xin Cai, Rong-Xia Geng and Guri L.V. Damu

Laboratory of Bioorganic & Medicinal Chemistry, School of Chemistry and Chemical Engineering, Southwest University, Chongqing 400715, P.R. China

Abstract: The research and development of organometallic supramolecular complexes as anticancer supramolecular drugs, which are aggregates mainly formed by one or more inorganic metal compounds with one or more either inorganic or organic molecules in general *via* coordination bonds, has been a quite rapidly developing, increasingly active and newly rising highlight interdisciplinary field. Numerous efforts have been directed toward organometallic supramolecular complexes as potential anticancer agents and the unprecedented progress has been made. This has opened up a wholly new and infinite space to create novel metal-based bioactive supermolecules. More importantly, metal-based complex supermolecules as potential anticancer agents with wide potential applications have become highlight topics in recent years, and are becoming increasingly useful and important in preventing and treating cancer diseases. In view of the rapid progress in organometallic complex anticancer supermolecules with rich variation of structural types, this work systematically reviewed the recent research and development of the whole range of metal-based supramolecular complexes as anticancer agents mainly since 2009. The perspectives of the foreseeable future and potential application of organometallic supramolecular complexes in cancer therapy were also presented. It is hoped that this review will serve as a stimulant for new thoughts in the quest for rational designs of more active and less toxic organometallic supramolecular complex anticancer drugs.

Keywords: Anticancer, cytotoxicity, metal complex, supramolecular drug, platinum, palladium, copper, cobalt.

***Address correspondence to Cheng-He Zhou:** Laboratory of Bioorganic & Medicinal Chemistry, School of Chemistry and Chemical Engineering, Southwest University, Chongqing 400715, P.R. China; Tel/Fax: +86-23-68254967; E-mail: zhouch@swu.edu.cn

Michelle Prudhomme (Ed)

1. INTRODUCTION

Cancer is one of the most formidable diseases in the world and has a significant social and economic impact on the human health care system. Despite modern advancements in diagnosis, prevention and therapy, this disease still affects millions of patients, diminishes the people's quality of life and also is one of the leading causes of death. An investigation from the World Health Organization (WHO) indicates that the number of patients suffering from cancer has continued to rise rapidly with years. The treatment of cancer is multimodal, involving an integrated employment of surgical techniques, radiation therapy, and chemotherapy. The anticancer agents in clinical use include antimetabolites that interfere with the synthesis or formation of nucleic acids, chemically reactive compounds such as alkylating agents, DNA-complexation agents, mitosis inhibitors, and hormones [1, 2]. Unfortunately, most of the agents are pro-apoptotic drugs, which are rather ineffective in combating apoptosis-resistant metastatic cancers [3, 4]. Great hopes are therefore being invested in molecules able to kill metastatic or highly invasive cancer cells by non-apoptotic means, notably for example pro-autophagic drugs. Meanwhile, efforts are also being made to discover and develop new types of compounds that may be able to selectively decrease the migration of cancer cells, notably metastatic cancer cells, and increase their sensitivity to cytotoxic drugs with either pro-apoptotic and/or pro-autophagic effects.

Among various types of anticancer drugs, metal-based supramolecular complexes have been paid special attention, since a large number of metal supramolecular complexes such as cisplatin and carboplatin are successfully marketed or have been in clinical trial in the treatment of various cancer diseases. Metal supramolecular complexes could be called metal complex supermolecules, which are aggregates mainly formed by one or more inorganic metal compounds with one or more either inorganic or organic molecules in general *via* the coordination bonds. Take the anticancer cisplatin *cis*-$[Pt(NH_3)_2Cl_2]$ for example, this drug was usually considered to be the inorganic metal supramolecular complex formed by one molecule of inorganic compound $PtCl_2$ and two NH_3 molecules through coordination bonds, this complex was an aggregate of three molecules formed through non-covalent bonds (here generally considered to be coordination bonds), therefore, cisplatin could be called inorganic complex supermolecule. Metal supramolecular complexes exhibited some specific functions and possessed wide potential application in chemistry, physics, materials, information and environmental sciences and so on [5-7]. Particularly, accompanied with the rapid expansion of supramolecular chemistry in pharmaceutical sciences, metal-based complexes as an important class of supermolecules in the research and development of new drugs have become increasingly active topics. Numerous efforts have been directed toward metal supramolecular complexes as potential medicinal agents, so far this field has been a quite rapidly developing, increasingly active and newly rising highlight interdiscipline. The unprecedented progress has been made [8, 9], and it has opened up a wholly new and infinite space to create novel metal-based bioactive supermolecules. More importantly, metal-based complex supermolecules as potential anticancer agents have been becoming increasingly useful and important since the discovery of cisplatin in the 1960's [10-12].

Metal ions exhibit a wide range of coordination numbers and geometries, which allow to organize the most different anions and organic ligands (with their chemical and biological properties) in more appropriate spatial distributions, affording better modalities of attack to the target molecules. Furthermore, the redox potential of metal can interact with the balanced cellular redox state, modify cell viability either directly or through the conversion of a rather inert compound into an activated one, and thus tune the inherent toxicity of drug [13, 14]. Taken together, it is of imperative to treat cancer with a series of chemically different active metal supramolecular complexes. This is desirable and provides an incentive for expanded research to discover a greater variety of new antitumor drugs. Additionally, the metal ions and the ligands can have a synergic effect. The metals can stabilize the ligands against possible enzymatic degradation before reaching the target while the coordination molecules can have a better hydrophilicity/hydrophobicity ratio than the free ligands, *etc.*

Furthermore, metal-based supramolecular complexes as anticancer drugs might be relatively convenient, cheap and easy for their preparation, and thus result in not only less expense, shorter time and larger possibility to some extent as clinic drugs for their successful research and development, but also better modalities of attack with rich variation of structural types to the target molecules in higher safety, lower toxicity, less adverse effect, higher bioavailability, better biocompatibility, fewer drug-resistances and better curative effects. These overwhelming advantages have been enormously paid special attention and therefore exhibited extensive potential as clinical drugs. This work systematically reviewed the recent research and development of the whole range of metal supramolecular complexes as anticancer drugs mainly since 2009. The perspectives of the foreseeable future and potential application of metal supramolecular complexes in cancer therapy were also presented. It is hoped that this review will serve as a stimulant for new thoughts in the quest for rational designs of more active and less toxic metal supramolecular complex anticancer drugs.

2. TRANSITION METAL SUPRAMOLECULAR COMPLEXES AS ANTICANCER AGENTS

Transition metal has always been a highlighted subject in the field of coordination chemistry due to its distinctive electronic structure. The existence of unpaired electron precipitates the metal to accept electron-donor through coordination, and the strong complexation of transition metal with various ligands by the coordination bonds forms the corresponding metal supramolecular complexes with wide potentials possibly used as conductors, magnetic materials, sensors, drugs, *etc*. It is especially noteworthy that the transition metal-based supramolecular complexes exert intriguing and broad biological activities, and this has motivated a vast amount of related work in cancer therapy. So far many transition metal-based supermolecules as drugs have been extensively used in clinic, some are being investigated in the clinical phase I or II trails, and more are as drugs' candidates in actively ongoing research and development.

2.1. Noble Metal-Based Supramolecular Complexes as Anticancer Agents

Noble metals, a rare expensive kind of transition metals, are of widely interest due to not only their good chemical stability but also their unique or irreplaceable properties such as wavelength selective plasmon absorption resonances, conductivity, catalytic activity, and potential wide applications in conventional and novel technologies (electronics, catalysts, including automotive, as well as the emerging area of fuel-cells *etc.*). In particular, the research and development of noble metal-based supramolecular complexes in the realm of medicine, has progressively become dominated, since the advent of the first inorganic metal supramolecular complex—cisplatin as an anticancer agent.

However, the spectrum of cancers that can be treated with platinum agents is narrow and the therapeutic efficacy suffers from side effects and resistance phenomena. These unresolved problems in platinum-based anti-cancer therapy have stimulated increasing efforts in the search for novel non-platinum-containing metal species as cytostatic agents. Up to now, many excellent achievements have been obtained. As examples, gold complexes have been evaluated in phase I and phase II trials. Some palladium complexes showed significant antitumor activity in normal tumor cells and lower resistance of tumor cells in clinical treatments as well as lower side effects. Noble metal-based supramolecular complexes as anticancer agents have shown wide potential in the prevention and treatment of cancers.

2.1.1. Platinum-Based Supramolecular Complexes as Anticancer Agents

The investigation and application of platinum-based supramolecular complexes as anticancer drugs have been developed vigorously and increased actively since 1969. Platinum complex cisplatin and its second-generation analogues, carboplatin and oxaliplatin, are the most widely used metal-based supramolecular anticancer drugs, and effective to many types of cancers including breast, ovarian carcinoma, colorectal, and metastatic cancers. The success of cisplatin supramolecular complex paved the way for the second- and third-generation platinum drugs, carboplatin and oxaliplatin. In order to improve biological activity, several approaches were considered, for example, the exchange of platinum centers by other metals, the connection of more than one platinum center, platinum complexes with *trans* geometry, and conjugation of metal drugs to proteins or other biomolecules as targeting concepts. Recent attentions have been focused on *trans*-platinum complexes, polyplatinum compounds, and platinum(IV) analogues [15-19]. The current anticancer researches on platinum supramolecular complexes could be categorized as *cis*-Pt(II/IV), *trans*-Pt(II/IV) and polynuclear ones.

(1) *cis*-Platinum(II) Supramolecular Complexes as Anticancer Agents

Cisplatin [*cis*-diamminedichloroplatinum(II)] is the flagship inorganic metal supramolecular complex for a series of platinum(II) antitumor agents employed in the treatment of a wide range of cancers [20]. Its cytotoxic mechanism of action involves intracellular exchange of the labile chloride ligands and ultimate coordination to "soft" biomolecular donor sites. *In vivo*, cisplatin is known to bind to multiple targets including DNA, RNA, proteins, and small-molecule ligands. The anticancer activity of cisplatin is attributed in part to the formation of inter- and intrastrand cross-links in DNA, which inhibits gene transcription and DNA replication, thereby blocking protein synthesis and cell proliferation. Although cisplatin is one of the most effective and commonly used agents to treat various types of human cancer, its clinical effectiveness has been limited by significant undesirable side effects, such as dose dependent, nephrotoxicity and neurotoxicity. Therefore, much attention has been paid to the design of new platinum(II)-based complex supermolecules, like replacing the labile chloride and stable amine ligands with other leaving groups such as cyclic and acyclic amines, to improve pharmacological properties and broad the range of antitumor activity with lower toxicity [21]. For example, in order to prompt the development of novel functionalized platinum complexes, selectively protected monohydroxy derivatives of glucose and galactose were etherified by ω-halo ethers and were transformed into their (diammine) platinum supramolecular complexes. In particular, complex **1** showed nearly the same activities on different tumor cell lines compared to the reference drug carboplatin [22-24].

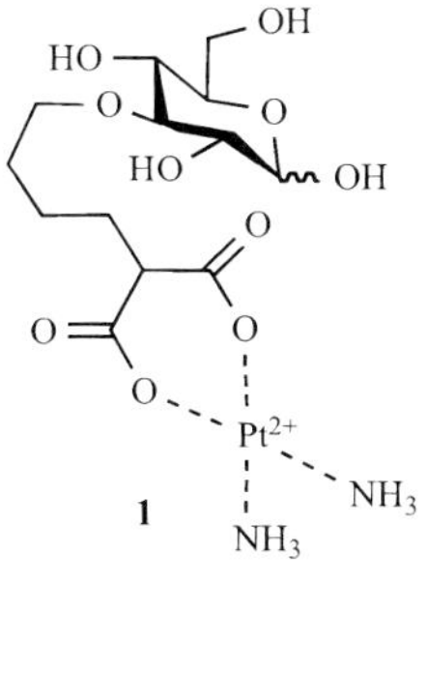

1

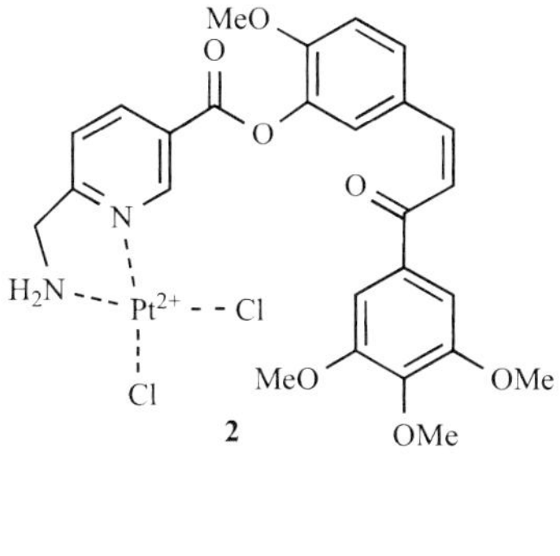

2

In recent years, much work has been done to remain the two leaving group chloride, and modify the NH_3 of N-donor to afford different monoamines, polyamines or N-heterocycle by taking different alkylating agents to replace H of NH_3. Carbobicyclic, estradiol or iminoether as ligands could also exhibit significant activities in overcoming some cancer or even cisplatin resistance cancer cell lines. After finding the analogue of (6-aminomethylnicotinate) dichloridoplatinum(II) and their esterified compounds showed tumor-specific and structure-dependent, Schobert *et al.* synthesized chalcone-platinum supramolecular complex **2**, which exhibited excellent tumor growth inhibition across a panel of 21 cell lines, similar in magnitude and cell line specificity to the activity of the free chalcone. Moreover, complex **2** could also prevent the regrowth of A427 non-small-cell lung cancer cells and 1411HP germ cell tumor cells more effectively than chalcone at low 0.1 μM concentration [25].

N-substituted cyclohexyldiamine platinum(II) supramolecular complexes **3a-c**, which enhanced drug efficiency and reduced toxicity to normal cells, exhibited significant activities compared to cisplatin and oxaliplatin. The IC_{50} value of complex **3** with *R,R* configuration was found to be 5 times lower than cisplatin and oxaliplatin in MCF-7 cells, while the IC_{50} value against MCF-10A cells was observed to be the order **3c** < **3b** < **3a**, in contrast with MCF-7 cells [26]. These results indicated that the configuration of the platinum(II) supramolecular complexes has obvious influence on the antiproliferative activities.

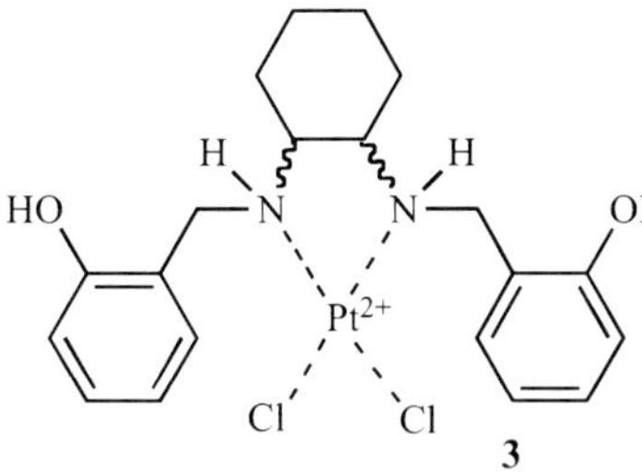

3

a, (R, R)
b, (S, S)
c, (R, S)

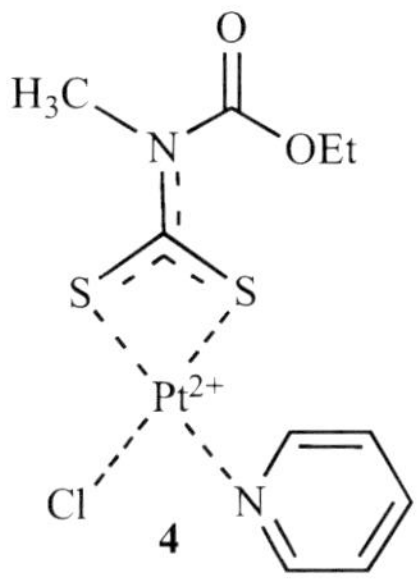

4

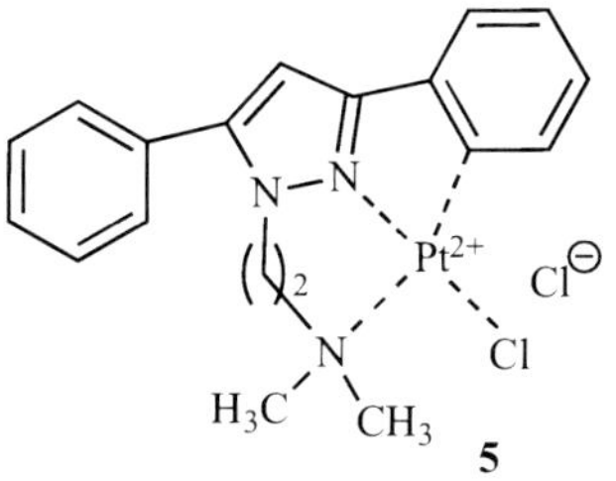

5

Interestingly, some researches revealed that compounds containing one Cl anion as leaving group and N(S)-donor derivatives could also display significant activities. Therefore, the studies of pattern *cis*-[PtCl(L)(L')(L″)] (L, L', L″ = amines, N(S)-heterocycle or thiocarbamide) attracted much attention. It was found that heterocyclic aromatic ligands such as pyridine, terpyridine and acridine exhibited highly cytotoxic activity against a variety of tumor cells, with AMD473 [*cis*-$PtCl_2(NH_3)$(2-methylpyridine)] as one of the most relevant examples, which entered clinical trials and have shown to be particularly helpful in the treatment of ovarian cancer resistant to carboplatin [27, 28]. For another, supramolecular complex [Pt(II)Cl(ESDT)(py)] **4** showed *in vitro* cytotoxic activity higher or, at least, comparable to cisplatin toward all the tested human tumor cell lines. The IC_{50} values reported for Daudi, LoVo, A549 and MeWo cells are particularly interesting since those cell lines represent tumor types intrinsically resistant to cisplatin. Supermolecule **4** was also tested on cisplatin-sensitive and -resistant (C13*) human ovarian carcinoma cells. Intriguingly, it induced a greater inhibition of cell growth than cisplatin on both parent lines, and a complete lack of cross-resistance in C13* cells was observed [29]. In the search of new metallodrugs avoiding toxicity and resistance, special attention has been paid to the replacement of one or both NH_3 ligands of cisplatin by other N-donor ligand(s). Complex **5** as the first example of pyrazole containing metal supermolecule, showed greater antitumoral *in vitro* potential than cisplatin against lung (A549) and breast (MDA MB 231 and MCF7) human cancer cell lines, and this result revealed that pyrazole ring played an important role in exerting anticancer activity [30]. The cytotoxic potencies of platinum complexes **6a-d** were also comparable to those of cisplatin in the cisplatin-sensitive ovarian carcinoma cell line CH1 and the intrinsically cisplatin-resistant colon carcinoma cell line SW480, and complex **6c** gave the best cytotoxicity (IC_{50} = 1.3–2.3 μM). It was found that the presence of iodide resulted in better antitumor activity than the corresponding bromide [31].

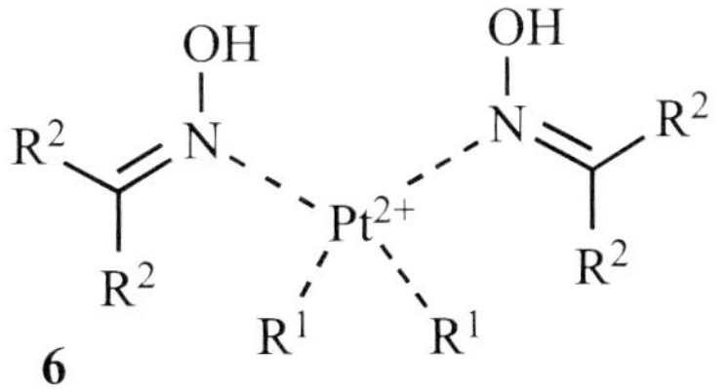

6

a, R^1 = Cl, R^2 = CH_3
b, R^1 = Br, R^2 = CH_3
c, R^1 = I, R^2 = CH_3
d, R^1 = Cl, R^2 = C_2H_5

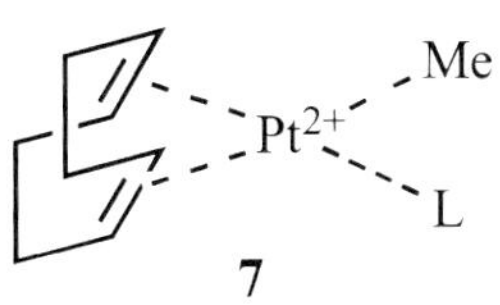

7

a, L = Cl
b, L =

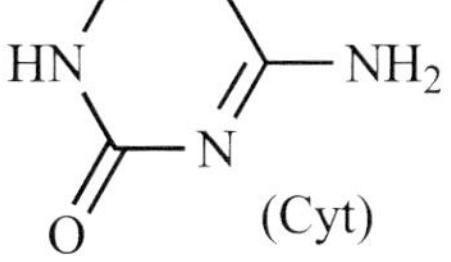

(Cyt)

Moreover, other ligands like lipophilic PPh_3, dipyridophenazine (dppz) and C-deprotonated 2-phenylpyridine were also investigated [32]. For example, platinum complexes [(COD)Pt(Me)Cl] **7a** (cyclooctadiene, COD) and [(COD)Pt(Me)(Cyt)](SbF_6) **7b** exhibited promising antiproliferative effects with IC_{50} values in the range of 8.3-17.5 μM. Compared to cisplatin, these values represent a good starting point for further drug development of COD complexes, probably leading to species with a more pronounced cytotoxicity profile. This preliminary bioactivity showed that replacement of at least one Cl of [(COD)$PtCl_2$] led to active agents [33].

Porphyrin-based platinum(II) supramolecular complex of chlorin **8** showed remarkable photocytotoxicity in HeLa cells at the concentration of 0.5 μM, while the corresponding porphyrin did not. Furthermore, the photocytotoxicity of complex **8** was significantly inhibited by addition of sodium azide, suggesting that $^1O_2$ was the major species causing cell death and also indicated that complex **8** could act as efficient $^1O_2$ generator due to the heavy-atom effect in a cellular microenvironment as well as in nonphysiological media [34].

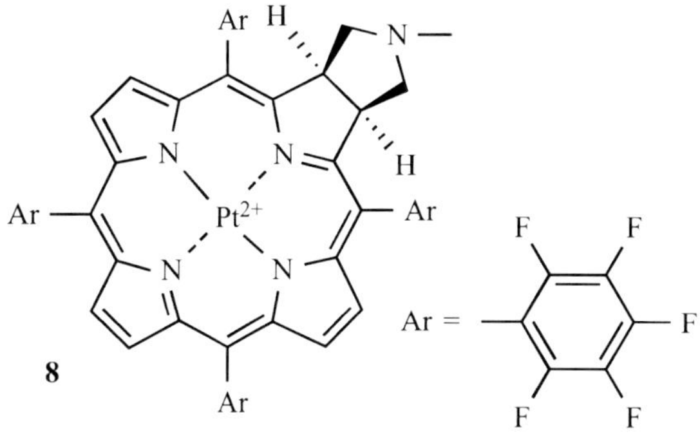

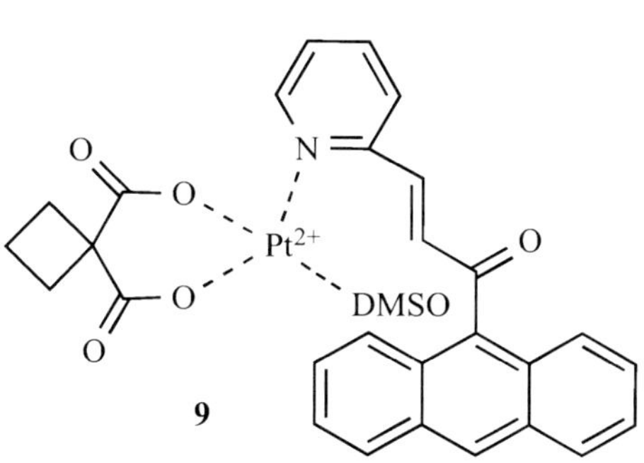

It was known that the anionic replacement of chloride in cisplatin by carboxylato-type leaving groups results in an improved water solubility and lower toxicity. Complex [Pt(A9pyp)(dmso)(cbdca)] **9**, in which cyclobutanedicarboxylate substituted two chloride of *cis*-[Pt(A9pyp)(dmso)Cl_2], showed much better cytotoxicity in A2780R than cisplatin as expected. This suggested that it might indeed have a broader range of antitumor activity than cisplatin. Moreover, these two compounds displayed higher activity than cisplatin in the A496 cells (renal cancer) and in the H226 cells (non-small lung cancer), while cisplatin exhibited moderate activity [35].

(2) *trans*-Platinum(II) Supramolecular Complexes as Anticancer Agents

One major problem with platinum-based supramolecular anticancer drugs is the development of cell resistance. Recent works have increasingly focused on the development of *trans*-platinum complexes, which were initially neglected after the *trans*-[$PtCl_2(NH_3)_2$] was found to have no cytotoxicity. In general, although the usefulness of *trans*-[$PtCl_2(NH_3)_2$] analogues were limited due to their low water solubility, other neutral ligands such as phosphines and thiolates were reported to show significant biological activity. It is now clear that substitution of NH_3 by a range of amines actually produces compounds with cytotoxicity significantly improved over the parent transplatin and in many cases equivalent to that of cisplatin [36].

The pattern of *trans*-[$PtCl_2$(L)(L′)] (L, L′ = amines, N-heterocycle or iminoethers) is considered to be investigated abundantly, and showed good activities against breast cancer, cisplatin-resistant cell lines and leukaemic. Besides the ligands of chiral diamines and planar heterocycles, some researches focused on the iminoether ligands because of their potential N-donor ligands and the nitrogen atom carrying a hydrogen atom suitable for hydrogen-bond formation.

Acetylpyridine platinum(II) supermolecules showed antiproliferative activity against most of the investigated cell lines. Supramolecular complex **10b** with 4-acetylpyridine was 2-4 times more potent cytotoxic agent than 3-acetylpyridine supermolecule **10a**, and overcame cisplatin resistance U2OScisR cells. It suggested that the difference in activity between **10a** and **10b** might be attributed to the positioning of the acetyl substituent on the pyridine ligand. Overall it might be expected that greater activity could be observed for *trans*-dichloridoplatinum(II) complexes with substituents on the *para* (4) rather than the *meta* (3) position [37].

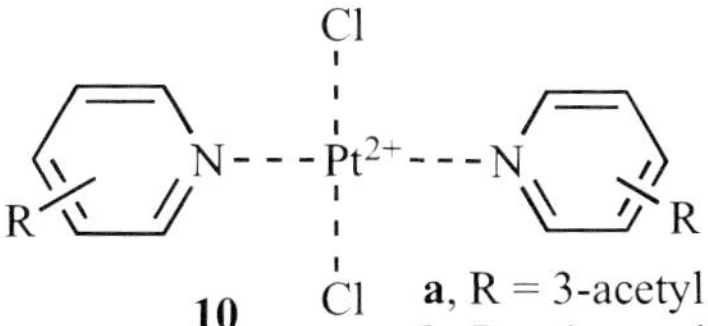

10 **a**, R = 3-acetyl
b, R = 4-acetyl

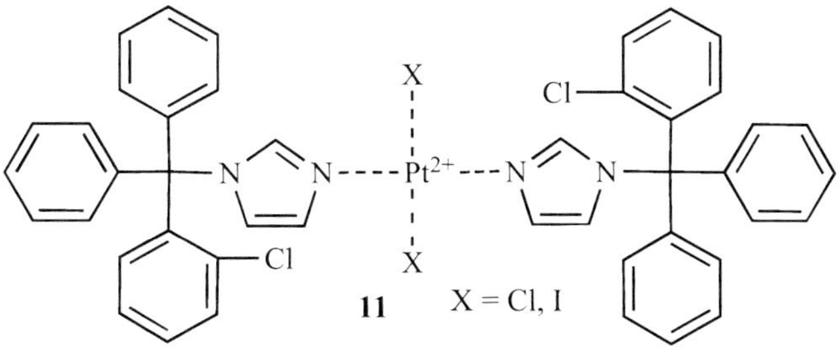

11 X = Cl, I

It is well known that clotrimazole is one of azole antifungal agents with significant curative effect on superficial fungal infection. Surprisingly, its platinum supramolecular complex **11**, formed by two clotrimazole molecules and one platinum dichloride molecule *via* coordination bonds, which interacted with the minor groove of DNA, showed growth inhibitory effects on MCF-7, SKBR-3, HT-29 and B16/BL6 with GI_{50} (50% growth inhibition) values in the 5-25 μM range [38]. To some extent, the researches have expanded the application of clotrimazole, and also represented a novel strategy to discovery and develop new platinum anticancer drugs by the use of other current drugs.

The complexes with formula *trans*-$[PtA_2(L)(L')]$ (A_2 = amines; L, L′ = carboxylate; N-heterocycle), especially the ligands of different isomers of 1,2-diaminocyclohexane (DACH) were found to exhibit superior *in vitro* anticancer activity against colorectal and human hepatocellular cancer cell lines, when compared with oxaliplatin, cisplatin, and carboplatin. The chiral supramolecular complexes of platinum were tested against a panel of human cancer cell lines, with a number of complexes displayed activity significantly greater than that of cisplatin (up to 100-fold increase in activity in the A-427 cell line). Further *in vitro* testing was conducted on the most active compound **12a** and its enantiomer **12b** to provide information about the mechanism of action. These complexes, which displayed activity in cisplatin resistant cell lines, have higher cellular uptake than cisplatin, and did not activate caspase-3 as cisplatin, indicating that these supramolecular complexes exhibited a different mechanism of action [39].

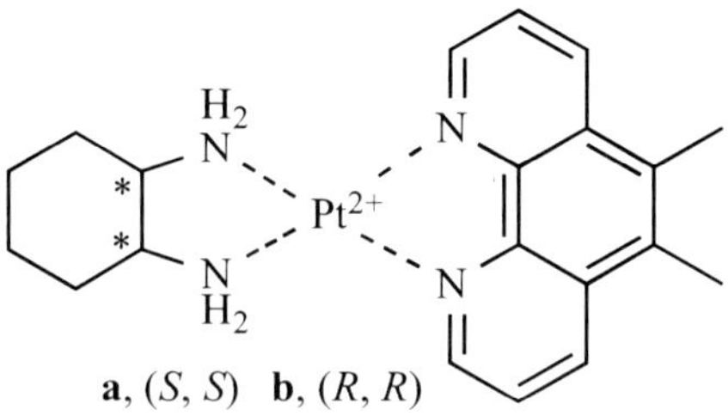

a, (*S*, *S*) **b**, (*R*, *R*)

12

(3) Polynuclear Platinum(II) Supramolecular Complexes as Anticancer Agents

Polynuclear platinum-based supermolecules containing polyamine linkers of variable chain length represent a novel class of antitumor agents with an activity profile distinctly different from that of mononuclear platinum drugs. Early studies indicated that dinuclear platinum supramolecular complexes in which the metal centers were separated by diaminoalkanes were more potent than cisplatin against murine leukemia cells, murine solid tumor cells as well as human tumor cells *in vitro*, and even had good activity against cisplatin-resistant cell lines [40].

Polyamine platinum supramolecular complexes **13a** (CT033) and **13b** (CT233) were derived from the structure of **13c** (BBR3005) and **13d** (BBR3571) respectively. Inclusion of an amine into the parent dinuclear complex **13c** to form **13a** significantly enhanced the cytotoxicity. Complex **13a** was approximately two fold less active than that reported for the corresponding dinuclear complex **13d**. Supermolecule **13b**, where the secondary ammonium ion has been converted into a quaternary ion through the addition of methyl group, was significantly less active than complex **13a**, but maintained its activity in the L1210/DDP cell line [41]. Moreover, another type which the two-platinum centers were linked by cycloamine has also been studied, like macrocyclic polyamine supramolecular complex **14**, whose cytotoxic activity against Hela has been tested and compared with cisplatin. At high concentration range (10^{-4}-10^{-6} M), the cytotoxicity of complex **14** was lower than cisplatin. However, the cytotoxicity of cisplatin was largely attenuated while that of complex **14** remained to be significant at low concentration range (10^{-7}-10^{-8} M) [42].

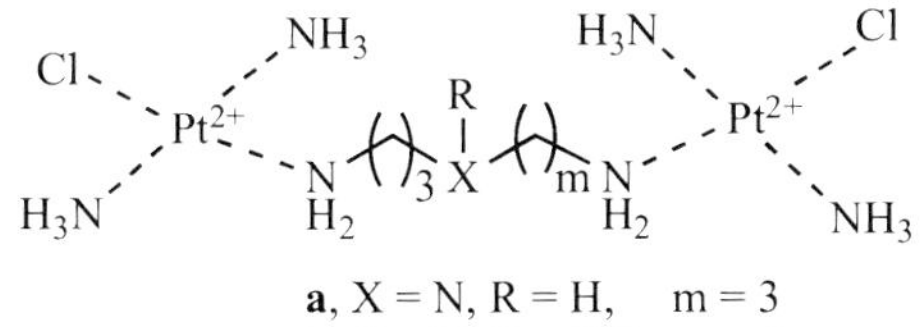

13 **a**, X = N, R = H, m = 3
b, X = N, R = CH_3, m = 3
c, X = C, R = H, m = 2
d, X = N, R = H, m = 4

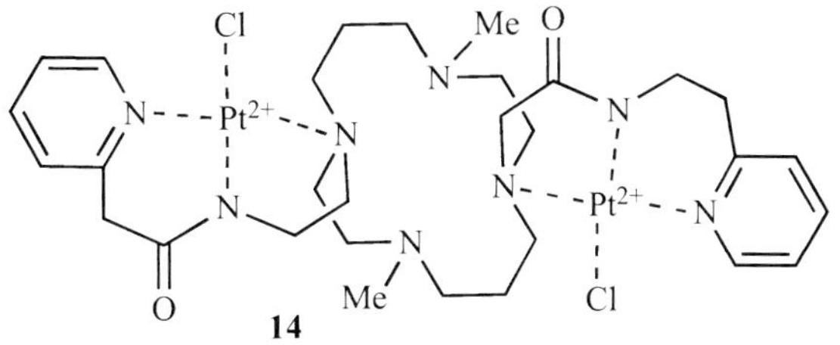

14

In the search for more stable polynuclear Pt(II) complexes to overcome the low stability against sulfur-containing biomolecules, Guo *et al.* reported several di- and tri-nuclear supramolecular complexes in which the Pt(II) centers are bridged by bulky aromatic linkers. The trinuclear supermolecule **15** maintained a relatively high antitumor activity at all the concentrations (10^{-4}-10^{-7} M) and demonstrated much higher *in vitro* cytotoxicity against the A-549 tumor cell line compared with cisplatin, while dinuclear platinum complexes, which one Pt nuclear was substituted by H exhibited no significant activity. This suggested that the third Pt center in trinuclear platinum complex **15** played an important role in the observed cytotoxic activity [43].

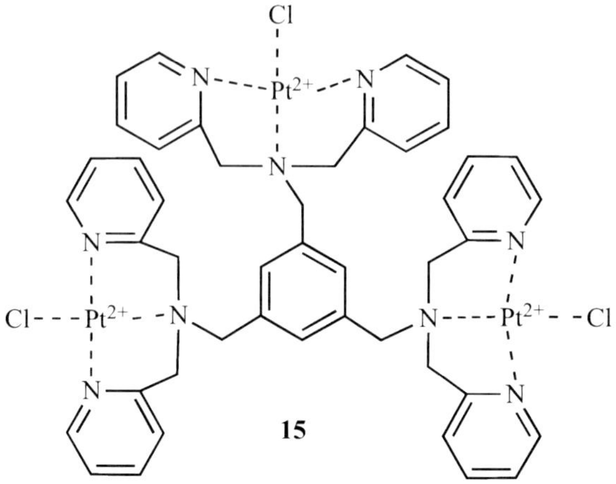

15

A similar structure "non-classical" trinuclear Pt(II) complex **16** with polydentate nitrogen ligand 2,4,6-tris(2-pyridyl)-1,3,5-triazine showed potent cytotoxic activity and reduced cell viability in a concentration-dependent manner against human HT29 colonerectal carcinoma, HepG2 hepatoma, MDA-MB-231 breast cancer and MG63 osteosarcoma cells, and was all higher than cisplatin. The new platinum supramolecular complex warranted further investigation into its antitumor activity against different types of tumors [44].

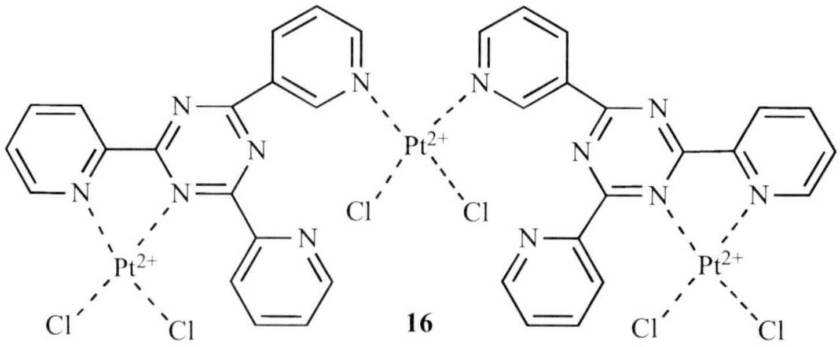

16

(4) Platinum(IV) Supramolecular Complexes as Anticancer Agents

Platinum(II) supramolecular complexes are widely used in cancer chemotherapy, but their efficacy against the majority of malignancies is limited. The reasons for this failure are a combination of uni- and multi-cellular resistance, toxicity, and poor whole-body or cellular pharmacokinetic profiles. Platinum(IV) supramolecular complexes, which have an octahedral structure, offer the opportunities to overcome some of these problems, and have a number of potential advantages over their platinum(II) analogues. In particular, the two extra ligand sites introduced by octahedral geometry and the high kinetic inertness make the complexes less reactive, and therefore will undergo fewer reactions on route to the tumor, resulting in fewer side effects and reducing drug loss due to deactivation. They also offer more possibilities for structural variation than Pt(II) complexes, allowing chemical and physical properties such as reduction potential and lipophilicity to be tuned. The axial ligands of platinum(IV) complexes offer a unique ability in drug design to modify the pharmacokinetic parameters of a prodrug in order to reduce side effects and increase activities.

At present, the pattern of $PtCl_2X_2(L)(L')$, in which X and L/L′ stand for amines and carboxylate or heterocycle, respectively, has been studied extensively. Since it is generally accepted that platinum(IV) supramolecular complexes act as prodrugs and that reduction to the corresponding platinum(II) compounds is crucial for the anticancer activity, a breakthrough was achieved with the carboxylation of transdihydroxidoplatinum(IV) complexes, yielding the first platinum(IV) drug satraplatin available for oral administration. Satraplatin was investigated in advanced phase III clinical trial in hormone refractory prostate cancer in combination with prednisone. The latest information from the 2009 American Society for Clinical Oncology (ASCO) Annual Meeting in Orlando, Florida showed that satraplatin has not been approved by FDA.

There has been a continuous interest in rationally designing polymeric nanocarriers of octahedral Pt(IV) complexes to improve targeting and reduce side effects because polymeric micelles have a superior thermodynamic and kinetic stability to low molecular weight surfactants. Platinum(IV) containing difunctional amine **17a** was evaluated using the sulforhodamine B (SRB) assay for its cytotoxicity. The toxicity assay showed that the Pt(IV) incorporated block copolymer micelles were comparable with the Pt(IV) cross-linker itself, while no toxicity was observed for the block copolymer [45]. Selectively targeting cancer tissue is one promising strategy to search for equally effective analogs that are better tolerated. Based on this, complex **17b** was designed by conjugating platinum(IV) to the cancer-targeting peptide chlorotoxin(CTX, TM601) to deliver cisplatin selectively to cancer cells, and the 1:1 Pt-CTX conjugate was characterized by mass spectrometry and gel electrophoresis. Like most platinum(IV) derivatives, the cytotoxicity of this conjugate was lower in cell culture than cisplatin, but greater than those of its Pt(IV) precursor and CTX in several cancer cell lines [46].

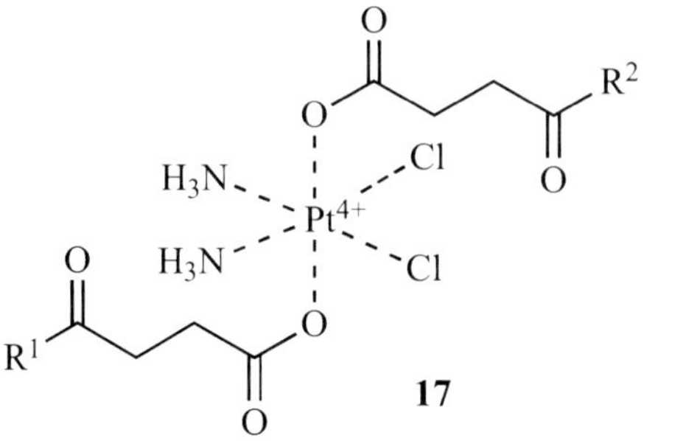

17

a, $R^1 = NH(CH_2)_2NH_2$, $R^2 = NH(CH_2)_2NH_2$
b, $R^1 = OH$, R^2 = NH-polypeptide

Considering the synthesized pyridine-2-thiolato and pyrimidine-2-thiolato platinum(II) complexes that showed significant anticancer activity, the interest for Pt(IV)-based supramolecular complexes, dinuclear Pt(IV) complexes **18a-c** were studied. Complex **18a** gave a significant *in vitro* anticancer activity, which was even higher than that of cisplatin. However, complex **18c** displayed the highest antiproliferative activity, which was found to be comparable or in the case of cisplatin resistant cell lines (DLD-1, 8505C) even higher than cisplatin, and seemed to be a very promising candidate for further *in vivo* or *in vitro* investigations on other cisplatin resistant cell lines [47].

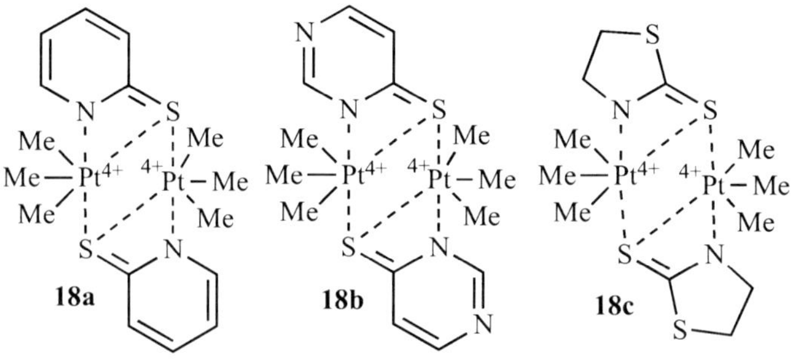

18a **18b** **18c**

2.1.2. Palladium-Based Supramolecular Complexes as Anticancer Agents

The successful exploitation and wide use of platinum complex supermolecules as anticancer drugs attracted great interests to investigate other noble metal supramolecular complexes. Very recently, a large number of researches have been dedicating to the discovery and development of novel non-platinum metal supramolecular antitumor agents including palladium-, ruthenium-, osmium-based complexes and so on, and many excellent achievements have been obtained.

Palladium(II)-based supramolecular complexes have also been a subject of extensive investigation on the basis of their structural and thermodynamic analogy with Pt(II) complexes. However, initial results were not very encouraging due to that Pd(II) complexes generally showed lower anticancer activity as well as higher toxicity than that of their Pt(II) analogues. A recent review has pointed out that such behavior may be related to the more labile nature of palladium(II) complexes, which undergo aquation and ligand exchange reactions 10^5 times faster than the corresponding Pt(II) complexes [48]. Consequently, rapid ligand exchanges were thought to diminish the possibility of Pd(II) complexes reaching the biological target unchanged and increase the risk of adverse effects on biochemical processes that occur in normal cells [49]. In order to overcome these problems, a considerable amount of studies, which can be seen in the recent reviews [50, 51], have suggested that employing robust chelating ligands to reduce the reactivity of the palladium center is a more convenient solution. As is known, palladium(II) is soft Lewis acids, and therefore could form stronger bonds with nitrogen or/and sulfur donor atoms (soft bases) than oxygen donors (hard bases). The compounds chelating metal ions *via* nitrogen donors are generally recognized as an overwhelming family in coordination chemistry, including amino acids, pyridines, pyrazoles, imidazoles and other N-heteraromatic derivatives.

Bis-amino acid esters could chelate Pd(II) to form stable *cis*-complexes **19a-d** through the couple of N atoms, which had lower cytotoxicity than their corresponding ligands although both of them exhibited moderate cytotoxic activities. Primary structure-activity relationships were also concluded, the sequence of activity was in correlation with the R substituent of ligand, with **19d**

> **19c** > **19b** > **19a**. The same order could be established when the lipophilicity of these ester groups were taken into account. Furthermore, the replacement of the central metal ion with Pt(II) significantly enhanced the cytotoxicity. It may provide a simple route to raise the cytotoxic activities of palladium(II) complexes by increasing lipophilicity of the ligands through changing the ester groups as well as the alkyl groups.

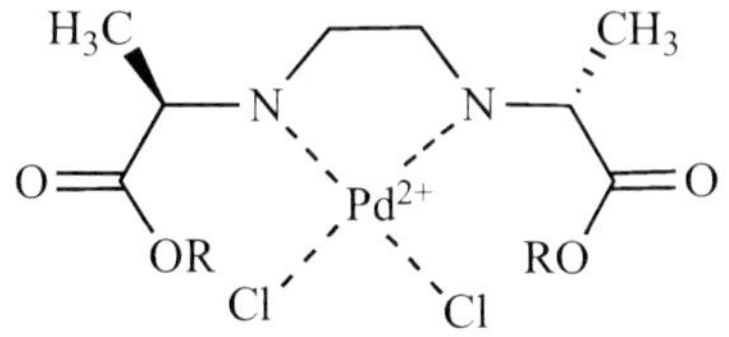

19
a, R = Bu-*i*
b, R = Pr-*i*
c, R = cyclopentyl
d, R = cyclohextyl

It has been proved that the chlorido group as well as oxalato ligand, considered to be very suitable leaving groups, are in favor of cytotoxicity of the platinum(II) complexes. Considering this fact, palladium(II) oxalato supramolecular complexes were prepared and found to exhibit pronounced anticancer activity. Palladium(II) oxalato complexes **20a-e** have been reported and showed significant cytotoxicity, the IC_{50} values especially for complexes **20c** and **20e** against human breast adenocarcinoma (MCF7) cancer cell line were rather lower than that of oxaliplatin and cisplatin [52].

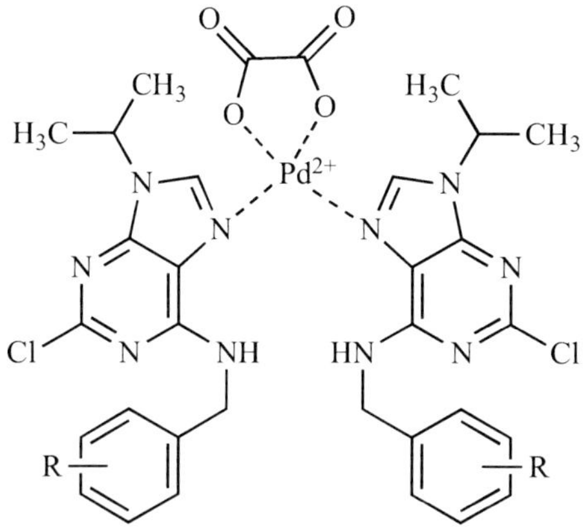

20
a, R = H
b, R = 4-OCH_3
c, R = 2,3-diOCH_3
d, R = 2,4-diOCH_3
e, R = 4-CH_3

The incorporation of carboxylic group to the methylene fraction of ligands based on bis(pyrazolyl) methane derivatives could produce bis(pyrazolyl)acetic acid (R_2bpza) ligands, which are assumed to improve water solubility of the resultant metal supramolecular complexes. However, their palladium(II) complexes **21a-b** give rather low anticancer activities against Chinese hamster ovary (CHO) cells. Substitution of complex **21** with L-cysteine, a molecule existing in the biological fluids likely to prevent these compounds from reaching targeted tumor cells, showed that the rate of substitution with sulfur-containing compounds was not the reason for the low anticancer activities [53].

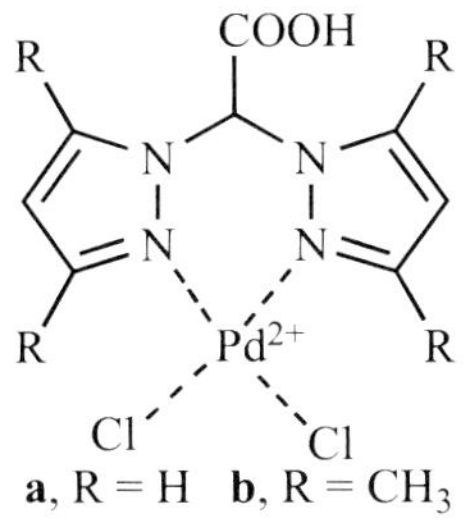

21

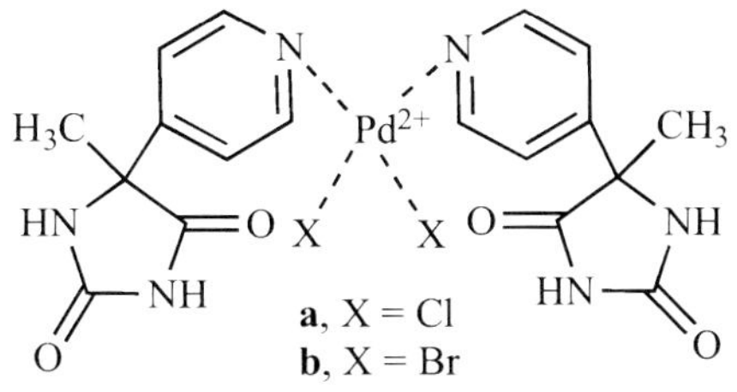

22

The biological activities of different pyridines depend on the substitution groups. The pyridine-derived Pd(II) supramolecular complexes involving imidazoldenedione **22** showed moderate cytotoxic effects, with the dichloro analogue more active [54], while *trans*-complexes containing phosphate ligand **23** did not seem to be promising potential anticancer agents as their cytotoxic activities was about 300 times lower than the reference drug cisplatin. In contrast, its Pt(II) *cis*-complex analogues displayed significant cytotoxic activity, indicating that the presence of bulky non-leaving phosphate ligands seemed to influence the specificity of interaction with cellular targets which gave a chance for the development of novel drugs with more specific toward cancer cells [55].

The introduction of thiosemicarbazone pharmacophores to the pyridine rings at ortho position could generate a sort of compounds as tridentate ligands as well. N (4)-tolyl thiosemicarbazones were proved to be highly active at nanomolar concentrations, much superior to cisplatin. Moreover, selenosemicarbazone, the analog of thiosemicarbazones, can be used as novel interesting ligands with potential antitumor activity as well. Cell cycle analysis of HeLa cells treated with complex **24** displayed that the Pd(II) induced cell cycle perturbations, and increased the number of hypodiploid cells, with fragmented DNA, indicating their ability to drive tumor cell apoptosis, comparable to reference compound CDDP [56].

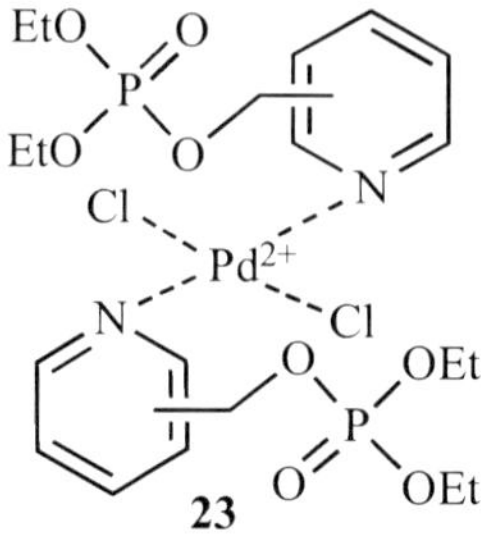

23

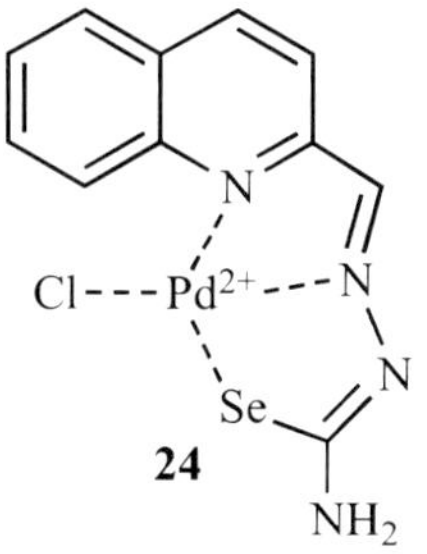

24

2.1.3. Gold -Based Supramolecular Complexes as Anticancer Agents

The application of gold in medicine could trace back to antiquity. Gold supramolecular complexes have definitely triggered an immense interest in the research for cancer chemotherapy starting from the discovery of auranofin **25**, which could inhibit *in vitro* proliferation of HeLa cervical. As a result, a relatively large number of gold-based supramolecular complexes with monovalence or trivalence state of gold were evaluated for antitumor activity and several excellent reviews of this subject are available [57-61].

(1) Gold(I) Supramolecular Complexes as Anticancer Agents

Prompted by the chrysotherapy for clinically treatment of rheumatoid arthritis, the research on gold-based supramolecular complexes has so far focused mainly on the monovalence state. Phosphine-containing gold (I) complexes have received special attention. Gold, as a 'soft' metal, can coordinate with sulphur or/and phosphorus atoms, regarded as 'soft' donors, and many investigations of phosphine gold(I) thiolates, *i.e.* auranofin **25** containing the linear P-Au-S arrangement, have been reported. The mechanism of anticancer activity was likely involving in the inhibition of thioredoxin reductase (TrxR) by binding of Au(I) to the selenocysteine residue of enzyme under loss of their ligands, indicated that the active species was the gold ion.

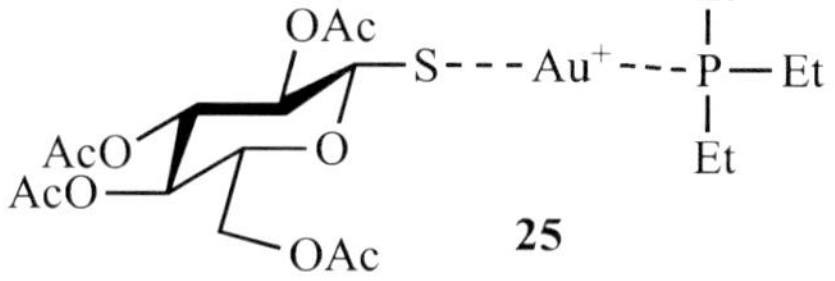

25

Consequently, the nature of ligands attached to the central gold atom is a valuable parameter for drug design. The previous structure-activity relationship study pointed out that phosphine ligand is an important factor for the biological potentiality, therefore, leaving the carbohydrate ligand of auranofin is the first choice for structural variations. A considerable amount of such phosphine-containing gold(I) complexes were reported to have outstanding antiproliferative potency and presented in the latest review.

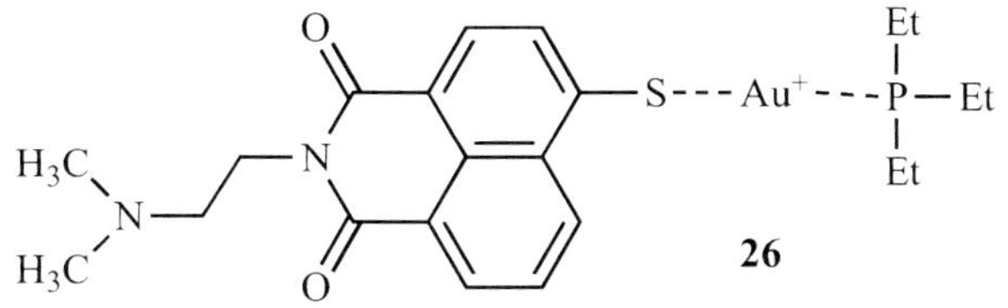

26

In recent studies, gold(I) supramolecular complex **26** containing a naphthalimide ligand deserved to be discussed with significant antiangiogenic effects *in vivo* in contrast to Et_3PAuCl, a precursor which was almost inactive. Additionally, biodistribution experiments demonstrated an efficient uptake of complex **26** into the nuclei, while the non-naphthalimide Et_3PAuCl showed much lower nuclear uptake. It may be speculated that the naphthalimide ligand might be a useful vector to facilitate transport of metals into the nucleus [62].

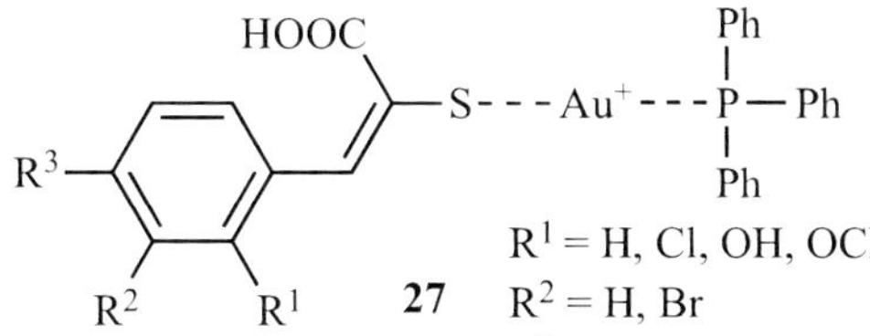

27 R^1 = H, Cl, OH, OCH_3
R^2 = H, Br
R^3 = H, OH, OCH_3

The replacement of carbohydrate with various sulfanylcarboxylic acids can afford the phosphine-based gold(I) supramolecular complex **27** with significant anticancer activity *in vitro*. The IC_{50} values were equal to or higher than that of cisplatin against human ovarian carcinoma cells A2780 and its cisplatin-resistant mutant A2780cis. Primary SAR study revealed that the anticancer potency mainly depended on the nature of the substituent, for instance, the complex of R^1 = OH and R^2 = R^3 = Br showed better cytotoxicity than that of cisplatin [63]. Given that salt formation could modify and optimize the properties and activities of pharmaceutical ingredients, the deprotonation of the carboxyl group in complex **27** with diisopropylamine and triethylamine as base could afford series of novel gold(I) phosphine complexes, respectively. The screening of the cytotoxic activity revealed that the use of diisopropylamine was in general the most effective approach, and its resulting complexes showed potent activity to the A2780cis cell line, with equal or lower IC_{50} values than that of complex **27** [64].

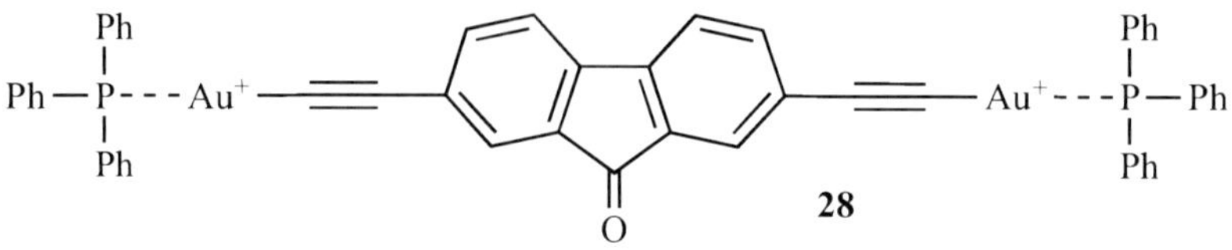

28

The dinuclear gold(I) supramolecular complex **28** containing a fluorenone group is of significance in which it exhibited noticeably potent cytotoxic activity on human cancer cells and provided an additional example of metal arylacetylide complexes with impressive antitumor activities, which are still very scarce. Importantly, the generation of ROS from the carbonyl group of the central ligand spacer is believed to be essential for its cytotoxicity. These findings provided a platform of organic skeleton for conjugation and also highlighted the prospect of acetylide derived gold (I) supermolecules as another promising lead for anticancer metallodrug development [65].

(2) Gold(III) Supramolecular Complexes as Anticancer Agents

The same as other metal-based supramolecular complexes, gold(I) complexes exhibit severe cardiotoxicity occurring after the accumulation of gold in body, making them unfavorable for clinical use. Nevertheless, the gold(III) supramolecular complexes, with their structural and electronic similarity to cisplatin and cisplatin-related antitumor drugs, represent a promising class of potential anticancer agents. However, researches on gold(III) complexes are relatively sparse because of their high electrochemical potential rendering them easily undergoing decomposition to gold(I) or colloidal gold in physiological buffer solutions, which conceivably may also lead to gold(I)-associated toxicity if used *in vivo*. Obviously, these problems can possibly be circumvented by forming stable gold(III) complexes.

Distinct from gold(I) compounds, the gold(III) ion generally features 'hard' atom donors such as nitrogen, oxygen and carbon, but also some species with Au-S bonds have been described. A huge number of studies on gold(III) complexes revealed that one or more multidentate nitrogen-donors could enhance their stability through experiencing reversible electrochemical reduction without decomposition. Pyridine-based gold(III) complexes **29a-d** were prepared and their cytotoxic activity was evaluated toward the human ovarian cancer A2780S cell line and its cisplatin-resistant subline. The results showed that the newly prepared complexes demonstrated remarkable anti-proliferative effects against both ovarian cancer cell lines being all more cytotoxic than cisplatin in the cisplatin-resistant cell line. The gold(III) complexes **29a** and **29b** bearing α-diiminic ligands, that differ only for the substituents on the oxazoline ring, manifested similar biological effects. In **29a** and **29b** the donor atoms are both iminic: one of the pyridine the other of the oxazoline ring. In **29c** and **29d**, the second nitrogen donor is in both case samidic; in **29d** an oxygen donor atom of an alkoxo group is further coordinated to the gold(III) center. Compound **29d** displayed remarkable stability toward reduction and is the most cytotoxic either in the cisplatin-sensitive and - resistant cell lines [66].

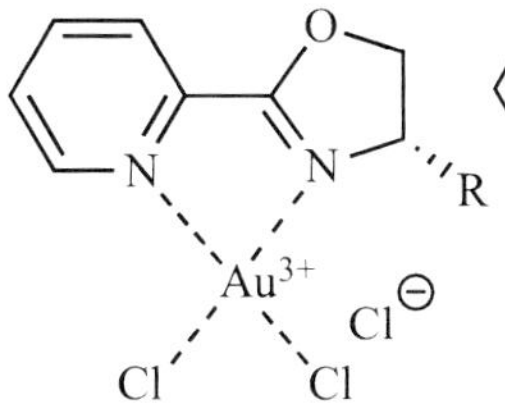

29

a, R = CH_2Ph

b, R = $CH(Me)_2$

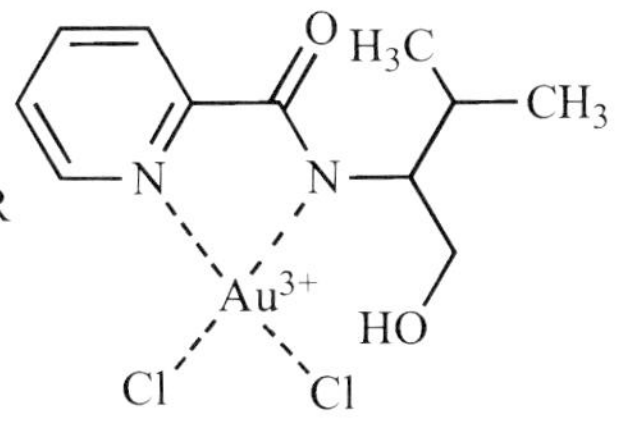

29c

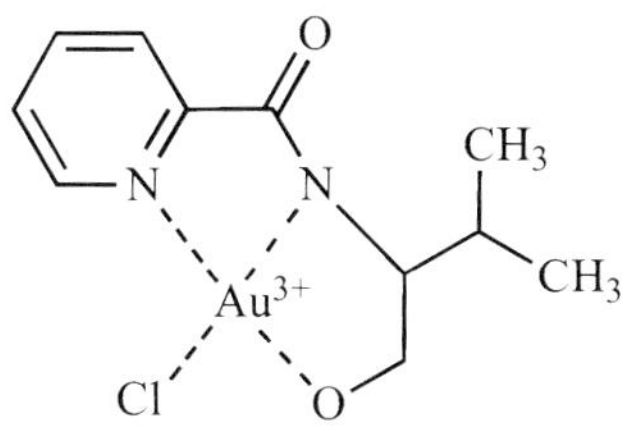

29d

Porphyrin ring can exert strong chelating effect to avoid demetalation, which provides a rigid ligand scaffold to stabilize gold(III) ion. Porphyrin-based gold(III) supramolecular complex **30** exhibited 100-fold higher potency than cisplatin in killing nasopharyngeal carcinoma (NPC) cells, including the cisplatin-sensitive and cisplatin-resistant variants. More importantly, weekly intraperitoneal injection of 3 mg/kg was more effective than the same dose of cisplatin in inducing tumor apoptosis *in vivo* and remarkably inhibited tumor growth without any noticeable side effect. Hence, the use of gold(III) porphyrin complexes may avoid gold(I)-induced cardiotoxicity and exert an advantage for clinical application [67].

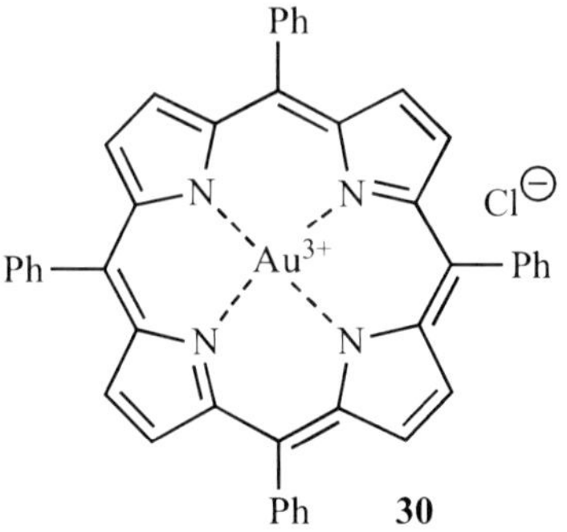

30

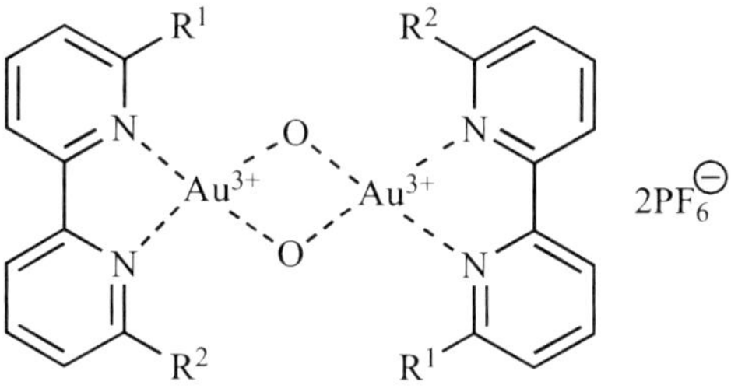

31 **a**, $R^1 = R^2 = H$
b, $R^1 = R^2 = CH_3$
c, $R^1 = H$, $R^2 = CH_2C(CH_3)_3$

Polypyridine is a class of more robust and frequently used ligand to chelate with various metal ions as well. Recently, several polypyridine-containing gold(III) complexes were developed and evaluated for the cell growth inhibition properties of a wide and common panel of human tumor cell lines. Notably, complex **31** turned out to be the best performers on tumor inhibition, with cytotoxic potency commonly ranging from micromolar even low to nanomolar concentration. Good-to-excellent tumor selectivity was additionally established, making them particularly attractive for further pharmacological evaluation. In contrast, complex **32**, although being the most cytotoxic, exhibited a very poor selectivity. The mechanisms of these gold(III)-based complexes in cell growth inhibition possibly involved in depressing histone deacetylase (HDAC), mammalian target of rapamycin (mTOR) or protein kinase C (PKC), acting on the proteasome or alternatively on DNA synthesis, which are profoundly different from those of platinum drugs (where DNA is the primary target). In any case, further work has to be warranted to validate these hypotheses [68].

Pyrazole rings, as core functional groups in the synthesis of different kinds of drugs, exhibit extensive pharmaceutical activities including anticancer property. Many reports have presented that the platinum complexes of pyrazoles and their derivatives possess significant cytotoxicity, while lower toxicity than cisplatin, suggesting that pyrazole-containing ligands could stabilize gold(III) centers and overcome complex instability under physiological conditions. Incorporating the substituted pyrazoles into the ring of pyridine linked by methylene at the 2- or 3-

position could gain two series of gold(III) complexes of totally distinct coordination modes. However, unlike the platinum complexes mentioned above, the bidentate cationic gold(III) supramolecular complex **33** and neutral monodentate supramolecular complex **34** both showed low cytotoxicity against HeLa cells [69].

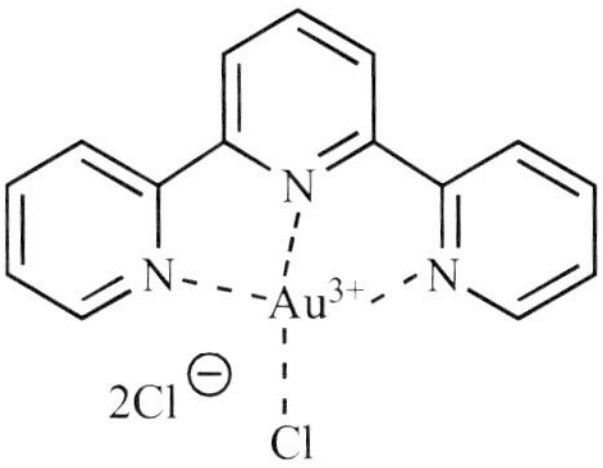

32

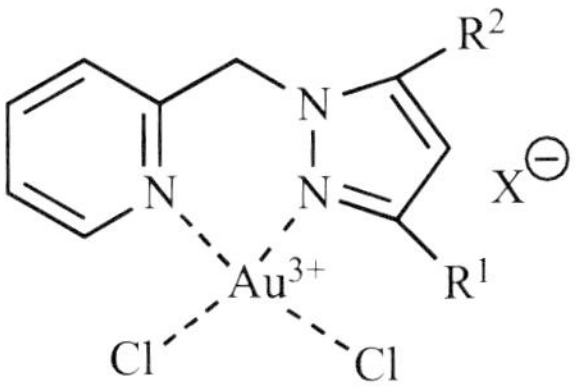

33 $R^1 = CH_3$, t-Bu, Ph, p-Tol
$R^2 = CH_3$, t-Bu, Ph, H
$X = AuCl_4$, Cl

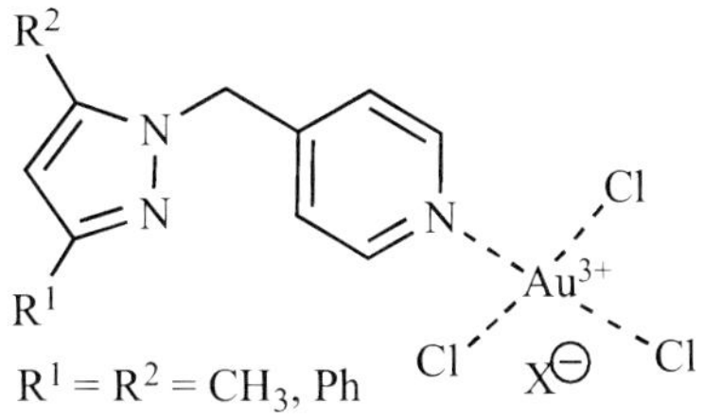

$R^1 = R^2 = CH_3$, Ph
34

The bis-thiosemicarbazone which coordinated with two different Au(III) atoms through the sulfur atoms as monodentate formed the cationic gold(III)-based supermolecule **35**. Its antitumor activity against the HeLa-299 cell line *in vitro* was slightly higher than that of cisplatin, whereas their maximum antiproliferative activities were similar. It indicated that gold(III) complexes of bis(thiosemicarbazone) ligands merit further investigations for treatment of neuroblastoma refractory to cisplatin chemotherapy [70].

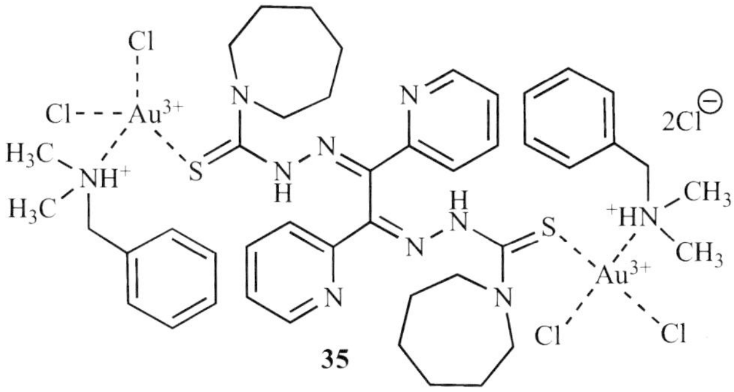

35

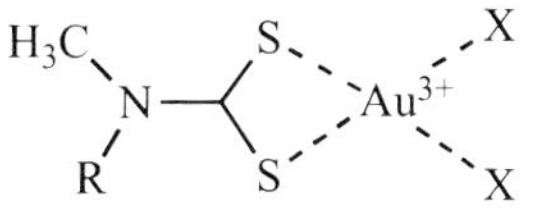

36 $R = CH_3$, CH_2COOCH_3
$X = Cl$, Br

Dithiocarbamate, employing the same coordination mode as the bisthiosemicarbazone presented above, can also stabilize gold(III) ion and the formation of supramolecular complex **36** stands out for its distinctive cytotoxicity *in vitro* on a panel of human tumor cell lines, much more potent even at nanomolar concentration with IC_{50} values about one- to four-fold lower than that of cisplatin. These cell lines include those intrinsically resistant to cisplatin, such as colon (LoVo) and non-small cells lung (A549) adenocarcinoma lines, suggesting a possible lack of cross-resistance with cisplatin for the gold(III) dithiocarbamato complexes, thus making them worthy of further preclinical investigations aiming at their recognition as suitable candidates for clinical trials [71].

2.1.4. Silver-Based Supramolecular Complexes as Anticancer Agents

Silver chemistry has attracted further substantial considerations in recent years to explore the versatility of silver(I) coordination polymers of unusual structures and useful properties, with particular focus on the helical structures, photouminescence and antimicrobial and antifungal properties [72, 73]. Apart from these, silver(I)-based supramolecular complexes as gold analogues have been evaluated for their antitumor activity recently.

Pyrimidine is an important component of nucleic acids and is frequently employed as building block in pharmaceutics for the synthesis of antiviral, anticancer, antibacterial and antifungal agents. Especially, the preparation of new transition metal complexes with pyrimidine derivatives is also a matter of interest. Sliver complex **37** was examined against the human breast cancer MDA-MB231 cell line in comparison with cisplatin as reference. Both [Pd(phen)(ahtp)]Cl and [Ag(ahtp)(PPh_3)(H_2O)] complexes exhibit remarkable growth inhibitory activities with mean values of 7.7 and 4.7 μM, respectively, while the IC value for *cis*-platin is 8.7 μM [74].

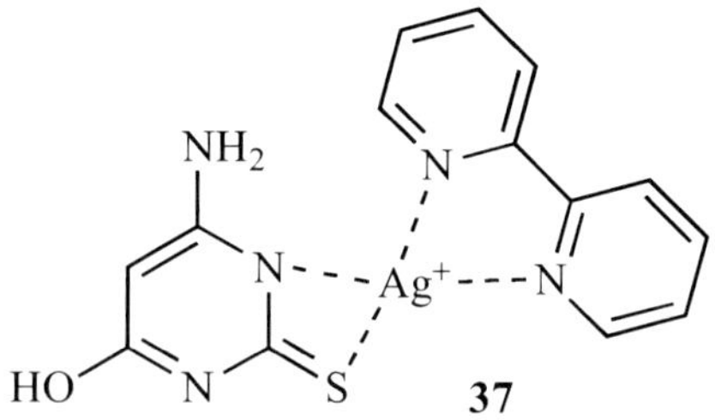

37

Recent studies indicated that some coumarin derivatives were capable of killing cancer cells by modulation of key biochemical pathways. The mixed silver(I) supramolecular complex **38** containing 4-oxy-3-nitro-coumarin and phenanthroline ligands exhibited better anti-proliferation in contrast with its related ligands, with almost 4 times more potent than cisplatin toward HepG2 cells functioning through an alteration in cell cycle progression. Additionally, there was no evidence that P-glycoprotein-mediated multi-drug resistance was likely to decrease antiproliferative activity. Taken together, complex **38** has showed to be a more potent antiproliferative agent capable of altering key biochemical events leading to cell death [75].

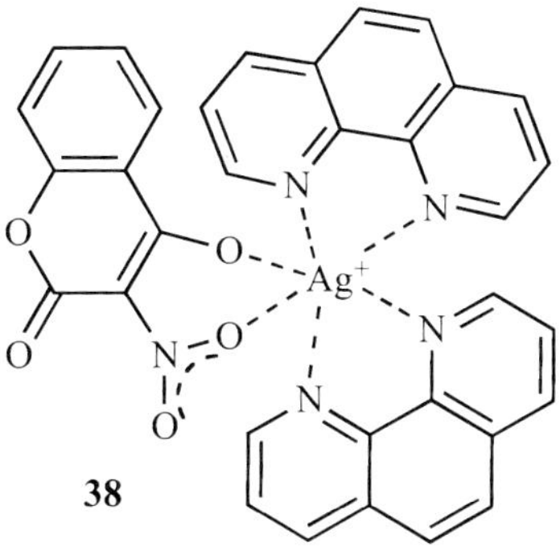

38

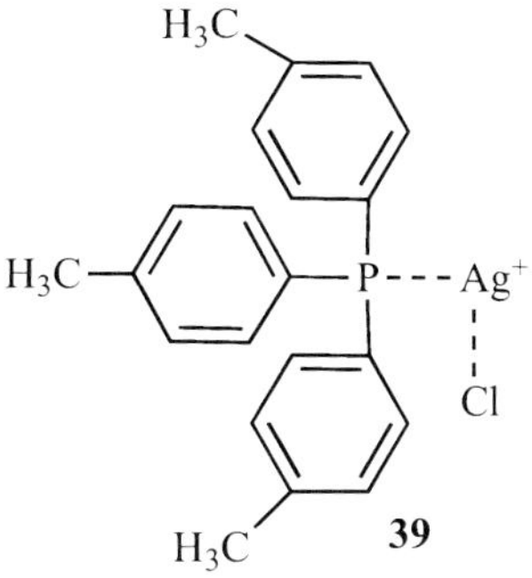

39

Phosphine-derived silver(I) supramolecular complexes of general formula [AgXLn] (L = tertiary phosphine, PR_3 (R = alkyl, aryl or H); n = 1-4; X = coordinating or non-coordinating anion) were systematically reviewed in 2009, which showed a rich variation of structural types. Reaction of silver(I) halides with tri(*p*-tolyl)phosphine (TPTP) in MeOH/MeCN solutions in 1:1 or 1:3 molar ratios can afford complexes of formula [AgCl(TPTP)] **39** or $[AgX(TPTP)_3]$ **40**, respectively. Among these, tetrahedral complexes **40b** and **40c** showed stronger

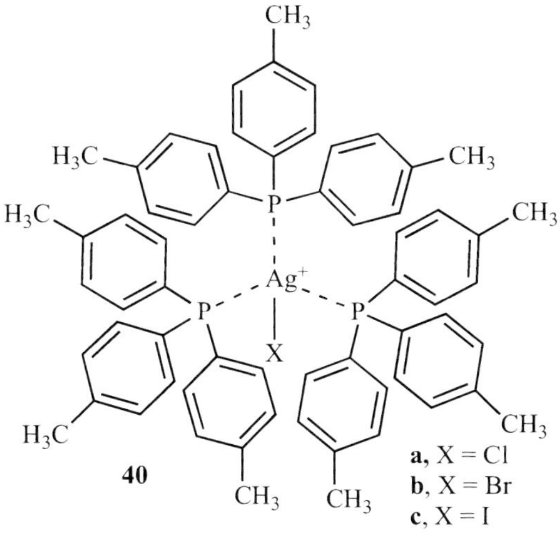

40

a, X = Cl
b, X = Br
c, X = I

cytotoxicity than that of complex **39** with the cubane structure. This may be explained by the aromaticity calculated at special positions located at the centre of the plane determined by the three nearest Ag atoms in case of complex **39**, which might give extra stability to this structure [76].

2.1.5. Ruthenium-Based Supramolecular Complexes as Anticancer Agents

Ruthenium(Ru)-derived complex supermolecules have less toxicity and higher water-solubility than cisplatin, giving them great potential as antitumor metallodrugs. With the development of supramolecular chemistry and medicine, some ruthenium complexes have been found to display a higher selectivity than platinum drugs [77-79], leading to reduce side effects [80]. Since early in the 1970s and 1980s, many reports have indicated the antitumor potential of ruthenium complexes [81]. For example, supermolecules **41** and **42** have already been applied in preclinical experiments. Very recently, Lay *et al.* has reviewed the ruthenium anticancer drugs in overall [82].

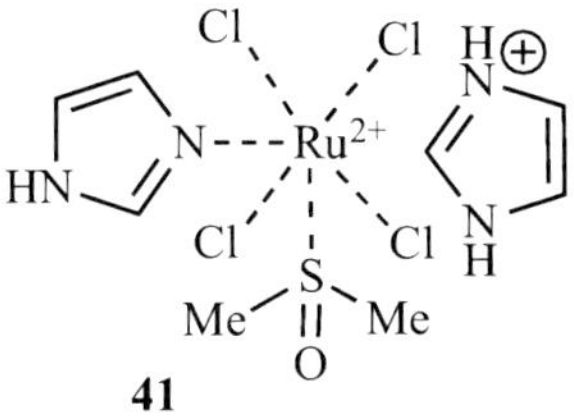

41

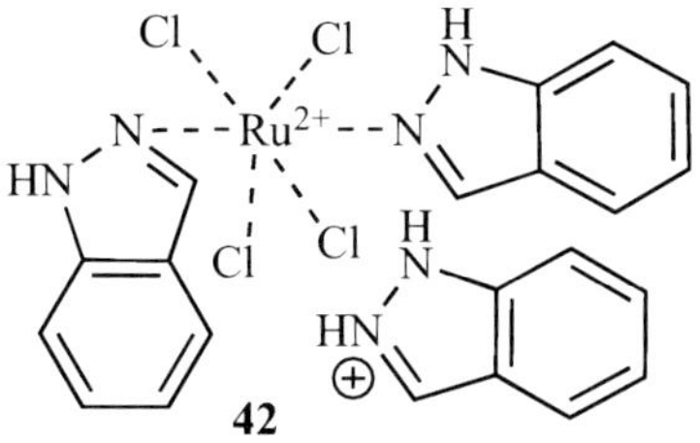

42

Thiazole ring with series of bioactivity could be coordinated with ruthenium to generate half-sandwich complexes which have currently attracted considerable attention in bioorganometallic chemistry due to their fine-tuning biological properties [83, 84]. Ruthenium thiazole **43** was evaluated for bioactivity against human ovarian cancer cell lines A2780 and A2780cisR (cisplatin-resistant), and also the interactions with plasmid DNA and the model protein ubiquitin were investigated. All the results displayed that the target complex **43** gave modest cytotoxicity towards human ovarian cancer cells, but with good antimetastatic activity on *in vivo* models [85].

Ruthenium arene supermolecules with sandwich structures can be easily functionalized to modulate the properties of complexes. Their anticancer activities

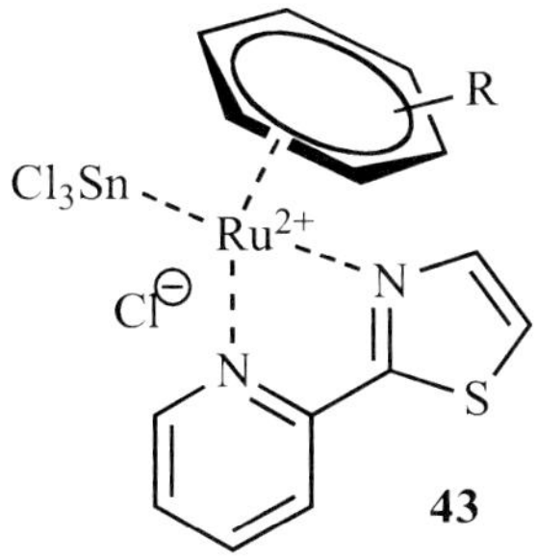

43

R = CH_3, $CH(CH_3)_2$

both *in vitro* and *in vivo* are very similar to that of the drug NAMI-A, such as good selectivity and anti-drug-resistance *in vivo*, and have been reviewed in 2009 [86]. For example, complex **44c** was the most active with the IC_{50} value of 24 μM in ovarian cancer cell line. The substituent on the aryl moiety of ligand appeared to influence the activity in all tested cell lines. Complexes **44c** and **44d** with electron withdrawing substituents exhibited a higher cytotoxic activity in CH1 cells than **44a**. In contrast, electron-donating substituents such as the methoxy groups in **44e** did not significantly influence the activity in CH1 cells, and were even disadvantageous in SW480 and A549 cells [87].

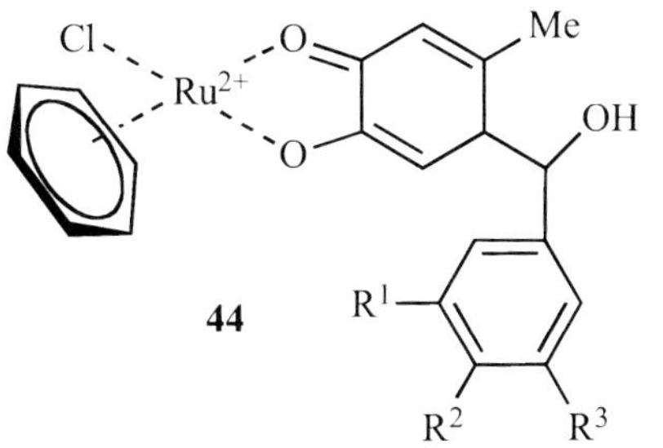

44

a, $R^1 = R^2 = R^3 = H$
b, $R^1 = R^3 = H$, $R^2 = NO_2$
c, $R^1 = R^3 = H$, $R^2 = F$
d, $R^1 = R^2 = H$, $R^3 = F$
e, $R^1 = R^2 = R^3 = OCH_3$

Phosphines as one of the most important classes of ligands were widely employed in organometallic and coordination chemistry. More recent interest has led to the development of metal-phosphine complexes for medicinal applications, and in which ruthenium ones have emerged as promising candidates. Organometallic Ru(II) complex **45** comprising lipophilic arene ligand and the hydrophilic pta ligand was around 3-fold more cytotoxic than its parent dichlorido complex. It was possible that this complex exerted its cytotoxic effect through non-covalent interactions and further studies will be necessary to evaluate its inhibition of relevant enzymes [88].

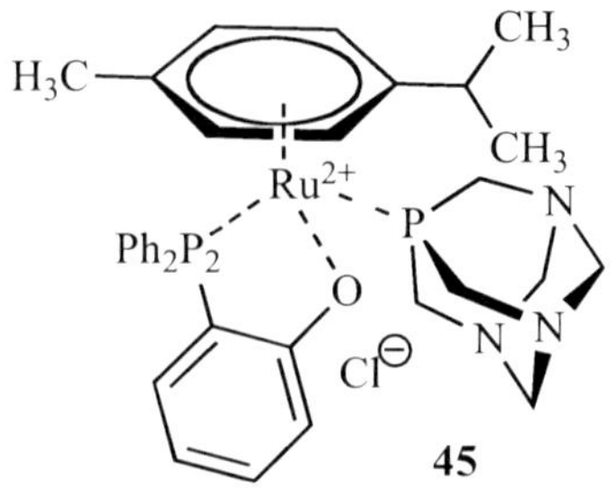

45

Considering multinuclear platinum anticancer complexes as a proven option to overcome resistance of established anticancer compounds, multinuclear Ru(II)-arene supermolecules which were linked by flexible chains of different length, have become highlighted. Multinuclear Ru(II)-based supermolecules **46a-d** displayed increased cytotoxicities in human cancer cells with the increasing length of linker. Especially, complex **46d** which was bound to natural doublehelical CT DNA, was markedly bound faster than cisplatin, and thus led more potent cytotoxicity than cisplatin [89].

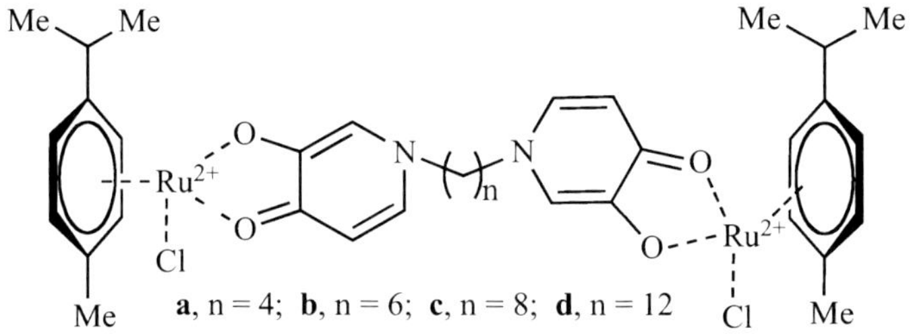

46

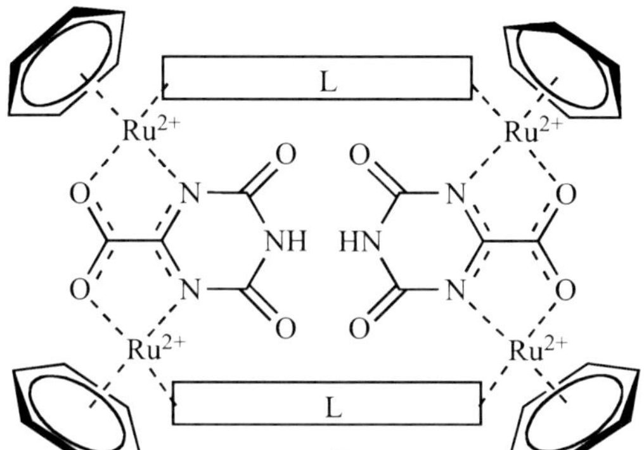

47

Ruthenium supramolecular complex **47** linked by 4,4′-bipyridine or 3,3-phenanthroline, exhibited highly significant antitumor activity, particularly towards the A2780cisR, and showed acquired resistance to cisplatin with IC_{50} values of 4.6 and 8.3 μM respectively, which gave rise to unusually low resistance factors values [90].

Ruthenium(II) and ruthenium(III) supramolecular complexes with R_2SO respectively, have showed significant antitumor activity against a wide range of preclinical tumor models including colorectal carcinomas and a variety of primary explanted human tumors *in vitro* and *in vivo* with low toxicity. Ruthenium(III) complexes are believed to behave as prodrugs, with low toxicity after activation by reduction to the corresponding Ru(II) supermolecules. For this reason, study of Ru(III) complexes is another way to reach the goal of anticancer activity. Taking Ru(III)-dithiocarbamato complex **48** as example, this ionic compound showed a reasonable cytotoxic activity *in vitro* towards all the tested cell lines with IC_{50} values resembling those recorded for the reference drug cisplatin [91].

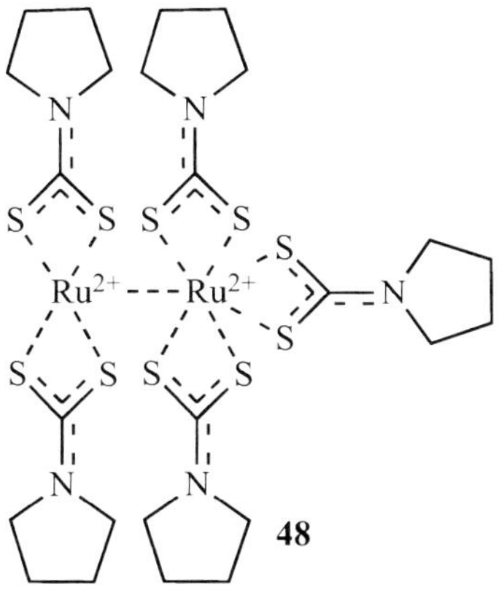

48

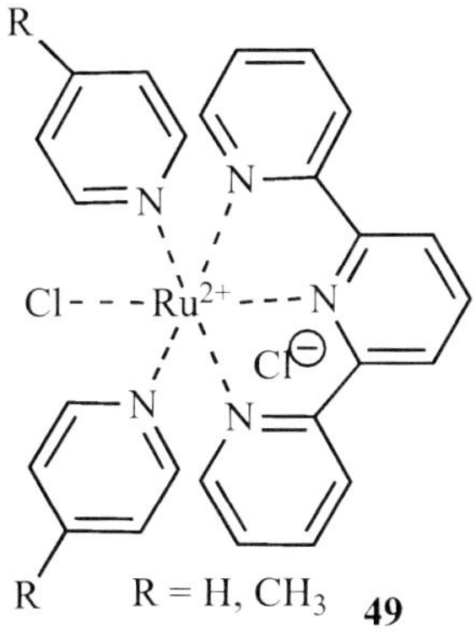

49

Ruthenium supramolecular complexes with polynitrogen chelating ligands constitute a relatively new group of anticancer agents. These complexes with six-coordinate, octahedral and highly water soluble have shown significant anticancer activity against a variety of cancer cell lines. For instance, ruthenium-based supermolecule **49** bearing 2,2'-bipyridine and 4-substituted pyridine was able to activate the P53-dependent, induced human hepatoma cells to undergo apoptosis and may have the potential for further development in cancer treatments [92].

Ruthenium supramolecular complexes involving tris(pyrazolyl)methane exhibited completely different antiproliferative properties against the MCF-7 (breast) and

HeLa (cervical) cancer cell lines with different solvents. Among these, the solvent complexes **50a** and **50b** showed no significant cytotoxicity under the conditions employed, while the phosphane complexes **50c-f** exhibited remarkable cytotoxic behavior, and were more active than cisplatin, even on the MCF-7 breast cancer cells which showed greater resistance towards cisplatin than the cervical cancer HeLa cell line. The different activity between the complex with monophosphane **50f** and those with chelate phosphanes **50c-e** was only marginal, suggested the linkage between donor atoms is not crucial. Likewise, chelate ring size did not appear to influence activity dramatically [93].

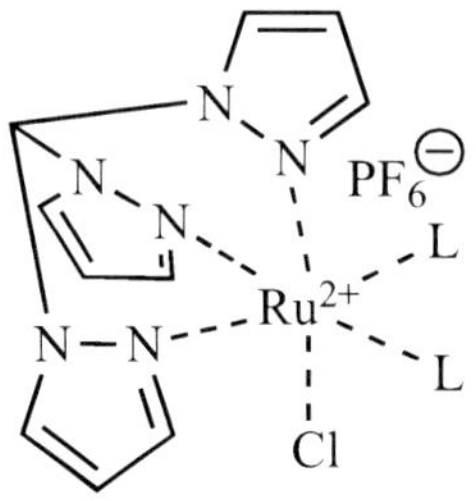

50
a, L = MeCN
b, L = DMSO
c, L = K^2-$Ph_2P(CH_2)_2PPh_2$
d, L = K^2-$Ph_2P(CH_2)_3PPh_2$
e, L = K^2-$Ph_2P(CH_2)_4PPh_2$
f, L = PPh_2Me

Complex **51** can exert interaction with human telomeric G-quadruplex DNA which is visually detected, and induce the guanine-rich single-strand oligomerd [$G_3(T_2AG_3)_3$] to form antiparallel G-quadruplex and have a moderate ability to stabilize G-quadruplex structures (ΔT_m = 11.2 °C). Furthermore, polymerase chain reaction-stop assay, telomerase repeat amplication protocol, and MTT assay demonstrated that the Ru-complex exhibited good inhibitory activity for

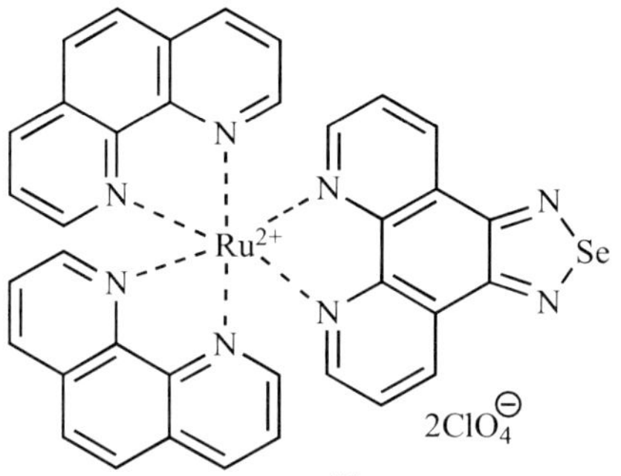

51

telomerase and cancer cells. The results suggested that Ru-complex might be a potential telomerase inhibitor for cancer chemotherapy [94].

Carbohydrates have been shown to play a central role in a variety of significant biological events. Meanwhile, the major focus of chiral carbohydrate ligand and the anticancer activity of the ruthenium carbonyl cluster complexes containing tribenzyl glucal ligand have prompted researchers to investigate them. Supermolecule **52** is a carbohydrate-based ruthenium cluster complex, obtained by the reaction of tribenzyl galactal with $Ru_3(CO)_{12}$ in benzene at reflux temperature, this novel structure was confirmed by a combination of FT-IR and NMR spectroscopy, mass spectrometry and elemental analysis. Ruthenium complex **52**, compared favorably to the activity of cisplatin, displayed good activity in all cell lines overall with the IC_{50} value rang of 25-40 μM in B-cell lymphoma, T-cell acute lymphoblastic leukemia, breast, ovarian, chronic myelogenous leukemia and prostate cancer cell lines [95].

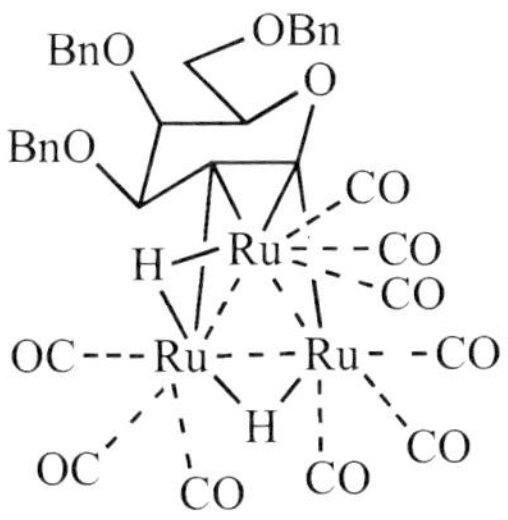

52

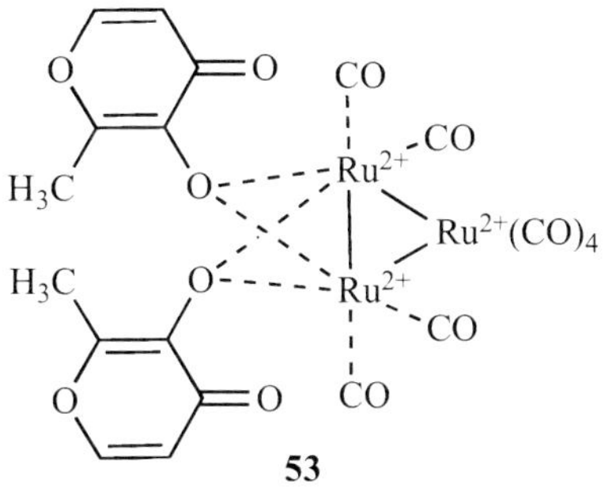

53

Innovative organometallic drugs are increasing in demand. Ruthenium-based compounds have attracted attention due to their promising anticancer activity and low toxicity. For ruthenium anticancer compounds, multiple biological pathways have been proposed including the inhibition of cysteine proteases and glutathione S-transferase(GST). DNA is not a primary target for ruthenium anticancer compounds because they bind more strongly to proteins than to DNA. The anticancer activity of compound **53** is 5–7 times more potent than cisplatin against the cancer cell lines K562 (CML), HT-29(colon) and HL-60(AML) [96].

Although phosphane ligands have been employed in cytotoxic compounds, only a few examples of phosphane-based Ru supramolecular complexes have been reported to show antitumor properties, and phosphanes remain a relatively unexplored class of ligands in a field mainly dominated by nitrogen-donor ligands. Based on this, a novel Ru(III) complex **54** was found to show high activity against both cell lines compared to cisplatin, and more importantly, without sensitivity towards cisplatin resistance present in the A2780R cells [97]. The ruthenium(III) complex **55** exhibited significant antitumor activity, its interaction with bovine serum albumin (BSA) indicated a probable secondary electrostatic interaction between the metal complex and the peptide [98].

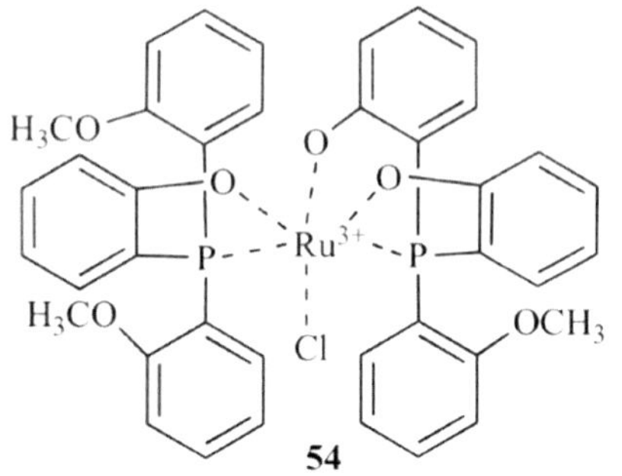

54

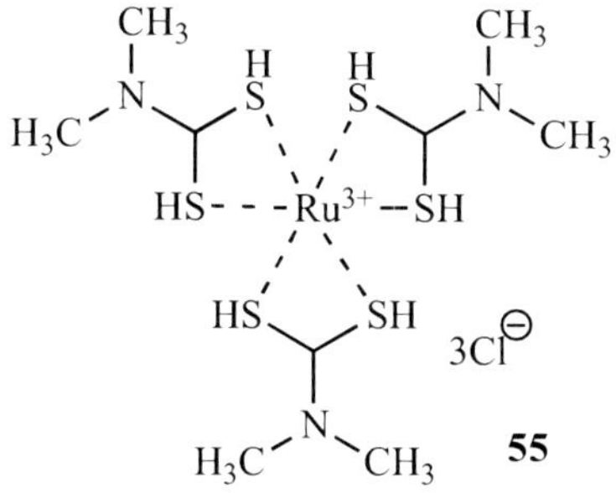

55

2.1.6. Rhodium-Based Supramolecular Complexes as Anticancer Agents

Since the antitumor activity of the inorganic complex cisplatin was discovered, the development of rhodium metal has become an active field of cytostatic drugs. Rhodium compounds, which were analogues to the corresponding platinum compounds, have attracted considerable attention in recent years [99]. Generally, rhodium compounds which have shown interesting antitumor properties can be classified into two sorts as monomeric and dimeric supramolecular complexes.

Both monomeric square planar Rh(I) and octahedral Rh(III) supramolecular complexes have shown significant antitumor properties. Recently, it is interesting to note that 1,4,7-trithiacyclononane alone showed no cytotoxic effect towards the human cancer cell lines MCF-7 and HT-29, but its rhodium-based supramolecular complexes with ligand 2,2′-bipyridine (bpy) (**56a**) and dipyrido[2,3-*a*:2′,3′-

c]phenazine (dppz) **56c** exhibited higher cytotoxicity towards MCF-7 and HT-29 cells with the IC_{50} value rang of 4.4-12.8 μM, with comparable activity to cisplatin. The observation in comparison to pyrazino[2,3-f]quinoxaline (tap) complex **(56b)** suggested that different mechanisms of action and target molecules may be involved in the ([9]aneS_3)Rh(III) complexes, depending on whether these contain either small or large polypyridyl ligands [100]. More interestingly, tris(pyrazolyl)methane-based rhodium (III) supermolecule (**57**) was potent cytotoxic agents (IC_{50} = 0.43, 0.37 μM) towards the human cancer cell lines MCF-7 and HT-29, which is much more potent than cisplatin and the ligand [101].

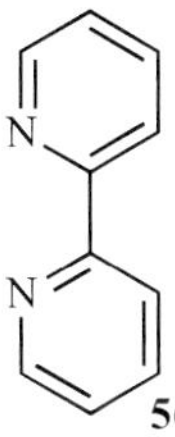
56a

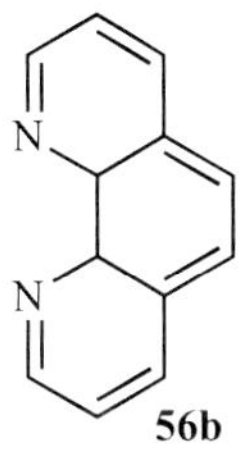
56b

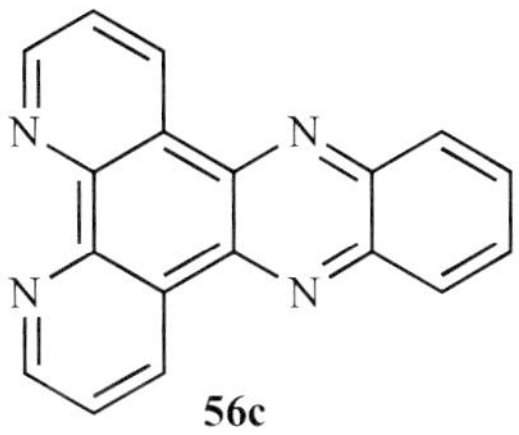
56c

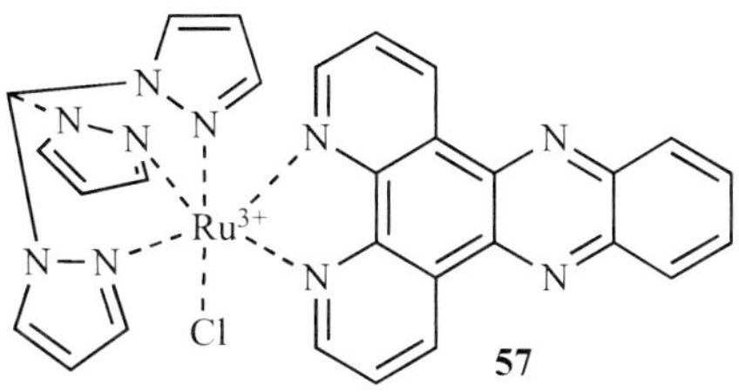
57

Di-rhodium supramolecular complexes with metal-metal bonds have also attracted much attention because of their considerable carcinostatic activity against various tumor cell lines. Researches revealed that di-rhodium derived supermolecules were favorably poised to bind to purine nucleobases and DNA. Moreover, direct DNA photo cleavage *in vitro* was affected by di-rhodium compounds in the presence of electron acceptors in solution or directly attached to the dirhodium core [102]. Also, it was found that the supramolecular complexes of di-rhodium with compound **58** and a series of aromatic heteroleptic diamines could potentially intercalate as well as covalently bind to DNA and exhibited a significant effect on inhibiting cell viability of the human cancer cells HeLa and COLO-316. The results demonstrated that the hydrophobicity of the compounds was correlated with their activity in both cell lines [103].

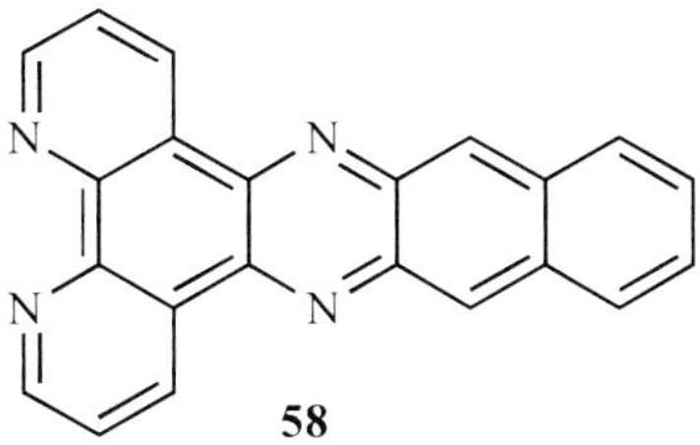
58

2.1.7. Osmium-Based Supramolecular Complexes as Anticancer Agents

Osmium, the heavier congener of ruthenium, and its complexes have a reputation for being either toxic (OsO_4) or substitution-inert Os(II) and Os(III) complexes, which therefore hamper their development as potential therapeutic agents. Sadler and co-workers synthesized some osmium(II) arene complexes with pronounced cytotoxicity that is comparable to the clinical drugs carboplatin and cisplatin, which provide an incentive for the further studies on osmium-based supramolecular complexes [104].

The investigation on the probable mode of action against tumor cells demonstrated that the Os(II) arene supermolecules are believed to interact with DNA in a similar manner to their ruthenium analogues, *i.e.* binding to N7 of guanine not only *via* combination bond but also by H-bonding and hydrophobic interaction triggered by the introduction of extended arene rings into the versatile structure of DNA. Interestingly, binding of Os(II) arenes to calf thymus DNA gives rise to a large unwinding of double-helical DNA, unlike cisplatin, which causes DNA bending. As a consequence, these osmium-based supermolecules do not display cross-resistance with cisplatin towards cancer cells, suggesting promise for addressing the problem of intrinsic or acquired resistance in chemotherapy [105, 106].

The incorporation of organic ligands into organometallic supermolecules may serve as an effective mean to increase solubility, bioavailability and preserve or even enhance their antitumor activity. Metal complexes with picolinamide ligands have been previously received attention owing to their relevance to peptide chemistry. These ligands are known to bind with metal ions as either neutral *N,O*-donors, or monoanionic *N,N*-donors with electron-donating or -withdrawing substituents on the phenyl ring, respectively. Sabine *et al.* confirmed that the different binding mode adopted by picolinamide derivatives in organometallic supermolecules could lead to distinct cytotoxicity. The *N,N*-coordinated Os(II) supramolecular complexes **59a-d** hydrolyzed rapidly, thus exhibited significant binding to guanine. Promising cytotoxic activity for Os(II)-based supermolecules followed the order **59b** >> **59c** > **59a** > **59d**, especially complex **59b** showed similar activity as cisplatin in HCT116 (colon) cell line and pronounced activity in the A2780cis (ovarian cisplatin resistant) cell line. In contrast, *N,O*-coordinated complex **59e** hydrolyzed slowly, did not bind to guanine or adenine, and therefore was nontoxic [107].

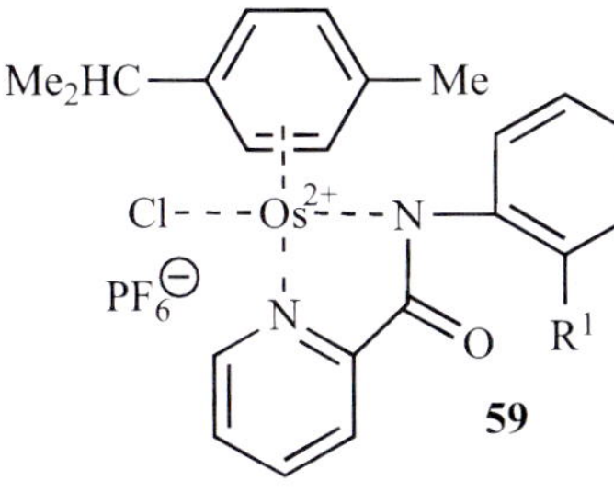

59

a, $R^1 = R^2 = F$
b, $R^1 = H$, $R^2 = NO_2$
c, $R^1 = NO_2$, $R^2 = H$
d, $R^1 = R^2 = OMe$

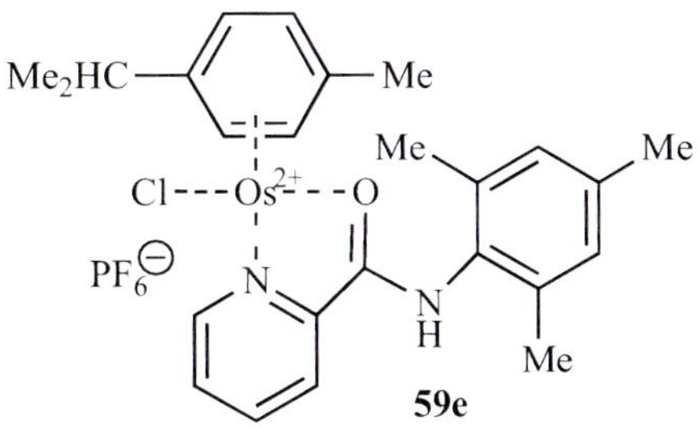

59e

Potential biological and medical applications of organometallic supramolecular complexes are hampered by a lack of knowledge of their aqueous solution chemistry. Data showed that the hydrolytic and aqueous solution chemistry of half-sandwich Os(II) arene complexes of the type [(η6-arene)Os(XY)Cl], in which XY means N,O-chelating ligands, can be tuned with XY chelating ligands to achieve cancer cell cytoxicity comparable to carboplatin. For example, chlorido osmium(II) arene complexes **60a** and **60c** showed comparable activities with cisplatin in A2780 (ovarian), HCT116 (colon), and even the cisplatin-resistant A2780cis (ovarian) cell line. Additionally, the inactivity of complex **60b** was attributed to the negative charge on its contrapuntal carboxylate substituent. These data illustrated how the chemical reactivity and cytotoxicity of osmium arene supermolecules can be controlled and "fine-tuned" by the use of steric and electronic effects of substituents on a chelating ligand to give Os(II) arene supermolecules with potent activity as cisplatin but different mechanism of action [108].

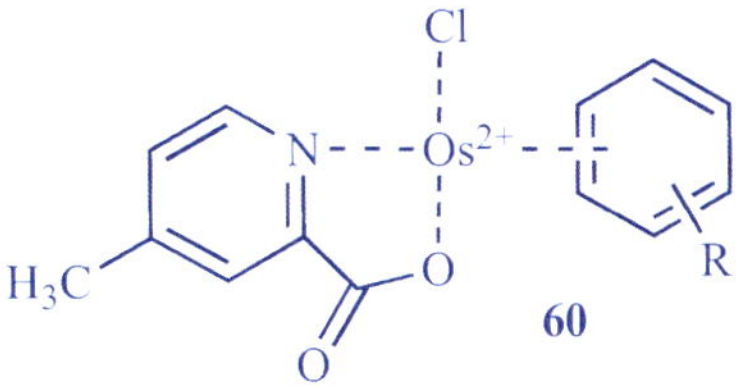

60

a, R = H
b, R = 1-CH_3-4-$CH(CH_3)_2$
c, R = C_6H_5

Encouragingly, some organometallic Os(II) arene complexes exerted promising *in vitro* cancer cell activity and their aqueous reactivity appeared to be tunable. Study showed that hydrophobicity (log*P*) values may be useful indicators of

A2780 cancer cell cytotoxicity for Os(II) arene complexes **60a-c**. Further work found that the arene ligand played an important role in cytotoxicity, the substitutions not only enhanced hydrophobicity and uptake by the cell, but also exhibited important part in the mechanism of cytotoxicity of the complexes. Complex **60c** gave the best anticancer activity [109].

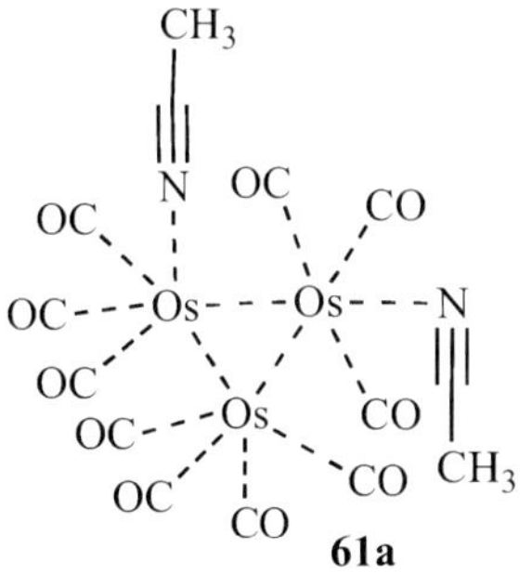

61a

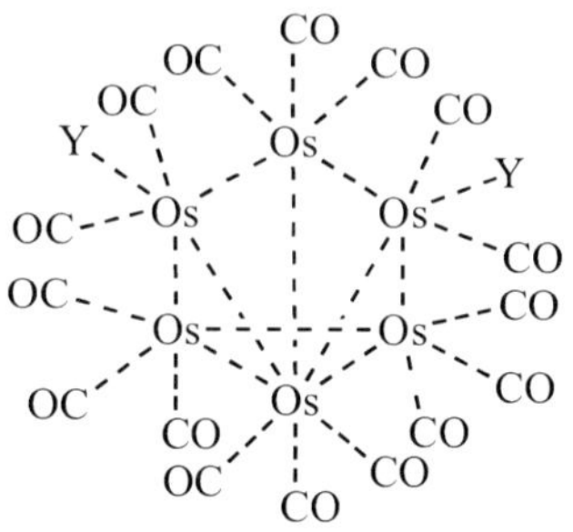

61b Y= CO, CH_3CN

Transition metal coordinating with carbon monoxide afforded the corresponding metal carbonyl supramolecular clusters, which may show potential applications in cancer therapy. The tri-osmium carbonyl supramolecular clusters **61a-b** showed appreciable cytotoxicity with supramolecular cluster **61b** to be most active with IC_{50} values as low as 6 μM, and more interestingly compound **61a** was the only one which was cytotoxic, albeit at a high treatment concentration, against the HT29 cells. Further studies on their mode of action with the MDA-MB-231 cell line pointed to the induction of apoptosis [110].

Noble metal-based supramolecular complexes as anticancer agents have extensively been explored and remarkable achievements have been obtained. More importantly, a lot of noble metal complex supermolecules especially platinum ones as drugs have successfully been developed and used in the defense of human health. Further researches of noble metals in coordination chemistry, organometallic chemistry and supramolecular chemistry inevitably result in more and more noble metal-based supramolecular complexes as effective clinical anticancer drugs. It is foreseeable that noble metal-based supramolecular complexes represent an important class of promising anticancer agents, their research and development will become increasingly active.

2.2. Non-Noble Metal-Based Supramolecular Complexes as Anticancer Agents

2.2.1. Titanium-Based Supramolecular Complexes as Anticancer Agents

Titanium-based supramolecular complexes have also been investigated extensively and consequently entered clinical practice in the field of non-platinum metal-based supermolecules with anticancer potency. Their chemical structures are restricted to two families, cyclopentadienyl (Cp) derived supramolecular complexes such as titanocene dichloride (Cp_2TiCl_2) **62**, and diketonato based titanium supermolecules, like budotitane [$(bzac)_2Ti(OEt)_2$] **63**. Most anticancer titanium complexes showed excellent activities against tumors in the gastrointestinal tract and activities towards breast, lung and skin (melanoma) cancers. Apart from their broad spectrum of activity, one appealing property is that they do not show common side effects of widely used cytostatic agents, *i.e.* emesis, alopecia or bone marrow impairment. These features make titanium-based supramolecular complexes interesting for combined therapy and further study. As a result, there have been several reviews available [111-113].

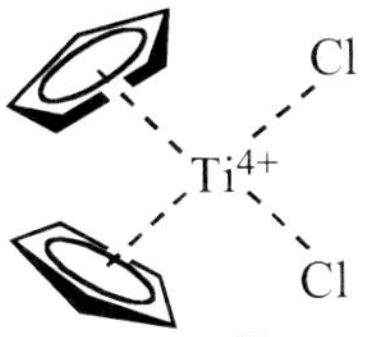

62

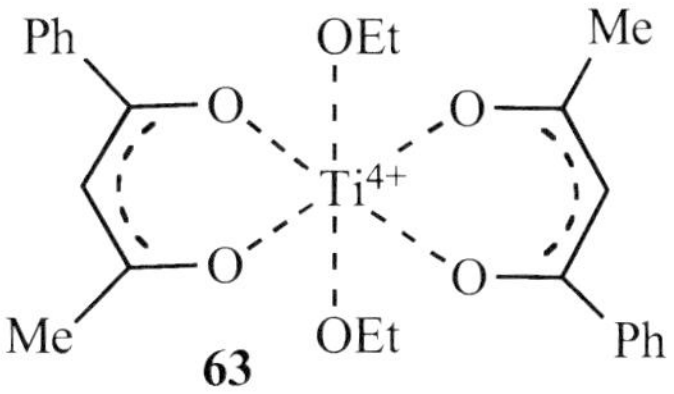

63

A novel discovery was made to further clarify the mechanism on anticancer action of titanocene dichloride, which demonstrated that titanocene dichloride **62** can inhibit tumour gelatinases in a dose-dependent manner. Binding experiments showed that cyclopentadiene-Ti(IV) moieties, resulting from titanocene dichloride at physiological pH, were bound mainly to different types of collagens and a lesser extent to casein or bovine serum albumin and then formed soluble and stable adducts. These results indicated that titanocene dichloride behaved as a competitive inhibitor against various proteolytic enzymes by binding to the substrate rather than to the enzyme active site. This property may be responsible for the antiangiogenic effect of titanocene dichloride and additionally contribute to its anticancer action [114].

Titanocene derived supermolecule **64a** was highly proliferative on MCF-7 cells even at low concentrations of 0.5 μM, thus behaved almost similarly to Cp_2TiCl_2. This proliferative effect was also observed in the presence of bovine serum albumin (BSA). Conversely, another titanocene derivative **64b** with *p*-methoxylbenzyl group has almost no effect even at 10 μM, whereas exhibited a significant dose dependent cytotoxic effect of up to 50% when incubated with BSA (20-50 μg/mL). This confirmed the crucial role played by the binding to serum proteins in the expression of the cytotoxicity *in vivo* of the titanocene complexes [115].

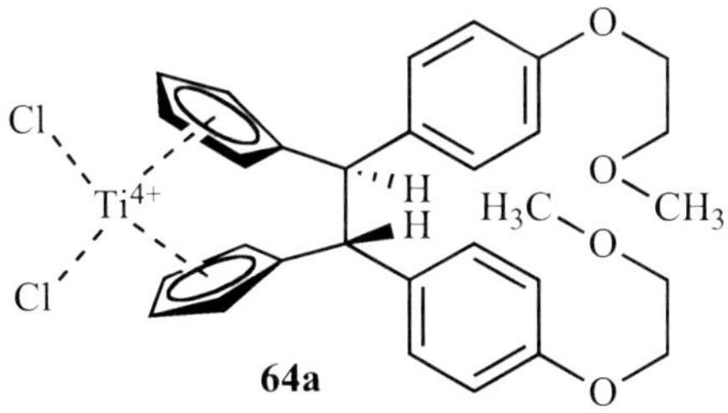

64a

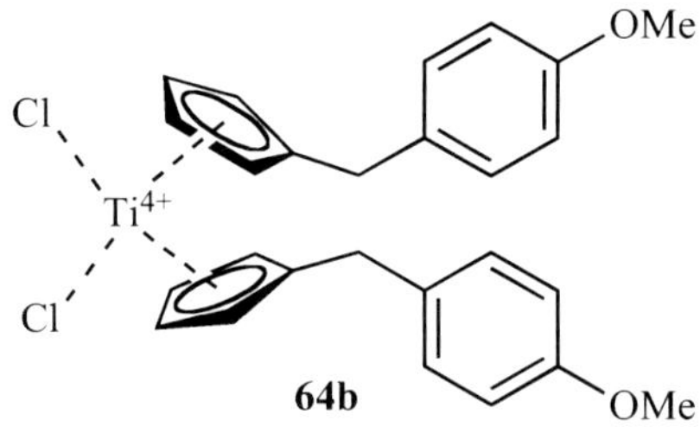

64b

Titanium supramolecular complexes **65a-b** can nearly exclusively kill the cells through apoptosis induction (above 90% apoptotic cell death), while metal-free ligands have no significant toxicity even with four times higher concentrations. Moreover, the IC_{50} values of the complexes are satisfactory as well with one order of magnitude higher than those of cisplatin. Complex **65b** was the first titanium-based supermolecule that combines high cytotoxicity with a selective induction of apoptosis [116].

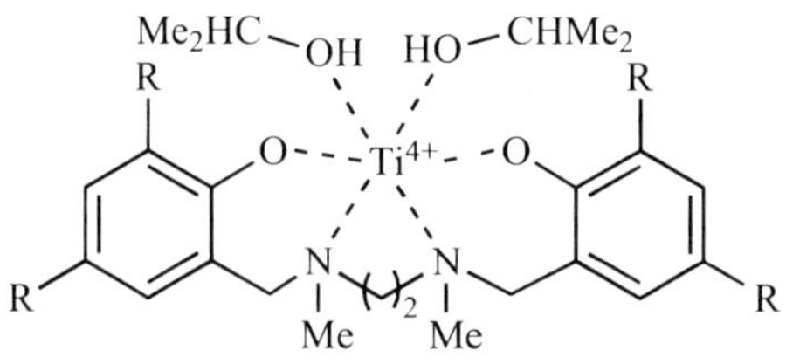

65 **a**, R = F **b**, R = Cl

2.2.2. Vanadium-Based Supramolecular Complexes as Anticancer Agents

Vanadium is a trace transition metal with relevant biological properties since it can interact with different biomolecules in its anionic and cationic forms. Studies on various cell lines revealed that vanadium exerts its antitumor effect through inhibition of cellular tyrosine phosphatases and/or activation of tyrosine phosphorylases. Both effects activate signal transduction pathways leading either to apoptosis and/or to activation of tumor suppressor genes. Furthermore, vanadium compounds may induce cell-cycle arrest and/or cytotoxic effects through DNA cleavage and fragmentation and plasma membrane lipoperoxidation.

Vanadocene was coordinated with bis(*p*-methoxybenzyl)cyclopentadienyl moiety to afford the corresponding supramolecular complexes **66b-c**, which yielded anti-tumour efficacy with IC_{50} values of 9.1 μM and 8.3 μM, respectively , while the complex **66a** exhibited an IC_{50} value of 3.0 μM against the LLC-PK cell line. This is particularly encouraging since complex **66a** was performing slightly better than cisplatin [117]. The analogue vanadocene supermolecule **66d** gave a superior IC_{50} value of 2.2 μM, which is an improvement upon its LLC-PK value, and proved to be the best compound of this series [118]. Another vanadyl supramolecular complex **67** containing dppz as potential DNA intercalating ligand also exhibited significant activity against HL-60 cells. The results showed that the percentage of necrotic dead cells was significantly higher for the vanadyl complex than for cisplatin, while the percentage of surviving cells being slightly higher for cisplatin than for V-dppz when both were administered at IC_{50} doses [119].

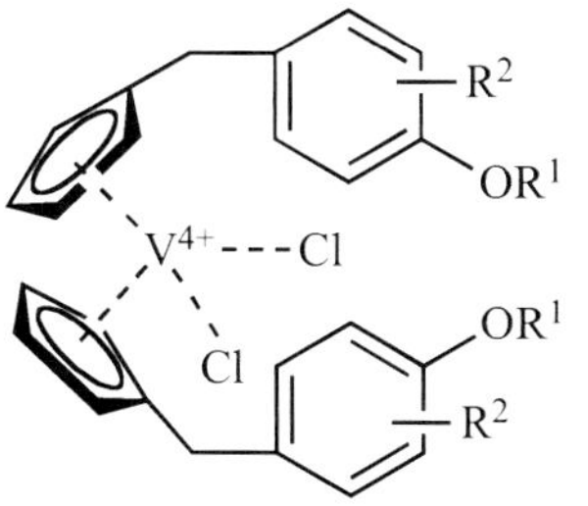

66
a, R^1 = Me, R^2 = 3-Me
b, R^1 = Me, R^2 = 3,5-diMe
c, R^1 = Me, R^2 = H
d, R^1 = CF_3, R^2 = H

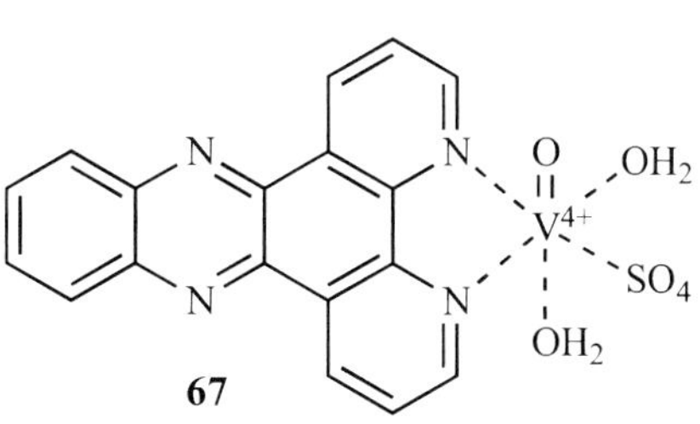

67

Researches in recent decades enriched our knowledge on the chemical and biochemical properties, as well as the mechanisms of systemic, cellular and molecular antitumor effects of vanadium compounds. The anticarcinogenic effects of vanadium, in combination to its low toxicity, established also by its administration in humans, suggested vanadium-based supermolecules as antineoplastic candidates against human cancer. New vanadium complexes with more potent and less toxic favor this perspective. However, a vast array of questions seeking immediate answers, demand more intensive basic and applied research in order vanadium supramolecular complexes to be established as a new class non-platinum group, effective antitumor agents.

2.2.3. Chromiun-Based Supramolecular Complexes as Anticancer Agents

Chromium(Cr) is ubiquitous in the environment, occurring naturally in soils, rocks and living organisms. Chromium exists in primarily two valence states, trivalent Cr(III) and hexavalent Cr(VI), with the latter primarily produced by anthropogenic sources. Chromium(III) is a micronutrient important in the biological activity (receptor binding) of insulin, and accordingly can be found in many dietary supplements. Furthermore, it was also found that Cr(III) supramolecular complex could inhibit the replication of DNA and RNA *in vitro*. For example, 5-iodopyrimidine-2,4(1H,3H)-dione derived complex $[Cr(HL)(OH)_2Cl]$ **68**, where HL is 5-iodouracil, showed higher inhibition on 3H-thymidine and 3H-uridine incorporation in DNA and RNA replication, respectively, at a dose of 5 μg/mL [120].

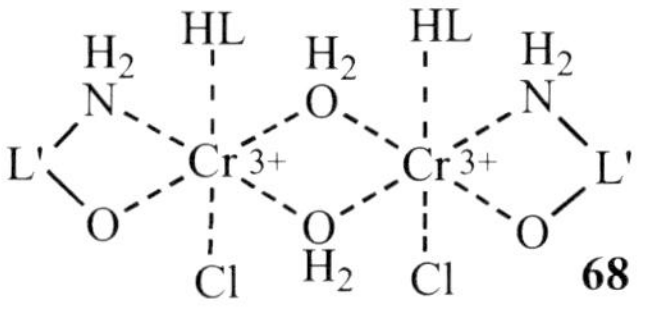

68

2.2.4. Manganese-Based Supramolecular Complexes as Anticancer Agents

Manganese is an essential micronutrient for all living things. In biology, manganese can work as acid-base catalysis in hydrolysis reactions carried out by carboxypeptidase, purple acid phosphatase, urease, arginase, *etc*., or be a redox catalysis of enzymes involved in oxygen metabolism, nitrogen fixation, radical formation, and have been reported to interact with G-quadruplex with some selectivity [121]. By now, manganese complexes with different ligands have been reported as anticancer agents. The most interesting ligands, such as Schiff base, porphyrin, thiosemicarbazone and flavonoids were taken as examples to explain their important effects on oncology.

Schiff base and its metal complex derivatives, especially heterocyclic amine family, have been an important field in drug research and development due to their broad bioactivities such as antitumor. Manganese(III)-salen supermolecule **69** showed the similar cytotoxicity and selectivity level to cisplatin, with the IC_{50} values ranging from 11 μM to 40 μM against malignant breast cells (MCF7). More importantly, several Mn(III)-salen complexes showed preferential cytotoxicity (2- to 5-fold) toward MCF7 over a non-malignant breast epithelial cell line (MCF10). Furthermore, treatment with active Mn(III)-salen and -salphen complexes induced release of cytochrome C from the mitochondria to cytosol which indicated the perturbance in mitochondrial membrane potential and the involvement of mitochondrial pathway of apoptosis [122]. Structure activity relationship demonstrated that the nature of substituents, bridging spacers and the central metal-ion are crucial factors in determining the apoptotic activities [123].

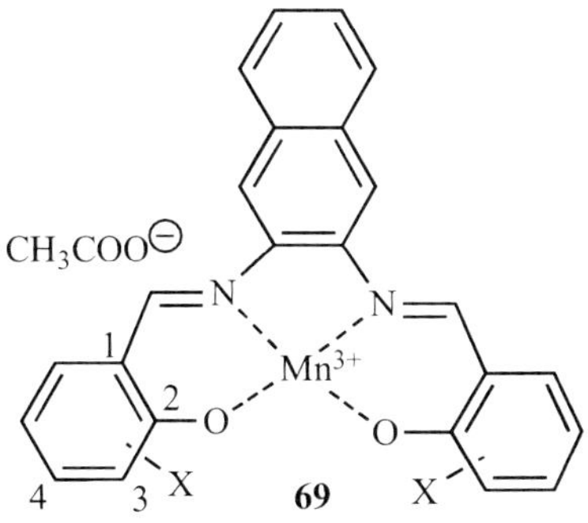

X = H, 3, 3'-OH, 4, 4'-OH, 5, 5' -OH, 3, 3'-OMe, 4, 4'-OMe, 5, 5'-OMe

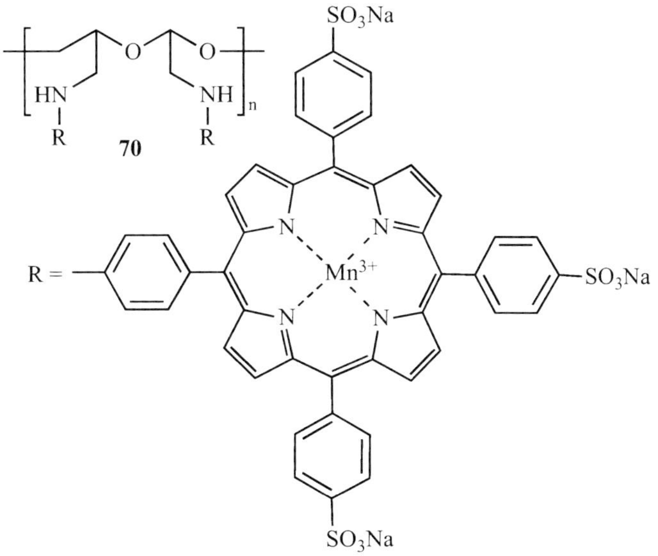

Porphyrin ring possessed the structural features of both macrocycles and multi-dentes. Porphyrins and their metalloporphyrins may give a lot of distinct physico-chemical properties and functions when changing substituent groups in porphyrin

ring, adjusting electron-donor ability of four nitrogen atoms, introducing different center metal ions, or changing different affinity of axial ligands. In recent years, porphyrin-based complexes as anticancer drugs have attracted wide interest. Porphyrin-based Mn(II) supermolecules, like complex **70** conjugated with dextran, also could exhibit high targeting specificity to tumor [124].

Flavonoids are important natural antioxidants and have been extensively studied because of their various biological activities. Most of flavonoids are good metal chelators due to their high superdelocalizability and conjugated system. Flavonoid-based Mn(II) supermolecule **71** was proved to possess higher growth inhibitory effects than free ligand and corresponding metal ions, and even more effective than the positive control cisplatin against the selected cell lines (A549, Hela, HepG2, SW620 and MDA-MB-435). The findings indicated that the antiproliferative effect of manganese supramolecular complex was associated with cellular apoptosis and cell cycle arrest and profits to the development of a new anticancer drug [125].

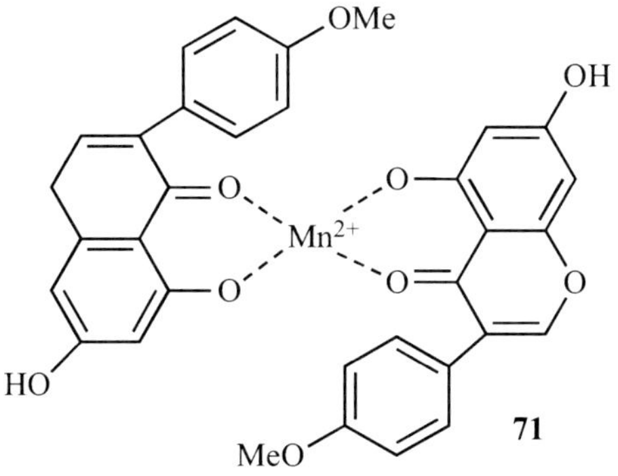

71

2.2.5. Iron-Based Supramolecular Complexes as Anticancer Agents

Iron, the earliest metal compounds to be studied in medicinal chemistry, plays essential roles in many biological systems, including oxygen delivery, energy metabolism, and anabolic processes, and is used to treat hypochromic anemia caused by iron deficiency [126]. Numerous studies *in vitro* and *in vivo* provide evidence that iron chelators may be effective antitumor agents. It is, therefore, an attractive target for chemotherapeutic compounds [127]. Effective chelators may be designed with preference for either Fe(II) or Fe(III). Iron(III)-specific chelators, the only trivalent metal of biological significance with properties unique in biological systems, are easier to design and form stronger supramolecular complexes than Fe(II) ones [128].

Thiosemicarbazones, which have a long history and broad spectrum of biological efficacy, are an important group for iron based supermolecules that showed potent and selective antitumor activity. Their abilities to bind iron and other metals are vital for their antiproliferative efficacy and elucidation of the structure-activity relationships is important to develop increasingly active and selective anticancer agents.

Bernhardt *et al.*, considering the previous work and the high antiproliferative activity of 3-aminopyridinecarbaldehyde thiosemicarbazone (3-AP, **72a**), generated the related 2-acetylpyridine thiosemicarbazone (HApT, **72b**) analogues to examine the influence of the methyl group at the imine carbon. Four of the six HApT chelators had potent antitumor activity (IC_{50}: 0.001-0.002 μM) and iron chelation efficacy that was similar to the most effective 2-benzoylpyridine thiosemicarbazone (HBpT, **72c**) and dipyridylketone thiosemicarbazone (HDpT, **72d**) ligands. This property made the HApT series to be one of the most potent antiproliferative agents [129].

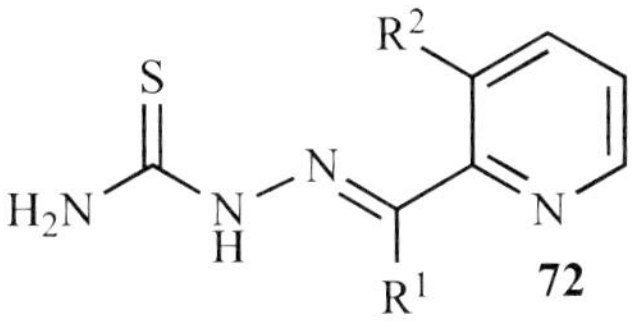

72

a, R^1= H, R^2 = NH_2
b, R^1= Me, R^2 = H
c, R^1= phenyl, R^2 = H
d, R^1= 2-pyridyl, R^2 = H

Curcumin-based iron supramolecular complexes **73-75** could cause plasmid DNA damage through releasing NO under UV irradiation and were toxic to B16-F10 cells *in vitro* with the LD_{50} values of 1 μM, 1 μM and 200 μM, respectively. Unfortunately, no synergistic cytotoxicity effect was noted in the treatments of the combinations of curcumin and DNICs, and complex **75** also reduced toxicity of curcumin. This study provides the basis for further investigation on the effects of combinations of curcumin and other NO donors [130].

Bis(salicylidene)-1,2-diaminocyclohexane (saldach) iron(III) supramolecular complex **76** displayed anticancer activity within a concentration range of 1 to 5 μM against MCF-7, MDA-MB 231 breast cancer and HT-29 colon carcinoma cells, and even more active than cisplatin at 5 μM. Significant inhibition of cell growth was caused at 1 μM only in the case of (R,R)-*trans*-[Fe(III)(saldach)Cl] complex against the MDA-MB 231 cell line. Antiproliferative effects depended on the presence of the central atom iron but were independent on the configuration at the saldach ligand [131]. Another salen-type iron (III) supramolecular complex involving heterocyclic *N*-donor ligands HL showed significant *in vitro* cytotoxicity against both K562 and MCF7 cell lines. Noticeably, complex **77** with the 5-aminotetrazolide anion displayed the most potent cytotoxicity with an IC_{50} of 6.4 mM against K562 [132].

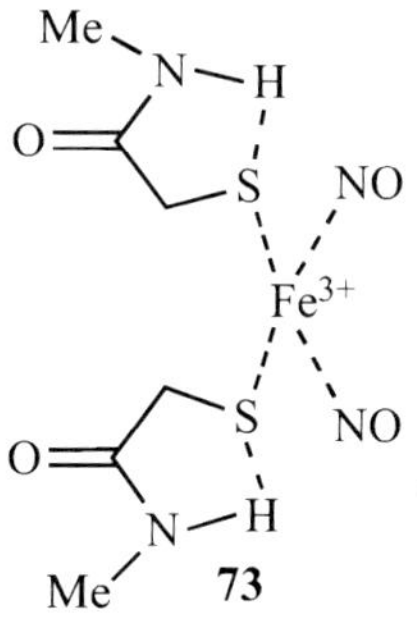

73

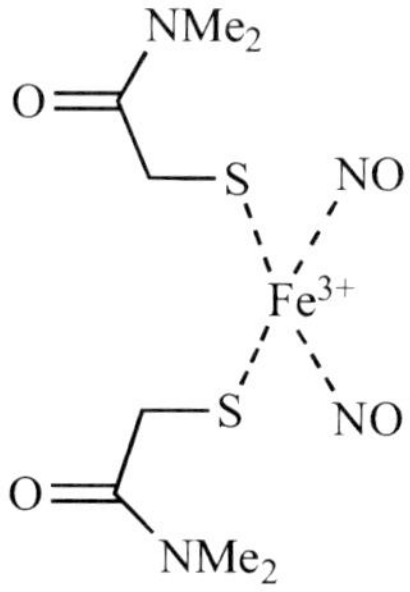

74

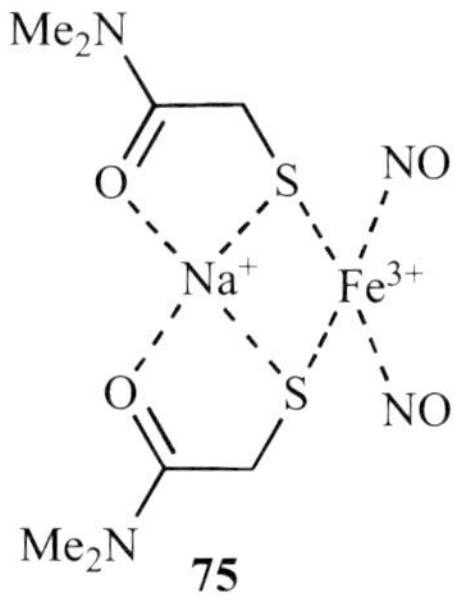

75

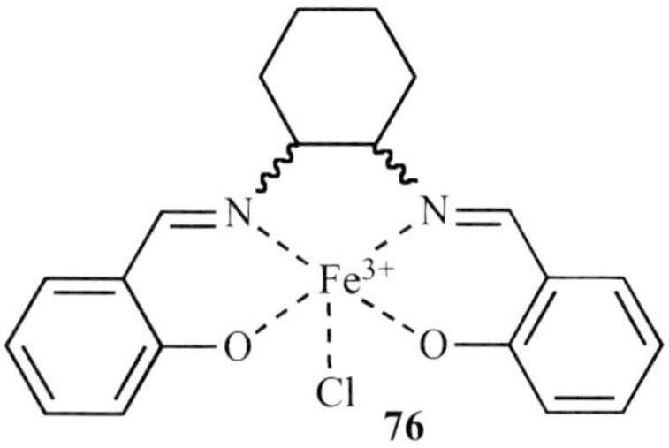

76

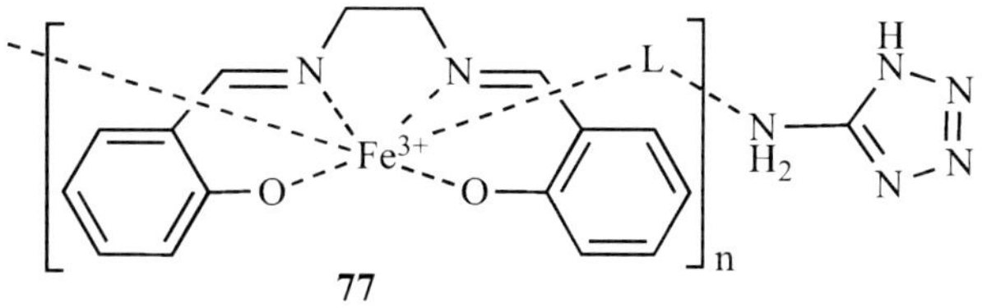

77

Finally, it must be pointed out that iron-based supramolecular complexes, like other anticancer agents, will affect both normal and neoplastic cells. However, the fact that iron complexes do inhibit the growth of a variety of tumors *in vivo* in animal studies and in clinical trials does demonstrate their selectivity and potential. Obviously, further studies are essential in order to examine the selectivity of new supermolecules against tumor cells compared to their normal counterparts. These studies may lead to the rational design of even more effective and selective agents for the treatment of neoplasia.

2.2.6. Cobalt-Based Supramolecular Complexes as Anticancer Agents

Cobalt is a natural trace element with the necessary component vitamin B_{12}. Although cobalt has redox-cycling activity and has been widely utilized in the development of DNA-acting metalloantibiotics, it shows carcinogenic properties at higher concentrations [133, 134].

Cobalt(III) supramolecular complexes have been described as hypoxia selective antitumor agents. This is based on the fact that main tumor cells that grow under anaerobic conditions develop resistance to chemotherapeutic agents. Cobalt(III) complexes might be reduced under hypoxic conditions to Co(II) species followed by loss of a neutral ligand. Based on this strategy, many Co(III) supramolecular complexes were synthesized and most of them showed hypoxic selectivity against repair-proficient tumor cells [135-138]. For example, the reduced forms of mononuclear Co(III) based supermolecule **78** presented high capacities to inhibit *S. cerevisiae* cell growth, with IC_{50} (0.50 mM for both complexes) lower than the cisplatin (0.6 mM) at the same time of exposure, and also promoted *S. cerevisiae* cells death at concentration higher than 0.5 mM, in a non-dose dependence. All these data indicated that Co(III) complexes showed great potential as possible bioreductively activated prodrugs, since their oxidized forms did not present expressive activities in promoting cell death and inhibiting cell growth, compared to their reduced forms [139].

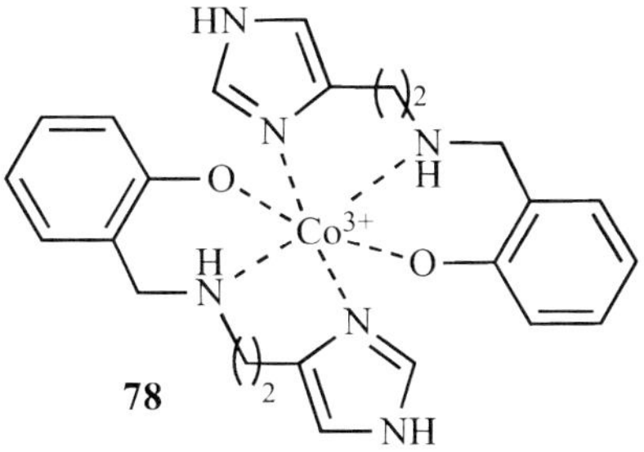

78

There has been tremendous interest in studies of cobalt complexes containing N_2O_2 Schiff base ligands to explore the interactions of metal complexes with DNA. Cobalt Schiff base **79** was successfully prepared by in situ method and the interactions with calf thymus DNA were investigated. The results revealed that there was no intercalative mode between DNA and cobalt(II) complex, and a strong electrostatic attraction between the anionic phosphate backbone of DNA and the cationic charge of the complex was highly suggested to exert the antitumor activity [140].

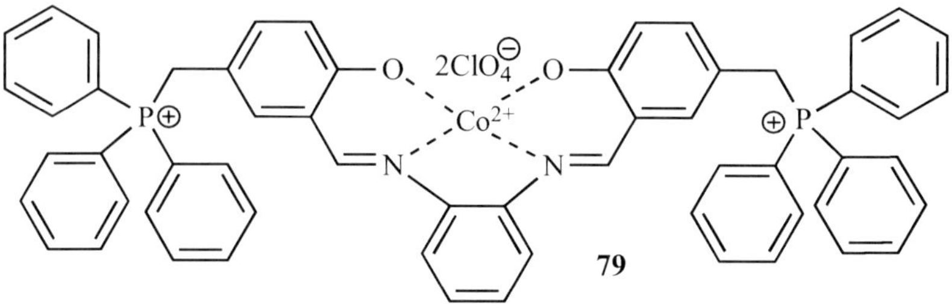

79

Mithramycin (plicamycin, Mith, **80**) is a member of the aureolic family of drugs isolated from *Streptomyces plicatus* and contains disaccharide and trisaccharide moieties that are connected to a chromophore aglycon *via* opposing O-glycosidicbonds, which has been used clinically to treat several types of cancer including testicular carcinoma, chronic myeloid leukemia (CML), and acute myeloid leukemia (AML). Structural analysis revealed that compound **80** should bind to the minor groove of DNA duplexes around GC-rich sequences and this binding was mediated by divalent metal ions such as Mg(II), Co(II) and Fe(II). Cobalt(II)-mediated dimeric Mith supramolecular complex was observed to be resistant to polyamine competition compared to the Fe(II)-mediated complexes. Although $(Mith)_2$-Co(II) exhibited the highest oxidative activity under physiological conditions, polyamines inhibited the DNA cleavage activity of the $(Mith)_2$-Co(II) in a concentration-dependent manner. Depletion of intracellular polyamines by methylglyoxal bis(guanylhydrazone) (MGBG) enhanced the sensitivity of A549 lung cancer cells to $(Mith)_2$-Co(II), most likely due to the decreased intracellular effect of polyamines on the action of (Mith)2-Co(II) [141]. This study suggested a novel method for enhancing the anticancer activity of DNA-binding metalloantibiotics through polyamine depletion.

Pyrophosphate is an important auxiliary ligand, which plays a key role in modifying reactivity, lipophilicity, and stabilizing specific oxidation states. Pyrophosphate-bridged Co(III) supramolecular complex **81** exhibited highly significant efficacy against the adriamycin-resistant ovarian cancer cell line A2780/AD with value as low as 160 pM. The underlying mechanism for such significant toxicity was based on DNA interactions, topoisomerase I enzyme inhibition and oxidative stress [142]. The results demonstrated a new class of prodrugs with significant potential for future development for the treatment of drug-resistant cancer cell lines.

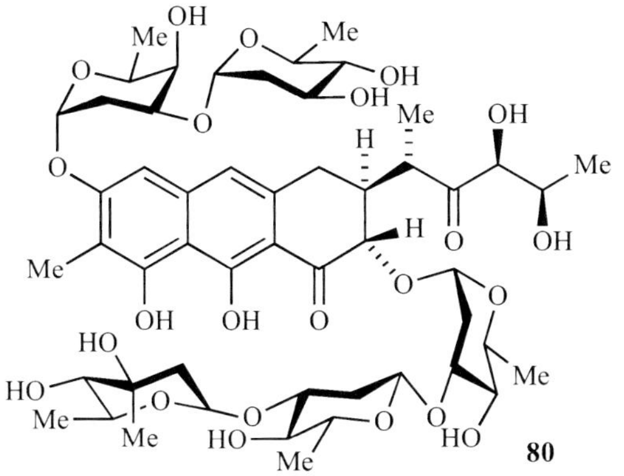

80

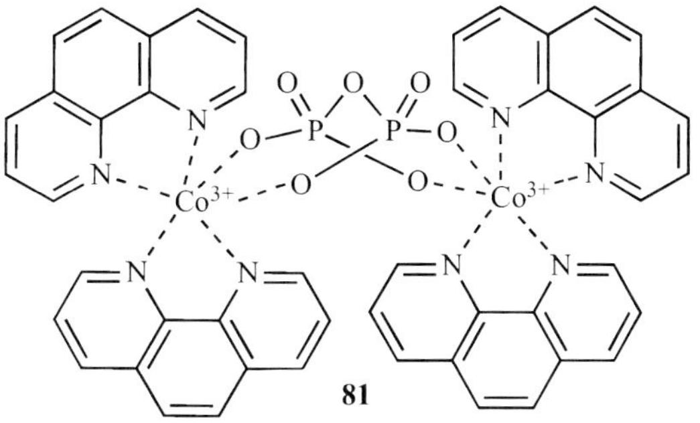

81

2.2.7. Nickel-Based Supramolecular Complexes as Anticancer Agents

Nickel is an essential element related to the life process. It can promote the absorption of iron element, the increase of red corpuscle as well as the syntheses of some amino-enzyme in the body [143]. The thermal denaturation studies have shown that nickel has a mild protection effect on DNA. Additionally, several DNA binding studies have indicated that Ni(II)-based supramolecular complexes displayed DNA intercalative behavior and DNA cleavage ability. The ligands can be an aromatic heterocyclic compound and often a Schiff base [144, 145]. Their capabilities are determined by several factors such as the planarity of ligand, atom type of ligand donor and the coordination geometry. With the understanding of the different binding modes of Ni(II) complexes, lots of new antitumor drugs toward specifically target DNA have been developed.

Metal supramolecular complexes of thiosemicarbazones are a class of compounds presenting some biological applications as antiviral, antibacterial and antitumour ones depending on the parent aldehyde, ketone and metal ion. S-Methyl-thiosemicarbazone derived nickel supramolecular complex **82**, whose cytotoxicity was significantly depended on the substituent position of aromatic rings, exhibited high cytotoxic activities against K562 and ECV304 human endothelial cell lines at low concentrations [146]. Nickel(II)-based supermolecule **83** with 2-quinolinecarboxaldehyde selenosemicarbazone showed induced cell cycle perturbations and increased hypodiploid cells, with fragmented DNA, comparable to the reference drug cisplatin.

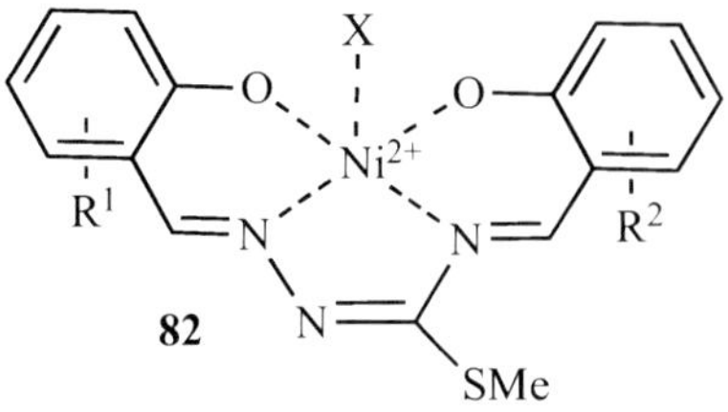

82

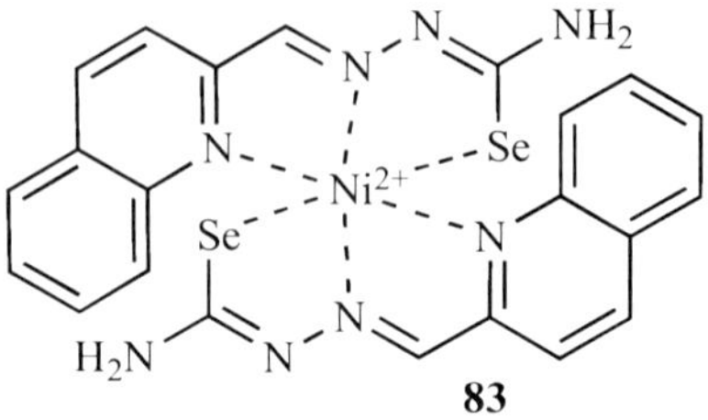

83

Previously, some work demonstrated that 4-quinolinecarboxylhydrazide exhibited pronounced anti-inflammatory and analgesic activity with quite low toxicity, while its nickel(II) supramolecular complex **84** showed significant cytotoxic activity against MFC cell lines. Moreover, it was also found that the complex bound to DNA *via* a groove binding mode could cleave pBR322 DNA, which was most succinctly illustrated by its considered cytotoxic activity against MFC cell lines [147, 148].

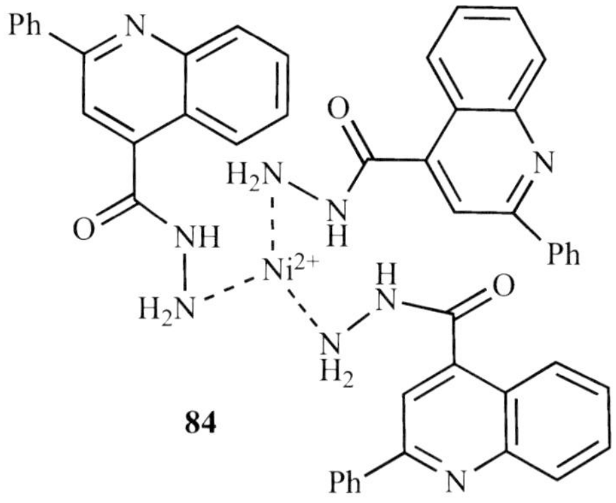

84

2.2.8. Copper-Based Supramolecular Complexes as Anticancer Agents

Copper, a kind of essential trace element in human body, involves in various vital movements and has significant effect on the living biological systems through chelation in its cation forms. Several excellent reviews concerning copper supramolecular complexes as potential anticancer agents are available since ligands coordinated with copper could elevate their activities, or even render the inactive ligands exhibiting obvious bioactivity [149-153].

Since aquated copper $[Cu(H_2O)_6]^{2+}$ was found toxicity to cells, much researches have been devoted to this type of copper complexes to develop novel molecules with excellent antitumor activity as potential clinical agents. Trigonal bipyramidal Cu(II) complex with a coordinated water molecule **85** gave better activity against neuroblastoma cells (IC_{50} = 377 μM) with recovery time 74 h, while exhibited weaker anti-ovarian cancer cell activity. Further researches demonstrated that this complex could not induce DNA strand scission, and additional work would be essenial to determine if DNA and/or proteins are targets for this metal complex in the cell [154].

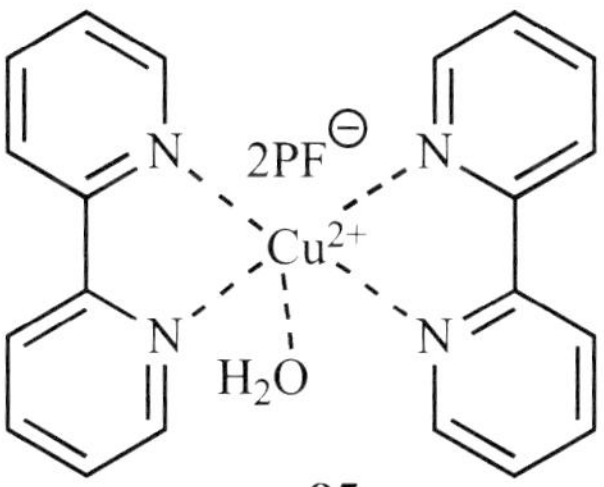

85

Schiff base and chelates are associated with lots of bioactivities such as antibacterial, antifungal and anticancer. The related researches on some metal(II) complexes of various Schiff bases have been conducted very well and are currently the most active area in the development of anticancer drugs. The cytotoxic study showed that the Cu(II) complex **86** had the best *in vitro* anticancer activity against both HT-29 (colon carcinoma) and MCF-7 (human breast adenocarcinoma) cells with activities of about a half (17.02 μM), and a fifth (9.78 μM) in comparison with cisplatin respectively [155].

The research on the metal supramolecular complex of active component in the *Chinese herb* was an effective way to find new anticancer compounds targeted DNA. A large number of investigations manifested that plant-derived polyphenolic compounds, generally recognized as nature antioxidants, also exhibited prooxidant properties under the presence of copper(II), and therefore led to mutation or cancer. Quercetin-based copper(II) supramolecular complex **87**, which was carried out with A549 cells in cytotoxicity experiments, confirmed its apoptosis-inducing activity, and demonstrated that the levels of survivin protein expression in A549 cells decreased, while the relative activity of caspase-3 increased significantly after treatment with compound **87**. These results suggested that the mechanisms of anticancer and apoptosis-inducing activities of the quercetin copper(II) complex should be involved in not only the oxidative DNA damage with generation of ROS but also its specific interaction with DNA [156].

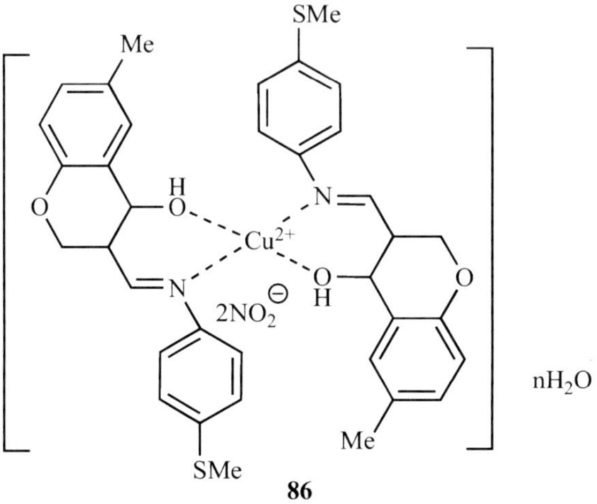

86

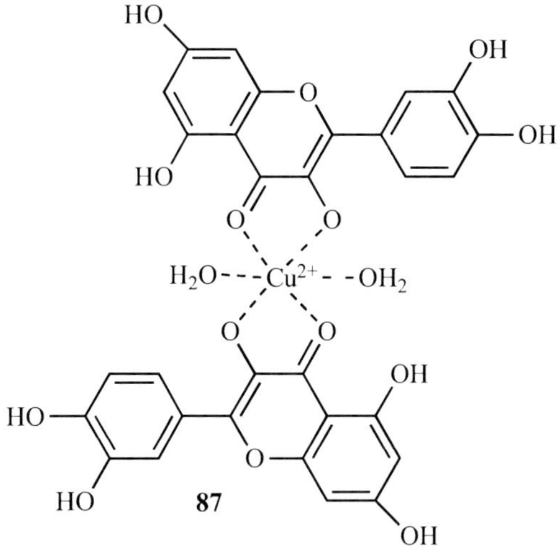

87

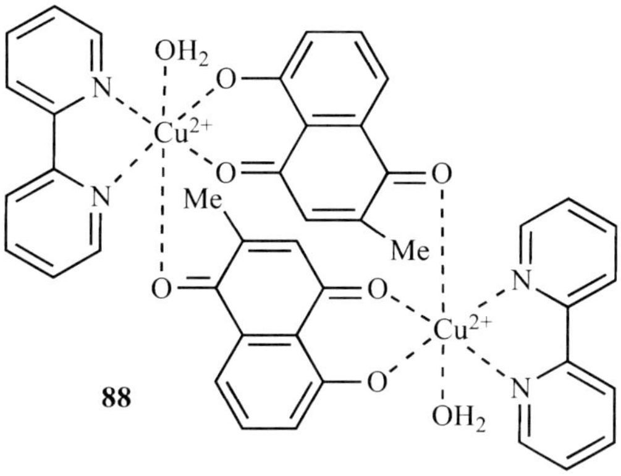

88

The anticancer traditional Chinese medicinal drug, plumbagin (PLN), was isolated from *Plumbago Zeylanica.* Its formation of copper(II) supramolecular complex enhanced cytotoxicity of free PLN, suggesting that metal ions in combination with plumbagin displayed synergy anticancer activity. The binding properties to DNA indicated that plumbagin-based copper(II) supermolecule **88** was non-covalent binding and mainly intercalated the neighboring base pairs of DNA [157].

Acetylsalicylic acid is generally used for the treatment of rheumatoid arthritis, whereas accompanying adverse effect was involved the formation of peptic ulcers. Interestingly, acetylsalicylic acid-derived copper(II) supramolecular complex was several times more active, and also exhibited appreciable anti-ulcer activity. The interaction between complex and DNA was observed as well and revealed that the occurrence of fragmentation of genomic DNA after incubation with copper(II) acetylsalicylate supermolecule, indicating that these drug substances might be responsible for cytotoxicity *in vivo* [158].

The success of metal-based supramolecular drugs is closely linked to the proper choice of the auxiliary ligand, which plays a key role in modifying reactivity, lipophilicity, and stabilizing specific oxidation states. Pyrophosphate ($P_2O_7^{4-}$), a polyphosphate anion, has been aroused considerable attention. Polyphosphates participate in diverse bioenergetic processes such as oxidative phosphorylation, oxidative decarboxylation (*e.g.* thiamine pyrophosphate), ATP production and energy storage. Given this, the first pyrophosphate-bridged Cu(II) complex **89** was prepared and displayed highly significant efficacy than that of cisplatin, toward the adriamycin-resistant ovarian cancer cell line A2780/AD [159].

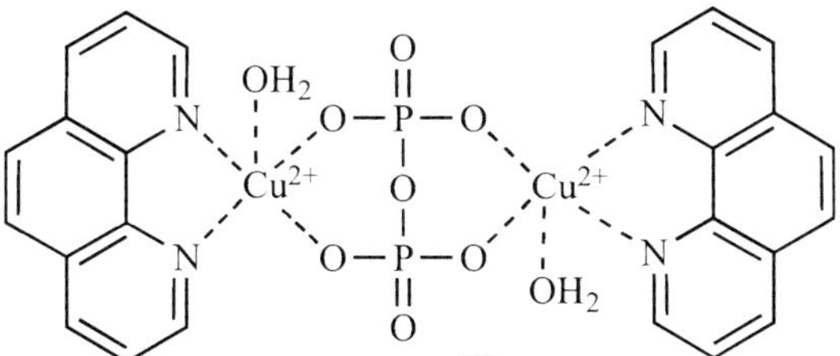

89

Recently, anticancer hybrid molecules which covalently combine an active therapeutic pharmacophore/agent to a biological carrier vector to diminish toxicity, enhance anti-proliferative activity and attribute some specificity have invoked interest. The synthesized hybrid copper complex **90** was tested in a multiple panel of hormonedependent (MCF-7, T47D), and hormone-independent (BT20 and MDA-MB231) breast cancer cell lines as well as androgen-independent prostate (PC3) cancer cell line. The metal complex gave low IC_{50} values, while against T47D it was even low to 5 μM. It was worthy to note that the platinum and cisplatin complexes gave weaker inhibition probably due to the presence of the identical planar geometries with '*cis*' placement of the chloro ligands and the donor atom set in cisplatin consists of NN atoms while it is NS atoms in case of present complexes [160].

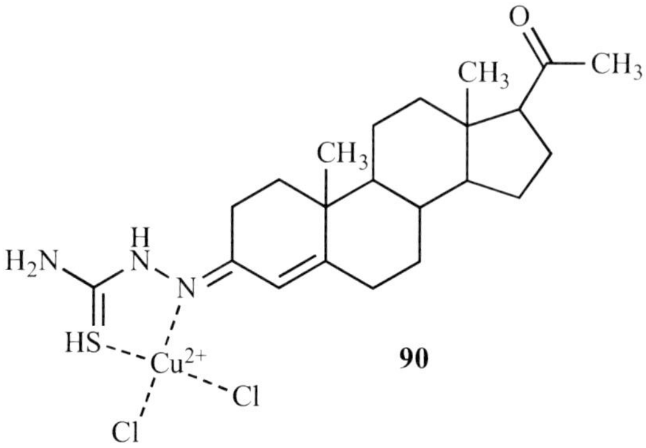

90

The synthesis and chemical investigation of thiosemicarbazones and their metal complexes are of considerable interest due to their potential for medicinal applications. A novel thiosemicarbazone from 2-acetonaphthone and its zinc, cobalt, and copper complexes displayed significant anticancer activity. Copper complex **91** was the most active complex with excellent activity against both cancer cell lines. For the 72 h exposure, the IC_{50} values are near 1 μM which is ten times as active as the zinc complex, five times as active as the cobalt complex for the HCT-116 cell line and than the etoposide drug comparison. Unfortunately, this complex with the lowest *in vitro* activity has the highest DNA binding constant [161].

As the interest in the development of antitumor molecules is astonishingly increasing, there is always a pursuit of designing compounds to combine with targeted organic compounds to inhibit specific enzymes because many anticancer drugs were either classic non-targeted coordination complexes or organic alkylating agents with serious side effects. Paullone copper complex **92** was prepared and evaluated against human cancer cell lines A549 (A), SW480 (B) and

CH1 (C). Experiment showed that the methyl substitution in position 15 of the Paullone ligand was favorable in terms of biological activity, as indicated by the lower IC_{50} values (0.053–0.54 μM) compared to those of hydrogen one (0.39–1.4 μM) [162].

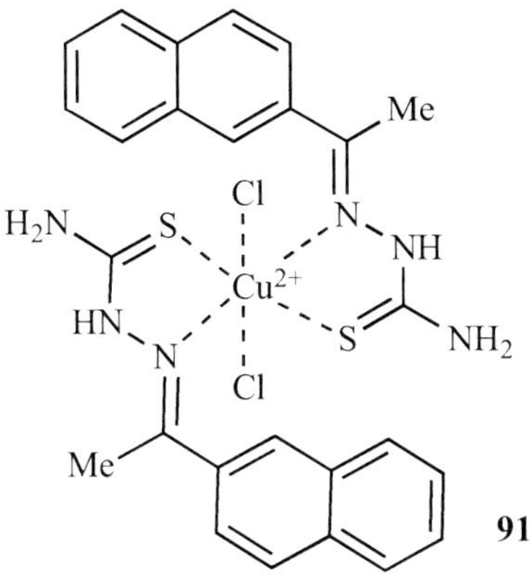

91

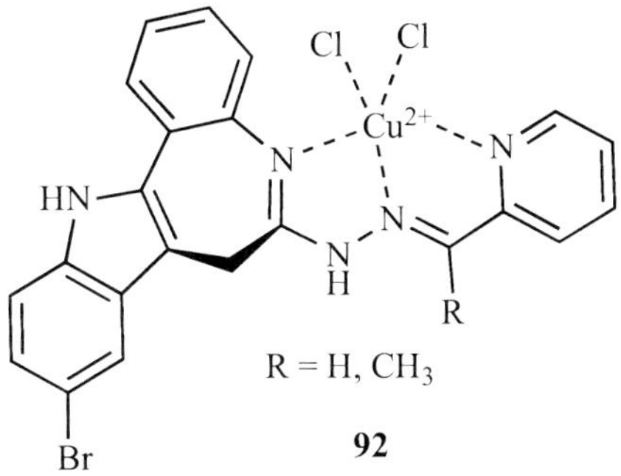

R = H, CH_3

92

Currently, photoactivated chemotherapy drugs have been attracted numerous attentions, which were expected to generate a reactive moiety on photoactivation in visible light, while the compound remains inactive in the dark. Copper(II) ion with a visible spectral band within the photo-dynamic therapy was chosen for the preparation of photoactivited metal complexes. Ferrocene-appended copper(II) complex **93** showed significantly better DNA photocleavage activity and enhanced cellular activity in HeLa cancer cells over its phenyl analogue. The results are of great importance toward developing the unexplored chemistry of metal-based photoactivated anticancer agents as clinical candidates which exerting DNA cleavage activity within the phototherapeutic spectral window [163].

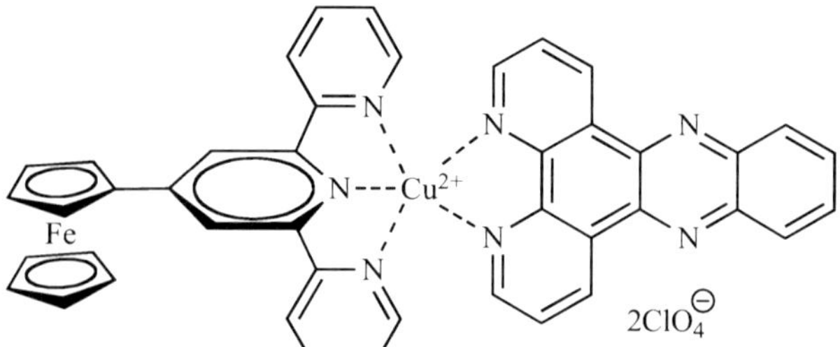

93

With the aim of improving clinical effectiveness, reducing general toxicity, and broadening the spectrum of activity. A series of novel copper(I) complexes of tris(2-cyanoethyl)phosphine were prepared and evaluated for cytotoxic potential against a panel of several human tumour cell lines. Complex **94** has shown high *in vitro* antitumour activity, especially toward lung and ovarian tumour hystotypes. Furthermore in isolated mitochondria for their ability to alter the most relevant mitochondrial pathophysiological parameters, this complex also showed noticeably respiration, coupling, ATP-synthetase activity and membrane potential [164].

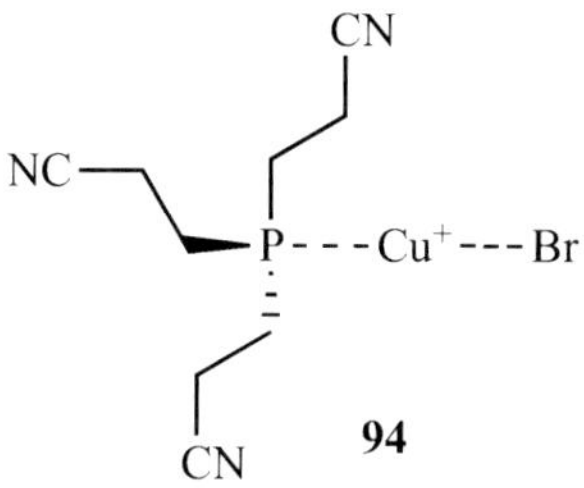

94

N-Heterocyclic carbenes (NHC) have been drawn special interest, since the first palladium (II)-NHC complex was proved to be superior to cisplatin as an antiproliferative agent against human promyelocytic leukaemia HL60 tumor cells. Very recently, N-heterocyclic carbenes derived copper(I) supramolecular complex **95** displayed comparable cytotoxicity with that of cisplatin on five different human cancer cell lines, including oral carcinoma KB, promyelocytic leukaemia HL60, breast cancer MCF-7 and MCF-7R as well as prostatic Cancer LNCaP. Unlike cisplatin, Cu(I)-NHC supermolecule arrests the cell cycle progression at the G1 phase and induces apoptosis at a lower concentration. More importantly, it is assumed that an aerobic radical process leading to a DNA strand break is responsible for the observed cytotoxicity [165].

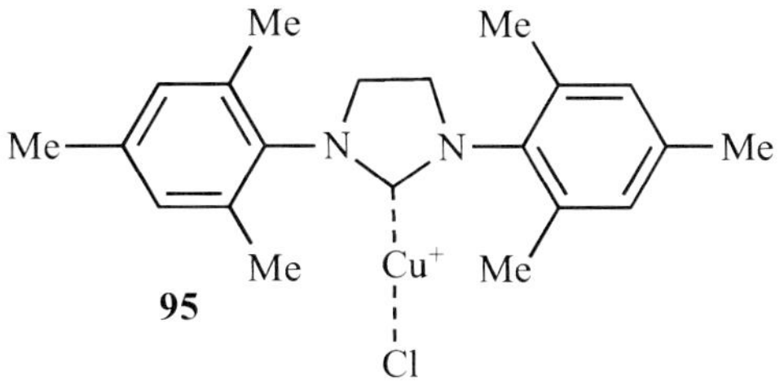

95

2.2.9. Zinc-Based Supramolecular Complexes as Anticancer Agents

Zinc, a member of the IIB group of metal, is essential for growth and developments and plays an important role in various biological systems. Epidemiologic studies suggested that zinc deficiency may be associated with increased risk of cancer [166]. Moreover, it is found that zinc protects against tumor necrosis factor (TNF) in a HSP70-dependent way, which could be helpful in developing a safer anticancer therapy with TNF/IFN-γ [167]. Therefore, the research with respect to the zinc supramolecular complexes as anticancer agents was beneficial for the invention of new anticancer drugs.

The photodynamic therapy (PDT) for treating tumors is particularly attractive because of its intrinsic dual selectivity. Among these, metal supramolecular complexes of photosensitisers were effective in PDT, such as the isopropylidene-protected glucosylated zinc(II) phthalocyanine **96a**. This complex showed excellent photocytotoxicity, which was particularly potent, having IC_{50} values as low as 0.03 μM. Another new zinc(II) di-α-substituted phthalocyanine

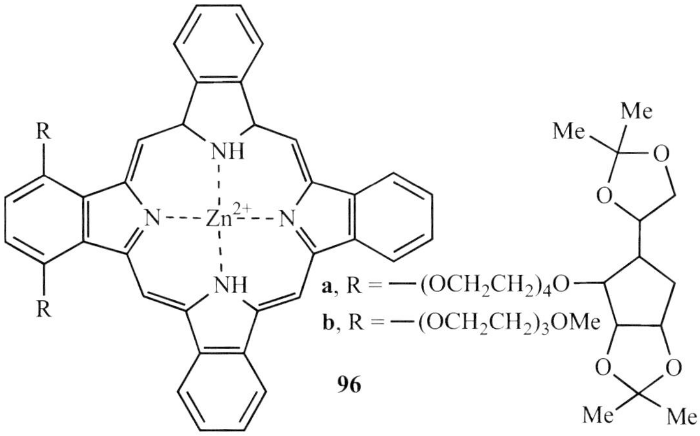

96

supermolecule **96b** was also highly cytotoxic towards HT29 human colorectal carcinoma and HepG2 human hepatocarcinoma cells, especially the complex **96b** with IC_{50} values as low as 0.06 μM against HepG2. The great photodynamic activities of these zinc(II)-based supermolecules can be attributed to their high cellular uptake and aggregation tendency in the biological media, leading to a high efficiency to generate reactive oxygen species inside the cells [168, 169].

DNA binding and cleavage are two critical events for gene mutation and carcinogenesis in biological systems. DNA targeting reagents may have great prospects as artificial nucleases, DNA structural probes or gene-selective drugs. Metalated terpyridine supermolecules are well documented for their high DNA affinity through intercalation, DNA nuclease activity and cytotoxicity. Recently, terpyridine based zinc(II) supramolecular complexes **97a** and **97b** were observed to demonstrate higher *in vitro* cytotoxicity than cisplatin against selected tumor cell lines (HeLa, MCF-7, HepG2 and PC-3). In particular, the complex **97b** was much cytotoxic, with about 10 times higher than its ligand against MCF-7 and PC-3 cell lines, indicating the crucial attribution of the metallization [170].

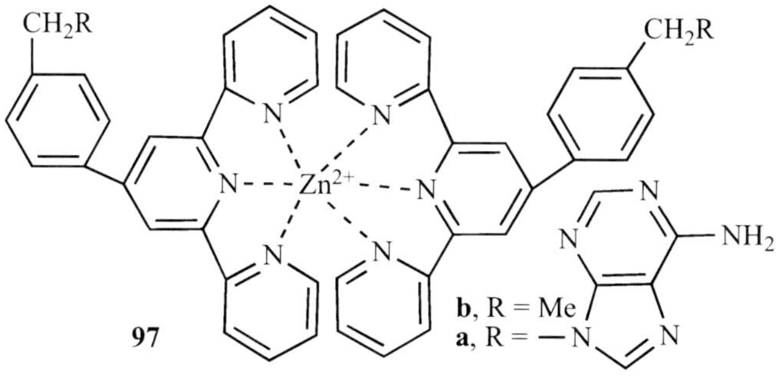

97

Xanthones have demonstrated multiple pharmacological properties, such as anti-oxidant, anti-inflammatory, anti-malarial and anti-cancer activities. Xanthone-based Zn(II) supramolecular complex **98** showed strong cytotoxic activities *in vitro* with IC_{50} values of 22.08 μM and 19.98 μM for the GLC-82 and SGC7901 cell lines, respectively, probably owing to the induction of DNA damage in cancer cells causing by the complex. This work may be helpful to the research of the anticancer mechanism of xanthones and the design of the new potent supramolecular anticancer drugs [171].

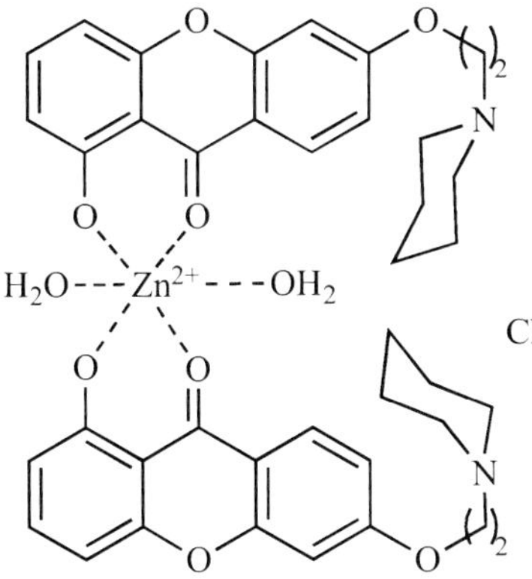

98

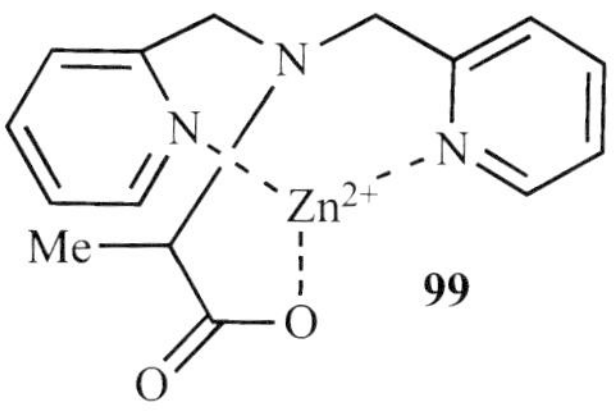

99

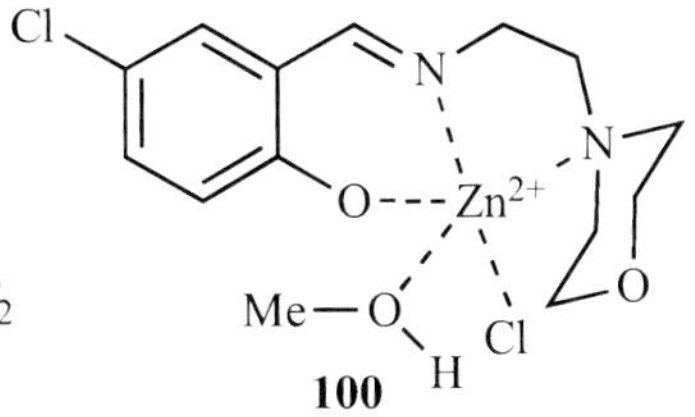

100

Zinc-di(picolyl)amine (DPA) complexes were employed as binding sites for histidine residues to study metalloenzyme function in bioinorganic chemistry. DPA-derived Zn(II) supermolecule **99** was active against the four cancer cells (MCF-7, ECA 109, A549, Hela), and the antitumor activity of zinc complexes was dependent on its binding to DNA [172].

Quercetin, a bioflavonoid widely distributed in fruits and vegetables, has been reported to exert multiple biological effects as an antioxidant and antitumor activity. Quercetin-based supramolecular complex, when copper was replaced by Zn(II) in example **87**, could cleave the DNA *via* hydrolytic pathway, which displayed much higher cytotoxic activities than that of quercetin alone in treatment of HepG2, SMMC7721 and A549 cells [173].

Many Schiff base complexes have provoked wide interest because they possess a diverses pectrum of biological and pharmaceutical activities, including antitumor and antioxidative properties. For instance, Zn(II) ion combining with the Schiff bases derived from salicylaldehydes and amides afforded zinc supramolecular complex **100**, which showed significant activity against K562, KB and Hep-G2, similar to 5-fluorouracil, compared with the ligand of no appreciable cytotoxicity [174].

2.2.10. Rhenium-Based Supramolecular Complexes as Anticancer Agents

The coordination behavior of $Re(CO)_3^+$ core has been extensively studied in supramolecular chemistry because its kinetic inertia and the three carbonyl donors serve to fix until three coordination sites about the metal, leaving available positions for ligands substitution with important applications for medical purposes like gene therapy and diagnostic radiopharmaceuticals for cell imaging utilization. Additionally, more attentions are paid to polypyridine complexes with $Re(CO)_3^+$ core in view of the interesting emission behaviors and efficient cellular uptake properties of luminescent polypyridine rhenium(I) supramolecular complexes.

β-Elemene, (1*S*, 2*S*, 4*R*) 1-methy-1-vinyl-2,4-diisopropenyl cyclohexane **101**, a natural sesquiterpene extracted from the *Traditional Chinese Herb Medicinal Material*, exhibited appreciable anticancer effects in human and murine tumor cells and had substantial clinical activity against various tumors without severe side effects. Recently, non-radioactive Re(I) based supermolecules with the 2,2'-dipicolylamine compounds derived from the β-elemene were reported to substantial decrease in IC_{50} values compared with the parent compound β-elemene, while their corresponding radioactive supramolecular complexes possessed good radioactive yield (above 90%) and radioactive chemical purity with Re-188 (above 95%), which provided the possibility to find a new kind of potential supramolecular radiopharmaceuticals [175].

The tyramine-derived 2,2'-dipicolylamine (DPAT) can chelate the $Re(CO)_3^+$ core in a different way as well, taking the tricarbonyl rhenium(I) polypyridine supramolecular complex **102b** for example. Moreover, DPAT-free complex **102a** was more cytotoxic than cisplatin toward the HeLa cells, with the complex **102b** more potent than the one **102a** in a 48 h incubation period. Furthermore, complex **102b** exhibited emission enhancement and lifetime extension upon binding of zinc(II) and cadmium(II) ions, suggesting the 2,2'-dipicolylamine unit can be utilized as the recognition site. It was the first luminescent transition metal supramolecular complexes that function as *in vitro* and *in vivo* probes for these two biologically and environmentally important metal ions [176].

The tremendous success for noble metal-based supramolecular complexes as anticancer drugs stimulated numerous efforts toward the focus on non-noble metal complex supermolecules as potential anticancer agents. So far some promising results have been found, in particularly titanium-, iron-, zinc- and copper-based supramolecular complexes have already showed good anticancer efficacy against some tumors. As the search for novel ligands and further study for mechanism of action, more and more non-noble metal supramolecular complexes as clinical anticancer agents will be obtained and are inevitable to play increasingly roles in the prevention and treatment of cancers.

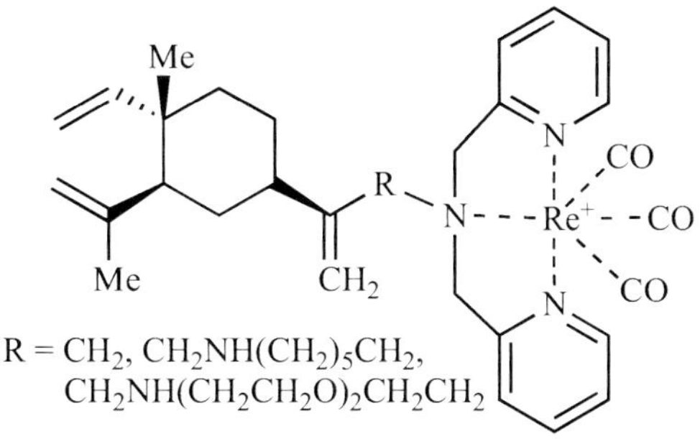

101

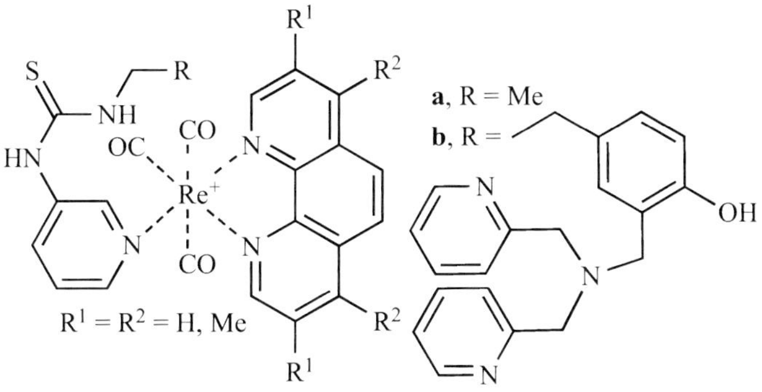

102

2.3. Lanthanide Series-Based Supramolecular Complexes as Anticancer Agents

Lanthanide compounds, for example with cerium as metal center, have been used for the treatment of cancer, and as anti-emetics due to favorable pharmacological properties [177, 178]. In addition, they have application in the treatment of burns and as phosphate binders against hyperphosphatemia. Very recently, Lanthanide series-based compounds have shown pronounced anticancer activity. The mode of action of anticancer-active lanthanides is related to their similarity to calcium. Ln(III) ions exhibit high affinity to Ca(II) binding sites in biomolecules because of their similar ionic radii, but are higher charged (HSAB principle). Therefore, such compounds are able to inhibit calcium fluxes, required for cell cycle regulation, but they can substitute not only for calcium but also for other metal ions such as Mg(II), Fe(III) and Mn(II) ions in proteins, leading to the inhibition of their functions. More importantly, the tumor-inhibiting activity of lanthanum is considerably enhanced by forming supramolecular complexes with various ligands. Lanthanide-based supramolecular complexes were gradually taken seriously in cancer prevention and treatment.

Phenanthroline with a large rigid aromatic ring is an important building ligand of supermolecules. Phenanthroline metal supramolecular complexes have become an important class of supermolecules for studying nucleic acid structure and design of nucleic acid secondary anti-cancer drugs, owing to their unique stability, redox, fluorescence lifetime as well as the excellent interaction with DNA. Phenanthroline La supramolecular complex KP772 **103** exerted potent activity against a wide range of tumor cell lines and a colon carcinoma xenograft model *in vivo* with comparable properties to cisplatin and methotrexate. Notably, long-term treatment of KBC-1 cells with KP772 led to a complete loss of drug resistance, and complementary studies showed that exposition of cells to subtoxic, stepwise increasing KP772 concentrations did not lead to acquired resistance. KP772 was expected to be active against multi-drug-resistant tumors, rendering it very interesting for further preclinical development [179]. Furthermore, cerium(III)-based phenanthroline supermolecule **104** showed excellent activity against tested

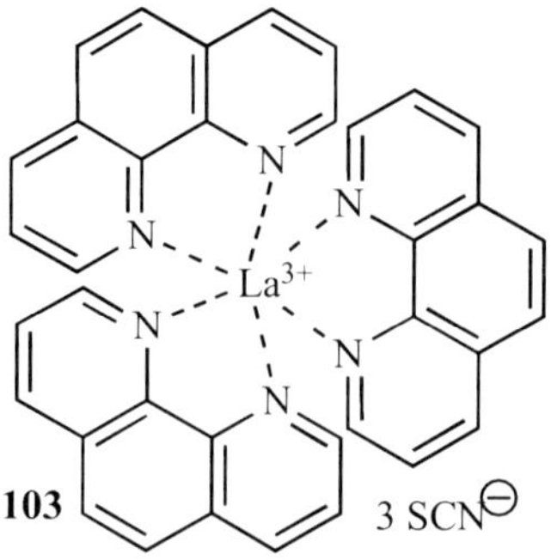

103

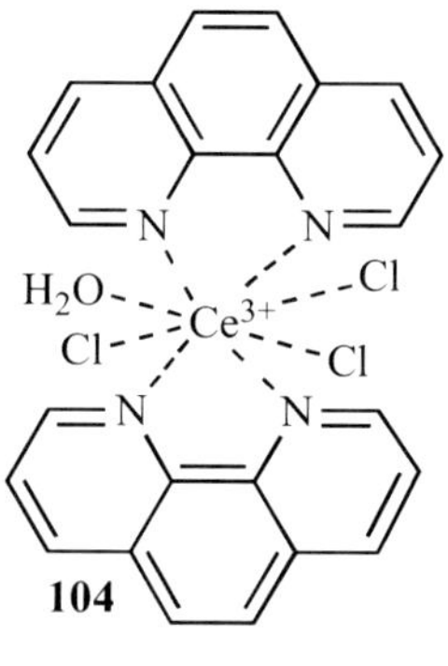

104

model systems with IC_{50} values 1.2-2.7 μM. Its mode of action may be very well based on interaction with cellular proteins (*e.g.* inhibition of metalloenzymes by Ce^{3+}) instead of permanent modification of the DNA as proposed for Pt-based chemotherapeutics [180].

Gadolinium-based supermolecules are most frequently used as magnetic resonance imaging (MRI) contrast agents because of their high magnetic moment, asymmetric electronic ground state, and potential for increased MRI intensity. The literature related to their anticancer activities is rare. Until recently, Arambula *et al.* reported that the new PEG-solubilized gadolinium texaphyrin (Gd-Tex) complex containing a malonate-Pt(NH_3)$_2$ moiety as well as gadolinium texaphyrinmalonate-Pt complex **105** could show similar active to that of carboplatin against A549 human lung cancer and A2780 human ovarian cancer cell lines, and displayed even greater efficacy against Pt-resistant 2780CP ovarian cell line than carboplatin [181].

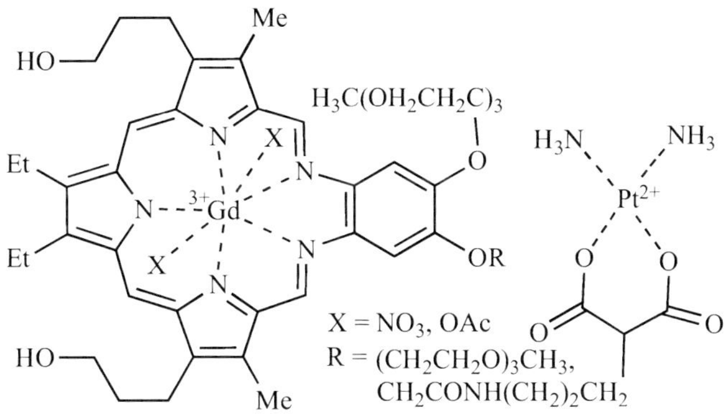

105

3. NON-TRANSITION METAL SUPRAMOLECULAR COMPLEXES AS ANTICANCER AGENTS

3.1. Gallium-Based Supramolecular Complexes as Anticancer Agents

Gallium is the second metal ion, after platinum, to be used in cancer treatment [182]. Its salts have been explored for their applicabilities as antineoplastic drugs for more than two decades, among which, citrated gallium nitrate (Ganite TM) is the first gallium complex approved for the treatment of hypercalcemia and bone cancer [81, 183]. However, their clinical experience has revealed unfavorable pharmacokinetic and toxicological properties. Fortunately, the formation of gallium based supermolecules with organic ligands by the coordination bonds, has been recognized as a promising strategy for creating tumor inhibiting therapeutics with a number of advantages over gallium salts regarding oral bioavailability

[184]. Therefore, more recently the researches on gallium complexes with diverse organic ligands as antitumor agents have been a renewed interesting field for the design of novel gallium-based drugs [185].

Hydroxyquinoline based gallium(III) supermolecule (KP46, **106**) has finished phase I trials with the outcome of promising tolerability and evidence of clinical activity in renal cell carcinoma [186]. Another study on KP46 suggested that gallium maltolate is a promising chemotherapeutic agent for the treatment of malignant melanoma and hepatocellular carcinoma (HCC). It showed dose-dependent antiproliferative activity in all four HCC cell lines after 6-day drug exposure (IC_{50} values range from 25-35 μM), and additionally induced apoptosis at 30 μM [187].

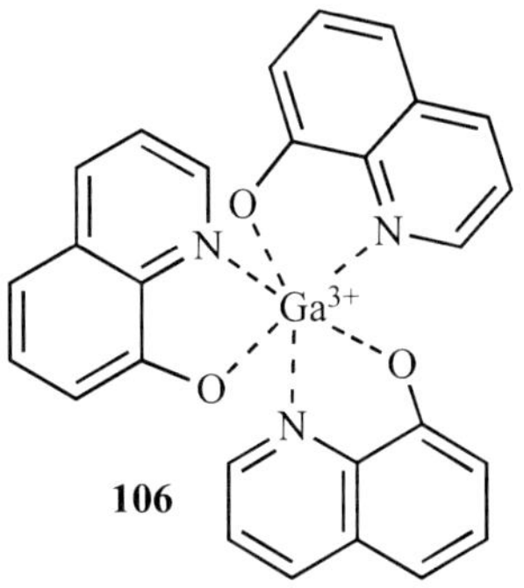

106

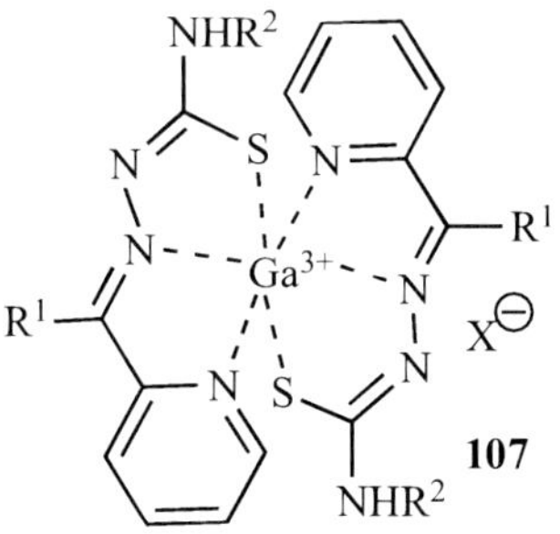

107

a, $R^1 = R^2 = Me$, $X = GaCl_4$
b, $R^1 = NH_2$, $R^2 = Me$, $X = NO_3$
c, $R^1 = NH_2$, $R^2 = Et$, $X = NO_3$

Many α-*N*-heterocyclic thiosemicarbazones and their metal complexes have been reported to exert tumor-inhibiting effects. Combination of gallium and thiosemicarbazones ligands seems to be a worthwhile task to obtain gallium-derived supermolecules as potential antitumor agents. Bis(2-acetylpyridine-4,4-dimethyl-3-thiosemicarbazonato-N,N,S) gallium(III) tetrachlorogallate (KP1089, **107a**) was the first representative of this class that has been assayed for antineoplastic activity in human tumor cell lines, and showed IC_{50} values in the low nanomolar range against ovarian (4 μM), mammary (SK-BR-3) and colon (SW480) carcinoma cells, though the values were similar to that of the ligand alone. Further test is undergoing to determine whether the gallium helps targeting the compound to gallium-avid cancer cells. Gallium supermolecules **107b-c** strongly increased the cytotoxic potential with 20-fold more potent than cisplatin against RT2 and T98 cells of IC_{50} values in the range of 0.81-9.57 and 3.6-11.30

μM, respectively. These compounds could probably activate apoptotic cell death pathways by mechanisms that are both dependent and independent of p53 [188].

Investigations concerning interactions of gallium complexes with amino acid derivatives have been limited during the past years. Recently, Gómez-Ruiz *et al.* reported that the novel gallium(III) supramolecular complexes containing *N*-phthaloyl derivatives of neutral amino acids such as glycine and alanine were observed against 8505C anaplastic thyroid cancer and DLD-1 colon carcinoma as well as A253 head and neck carcinoma. However, the studied carboxylic acids showed no proliferative activity, and their complex **108** presented very similar cytotoxic activity against all the tested cancer cell lines with IC_{50} values in the range of 5-25 μM, higher efficacy than the gallium(III) nitrate. In addition, DNA laddering method showed that treatment of the studied cell lines with IC_{90} doses of complex **108** resulted in the induction of apoptotic mode of cell death [189].

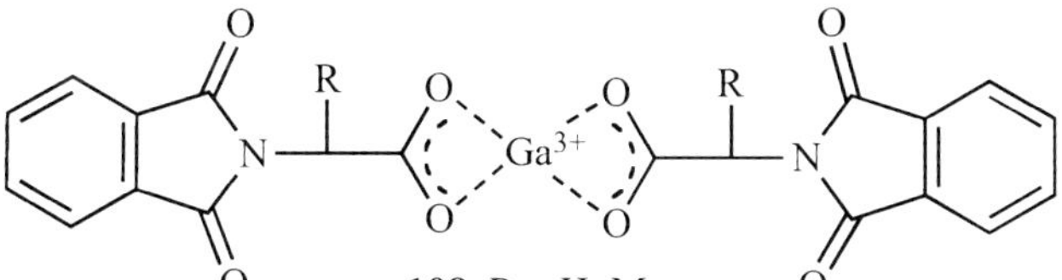

108, R = H, Me

The above discussions have shown a renewed interest in exploring gallium based supramolecular complexes in a host of malignancies, especially lymphoma and bladder cancer. However, the detailed mechanisms of action of gallium complexes are not completely defined. Further investigation of the underlying mechanisms along with optimizing the structural components of gallium based supermolecules will be helpful to improve the therapeutic index of gallium.

3.2. Organotin-Based Supramolecular Complexes as Anticancer Agents

Organotin compounds had been received an increasing interest, mainly due to their industrial, agricultural, and biological applications as early as last 50-70 years [190]. A large number of organotin-based supramolecular complexes have been synthesized and tested *in vitro* and *in vivo*, firstly, against murine leukemia cell lines and, after that, against different panels of human cancer cell lines and these data have been included in recent comprehensive reviews as well as the action mode of organotins in cancer chemotherapy [191-193].

Organotin(IV) complexes with carboxylates as ligands have been widely investigated for their antiproliferative properties and have become the most potential class of organotin supermolecules as anticancer agents. These antitumor data have been included in review articles [194-196] and book chapters [197].

Recent research found that organotin(IV) supermolecules with phenylethanoate moieties showed excellent anticancer activities. Supramolecular complex **109** showed significant anticancer activity with IC_{50} values between 2.53 μg/mL and 7.92 μg/mL, which was similar to the standard drug doxorubicin [198, 199]. Organotin(IV) complex of benzoic acid derivative **110** showed high activity against Hela cell lines with the IC_{50} values of 2.3 μg/mL, lower than that of cisplatin (IC_{50} = 3.50 μg/mL). Further study on the antitumor effects of these supermolecules is highly recommended [200].

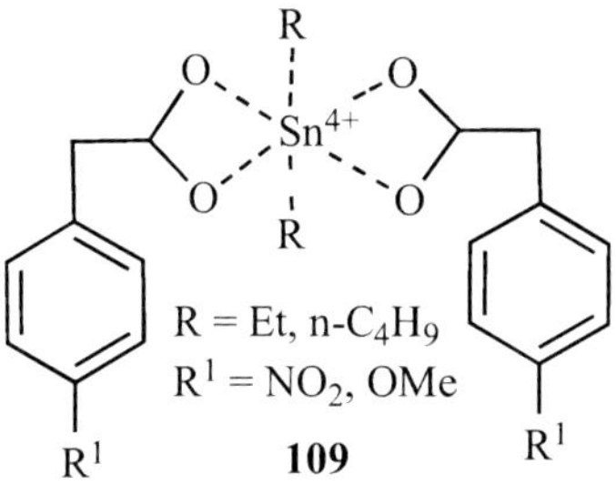

109

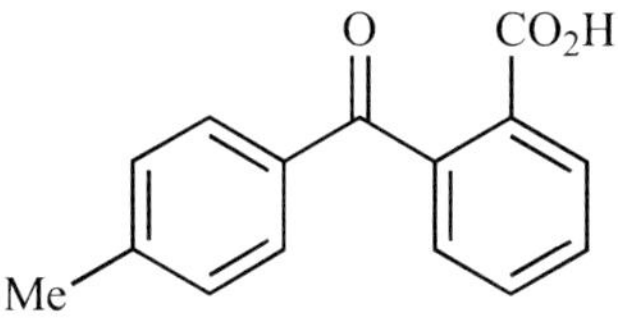

110

Iminodiacetic acid is a potential tridentate and its organotin complex **111** exhibited relatively higher inhibitory effect than cisplatin against three tumor cell lines (P388, HL-60 and A-549) for the experimental concentration range (10^{-4}-10^{-7} M). The results suggested that the organotin supermolecules of iminodiacetic acid were expected to use as potent antitumor agents [201].

Literatures indicated that the introduction of aminoglucosyl group would kill the tumor cells while being less toxic to normal cells in human body. It was found that the dibutyltin supramolecular complex of aminoglucosyl derivative **112** possessed rather high cytotoxicity to P388, HL-60, A549 as well as BEL-7402 tumor cell lines, but unfortunately it also had hematopoietic cell toxicity at 10^{-6} M even with amino glucose [202].

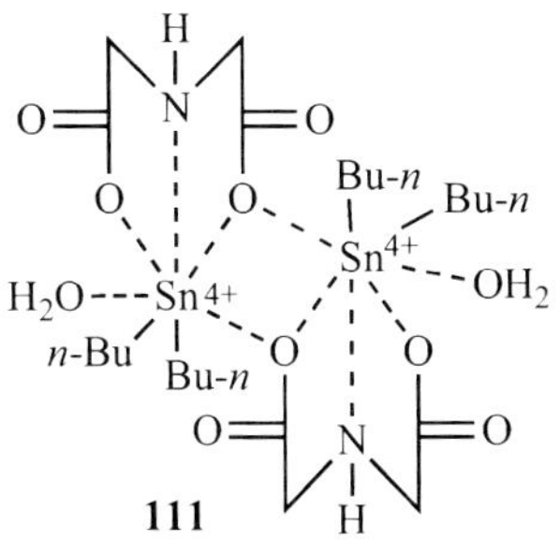

111

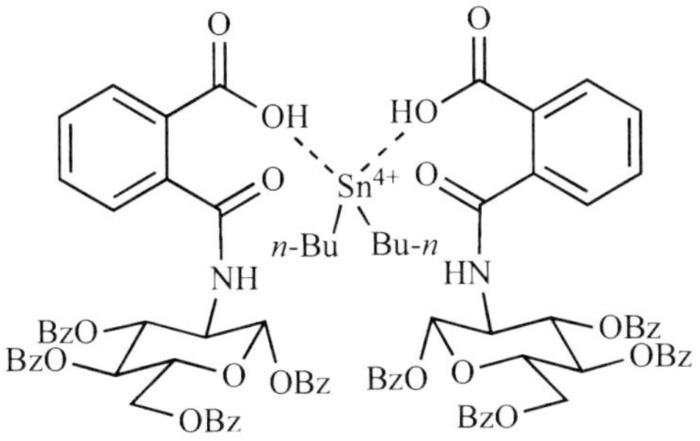

112

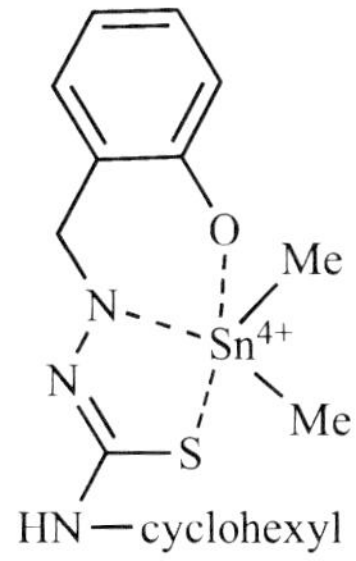

113

Thiosemicarbazone-based organotin supermolecules have been the research hotspots in the realm of medicine. Very recently, a novel rationally designed organotin complex (D4-t, **113**) bearing 4-cyclohexyl thiosemicarbazone ligand was observed to be able to reduce tumor mass without severe toxicity at the dose of 5 mg/kg and inhibited the synthesis of DNA in S-180 tumor cells in comparison to Platin10 and ConA. Additionally, the complexes had the lymphocyte activation property and stimulated immune response of the lymphoid cells, which in turn expressed the antitumor activity and therefore indicated promising therapeutic potential of D4-t [203].

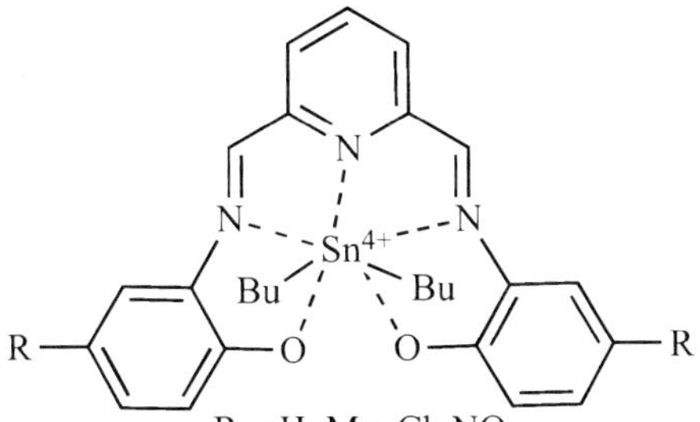

R = H, Me, Cl, NO_2

114

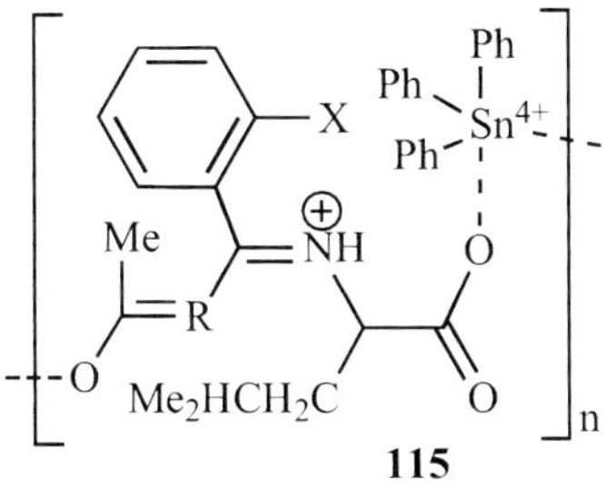

115

Schiff base, containing aromatic heterocycle with three nitrogen atoms, as well as their corresponding metal complexes showed significant biological activities, which received considerable attention. Especially metal complexes containing oxygen and nitrogen donor Schiff bases, possess unusual configuration and structural liability, and are sensitive to molecular environment. For instance, heptacoordinate tin(IV) supermolecule **114** derived from pyridine Schiff base, showed varied antiproliferative activity against six tumor cell lines including HTC-15, MCF7, K-562, U251, PC-3 and SKLU-1, with the IC_{50} values lower than that of cisplatin [204]. Noticeably, the amino acetate functionalized Schiff base organotin(IV) complex **115** was found to be more cytotoxic for A498, EVSA-T, H226, IGROV, M19 MEL, MCF7 and WIDR human tumor cell lines than doxorubicin, cisplatin, 5-fluorouracil and etoposide with an ID_{50} value of around 35 ng/mL [205].

Organotin supermolecule **116a** with sulfur donor ligand resulted significantly more active than parental compound **116b** with IC_{50} values in the range 0.16-1.8 μM against a panel of human cancer cell lines. Toxicity studies *in vivo*, after *i.v.* administration of escalating concentrations of **116a**, provided the identification of the maximal tolerated dose (3.5 mg/kg) which was employed as therapeutic dose in clinical use. Preliminary results, in transplanted murine tumor models, revealed that both the P388 myelomonocytic leukemia and the B16-F10 melanoma were inhibited about 96% in their tumor volume at day 11. Additional studies were mandatory to unravel the mechanism of action for **116a** as potential antitumor drug [206].

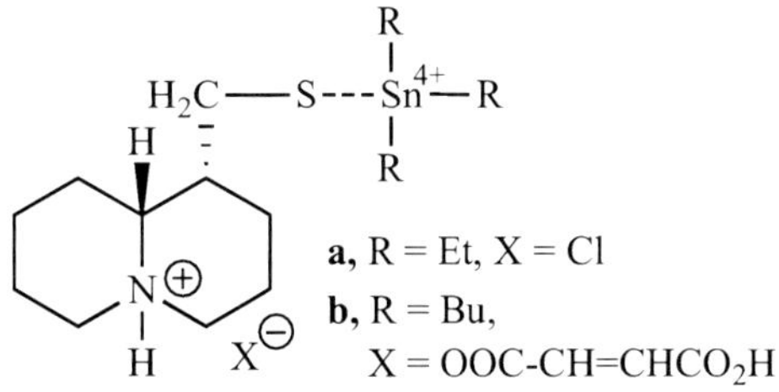

116

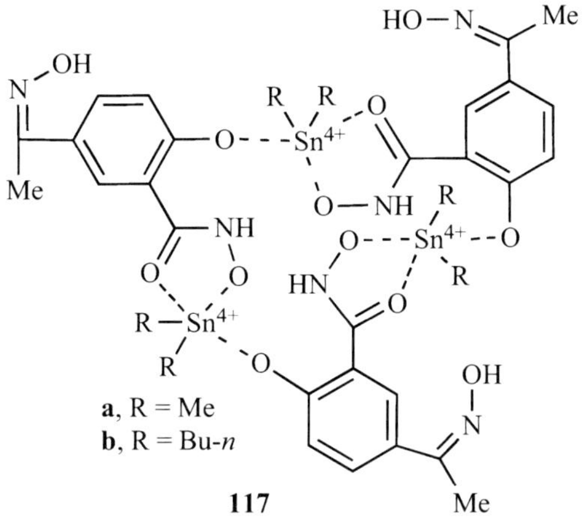

117

Apart from the discussed ligands above, cyclopentadienyl or oximehydroxamate organotin(IV) complexes could also present higher cytotoxicity than cisplatin. Complex **117a** displayed the high cytotoxic activity against all tested cancer cells, with IC_{50} values from 0.037 μM to 0.085 μM [207]. Another representative was complex **117b**, the first organotin(IV) supermolecule with oximehydroxamate, exhibited strong *in vitro* cytotoxic activity than cisplatin. This good anticancer activity may be related to the particularly promising coordinating properties of ligand to increase the water solubility in the presence of hydrophilic HON and HO moieties [208].

4. CONCLUSIONS AND OUTLOOKS

Organometallic supramolecular complexes as anticancer drugs have extensively been investigated and are becoming an increasingly active and newly rising interdisciplinary. Organometallic supramolecular drugs have been playing positive roles in treatment of cancer diseases with enhancing effectively the stability and safety, decreasing the toxicity and adverse effect, overcoming multidrug resistance, and elevating the drug-targeting, the biocompatibility as well as bioavailability and so on. All of these properties could greatly improve the therapeutic efficacy of drugs in the ultimate. Importantly, more and more organometallic supramolecular complexes have been used as clinical antitumor drugs and become anticancer candidates, and have shown enormous potential in ongoing research of antitumor drugs. Moreover, organometallic supramolecular drugs are relatively convenient, cheap and easy for their preparation with a large scale, might thus spend less expense, take shorter time and have larger possibility with rich variation of structural types as clinic drugs to some extent for their successful research and development. It was especially noteworthy that the rapid progress of scientific technology has highly promoted the developments of anticancer agents like newly appeared photoactivated drugs in theory and practice. All these virtues have been powerfully encouraging numerous researchers to engage in the research and development of novel metal-based supramolecular antitumor drugs. As predicting, it is inevitable that the research and development of metal supramolecular complexes as anticancer drugs will become increasingly active in future.

Currently, much important progress has been made in the research of organometallic complex supermolecules as anticancer drugs. However, most of them are to relieve suffering of patients, not to have cancer cured yet. In addition, unfortunately, the widespread and efficacious use of these agents is limited severely by the development of drug resistance in tumor cells, their severe toxicity and a narrow therapeutic spectrum. Therefore it should be fairly said that the research of organometallic supramolecular complexes was still in their developing stage. With the further expansion of supramolecular chemistry and the deep investigation of the supramolecular drugs, the research and development of organometallic complex supermolecules as anticancer drugs will be consequentially further extended. The important topic area to research in the future might mainly include the following eight aspects:

(1) Continuing using inorganic metal compounds including inorganic drugs with organic molecules to prepare organometallic supramolecular complexes with anticancer potential, further main expansion to possibly employ predominantly novel anticancer organic compounds as ligands due to their relatively low toxicity in general when compared to inorganic compounds;

(2) Researches on new organometallic supramolecular complexes of current organic drugs including anticancer and non-anticancer ones as ligands with metal and/or inorganic (or metallorganic) drugs with the view to expand the potential new application of these well-known drugs;

(3) Design and synthesis of organic ligands with poly-coordination sites such as poly-nitrogen and poly-sulphur ones *etc.* as well as their researches of coordination behavior, in order to form polymetal supramolecular complexes possibly having poly-active sites;

(4) Researches of photoactivated chemotherapy drugs to develop a new generation of metal-based anticancer agents to reduce adverse effect and enhance targeting;

(5) Developments of organometallic supramolecular complex of active component in the *Chinese herb* as natural agents to find new anticancer compounds targeted DNA with low toxicity;

(6) Researches in the solubility, stability, drug dissolution, selectivity as well as safety of organometallic supramolecular drugs themselves;

(7) Continuing investigating the action mechanism of organometallic supramolecular drugs;

(8) Studies on structure-activity relationships of organometallic supramolecular drugs.

With the further expansion of organometallic supramolecular chemistry and its extensive extention in pharmaceutical sciences, as well as the ongoing progress of cell biology, molecular biology, pharmaceutics, materials science, medicine and other disciplines, it is inevitable that more and more workers will engage in the research and development of metal-based supramolecular complexes as anticancer drugs. More and more organometallic supramolecular anticancer drugs with good efficacy, low toxicity and good pharmacokinetics properties will be used in clinic and make remarkable contributions for the protection of human health.

CONFLICT OF INTEREST

The authors declare that there is no conflict of interest.

ACKNOWLEDGEMENTS

This work was partially supported by National Natural Science Foundation of China [No. 21172181, 81250110089 (The Research Fellowship for International Young Scientists from International (Regional) Cooperation and Exchange Program)], the key program from Natural Science Foundation of Chongqing (CSTC2012jjB10026), the Specialized Research Fund for the Doctoral Program of Higher Education of China (SRFDP 20110182110007) and the Fundamental Research Funds for the Central Universities (XDJK2011D007, the key program XDJK2012B026).

DISCLOSURE

This e-Book chapter is an updated version of the review article entitled "Recent Researches in Metal Supramolecular Complexes as Anticancer Agents" published in *Anti-Cancer Agents in Medicinal Chemistry*, **2010**, *10*(5), 371-395.

REFERENCES

[1] Foye, W.O. *Cancer Chemotherapeutic Agents.*; American Chemical Society, Washington, DC, **1995**.

[2] Hellmann, K.; Carter, S.K. *Fundamentals of Cancer Chemotherapy*, McGraw-Hill, New York, **1987**.

[3] Lefranc, F.; Facchini, V.; Kiss, R. Proautophagic drugs: a novel means to combat apoptosis-resistant cancers, with a special emphasis on glioblastomas. *Oncologist*, **2007**, *12,* 1395-1403.

[4] Uzzo, R.G.; Haas, N.B.; Crispen, P.L.; Kolenko, V.M. Mechanisms of apoptosis resistance and treatment strategies to overcome them in hormone-refractory prostate cancer. *Cancer*, **2008**, *112*, 1660-1671.

[5] Chang, J.J.; Wang, Y.; Zhang, H.Z.; Zhou, C.H.; Geng, R.X.; Ji, Q.G. Recent advances in researches of triazole-based supramolecular chemistry and medicinal drugs. *Chem. J. Chin. Univ.*, **2011**, *32*, 1970-1985(in Chinese).

[6] Zhou, C.H.; Wang, Y. Recent researches in triazole compounds as medicinal drugs. *Curr. Med. Chem.*, **2012**, *19*, 239-280.

[7] Wang, Y.; Zhou, C.H. Recent advances in the researches of triazole compounds as medicinal drugs. *Sci. Sinca Chim.*, **2011**, *41*, 1429-1456(in Chinese).

[8] Zhou, C.H.; Gan, L.L.; Zhang Y.Y.; Zhang, F.F.; Wang G.Z.; Jin, L.; Geng, R.X. Review on supermolecules as chemical drugs. *Sci. China Ser. B-Chem.*, **2009**, *52*, 415-458.

[9] Zhou, C.H.; Zhang, F.F.; Gan, L.L.; Zhang Y.Y.; Geng, R.X. Research in supramolecular chemical drugs. *Sci. China Ser. B-Chem.*, **2009**, *39*, 208-252 (in Chinese).

[10] Hartinger, C.G.; Phillips, A.D.; Nazarov, A.A. Polynuclear Ruthenium, Osmium and Gold Complexes. The quest for innovative anticancer chemotherapeutics. *Curr. Top. Med. Chem.*, **2011**, *11*, 2688-2702.

[11] Turel, I.; Kljun, J. Interactions of metal ions with DNA, its constituents and derivatives, which may be relevant for anticancer research. *Curr. Top. Med. Chem.*, **2011**, *11*, 2661-2687.

[12] Zhang, J.; Zhang, F.; Li, H.; Liu, C.; Xia, J.; Ma, L.; Chu, W.; Zhang, Z.; Chen, C.; Li, S.; Wang, S. Recent progress and future potential for metal complexes as anticancer drugs targeting G-quadruplex DNA. *Curr. Med. Chem.*, **2012**, *19*, 2957-2975.

[13] Meléndez, E. Bioorganometallic chemistry of molybdenocene dichloride and its derivatives. *J. Organomet. Chem.*, **2012**, *706-707*, 4-12.

[14] Garbutcheon-Singh, K.B.; Grant, M.P.; Harper, B.W.; Krause-Heuer, A.M.; Manohar, M.; Orkey, N.; Aldrich-Wright, J.R. Transition metal based anticancer drugs. *Curr. Top. Med. Chem.*, **2011**, *11*, 521-542.

[15] Mendoza-Ferri, M.G.; Hartinger, C.G.; Mendoza, M.A.; Groessl, M.; Egger, A.E.; Eichinger, R.E.; Mangrum, J.B.; Farrell, N.P.; Maruszak, M.; Bednarski, P.J.; Klein, F.; Jakupec, M.A.; Nazarov, A.A.; Severin, K.; Keppler, B.K. Transferring the concept of multinuclearity to ruthenium complexes for improvement of anticancer activity. *J. Med. Chem.*, **2009**, *52,* 916-925.

[16] Klein, A.V.; Hambley, T.W. Platinum drug distribution in cancer cells and tumors. *Chem. Rev.*, **2009**, *109*, 4911-4920.

[17] Baskerville-Abraham, I.M.; Boysen, G.; Troutman, J.M.; Mutlu, E.; Collins, L.; deKrafft, K.E.; Lin, W.; King, C.; Chaney, S.G.; Swenberg, J.A. Development of an ultraperformance liquid chromatography/mass spectrometry method to quantify cisplatin 1,2 intrastrand guanine-guanine adducts. *Chem. Res. Toxicol.*, **2009**, *22*, 905-912.

[18] Ho, Y.P.; Au-Yeung, S.C.F.; To, K.K.W. Platinum-based anticancerAgents: Innovative design strategies and biological perspectives. *Med. Res. Rev.*, **2003**, *23*, 633-655.

[19] Pasqua, A.J.D.; Centerwall, C.R.; Kerwood, D.J.; Dabrowiak, J.C. Formation of carbonato and hydroxo complexes in the reaction of platinum anticancer drugs with carbonate. *Inorg. Chem.*, **2009**, *48*, 1192-1197.

[20] Arnesano, F.; Natile. G. Mechanistic insight into the cellular uptake and processing of cisplatin 30 years after its approval by FDA. *Coord. Chem. Rev.*, **2009**, *253*, 2070-2081.

[21] Łakomska, I. Molecular structure and antitumor activity of platinum(II) complexes containing purine analogs. *Inorg. Chim. Acta*, **2009**, *362*, 669-681.

[22] Möker, J.; Thiem, J. Synthesis of novel gluco- and galacto-functionalized platinum complexes. *Eur. J. Org. Chem.*, **2009**, *28*, 4842-4847.

[23] Alama, A.; Tasso, B.; Novelli, F.; Sparatore, F. Organometallic compounds in oncology: implications of novel organotins as antitumor agents. *Drug Discov. Today*, **2009**, *14*, 500-508.

[24] Hostetter, A.A.; Chapman, E.G.; DeRose, V.J. Rapid cross-linking of an RNA internal loop by the anticancer drug cisplatin. *J. Am. Chem. Soc.*, **2009**, *131*, 9250-9257.

[25] Schobert, R.; Biersack, B.; Dietrich, A.; Knauer, S.; Zoldakova, M.; Fruehauf, A.; Mueller, T. Pt(II) complexes of a combretastatin A-4 analogous chalcone: Effects of conjugation on cytotoxicity, tumor specificity, and long-term tumor growth suppression *J. Med. Chem.*, **2009**, *52*, 241-246.

[26] Jian, G.; Liu, Y.G.; Zingaro, R.A. Cytotoxic activities, cellular uptake, gene regulation, and optical imaging of novel platinum(II) complexes. *Chem. Res. Toxicol.*, **2009**, *22*, 1705-1712.

[27] Tian, T.; Mutikainen, I.; Wezel, G.P.; Aliaga-Alcalde, N.; Reedijk, J. Chemical, structural and biological studies of *cis*-[Pt(3-Acpy)$_2$Cl$_2$]. *J. Inorg. Biochem.*, **2009**, *103*, 1221-1227.

[28] Eryazici, I.; Moorefield, C.N.; Newkome, G.R. Square-planar Pd(II), Pt(II), and Au(III) terpyridine complexes: their syntheses, physical properties, supramolecular constructs, and biomedical activities. *Chem. Rev.*, **2008**, *108*, 1834-1895.

[29] Ronconi, L.; Fregona, D. The Midas touch in cancer chemotherapy: from platinum- to gold-dithiocarbamato complexes. *Dalton Trans.*, **2009**, 10670-10680.

[30] Quirante, J.; Ruiz, D.; Gonzalez, A.; López, C.; Cascante, M.; Cortés, R.; Messeguer, R.; Calvis, C.; Baldomà, L.; Pascual, A.; Guérardel, Y.; Pradines, B.; Font-Bardía, M.; Calvet, T.; Biot, C. Platinum(II) and palladium(II) complexes with (N,N′) and (C,N,N′)$^-$ ligands derived from pyrazole as anticancer and antimalarial agents: synthesis, characterization and *in vitro* activities. *J. Inorg. Biochem.* **2011**, *105*, 1720-1728.

[31] Scaffidi-Domianello, Y.Y.; Meelich, K.; Jakupec, M.A.; Arion, V.B.; Kukushkin, V.Y.; Galanski, M.; Keppler, B.K. Novel *cis*- and *trans*-configured bis(oxime)platinum(II) complexes: synthesis, characterization, and cytotoxic activity. *Inorg. Chem.*, **2010**, *49*, 5669-5678.

[32] Arnesano, F.; Boccarelli, A.; Cornacchia, D.; Nushi, F.; Sasanelli, R. Coluccia, M.; Natile, G. Mechanistic insight into the inhibition of matrix metalloproteinases by platinum substrates. *J. Med. Chem.*, **2009**, *52*, 7847-7855.

[33] Butsch, K.; Elmas, S.; Gupta, N.S.; Gust, R.; Heinrich, F.; Klein, A.; Mering, Y.; Neugebauer, M.; Ott, I.; Schafer, M.; Scherer, H.; Schurr, T. Organoplatinum(II) and -palladium(II) complexes of nucleobases and their derivatives. *Organomet.*, **2009**, *28*, 3906-3915.

[34] Obata, M.; Hirohara, S.; Tanaka, R.; Kinoshita, I.; Ohkubo, K.; Fukuzumi, S.; Tanihara, M.; Yano, S. *In vitro* heavy-atom effect of palladium(II) and platinum(II) complexes of pyrrolidine-fused chlorin in photodynamic therapy. *J. Med. Chem.*, **2009**, *52*, 2747-2753.

[35] Marqués-Gallego, P.; Contaldi, S.; Dulk, H.; Monari, M.; Brouwer, J.; Jaehde, U.; Kalayda, G.V.; Reedijk, J. Relevance of the leaving group for antitumor activity of new platinum(II) compounds containing anthracene derivatives as a carrier ligand. *J. Inorg. Biochem.*, **2009**, *103*, 1602-1608.

[36] Sheena M. Aris, Nicholas P. Farrell. Towards antitumor active *trans*-platinum compounds. *Eur. J. Inorg. Chem.*, **2009**, 1293-1302.

[37] Rakić, G.M.; Grgurić-šipka, S.; KaluCerović, G.N.; Gómez-Ruiz, S.; Bjelogrlić, S.K.; Radulović, S.S.; Tešić, Ž.L. Novel *trans*-dichloridoplatinum(II) complexes with 3- and 4-acetylpyridine: Synthesis, characterization, DFT calculations and cytotoxicity. *Eur. J. Med. Chem.*, **2009**, *44*, 1921-1925.

[38] Navarro, M.; Higuera-Padilla, A.R.; Arsenak, M.; Taylor, P. Synthesis, characterization, DNA interaction studies and anticancer activity of platinum-clotrimazole complexes. *Transition Met. Chem.*, **2009**, *34*, 869-875.

[39] Krause-Heuer, A.M.; Gr€unert, R.; K€uhne, S.; Buczkowska, M.; Wheate, N.J.; Pevelen, D.D.L.; Boag, L.R.; Fisher, D.M.; Kasparkova, J.; Malina, J.;. Bednarski, P.J; Brabec, V.; Aldrich-Wright, J.R. Studies of the mechanism of action of platinum(II) complexes with potent cytotoxicity in human cancer cells. *J. Med. Chem.*, **2009**, *52*, 5474-5484.

[40] Jr, R.A.C.; Woster, P.M. Recent advances in the development of polyamine analogues as antitumor agents. *J. Med. Chem.*, **2009**, *52*, 4551-4573.

[41] Zhao, Y.J.; Bali, M.S.; Cullinane, C.; Day, A.I.; Collins, J.G. Synthesis, cytotoxicity and cucurbituril binding of triamine linked dinuclear platinum complexes. *Dalton Trans.*, **2009**, *26*, 5190-5198.

[42] Xu, Z.H.; Zhang, Y.M.; Xue, Z.Q.; Yang, X.L.; Wu, Z.Y.; Guo, Z.J. DNA-binding property and antitumor activity of a cyclam bridged dinuclear platinum(II) complex. *Inorg. Chim. Acta*, **2009**, *362*, 2347-2352.

[43] Zhu, J.H.; Zhao, Y.M.; Zhu, Y.Y.; Wu, Z.Y.; Lin, M.X.; He, W.J.; Wang, Y.; Chen, G.J.; Dong, L.; Zhang, J.F.; Lu, Y.; Guo, Z.J. DNA cross-linking patterns induced by an antitumor-active trinuclear platinum complex and comparison with its dinuclear analogue. *Chem. Eur. J.*, **2009**, *15*, 5245-5253.

[44] Rubino, S.; Portanova, P.; Girasolo, A.; Calvaruso, G.; Orecchio, S.; Stocco, G.C. Synthetic, structural and biochemical studies of polynuclear platinum(II) complexes with heterocyclic ligands. *Eur. J. Med. Chem.*, **2009**, *44*, 1041-1048.

[45] Duong, H.T.T.; Huynh, V.T.; Souza, P.; Stenzel, M.H. Core-cross-linked micelles synthesized by clicking bifunctional Pt(IV) anticancer drugs to isocyanates. *Biomacromolecules*, **2010**, *11*, 2290-2299.

[46] Graf, N.; Mokhtari, T.E.; Papayannopoulos, I.A.; Lippard, S.J. Platinum(IV)-chlorotoxin(CTX) conjugates for targeting cancer cells. *J. Inorg. Biochem.*, **2012**, *110*, 58-63.

[47] Vetter, C.; Kaluderović, G.N.; Paschke, R.; Gómez-Ruiz, S.; Steinborn, D. Synthesis, structures and *in vitro* cytotoxicity studies of platinum(IV) complexes with N,S and S,S heterocyclic ligands. *Polyhedron*, **2009**, *28*, 3699-3706.

[48] Garoufis, A.; Hadjikakou, S.K.; Hadjiliadis, N. Palladium coordination compounds as anti-viral, anti-fungal, anti-microbial and anti-tumor agents. *Coord. Chem. Rev.*, **2009**, *253*, 1384-1397.

[49] Zmejkovski, B.B.; KaluCerović, G.N.; Gómez-Ruiz, S.; Žižak, Ž.; Steinborn, D.; Schmidt, H.; Paschke, R.; Juranić, Z.D.; Sabo, T.J. Palladium(II) complexes with R2edda-derived ligands. Part II. Synthesis, characterization and *in vitro* antitumoral studies of R2eddip esters and palladium(II) complexes. *Eur. J. Med. Chem.*, **2009**, *44*, 3452-3458.

[50] Quiroga, A.G.; Ranninger, C.N. Contribution to the SAR field of metallated and coordination complexes studies of the palladium and platinum derivatives with selected thiosemicarbazones as antitumoral drugs. *Coord. Chem. Rev.*, **2004**, *248*, 119-133.

[51] Gao, E.; Liu, C.; Zhu, M.C.; Lin, H.K.; Wu, Q.; Liu, L. Current development of Pd(II) complexes as potential antitumor agents. *Anti-Cancer Agents Med. Chem.*, **2009**, *9*, 356-368.

[52] Štarha, P.; Trávníček, Z.; Popa, I. Synthesis, characterization and *in vitro* cytotoxicity of the first palladium(II) oxalato complexes involving adenine-based ligands. *J. Inorg. Biochem.*, **2009**, *103*, 978-988.

[53] Keter, F.K.; Ojwach, S.O.; Oyetunji, O.A.; Guzei, I.A.; Darkwa, J. Bis(pyrazolyl) palladium(II), platinum(II) and gold(III) complexes: Syntheses, molecular structures and substitution reactions with L-cysteine. *Inorg. Chim. Acta*, **2009**, *362*, 2595-2602.

[54] Bakalova, A.; Varbanov, H.; Buyukliev, R.; Momekov, G.; Ivanov, D. Palladium (II) complexes with 5-methyl-5-(4-pyridyl)- 2,4-imidazoldenedione: Synthesis, thermogravimetric and cytotoxic investigation. *J. Therm. Anal. Calorim.*, **2009**, *95*, 241-246.

[55] Kalinowska-Lis, U.; Szmigiero, L.; Studzian, K.; Ochocki, J. Cytotoxic activity and chemical reactivity of *cis*-platinum(II) and *trans*-palladium(II) complexes with diethyl (pyridinylmethyl) phosphates. *Eur. J. Med. Chem.*, **2009**, *44*, 660-664.

[56] Gligorijevic, N.; Todorovic, T.; Radulovic, S. Synthesis and characterization of new Pt(II) and Pd(II) complexes with 2-quinolinecarboxaldehyde selenosemicarbazone : Cytotoxic activity evaluation of Cd(II), Zn(II), NI(II), Pt(II) and Pd(II) complexes with heteroaromatic selenosemicarbazones. *Eur. J Med. Chem.*, **2009**, *44*, 1623-1629.

[57] Tiekink, E.R.T. Gold derivatives for the treatment of cancer. *Crit. Rev. Oncol.*, **2002**, *42*, 225-248.

[58] Espósito, B.P.; Najjar, R. Interactions of antitumoral platinum-group metallodrugs with albumin. *Coord. Chem. Rev.*, **2002**, *232*, 137-149.

[59] McKeage, M.J.; Maharaj, L.; Berners-Price, S.J. Mechanisms of cytotoxicity and antitumor activity of gold(I) phosphine complexes: the possible role of mitochondria. *Coord. Chem. Rev.*, **2002**, *232*, 127-135.

[60] Barnard, P.J.; Berners-Price, S.J. Targeting the mitochondrial cell death pathway with gold compounds. *Coord. Chem. Rev.*, **2007**, *251*, 1889-1902.

[61] Ott, I. On the medicinal chemistry of gold complexes as anticancer drugs. *Coord. Chem. Rev.*, **2009**, *253*, 1670-1681.

[62] Ott, I.; Qian, X.H.; Xu, Y.F.; Vlecken, D.H. W.; Marques, I.J.; Kubutat, D.; Will, J.; Sheldrick, W.S.; Jesse, P.; Prokop, A.; Bagowski, C.P.A Gold(I) phosphine complex

containing a naphthalimide ligand functions as a TrxR inhibiting antiproliferative agent and angiogenesis inhibitor. *J. Med. Chem.*, **2009**, *52*, 763-770.

[63] Barreiro, E.; Casas, J.S.; Couce, M.D.; Sánchez, A.; Sánchez-Gónzalez, A.; Sordo, J.; Varela, J.M.; López, E.M.V. *J. Inorg. Biochem.*, **2008**, *102*, 184-192.

[64] Barreiro, E.; Casas, J.S.; Couce, M.D.; Sánchez, A.; Sánchez-González, A.; Sordo, J.; Varela, J.M.; López, E.M.V. Synthesis, structure and cytotoxicity studies of diisopropylammonium and triethylammonium salts of triphenylphosphinegold(I) sulfanylcarboxylates. *J. Inorg. Biochem.*, **2009**, *103*, 1023-1032.

[65] Chui, C.H.; Wong, R.S.M.; Gambari, R.; Cheng, G.Y.M.; Yuen, M.C.W.; Chan, K.W.; Tong, S.W.; Lau, F.Y.; Lai, P.B.S.; Lama, K.H.; Ho, C.L.; Kan, C.W.; Leung, K.S.Y.; Wong, W.Y. Antitumor activity of diethynylfluorene derivatives of gold(I). *Bioorg. Med. Chem.*, **2009**, *17*, 7872-7877.

[66] Maiore, L.; Cinellu, M.A.; Nobili, S.; Landini, I.; Mini, E.; Messori. L.; Gabbiani, C. Gold(III) complexes with 2-substituted pyridines as experimental anticancer agents:Solution behavior, reactions with model proteins, antiproliferative properties. *J. Inorg. Biochem.*, **2012**, *108*, 123-127.

[67] To, Y.F.; Sun, R.W.Y.; Chen, Y.X.; Chan, V.S.F.; Yu, W.Y.; Tam, P.K.H.; Che, C.M.; Steve Lin, C.L. Gold(III) porphyrin complex is more potent than cisplatin in inhibiting growth of nasopharyngeal carcinoma *in vitro* and *in vivo*. *Int. J. Cancer*, **2009**, *124*, 1971-1979.

[68] Casini, A.; Kelter, G.; Gabbiani, C.; Cinellu, M.A.; Minghetti, G.; Fregona, D.; Fiebig, H.H.; Messori, L. Chemistry, antiproliferative properties, tumor selectivity, and molecular mechanisms of novel gold(III) compounds for cancer treatment: a systematic study. *J. Biol. Inorg. Chem.*, **2009**, *14*, 1139-1149.

[69] Segapelo, T.V.; Guzei, I.A.; Spencer, L.C.; Zyl, W.E.V.; Darkwa, J. (Pyrazolylmethyl) pyridine platinum(II) and gold(III) complexes: Synthesis, structures and evaluation as anticancer agents. *Inorg. Chim. Acta*, **2009**, *362*, 3314-3324.

[70] Castiñeiras, A.; Dehnen, S.; Fuchs, A.; García-Santos, I.; Sevillano, P. Stabilization of gold(I) and gold(III) complexes by pyridil bis{3-hexamethylene -iminylthiosemicarbazone}: spectroscopic, structural and computational study. *Dalton Trans.*, **2009**, 2731-2739.

[71] Aldinucci, D.; Ronconi, L.; Fregona, D. Groundbreaking. gold(III) anticancer agents. *Drug Discov. Today*, **2009**, *14*, 21-22.

[72] Meijbooma, R.; Bowen, R.J.; Berners-Price, S.J. Coordination complexes of silver(I) with tertiary phosphine and related ligands. *Coord. Chem. Rev.*, **2009**, *253*, 325-342.

[73] Hindi, K.M.; Panzner, M.J.; Tessier, C.A.; Cannon, C.L.; Youngs, W.J. The medicinal applications of imidazolium carbene-metal complexes. *Chem. Rev.*, **2009**, *109*, 3859-3884.

[74] Elsayed, S.A.; Jean-Claude, B.J.; Butler, I.S.; Mostafa, S.I. Synthesis, structural characterization and anticancer activity of some new complexes of 6-amino-4-hydroxy-2-thiopyrimidine. *J. Mol. Struct.*, **2012**, *1028*, 208-214.

[75] Thati, B.; Noble, A.; Creaven, B.S.; Walsh, M.; McCann, M.; Devereux, M.; Kavanagh, K.; Egan, D.A. Role of cell cycle events and apoptosis in mediating the anti-cancer activity of a silver(I) complex of 4-hydroxy-3-nitro-coumarin- bis(phenanthroline) in human malignant cancer cells. *Eur. J. Pharm.*, **2009**, *602*, 203-214.

[76] Zartilas, S.; Hadjikakou, S.K.; Hadjiliadis, N.; Kyros, N.K.L.; Kubicki, M.; Baril, M.; Butler, I.S.; Karkabounas, S.; Balzarini, J. Tetrameric 1:1 and monomeric 1:3 complexes of

silver(I) halides with tri(p-tolyl)-phosphine: a structural and biological study. *Inorg. Chim. Acta*, **2009**, *362*, 1003-1010.

[77] Mendoza-Ferri, M.G.; Hartinger, C.G.; Mendoza, M.A.; Groessl, M.; Egger, A.E.; Eichinger, R.E.; Mangrum, J.B.; Farrell, N.P.; Maruszak, M.; Bednarski, P.J.; Klein, F.; Jakupec, M.A.; Nazarov, A.A.; Severin, K. Keppler, B.K. Transferring the concept of multinuclearity to ruthenium complexes for improvement of anticancer activity. *J. Med. Chem.*, **2009**, *52*, 916-925;

[78] Kandioller, W.; Hartinger, C.G.; Nazarov, A.A.; Kuznetsov, M.L.; John, R.O.; Bartel, C.; Jakupec, M.A.; Arion, V.B.; Keppler, B.K. From pyrone to thiopyrone ligands-rendering maltol-derived ruthenium(II)-arene complexes that are anticancer active *in vitro*. *Organomet.*, **2009**, *28*, 4249-4251.

[79] Bugarcic, T.; Habtemariam, A.; Deeth, R.J.; Fabbiani, F.P.A.; Parsons, S.;. Sadler, P.J. Ruthenium(II) arene anticancer complexes with redox-active diamine ligands. *Inorg. Chem.*, **2009**, *48*, 9444-9457.

[80] Ott, I.; Gust, R. Non platinum metal complexes as anti-cancer drugs. *Arch. Pharm. Chem. Life Sci.*, **2007**, *340*, 117-126.

[81] Clarke, M.J.; Zhu, F.C.; Frasca, D.R. Non-platinum chemotherapeutic metallo pharmaceuticals. *Chem. Rev.*, **1999**, *99*, 2511-2533.

[82] Levina, A.; Mitra, A.; Lay, P.A. Recent developments in ruthenium anticancer drugs. *Metallomics*, **2009**, *1*, 458-470.

[83] Cui, S.F.; Zhou, C.H.; Geng, R.X.; Ji, Q.G. Recent advances in the researches of thiazole compounds as enzyme and acceptor inhibitors. *Chin. J. Biochem. Pharm.*, **2012**, *33*, 311-315(in Chinese).

[84] Kashyap, S.J.; Garg, V.K.; Sharma, P.K.; Kumar, N.; Dudhe, R.; Gupta, J.K. Thiazoles: having diverse biological activities. *Med. Chem. Res.,* **2012**, *21*, 2123-2132.

[85] Gras, M.; Therrien, B.; Süss-Fink, G.; Casini, A.; Edafe, F.; Dyson, P.J. Anticancer activity of new organo-ruthenium, rhodium and iridium complexes containing the 2-(pyridine-2-yl)thiazole N,N-chelating ligand. *J. Organomet. Chem.*, **2010**, *695*, 1119-1125.

[86] Renfrew, A. Ruthenium(II) arene compounds as versatile anticancer agents. *Chimica*, **2009**, *63*, 217-219.

[87] Kandioller, W.; Hartinger, C.G.; Nazarov, A.A.; Kasser, J.; John, R.; Jakupec, M.A.; Arion, V.B.; Dyson, P.J.; Keppler, B.K. Tuning the anticancer activity of maltol-derived ruthenium complexes by derivatization of the 3-hydroxy-4-pyrone moiety. *J. Org. Chem.*, **2009**, *694*, 922-929.

[88] Renfrewa, A.K.; Egger, A.E.; Scopelliti, R.; Hartinger, C.G.; Dyson, P.J. Synthesis and characterisation of the water soluble bis-phosphine complex [Ru(η^6-cymene)(PPh_2(*o*-C_6H_4O)-κ^2-*P,O*)(pta)]$^+$ and an investigation of its cytotoxic effects. *C. R. Chimie*, **2010**, *13*, 1144-1150.

[89] Olga, N.; Alexey, A.N.; Christian, G.H.; Bernhard, K.K.; Viktor B. DNA interactions of dinuclear RuII arene antitumor complexes in cell-free media. *Biochem. Pharmacol.*, **2009**, *77*, 364-374.

[90] Linares, F.; Galindo, M.A.; Galli, S.; Romero, M.A.; Navarro, J.A.R.; Barea, E. Tetranuclear coordination assemblies based on half-sandwich ruthenium(II) complexes: noncovalent binding to DNA and cytotoxicity. *Inorg. Chem.*, **2009**, *48*, 7413-7420.

[91] Giovagnini, L.; Mancinetti, E.; Ronconi, L.; Sitran, S.; Marchiò, L.; Castagliuolo, I.; Brun, P.; Trevisan, A.; Fregona, D. Preliminary chemico-biological studies on Ru(III) compounds

with S-methyl pyrrolidine/dimethyl dithiocarbamate. *J. Inorg. Biochem.*, **2009**, *103*, 774-782.

[92] Wang, Y.H.; Cheng, C.C.; Lee, W.J.; Chiou, M.L.; Pai, C.W.; Wen, C.C.; Chen, W.L.; Chena, Y.H. A novel phenotype-based approach for systematically screening antiproliferation metallodrugs. *Chem. Biol. Interact.*, **2009**, *182*, 84-91.

[93] Walker, J.M.; McEwan, A.; Pycko, R.; Tassotto, M.L.; Gottardo, C.; Thng, J.; Wang, R.; Spivak, G.J. [Tris(pyrazolyl)methane]ruthenium complexes capable of inhibiting cancer cell growth. *Eur. J. Inorg. Chem.*, **2009**, *31*, 4629-4633.

[94] Li, Q.; Sun, D.D.; Zhou, Y.H.; Liu, D.; Zhang, Q.L.; Liu, J. Anticancer activity of novel ruthenium complex with 1,10-phenanthrolineselenazole as potent telomeric G-quadruplex inhibitor. *Inorg. Chem. Commun.*, **2012**, *20*, 142-146.

[95] Reddy, V.D.; Dayal, D.; Cosenza, S.C.; Reddy, M.V.R.; Jr., W.C.P.; Adams, R. Glycal-ruthenium carbonyl clusters: Syntheses, characterization, and anticancer activity. *J. Organomet. Chem.*, **2009**, *694*, 959-967.

[96] Reddy, V.D.; Dayal, D.; David J.; Szalda, S.; Cosenza, C.; Ramana, R.M.V. Syntheses, structures, and anticancer activity of novel organometallic rutheniume-maltol complexes. *J. Organomet. Chem.*, **2012**, *700*, 180-187.

[97] Van Rijn, J.A.; Marqu'es-Gallego, P.; Reedijk, J.; Lutz, M.; Spek, A.L.; Bouwman, E. A novel ruthenium(III) complex with a tridentate dianionic P,O,O-ligand showing high cytotoxic activity. *Dalton Trans.*, **2009**, 10727-10730.

[98] Nagy, E.M.; Nardon, C.; Giovagnini, L.; Marchiò, L.; Trevisan, A.; Fregona, D. Promising anticancer mono- and dinuclear ruthenium(III) dithiocarbamato complexes: systematic solution studies. *Dalton Trans.*, **2011**, *40*, 11885-11895.

[99] Katsaros, N.; Anagnostopoulou, A. Rhodium and its compounds as potential agents in cancer treatment. *Crit. Rev. Oncolo.*, **2002**, *42*, 297-308.

[100] Bieda, R.; Ott, I.; Dobroschke, M.; Gust, A.P.R.; Sheldrick, W.S. Structure-activity relationships and DNA binding properties of apoptosis inducing cytotoxic rhodium(III) polypyridyl complexes containing the cyclic thioether [9]aneS3. *J. Inorg. Biochem.*, **2009**, *103*, 698-708.

[101] Bieda, R.; Ott, I.; Gust, R.; Sheldrick, W.S. Cytotoxic rhodium(III) polypyridyl complexes containing the tris(pyrazolyl)methane coligand: Synthesis, DNA binding properties and structure-activity relationships. *Eur. J. Inorg. Chem.*, **2009**, *25*, 3821-3831.

[102] Chifotides, H.T.; Dunbar K.R. Interactions of metal-metal-bonded antitumor active complexes with DNA fragments and DNA. *Acc. Chem. Res.*, **2005**, *38*, 146-156.

[103] Aguirre, J.D.; Angeles-Boza, A.M.; Chouai, A.; Turro, C.; Pellois, J.P.; Dunbar, K.R. Anticancer activity of heteroleptic diimine complexes of dirhodium: a study of intercalating properties, hydrophobicity and in cellulo activity. *Dalton Trans.*, **2009**, *48*, 10806-10812.

[104] Peacock, A.F.A.; Sadler, P.J. Medicinal organometallic chemistry: Designing metal arene complexes as anticancer agentss. *Chem. Asian J.*, **2008**, *3*, 1890-1899.

[105] Kostrhunova, H.; Florian, J.; Novakova, O.; Peacock, A.F.A.; Sadler, P.J.; Brabec, V. DNA interactions of monofunctional organometallic osmium(II) antitumor complexes in cell-free media. *J. Med. Chem.*, **2008**, *51*, 3635-3643.

[106] Rijt, S.H.; Sadler, P.J. Current applications and future potential for bioinorganic chemistry in the development of anticancer drugs. *Drug Discov. Today*, **2009**, *14*, 1089-1097.

[107] Rijt, S.H.; Hebden, A.J.; Amaresekera, T.; Deeth, R.J.; Clarkson, G.J.; Parsons, S.; McGowan, P.C.; Sadler, P.J. Amide linkage isomerism as an activity switch for

organometallic osmium and ruthenium anticancer complexes. *J. Med. Chem.*, **2009**, *52*, 7753-7764.

[108] Rijt, S.H.; Peacock, A.F.A.; Johnstone, R.D.L.; Parsons, S.; Sadler, P.J. Organometallic osmium(II) arene anticancer complexes containing picolinate derivatives. *Inorg. Chem.*, **2009**, *48*, 1753-1762.

[109] Rijt, S.H.; Mukherjee, A.; Pizarro, A.M.; Sadler, P.J. Cytotoxicity, hydrophobicity, uptake, and distribution of Osmium(II) anticancer complexes in ovarian cancer cells. *J. Med. Chem.*, **2010**, *53*, 840-849.

[110] Kong, K.V.; Leong, W.K.; Lim, L.H.K. Induction of apoptosis by hexaosmium carbonyl clusters. *J. Organomet. Chem.*, **2009**, *694*, 834-839.

[111] Tshuva, E.Y.; Ashenhurst, J.A. Cytotoxic titanium(IV) complexes: Renaissance. *Eur. J. Inorg. Chem.*, **2009**, *15*, 2203-2218.

[112] Kostova, I. Titanium and vanadium complexes as anticancer agents. *Anti-Cancer Agents Med. Chem.*, **2009**, *9*, 827-842.

[113] Tshuva, E.Y.; Peri, D. Modern cytotoxic titanium(IV) complexes: Insights on the enigmatic involvement of hydrolysis. *Coord. Chem. Rev.*, **2009**, *253*, 2098-2115.

[114] Pavlaki, M.; Debeli, K.; Triantaphyllidou, I.E.; Klouras, N.; Giannopoulou, E.; Aletras, A.J. A proposed mechanism for the inhibitory effect of the anticancer agent titanocene dichloride on tumour gelatinases and other proteolytic enzymes. *J. Biol. Inorg. Chem.*, **2009**, *14*, 947-957.

[115] Vessières, A.; Plamont, M.A.; Cabestaing, C.; Claffey, J.; Dieckmann, S.; Hogan, M.; Müller-Bunz, H.; Strohfeldt, K.; Tacke, M. Proliferative and anti-proliferative effects of titanium- and iron-based metallocene anti-cancer drugs. *J. Organomet. Chem.*, **2009**, *694*, 874-879.

[116] Immel, T.A.; Debiak, M.; Groth, U.; Brkle, A.; Huhn, T. Highly selective apoptotic cell death induced by Halo-Salane titanium complexes. *Chem. Med. Chem.*, **2009**, *4*, 738-741.

[117] Gleeson, B.; Claffey, J.; Hogan, M.; Müller-Bunz, H.; Wallis, D.; Tacke, M. Novel benzyl-substituted vanadocene anticancer drugs. *J. Organomet. Chem.*, **2009**, *694*, 1369-1374.

[118] Gleeson, B.; Claffey, J.; Deally, A.; Hogan, M.; Méndez, L.M.M.; Müller-Bunz, H.; Patil, S.; Wallis, D.; Tacke, M. Synthesis and cytotoxicity studies of fluorinated derivatives of vanadocene Y. *Eur. J. Inorg. Chem.*, **2009**, *19*, 2804-2810.

[119] Benítez, J.; Guggeri, L.; Tomaz, I.; Pessoa, C.; Moreno, V.; Lorenzo, J.; Avilés, F.X.; Garat, B.; Gambino, D. A novel vanadyl complex with a polypyridyl DNA intercalator as ligand: A potential anti-protozoa and anti-tumor agent. *J. Inorg. Biochem.*, **2009**, *103*, 1386-1394.

[120] Singh, V.P.; Singh, S.; Narang, K.K.; Bhattacharya, D. Aluminium(III), chromium(III) and iron(III) complexes with 5-iodouracil and 5-iodouracil- histidine and their antitumour activity. J. *Enzym. Inhib. Med. Chem.*, **2009**, *24*, 105-111.

[121] Haas, K.L.; Franz, K.J. Application of metal coordination chemistry to explore and manipulate cell biology. *Chem. Rev.*, **2009**, *109*, 4921-4960.

[122] Ansari, K.I.; Grant, J.D.; Kasiri, S.; Woldemariam, G.; Shrestha, B.; Mandal, S.S. Manganese(III)-salens induce tumor selective apoptosis in human cells. *J. Inorg. Biochem.*, **2009**, *103*, 818-826.

[123] Ansari, K.I.; Grant, J.D.; Kasiri, S.; Mandal, S.S. Apoptosis and anti-tumour activities of manganese(III)-salen and -salphen complexes. *Dalton Trans.*, **2009**, *40*, 8525-8531.

[124] Zhang, Z.; He, R.; Yan, K.; Guo, Q.N.; Lu, Y.G.; Wang, X.X.; Lei, H.; Li, Z.Y. Synthesis and *in vitro* and *in vivo* evaluation of manganese(III) porphyrin-dextran as a novel MRI contrast agent. *Bioorg. Med. Chem. Lett.*, **2009**, *19*, 6675-6678.

[125] Chen, X.; Tang, L.J.; Sun, Y.N.; Qiu, P.H.; Liang, G. Syntheses, characterization and antitumor activities of transition metal complexes with isoflavone. *J. Inorg. Biochem.*, **2010**, *104*, 379-384.

[126] Schwietert, C.W.; McCue, J.P. Coordination compounds in medicinal chemistry. *Coord. Chem. Rev.*, **1999**, *184*, 67-89.

[127] Pahl, P.M.B.; Horwitz, L.D. Cell permeable iron chelators as potential cancer chemotherapeutic agents. *Cancer Investig.,* **2005**, *23*, 683-691,.

[128] Buss, J.L.; Greene, B.T.; Turner, J.; Torti, F.M.; Torti, S.V. Iron chelators in cancer chemotherapy. *Curr. Top. Med. Chem.,* **2004**, *4*, 1623-1635.

[129] Richardson, D.R.; Kalinowski, D.S.; Richardson, V.; Sharpe, P.C.; Lovejoy, D.B.; Islam, M.; Bernhardt, P.V. 2-Acetylpyridine thiosemicarbazones are potent iron chelators and antiproliferative agents: redox activity, iron complexation and characterization of their antitumor activity. *J. Med. Chem.*, **2009**, *52*, 1459-1470.

[130] Wen, Y.D.; Ho, Y.L.; Shiau, R.J.; Yeh, J.K.; Wu, J.Y.; Wang, W.L.; Chiou, S.J. Synergistic antitumor effect of curcumin and dinitrosyl iron complexes for against melanoma cells. *J. Organomet. Chem.*, **2010**, *695*, 352-359.

[131] Hille, A.; Gust, R. Relationship between anticancer activity and stereochemistry of saldach ligands and their iron(III) complexes. *Arch. Pharm. Chem. Life Sci.*, **2009**, *342*, 625-631.

[132] Herchel, R.; Sindelǎr, Z.; Tŕavnı̌cek, Z.; Zbǒril, R.; Vańco, J. Novel 1D chain Fe(III)-salen-like complexes involving anionic heterocyclic N-donor ligands. Synthesis, X-ray structure, magnetic, 57Fe M¨ossbauer, and biological activity studies. *Dalton Trans.*, **2009**, *44*, 9870-9880.

[133] Galanis, A.; Karapetsas, A.; Sandaltzopoulos, R. Metal-induced carcinogenesis, oxidative stress and hypoxia signaling. *Mutat. Res.*, **2009**, *674*, 31-35.

[134] Ming, L.J. Structure and function of "metalloantibiotics. *Med. Res. Rev.*, **2003**, *23*, 697-762.

[135] Chen, Y.; Hu, L.Q. Design of anticancer prodrugs for reductive activation. *Med. Res. Rev.*, **2009**, *29*, 29-64.

[136] Naura, A.S.; Sharma, R. Studies on mode of action of hexaammine Co(III) chloride against diethylnitrosamine-induced hepatocarcinogenesis in mice. *J. Biochem. Mol. Toxic.* **2009**, *23*, 193-201.

[137] Erwin, R.; Vladimir, B.A.; Bernhard, K.K.; Armando, J.L.P. Electron-transfer activated metal-based anticancer drugs. *Inorg. Chim. Acta*, **2008**, *361*, 1569-1583.

[138] Nagababua, P.; Latha, J.N.L.; Rajesh, M.; Satyanarayana, S. DNA-binding and cytotoxicity of the cobalt(III) ethylenediamine pyrazole complex $[Co(en)_2(pyz)_2]^{3+}$. *J. Iran. Chem. Soc.*, **2009**, *6*, 145-152.

[139] Elizabeth, T.S.; Lidiane C.C.; Frederico, A.V.C.; Lorenzo, C.V.; Carlos, B.P.; Marcos D.P.; Sérgio P.M.; Marciela, S. Synthesis, characterization and biological activities of mononuclear Co(III) complexes as potential bioreductively activated prodrugs. *J. Inorg. Biochem.*, **2009**, *103*, 1355-1365.

[140] Shahabadi, N.; Kashanian, S.; Darabi, F. DNA binding and DNA cleavage studies of a water soluble cobalt(II) complex containing dinitrogen Schiff base ligand: the effect of metal on the mode of binding. *Eur. J. Med. Chem.*, **2010**, *45*, 4239-4245.

[141] Hou, M.H.; Lu, W.J.; Huang, C.Y.; Fan, R.J.; Yuann, J.M.P. Effects of polyamines on the DNA-reactive properties of dimeric mithramycin complexed with cobalt(II): implications for anticancer therapy. *Biochem.*, **2009**, *48*, 4691-4698.

[142] Oluwatayo, F.I.; Elizabeth, M.H.; Wayne, O.; Robert, P.D. Pyrophosphate-bridged complexes with picomolar toxicity. *J. Inorg. Biochem.*, **2009**, *103*, 1254-1264.

[143] Barone, G.; Gambino, N.; Ruggirello, A.; Silvestri, A.; Terenzi, A.; Liveri, V.T. Spectroscopic study of the interaction of Ni(II)-5-triethyl ammonium methyl salicylidene ortho-phenylendiiminate with native DNA. *J. Inorg. Biochem.*, **2009**, *103*, 731-737.

[144] Buschini, A.; Pinelli, S.; Pellacani, C.; Giordani, F.; Ferrari, M.B.; Bisceglie, F.; Giannetto, M.; Pelosi, G.; Tarasconi, P. Synthesis, characterization and deepening in the comprehension of the biological action mechanisms of a new nickel complex with antiproliferative activity. *J. Inorg. Biochem.*, **2009**, *103*, 666-677.

[145] Wang, B.D.; Yang, Z.Y.; Lü, M.H.; Hai, J.; Wang, Q.; Chen, Z.N. Synthesis, characterization, cytotoxic activity and DNA binding Ni(II) complex with the 6-hydroxy chromone-3-carbaldehyde thiosemicarbazone. *J. Organomet. Chem.*, **2009**, *694*, 4069-4075.

[146] Atasever, B.; Ülküseven, B.; Bal-Demirci, T.; Erdem-Kuruca, S.; Solakoğlu, Z. Cytotoxic activities of new iron(III) and nickel(II) chelates of some S-methyl-thiosemicarbazones on K562 and ECV304 cells. *Invest. New Drugs*, **2010**, *28*, 421-432.

[147] Bruijnincx, P.C.A.; Sadler, P.J. New trends for metal complexes with anticancer activity. *Curr. Opinion Chem. Bio.*, **2008**, *12*, 197-206.

[148] Xi, P.X.; Xu, Z.H.; Chen, F.J.; Zeng, Z.Z.; Zhang, X.W. Study on synthesis, structure, and DNA-binding of Ni, Zn complexes with 2-phenylquinoline-4-carboylhydrazide. *J. Inorg. Biochem.*, **2009**, *103*, 210-218.

[149] Tardito, S.; Marchiò, L. Copper compounds in anticancer strategies. *Curr. Med. Chem.*, **2009**, *16*, 1325-1348.

[150] Chen, D.; Milacic, V.; Frezza M.; Dou, Q.P. Metal complexes, their cellular targets and potential for cancer therapy. *Curr. Pharm. Design.*, **2009**, *15*, 777-791.

[151] Wadas, T.J.; Wong, E.H.; Weisman, G.R.; Anderson, C.J. Copper chelation chemistry and its role in copper radiopharmaceuticals. *Curr. Pharm. Design*, **2007**, *13*, 3-16.

[152] Xie, H.Q.; Kang, Y.J. Role of copper in angiogenesis and its medicinal implications. *Curr. Med. Chem.*, **2009**, *16*, 1304-1314.

[153] Wang, T.; Guo, Z.J. Copper in medicine: Homeostasis, chelation therapy and antitumor drug design. *Curr. Med. Chem.,* **2006**, *13*, 525-537.

[154] Shi, Y.; Toms, B.B.; Dixit, N.; Kumari, N.; Mishra, L.; Goodisman, J.; Dabrowiak, J.C. Cytotoxicity of Cu(II) and Zn(II) 2,2′-bipyridyl complexes: dependence of IC_{50} on recovery time. *Chem. Res. Toxicol.*, **2010**, *23*, 1417-1426.

[155] Amoke, O.A. Synthesis, characterization, *in vitro* antibacterial and anticancer studies on some metal(II) complexes of (methylsulfanyl) chromenol Schiff base. *Elixir Appl. Chem.*, **2011**, *39*, 4827-4831.

[156] Tan, J.; Wang, B.C.; Zhu, L.C. DNA binding and oxidative DNA damage induced by a quercetin copper(II) complex: potential mechanism of its antitumor properties. *J. Biol. Inorg. Chem.*, **2009**, *14*, 727-739.

[157] Chen, Z.F.; Tan, M.X.; Liu, L.M.; Liu, Y.C.; Wang, H.S.; Yang, B.; Peng, Y.; Liu, H.G.; Liang, H.; Orvigd, C. Cytotoxicity of the traditional chinese medicine (TCM) plumbagin in its copper chemistry. *Dalton Trans.*, **2009**, 10824-10833.

[158] Iqbal, M.S.; Mughal, M.S.; Arif, R.; Fatima, S.; Sher, M. An *in vitro* study of the interaction of copper(II) salicylates with genomic DNA using gel electrophoresis and gel permeation chromatography. *Chromatographia.*, **2009**, *70*, 1659-1663.

[159] Ikotun, O.F. Higbee, E.M.; Ouellette, W.; Doyle, R.P. Pyrophosphate-bridged complexes with picomolar toxicity. *J. Inorg. Biochem.*, **2009**, *103*, 1254-1264.

[160] Adsule, S.; Banerjee, S.; Ahmed, F.; Padhye, S.; Sarkar, F.H. Hybrid anticancer agents: sothiocyanate-progesterone conjugates as chemotherapeutic agents and insights into their cytotoxicities. *Bioorg. Med. Chem. Lett.*, **2010**, *20*, 1247-1251.

[161] LeBlanc, M.-A.; Gonzalez-Sarrías, A.; Beckford, F.A.; Canisius Mbarushimana, P.; Seeram, N.P. Coordination chemistry of polyaromatic thiosemicarbazones 2: synthesis and biological activity of Zinc, Cobalt, and Copper Complexes of 1-(Naphthalene-2-yl)ethanone thiosemicarbazone. *Inter. J. Inorg. Chem.*, **2011**, *2011*, 1-8.

[162] Primik, M.F.; Muhlgassner, G.; Jakupec, M.A.; Zava, O.; Dyson, P.J.; Arion, V.B.; Keppler, B.K. Highly cytotoxic Copper(II) complexes with modified paullone ligands. *Inorg. Chem.*, **2010**, *49*, 302-311.

[163] Maity, B.; Roy, M.; Banik, B.; Majumdar, R.; Dighe, R.R.; Chakravarty, A.R. Ferrocene-promoted photoactivated DNA cleavage and anticancer activity of terpyridyl copper(II) phenanthroline complexes. *Organometallics*, **2010**, *29*, 3632-3641.

[164] Zanella, A.; Gandin, V.; Porchia, M.; Refosco, F.; Tisato, F.; Sorrentino, F.; Scutari, G.; Rigobello, M.P.; Marzano, C. Cytotoxicity in human cancer cells and mitochondrial dysfunction induced by a series of new copper(I) complexes containing tris(2-cyanoethyl)phosphines. *Invest. New Drugs*, **2011**, *29*, 1213-1223.

[165] Teyssot, M.L.; Jarrousse, A.S.; Beaudoin, C.; Nolan, S.P.; Morel, L.; Gautier, A. Toxicity of copper(I)-NHC complexes against human tumor cells: Induction of cell cycle arrest, apoptosis, and DNA cleavage. *Chem. Eur. J.*, **2009**, *15*, 314-318.

[166] Prasad; A.S.; Kucuk, O. Zinc in cancer prevention. *Cancer Metastasis Rev.*, **2002**, *21*, 291-295.

[167] VanMolle, W.; VanRoy, M.; Bogaert, T.V.; Dejager, L.; Lint, P.V.; Vanlaere, I.; Sekikawa, K.; Kollias, G.; Libert, C. Protection of zinc against tumor necrosis factor-induced lethal inflammation dependson heat shock protein 70 and allows safe antitumor therapy. *Cancer Res.*, **2007**, *67*, 7301-7307.

[168] Liu, J.Y.; Lo, P.C.; Fongb, W.P.; Dennis, K.P.N. Effects of the number and position of the substituents on the *in vitro* photodynamic activities of glucosylated zinc(II) phthalocyanines. *Org. Biomol. Chem.*, **2009**, *7*, 1583-1591.

[169] Liu, J.Y.; Lo, P.C.; Jiang, X.J.; Fongb, W.P.; Dennis, K.P.N. Synthesis and *in vitro* photodynamic activities of di-α-substituted zinc(II) phthalocyanine derivatives. *Dalton Trans.*, **2009**, *7*, 4129-4135.

[170] Jiang, Q.; Zhu, J.H.; Zhang, Y.M.; Xiao, N.; Guo, Z.J. DNA binding property, nuclease activity and cytotoxicity of Zn(II) complexes of terpyridine derivatives. *Biometals*, **2009**, *22*, 297-305.

[171] Wang, H.F.; Shen, R.; Tang, N. Synthesis and characterization of the Zn(II) and Cu(II) piperidinyl isoeuxanthone complexes: DNA-binding and cytotoxic activity. *Eur. J. Med. Chem.*, **2009**, *44*, 4509-4515.

[172] Huang, J.; Chen, Q.Y.; Wang, L.; Yun, F.H.; Jian, L.B. Synthesis, interaction with DNA and antitumor activities of zinc(II) complexes with substituted di(picolyl)amines. *Chin. J. Inorg. Chem.*, **2009**, *25*, 1077-1083.

[173] Tan, J.; Wang, B.C.; Zhu, L.C.; DNA binding, cytotoxicity, apoptotic inducing activity, and molecular modeling study of quercetin zinc(II) complex. *Bioorg. Med. Chem.*, **2009**, *17*, 614-620.

[174] Shi, L.; Mao, W.J.; Yang, Y.; Zhu, H.L. Synthesis, characterization, and biological activity of a Schiff-base Zn(II) complex. *J. Coord. Chem.*, **2009**, *62*, 3471-3477.

[175] Ren, Y.F.; Sun, Y.H.; Cheng, K.M.; Liu, G.F.; Shen, Y.M. Synthesis and radiolabelling of $Re(CO)_3$-belemene derivatives as potential therapeutic radiopharmaceuticals. *J. Label Compd. Radiopharm.*, **2009**, *52*, 139-145.

[176] Louie, M.W.; Liu, H.W.; Lam, M.H.C.; Lau, T.C.; Lo, K.K.W. Novel luminescent tricarbonylrhenium(I) polypyridine tyramine-derived dipicolylamine complexes as sensors for zinc(II) and cadmium(II) ions. *Organomet.*, **2009**, *28*, 4297-4307.

[177] Jakupec, M.A.; Untried, P.; Keppler, B.K. Pharmacological properties of cerium compounds. *Rev. Physiol. Biochem. Pharmacol.*, **2005**, *153*, 101-111.

[178] Fricker, S.P. The therapeutic application of lanthanides. *Chem. Soc. Rev.*, **2006**, *35*, 524-533.

[179] Biba, F.; Groessl, M.; Egger, A.; Roller, A.; Hartinger, C.G.; Keppler, B.K. New insights into the chemistry of the antineoplastic lanthanum complex tris(1,10-phenanthroline)-tris(thiocyanato-κN)lanthanum(III) (KP772) and its interaction with biomolecules. *Eur. J. Inorg. Chem.*, **2009**, *28*, 4282-4287.

[180] Biba, F.; Groessl, M.; Egger, A.; Jakupeca, M.A.; Keppler, B.K. A novel cytotoxic cerium complex: aquatrichloridobis(1,10-phenanthroline)cerium(III) (KP776). Synthesis, characterization, behavior in H2O, binding towards biomolecules, and antiproliferative activity. *Chem. Biodiversity*, **2009**, *6*, 2153-2165.

[181] Arambula, J.F.; Sessler, J.L.; Fountain, M.E.; Wei, W.H.; Magda, D.; Siddik, Z.H. Gadolinium texaphyrin (Gd-Tex)-malonato-platinum conjugates: Synthesis and comparison with carboplatin in normal and Pt-resistant cell lines. *Dalton Trans.*, **2009**, *48*, 10834-10840.

[182] Collery, P.; Keppler, B.; Madoulet, C.; Desoize, B. Gallium in cancer treatment. *Crit. Rev. Oncol. Hemat.*, **2002**, *42*, 283-296.

[183] Gielen, M.; Tiekink, E.R.T. *Metallotherapeutic drugs and metal-based diagnostic agents*, Wiley & Sons: New York, **2005**.

[184] Jakupec, M.A.; Keppler, B.K.; in: *Metal Ions in Biological Systems*, A. Siegel, H. Siegel (Eds.), Dekker, New York, **2004**; Vol. *42*, pp. 425-462.

[185] Bandoli, G.; Dolmella, A.; Tisato, F. Mononuclear six-coordinated Ga (III) complexes: A comprehensive survey, *Coord. Chem. Rev.*, **2009**, *253*, 56-77.

[186] Timerbaev, A.R. Advances in developing tris(8-quinolinolato)gallium(III) as an anticancer drug: critical appraisal and prospects. *Metallomics*, **2009**, *1*, 193-198.

[187] Valiahdi, S.M.; Heffeter, P.; Jakupec, M.A.; Marculescu, R.; Berger, W.; Rappersberger, K.; Keppler, B.K. The gallium complex KP46 exerts strong activity against primary explanted melanoma cells and induces apoptosis in melanoma cell lines. *Melanoma Res.*, **2009**, *19*, 283-293.

[188] Mendes, I.C.; Soares, M.A.; Santos, R.G.; Pinheiro, C.; Beraldo, H. Gallium(III) complexes of 2-pyridineformamide thiosemicarbazones: Cytotoxic activity against malignant glioblastoma, *Eur. J. Med. Chem.*, **2009**, *44*, 1870-1877.

[189] Gómez-Ruiz, S.; Gallego, B.; Kaluderović, M.R.; Kommera, H.; Hey-Hawkins, E.; Paschke, R.; Kaluderović, G.N. Novel gallium(III) complexes containing phthaloyl

derivatives of neutral aminoacids with apoptotic activity in cancer cells. *J. Organomet. Chem.*, **2009**, *694*, 2191-2197.

[190] Vasiliki, V.; Maria, B.C. Chemical aspects of organotin derivatives of beta-diketones, quinonoids, steroids, and some currently used drugs: A review of the literature with emphasis on the medicinal potential of organotins. *Syn. Reactivity Inorg. Met. Org. Nan. Met. Chem.*, **2007**, *37*, 507-525.

[191] Hadjikakou, S.K.; Hadjiliadis, N. Antiproliferative and anti-tumor activity of organotin compounds. *Coord. Chem. Rev.*, **2009**, *253*, 235-249.

[192] Nath, M.; Pokharia, S.; Yadav, R. Organotin(IV) complexes of amino acids and peptides. *Coord. Chem. Rev.*, **2001**, *215*, 99-149.

[193] Carraher, C.E.; Deborah, S.L. *Organotin Macromolecules as Anti-Cancer Drugs, Metal- and Metalloid- Containing Macromolecules*. John Wiley & Sons, New York, **2004**.

[194] Saxena, A.K.; Huber, F. Organotin compounds and cancer chemotherapy. *Coord. Chem. Rev.*, **1989**, 95: 109-123.

[195] Gielen, M. Tin-based antitumor drugs. *Coord. Chem. Rev.*, **1996**, *151*, 41-51.

[196] Pellerito, L., Nagy, L. Organotin(IV) complexes formed with biologically active ligands: equilibrium and structural studies, and some biological aspects. *Coord. Chem. Rev.*, **2002**, *224*, 111-150.

[197] Gielen, M.; Tiekink, E.R.T.; in: M. Gielen, E.R.T. Tiekink (Eds.), *Tin Compounds and their Therapeutic Potential in Metallotherapeutic Drugs and Metal-Based Diagnostic Agents: The Use of Metals in Medicine*, JohnWiley & Sons, Ltd., **2005**.

[198] Muhammad, N.; Shah, A.; Shuja, S.; Ali, S.; Qureshi, R.; Meetsma, A.; Tahir, M.N. Organotin(IV) 4-nitrophenylethanoates: Synthesis, structural characteristics and intercalative mode of interaction with DNA. *J. Organomet. Chem.*, **2009**, *694*, 3431-3437.

[199] Muhammad, N.; Ali, S.; Meetsma, A.; Shaheen, F. Organotin(IV) 4-methoxyphenyl-ethanoates: Synthesis, spectroscopic characterization, X-ray structures and *in vitro* anticancer activity against human prostate cell lines (PC-3). *Inorg. Chim. Acta*, **2009**, *362*, 2842-2848.

[200] Kang, W.L.; Wu, X.Y.; Huang, J.B. Synthesis, crystal structure and biological activities of four novel tetranuclear di-organotin(IV) carboxylates. *J. Organomet. Chem.*, **2009**, *694*, 2402-2408.

[201] Siddiqi. Z.A.; Shahid, M; Kumar, S; Khalid, M; Noor, S. Synthesis, crystal structure and *in vitro* antitumor activity of carboxylate bridged dinuclear organotin(IV) complexes. *J. Organomet. Chem.*, **2009**, *694*, 3768-3774.

[202] Li, W.; Zhang, Z.W.; Ren, S.M.; Sibiri, Y.; Massin, D.P.; Jiang, T.; Synthesis and antitumor activity of novel dibutyltin carboxylates of aminoglucosyl derivatives. Chem. Biol. *Drug. Des.*, **2009**, *73*, 682-686.

[203] Sen, A.; Chaudhuri, T.K. Synthesis and evaluation of dimethyl tin 4-cyclohexyl thiosemicarbazone as a novel antitumor agent. *Exp. Oncol.*, **2009**, *31*, 22-26.

[204] González, A.; Gómez, E.; Cortés-lozada, A.; Hernández, S.; Ramírez-apan, T.; Nieto-camacho, A. Heptacoordinate tin(IV) compounds derived from pyridine schiff bases: synthesis, characterization, *in vitro* cytotoxicity, anti-inflammatory and antioxidant activity. *Chem. Pharm. Bull.*, **2009**, *57*, 5-15.

[205] Basu, T.S.; Basu, S.; Vos, D.; Linden, A. Amino acetate functionalized schiff base organotin(IV) complexes as anticancer drugs: synthesis, structural characterization, and *in vitro* cytotoxicity studies. *Invest. New Drugs*, **2009**, *27*, 419-431.

[206] Alama, A.; Viale, M.; Cilli, M.; Bruzzo, C.; Novelli, F.; Tasso, B.; Sparatore, F. *In vitro* cytotoxic activity of tri-n-butyltin(IV)lupinylsulfide hydrogen fumarate (IST-FS 35) and preliminary antitumor activity *in vivo*. *Invest. New Drugs*, **2009**, *27*, 124-130.

[207] Gómez-Ruiz, S.; Prashar, S.; Walther, T.; Fajardo, M.; Steinborn, D.; Reinhard, P.; Kaluderović, G.N. Cyclopentadienyltin(IV) derivatives: synthesis, characterization and study of their cytotoxic activities. *Polyhedron*, **2010**, *29*, 16-23.

[208] Gajewska, M.; Luzyanin, K.V.; Li, Q.S.; Cui, J.R.; Pombeiro, A.J.L. Cyclic trinuclear diorganotin(IV) complexes - the first tin compounds bearing oximehydroxamate ligands: Synthesis, structural characterization and high *in vitro* cytotoxicity. *Eur. J. Inorg. Chem.*, **2009**, *25*, 3765-3769.

CHAPTER 3

Perspective Gold(III)-Dithiocarbamato Anticancer Therapeutics: Learning from the Past, Moving to the Future

Luca Ronconi, Chiara Nardon, Giulia Boscutti and Dolores Fregona*

The Biomedicinal Chemistry Research Group, Department of Chemical Sciences, University of Padova, Padova, Italy

Abstract: The unquestionable therapeutic success of the anticancer drug cisplatin and its second and third generation analogues has triggered, during the past fifty years, the development of several metal-based potential chemotherapeutic agents, most of which have unfortunately failed to enter clinical trials. In this context, since the late 1990s, the *Biomedicinal Chemistry Research Group* at the University of Padova (Italy) has been making quite an effort to design a number of metal-dithiocarbamato derivatives that were expected, at least in principle, to resemble the main features of cisplatin together with higher activity, improved selectivity and bioavailability, and reduced side-effects. Among all, some selected gold(III) complexes have been showing outstanding *in vitro* and *in vivo* antitumor properties and negligible (or even no) acute and renal toxicity, compared to the reference clinically-established platinum drugs.

Starting from the rationale behind such investigations, results achieved to date are here summarized, focusing on the in-depth mechanistic studies that have been providing insights into the mechanism of action of this class of metal compounds. New prospects opened up by these anticancer agents, including the latest development of "second generation" gold-based peptidomimetics for the targeted chemotherapy, are also illustrated and discussed.

Keywords: Gold, dithiocarbamate, anticancer activity, metallodrug, proteasome inhibitor, nephrotoxicity, peptidomimetic, drug delivery, targeted chemotherapy.

INTRODUCTION

The medicinal applications of metal ions have been widely recognized in the treatment of various diseases, including cancer. The accidental discovery of the anticancer properties of cisplatin (*cis*-dichloridodiamminoplatinum(II), *cis*-

***Address correspondence to Dolores Fregona:** Department of Chemical Sciences, University of Padova, *Via* F. Marzolo 1, Padova 35131, Italy; Tel: +39 (0)49 8275159; Fax: +39 (0)2 700500560; E-mail: dolores.fregona@unipd.it

Michelle Prudhomme (Ed)

[$Pt^{II}Cl_2(NH_3)_2$]) in the mid-1960s [1], has triggered the development of both alternative platinum- [2] and other metal-based [3,4] compounds. Metal complexes have shown interesting preclinical and clinical results as antitumor drugs and platinum compounds are well-established in current cancer chemotherapy. At present, cisplatin is one of the most effective drugs employed to treat testicular and, in combination with other chemotherapeutic agents, ovarian, non-small-cells lung, small-cells lung, bladder, cervical, brain and breast cancer [5]. Anyway, all drugs have drawbacks, and cisplatin is no exception. In fact, its high effectiveness is severely hindered by some severe side-effects (such as nausea, alopecia, ototoxicity, neurotoxicity, myelosuppression and nephrotoxicity) as well as by tumor resistance (either intrinsic or acquired during cycles of therapy) [6]. Therefore, much of the early efforts in designing new platinum drugs was aimed at making cisplatin-based therapy safer to patients, in particular by lessening or removing unpredictable and severe side-effects, providing oral bioavailability, and overcoming resistance. Attempts to mitigate drawbacks have prompted chemists to synthesize a variety of second and third generation analogues, but only a handful of metal compounds where shown to be suitable for clinical use and, consequently, achieved marketing approval for human use. Remarkably, all contain a platinum center and are commonly known as carboplatin (global), oxaliplatin (global), nedaplatin (Japan), lobaplatin (China) and heptaplatin (South Korea) [7].

The development of novel metallodrugs with a pharmacological profile different from that of the clinically-established platinum drugs is a major goal of modern medicinal chemistry and drug design. Owing to the intrinsic nature of metal centers, peculiar coordination modes and kinetic properties, metallodrugs function through mechanisms that cannot be mimicked by organic agents, that is, they affect cellular processes such as cellular division and carcinogenic reactions in different ways. The latest approaches focus on complexes with tumor-targeting properties, thereby maximizing the impact on cancer cells and minimizing the occurrence of adverse side-effects, and on complexes with biologically-active ligands [8,9].

Among the non-platinum antitumor agents, gold compounds are currently gaining ground as a new class of chemotherapeutics owing to their strong tumor cell growth inhibiting effects generally achieved by exploiting non-cisplatin-like pharmacodynamic and pharmacokinetic properties and mechanisms of action [10]. Up to date, late-stage rheumatoid arthritis has been treated with various gold drugs, including aurothioglucose (solganal), aurothiomalate (myocrisin), aurothiosulfate (sanocrysin), aurothiopropanol sulfonate (allocrysin), and triethylphosphino-gold(I)tetraacetylthioglucose (auranofin) (Fig. **1**). The application of gold complexes, especially gold(I) derivatives, in medicine has been called "chrysotherapy" and aims at reducing inflammation and disease progression in patients [11,12].

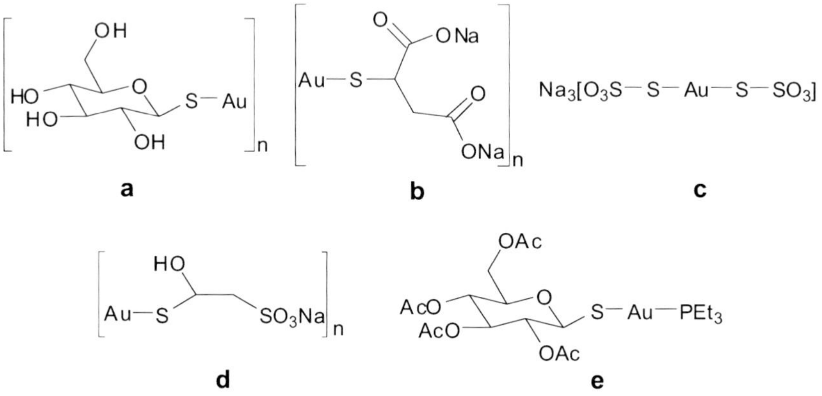

Fig. (1). Clinically-established gold(I) antiarthritic drugs: solganal (**a**), myocrisin (**b**), sanocrysin (**c**), allocrysin (**d**), and auranofin (**e**).

Owing to their traditional use in medicine for the treatment of rheumatoid arthritis [13], gold compounds are natural candidates as potential alternatives to platinum drugs. In fact, their antiarthritic activity arises from the well-known immunosuppressive and antiinflammatory actions thus establishing, at least in principle, a connection between the two therapies [14]. For example, auranofin (Fig. **1e**) is of special interest since it can be administered orally, in contrast to the other marketed gold(I) salts usually injected. Experimental research revealed that, together with its antiarthritic properties, it showed promising *in vitro* cytotoxic activity as well, but further evaluation as potential anticancer agent was dismissed because of its relatively poor effectiveness on *in vivo* tumor models [15].

The spectrum of gold complexes with reported cell growth inhibiting properties comprises a number of different ligands coordinated to the metal ion either in the

+1 or +3 oxidation states. Based on the wide structural variety of the investigated ligands, a unique mode of action or pharmacological profile for gold complexes is unlikely to exist, and several biological targets, other than intracellular DNA (generally recognized as the major biological target of cisplatin and its analogues [16]) have to be considered to elucidate the pharmacology of gold-based metallodrugs. Gold(III) complexes show chemical features that are very close to those of clinically-established platinum(II) complexes, such as the preference for square-planar coordination and the typical d^8 electronic configuration, making them very attractive for testing as antineoplastic drugs. Surprisingly, despite the strict similarity, little literature (compared to platinum compounds) exists on the use of gold(III) complexes as anticancer agents, the lower amount of data probably due to their high reducing potential and relatively poor stability, thus making their use rather problematic under physiological conditions.

In this context, during the last decade, a number of gold(III)-dithiocarbamato derivatives have been designed and tested by our research group as potential anticancer agents, showing promising and outstanding properties [17], thus justifying the need to carry out further in-depth biological and mechanistic studies. Up-to-date results are here summarized and discussed.

WHY DITHIOCARBAMATES?

As previously reminded, nephrotoxicity (*i.e.* kidney toxicity) is a major limiting factor for the use of cisplatin and related platinum-based therapeutics in the clinic. It may result from either too high administered doses or accumulation of platinum in the body. The effects of cisplatin on renal functions are not fully understood yet, but recent studies have provided new insights into the mechanism of cisplatin-induced nephrotoxicity, especially on the signaling pathways leading to tubular cells death and inflammation. It has been hypothesized that renal failure may be induced by platinum binding to, and consequent inactivation of, thiol-containing renal enzymes [18,19]. Sulfur-containing biomolecules, such as cysteine, methionine, glutathione, metallothionein and albumin, play a significant role in platinum anticancer chemotherapy because of their high affinity to platinum(II) ion. Sulfur is involved in the entire metabolic process of platinum drugs, including reactions prior to cellular uptake and deactivation prior to DNA binding. Although the role of sulfur compounds is still controversial, the interaction between sulfur-containing biomolecules and platinum drugs is generally believed to have negative effects on the therapeutic effectiveness since it has been associated with drug detoxification, nephrotoxicity and resistance. Strong and irreversible binding of cisplatin to intracellular thiolato ligands is considered as a major inactivation step, and reactions with sulfur donors present in peptides and proteins are believed to alter the conformation of the proteins themselves, and lead to changes in their biological activity, especially when enzymatic processes are affected [20].

Thus, a number of thiol-based and sulfur-containing nucleophiles have been tested as chemoprotectants to modulate cisplatin nephrotoxicity [21,22]. Two main issues must be taken into account for the development of chemoprotectants: (1) the selective protection of human normal cells, and (2) the addition of no or little toxicity. For this reason, most of the potential modulators of cisplatin toxicity were based on the endogenous defense system for electrophiles, the tripeptide glutathione. Many sulfur-based chemoprotectants were tested (Fig. **2**), and some showed promising for clinical use. However, a selective protection of normal tissues without inhibition of the anticancer activity was proved challenging.

In this regard, positive outcomes were achieved with sodium diethyldithiocarbamate (DEDTNa, Fig. **2c**). In fact, it was shown to provide protection against renal, gastrointestinal and bone marrow toxicity induced by cisplatin without decreasing its antitumor activity [23]. The chemoprotective effect results from the capability to remove platinum from the thiol groups of proteins without reversal of platinum-DNA adducts, widely recognized as responsible for its antitumor activity. Platinum-DNA adducts were shown to decrease by *ca.* 50% upon treatment with DEDTNa soon after cisplatin administration, causing a loss of therapeutic effect, whereas no change in anticancer activity was observed when DEDTNa was administered 3 h after the drug. This behavior is due to the fact that, when DEDTNa is administered soon after cisplatin, it reacts immediately with the drug causing its inactivation. Conversely, when administered 3 h later, cisplatin has already reacted with DNA, and the dithiocarbamate cannot cleave platinum-DNA adducts, whereas it is able to chelate and remove platinum from a variety of other sulfur-containing molecules, making it again available for further interactions with DNA. Thus, the accurate use and dosing of DEDTNa as chemoprotectant reduces nephrotoxicity of cisplatin chemotherapy without decreasing its antitumor properties [24]. Nevertheless, the overall nephroprotective benefits of DEDTNa are somewhat limited by the acute toxicity profile of dithiocarbamates themselves. In fact, potential human health hazards associated with free (*i.e.* not coordinated) dithiocarbamates is still being investigated, including genotoxicity [25].

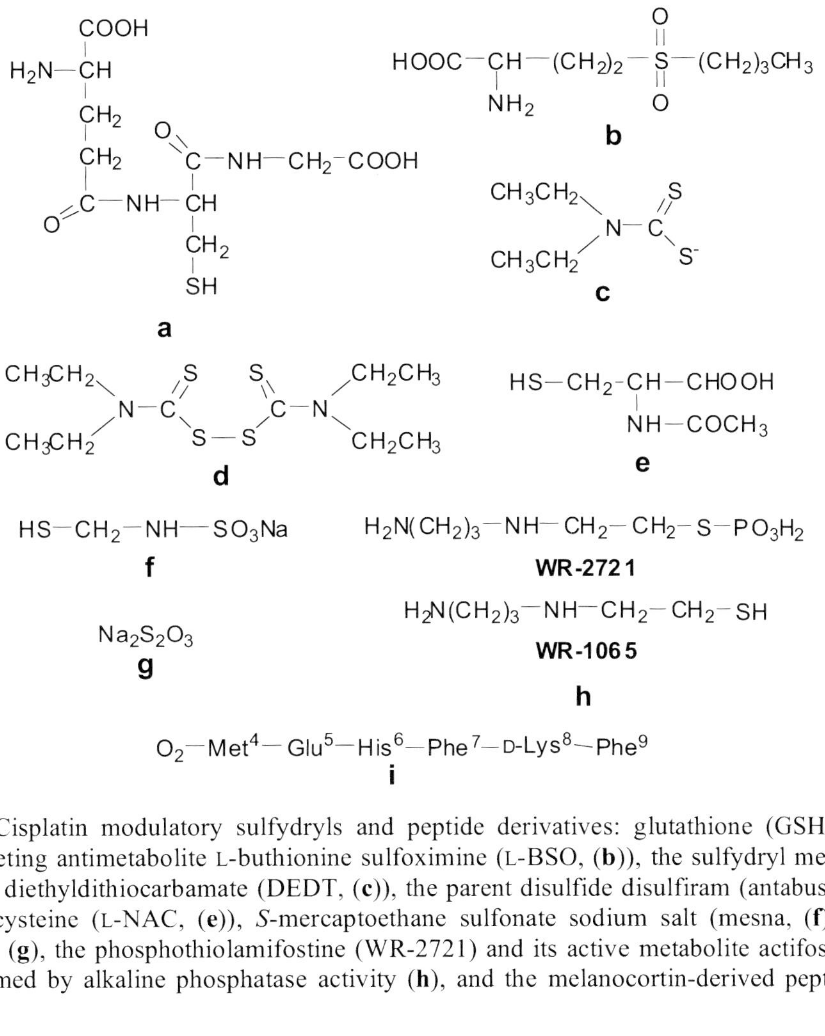

Fig. (2). Cisplatin modulatory sulfydryls and peptide derivatives: glutathione (GSH, (**a**)), the GSH-depleting antimetabolite L-buthionine sulfoximine (L-BSO, (**b**)), the sulfydryl metabolite of disulfiram diethyldithiocarbamate (DEDT, (**c**)), the parent disulfide disulfiram (antabuse, (**d**)), *N*-acetyl- L-cysteine (L-NAC, (**e**)), *S*-mercaptoethane sulfonate sodium salt (mesna, (**f**)), sodium thiosulfate (**g**), the phosphothiolamifostine (WR-2721) and its active metabolite actifostine (WR-1065) formed by alkaline phosphatase activity (**h**), and the melanocortin-derived peptide ORG-2766 (**i**).

On the basis of these considerations, we have been designing a number of metal-dithiocarbamato complexes potentially able to combine the cytotoxic activity of the metal centers (*e.g.* Pt(II) [26-34], Pd(II) [26,27,30,31,34-36], Au(III) [37,38], Ru(II/III) [39-41], Zn(II) [42,43], Cu(II) [42,44]) with the lack of nephrotoxicity. The rationale of our strategy is based on the chemical features of the dithiocarbamato moiety (–$NCSS^-$). Dithiocarbamates are bidentate chelating ligands and, upon coordination to a metal ion, the resulting complexes are expected to be quite stable due to the so-called "chelate effect", and possible decomposition with subsequent loss of the dithiocarbamato ligand is unlikely to occur. Moreover, the solubility properties of the metal-dithiocarbamato derivatives may be, at least in principle, modulated by modifying the organic chain of the dithiocarbamate. As concerns square-planar complexes, the presence of a chelating dithiocarbamate should make the coordination of additional *S*-donor ligands (*e.g.* methionine and cysteine residues) *trans* to the NCSS moiety less favorable because of the rather strong *trans*-influencing effect of the dithiocarbamato sulfur atoms, thus potentially avoiding the interaction of the metal center with thiol-containing renal enzymes and, consequently, reducing nephrotoxic side-effects [45].

ONCE UPON A TIME: "FIRST GENERATION" GOLD-DITHIOCARBAMATO ANTICANCER AGENTS

As a natural starting point, we first designed a number of platinum(II)- and, owing to the strict similarity, palladium(II)-dithiocarbamato derivatives, some of which were proved promising in terms of both higher antitumor activity and lack of nephrotoxicity compared to the reference drug cisplatin [37]. Unfortunately, despite these encouraging results, long synthetic routes, poor water solubility and inadequate (for pharmacological purposes) stability under physiological conditions were the major drawbacks, so their further evaluation as potential anticancer agents was dismissed.

In order to overcome the above mentioned issues, we have been exploring alternative ways, the most promising being the design of dithiocarbamato derivatives of metals other than platinum and palladium. In particular, we have synthesized a number of gold(III)-dithiocarbamato derivatives of the type [$Au^{III}X_2$(dtc)] (X = Cl, Br; dtc = various dithiocarbamato ligands) that have been designed in such a way to reproduce very closely the main features of cisplatin (Fig. **3**).

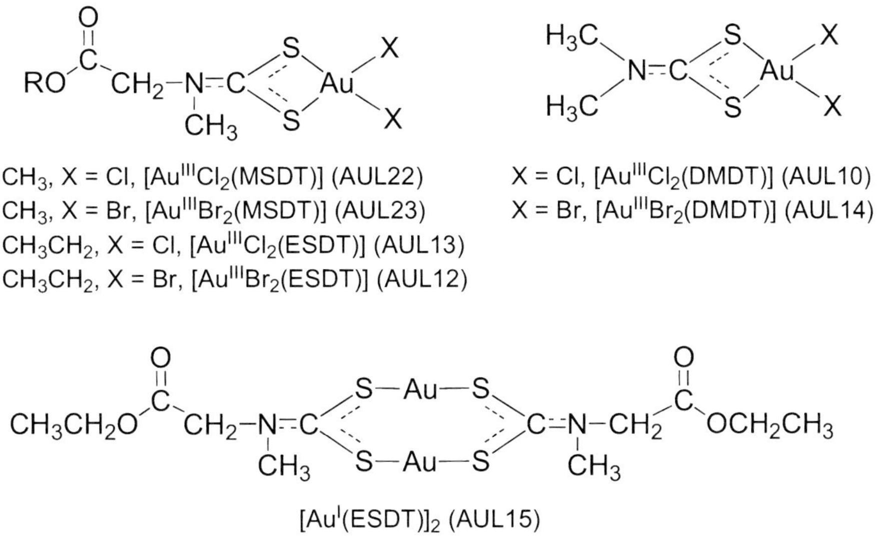

Fig. (3). Selected gold-dithiocarbamato derivatives: X = Cl, Br; DMDT = *N,N*-dimethyldithiocarbamate ($(CH_3)_2NCSS^-$); MSDT = methylsarcosinedithiocarbamate ($CH_3O(O)CCH_2N(CH_3)CSS^-$); ESDT = ethylsarcosinedithiocarbamate ($CH_3CH_2O(O)CCH_2N(CH_3)CSS^-$).

As regards the sarcosine derivatives, the choice of the ligands was not accidental. In fact, sarcosinedithiocarbamate pretreatment was shown to increase the therapeutic effectiveness of the clinically established antineoplastic drugs doxorubicin, methotrexate, teniposide and mitoxontrone in leukemia L1210 [46]. Esterification of the carboxylic group was proved necessary because it was shown that analogues containing a free carboxylate function are not active [47]. Moreover, the use of different ester moieties could allow modulation of the solubility properties of the resulting compounds.

All the gold complexes have been fully characterized by means of several techniques, confirming that coordination of the dithiocarbamato ligand takes place in a near square-planar geometry through the sulfur-donating atoms, the NCSS moiety coordinating the metal center in a bidentate symmetrical mode and lying in the same plane, and the remaining coordination positions being occupied by two *cis*-halogen atoms (Fig. **4**).

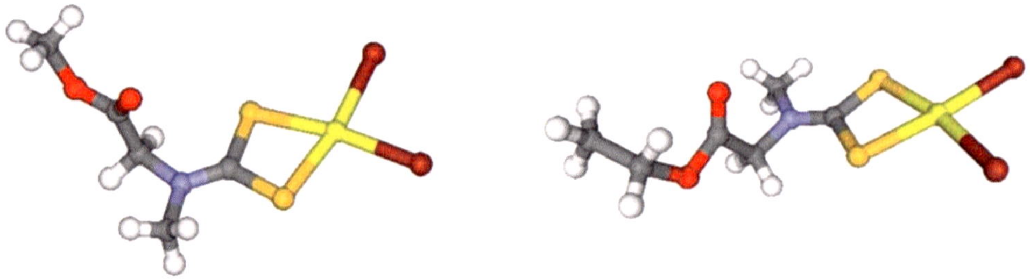

[$Au^{III}Br_2$(MSDT)] (AUL23) **[$Au^{III}Br_2$(ESDT)] (AUL12)**

Fig. (4). X-ray crystal structures of [$Au^{III}Br_2$(MSDT)] (AUL23) and [$Au^{III}Br_2$(ESDT)] (AUL12).

In Vitro Cytotoxic Activity

From comparative *in vitro* cytotoxicity studies on Pt(II)-, Pd(II)-, and Au(III)-MSDT derivatives on human squamous cervical adenocarcinoma (HeLa) cells and human leukemic promyelocytes (HL60), gold(III) complexes resulted to be significantly more active (in terms of IC_{50} values, that is, the drug concentration required for 50% inhibition of cell growth *in vitro* compared to the control) than both cisplatin and the platinum(II) and palladium(II) counterparts tested under the same experimental conditions (IC_{50} *ca.* 1 μM *vs ca.* 2, >15, and 5 μM, respectively), inducing apoptosis especially in HL60 cells [48]. [$Au^{III}X_2$(MSDT)]-type compounds were also tested on a panel of acute myelogenous leukemia cell lines, representing different French-American-British subtypes, and toward the Philadelphia-positive (K562) cells [49]. Compared to the corresponding palladium(II) analogues [36] they showed to inhibit cell growth in all the tested myeloid cell lines with IC_{50} values *ca.* ten-fold lower than the reference drug. Moreover, after short exposure (18 h), [$Au^{III}X_2$(MSDT)]-type compounds induced strong and rapid apoptosis accompanied by downregulation of the antiapoptotic molecule Bcl-2 and upregulation of the proapoptotic molecule Bax, whereas cisplatin did not. Finally, after longer exposure (72 h), they were proved to induce only modest cell cycle perturbations but high DNA fragmentation, whereas classical platinum(II) complexes are known to promote characteristic cell cycle alterations resulting in increased G_2M cell fraction [50]. Therefore, [$Au^{III}X_2$(MSDT)] derivatives are able to promote early apoptosis and membrane damage to a much greater extent than cisplatin, suggesting a different mechanism of action.

On account of these encouraging results, we developed other gold(III)-dithiocarbamato derivatives, namely [$Au^{III}Cl_2$(DMDT)], [$Au^{III}Br_2$(DMDT)], [$Au^{III}Cl_2$(ESDT)] and [$Au^{III}Br_2$(ESDT)] (from now on referred to as AUL10, AUL14, AUL13 and AUL12, respectively). These compounds were proved to be much more cytotoxic *in vitro* than cisplatin even toward human tumor cell lines intrinsically resistant to cisplatin itself, such as Daudi, MeWo, LoVo and A549 cells. Moreover, they appeared to be equally active on cell lines made resistant to cisplatin treatment, compared to the corresponding cisplatin-sensitive parent cell lines, ruling out the occurrence of cross-resistance phenomena (Table **1**) [51a]. Such evaluation has been recently extended to *t*-butylsarcosinedithiocarbamato gold(III) analogues, confirming the potential of this class of metallodrugs [51b].

In order to get further insights into the ability of the investigated gold(III) complexes to overcome resistance to cisplatin, their capability to inhibit DNA synthesis in tumor cells that had acquired resistance to cisplatin *in vivo* has been investigated [52]. In this regard, a comparison of the inhibitory effect of AUL12 and cisplatin toward murine leukemia cisplatin-sensitive L1210 and -resistant L1210-R cells is reported in Fig. (**5**). Remarkably, AUL12 induces a dramatic inhibition of DNA synthesis in both cell lines at comparable levels, whereas cisplatin does not. These results, confirming the circumvention of cisplatin resistance, are particularly interesting since L1210-R cells, contrarily to the resistant sublines previously tested, acquired their resistance *in vivo*, thus evading all the host defense mechanisms.

Solution Chemistry and DNA Binding Affinity

Although still under debate, the commonly accepted mechanism of action of cisplatin involves its uptake into the cell followed by hydrolysis in the cytoplasm, favored by low Cl^- concentrations (4-20 mM), leading to the positively charged aquo species that may reach the nucleus and react with DNA, acknowledged as its ultimate biological target [53]. In this regard, the behavior under physiologically-relevant conditions as well as the DNA binding properties of some selected gold(III)-dithiocarbamato complexes have been investigated [52].

Table 1. *In vitro* cytotoxic activity over 24 h of Au(III)-dithiocarbamato derivatives $[Au^{III}Cl_2(DMDT)]$ (AUL10), $[Au^{III}Br_2(DMDT)]$ (AUL14), $[Au^{III}Cl_2(ESDT)]$ (AUL13) and $[Au^{III}Br_2(ESDT)]$ (AUL12), and the reference drug cisplatin tested under the same experimental conditions toward selected human tumor cell lines: human squamous cervical adenocarcinoma (HeLa), human leukemic promyelocytes (HL60), human Burkitt's lymphoma (Daudi), human malignant melanoma (MeWo), human colon adenocarcinoma (LoVo), human non-small-cells lung adenocarcinoma (A549), human ovarian carcinoma cisplatin-sensitive (2008) and cisplatin-resistant (C13*), human squamous cervix carcinoma cisplatin-sensitive (A431) and cisplatin-resistant (A431-R), human osteosarcoma cisplatin-sensitive (U2OS) and cisplatin-resistant (U2OS-R) cells. Data are expressed in terms of $IC_{50} \pm$ S.D. (standard deviation) values (μM)

Cell Line	Compound				
	AUL10	AUL14	AUL13	AUL12	Cisplatin
HeLa	2.10 ± 0.01	3.50 ± 0.01	8.2 ± 0.2	7.6 ± 0.2	15.6 ± 0.4
HL60	$(0.80 \pm 0.01) \times 10^{-2}$	$(0.70 \pm 0.01) \times 10^{-2}$	0.43 ± 0.09	0.14 ± 0.02	25.6 ± 0.3
Daudi	$(0.10 \pm 0.01) \times 10^{-2}$	$(0.10 \pm 0.01) \times 10^{-2}$	4.65 ± 0.09	5.8 ± 0.2	95 ± 1
MeWo	2.0 ± 0.3	$(0.10 \pm 0.01) \times 10^{-2}$	12.5 ± 0.9	10.0 ± 0.9	48 ± 2
LoVo	$(2.40 \pm 0.04) \times 10^{-2}$	3.8 ± 0.1	7.6 ± 0.2	7.9 ± 0.1	56 ± 2
A549	$(0.35 \pm 0.01) \times 10^{-2}$	0.41 ± 0.03	4.73 ± 0.04	9.6 ± 0.2	35 ± 1
2008	$(0.20 \pm 0.01) \times 10^{-2}$	30.0 ± 0.1	49.3 ± 0.1	16.5 ± 0.4	43.2 ± 0.4
C13*	$(0.10 \pm 0.01) \times 10^{-2}$	21.8 ± 0.2	23.8 ± 0.1	$(0.10 \pm 0.01) \times 10^{-2}$	556 ± 3
A431	$(1.20 \pm 0.01) \times 10^{-2}$	1.8 ± 0.1	0.29 ± 0.01	$(1.50 \pm 0.01) \times 10^{-2}$	77.4 ± 0.4
A431-R	$(0.20 \pm 0.01) \times 10^{-2}$	2.8 ± 0.2	0.43 ± 0.03	$(0.10 \pm 0.01) \times 10^{-2}$	382 ± 3
U2OS	4.8 ± 0.3	18 ± 1	5.8 ± 0.4	0.49 ± 0.09	35 ± 2
U2OS-R	6.4 ± 0.1	13 ± 1	5.2 ± 0.2	0.24 ± 0.09	84 ± 3

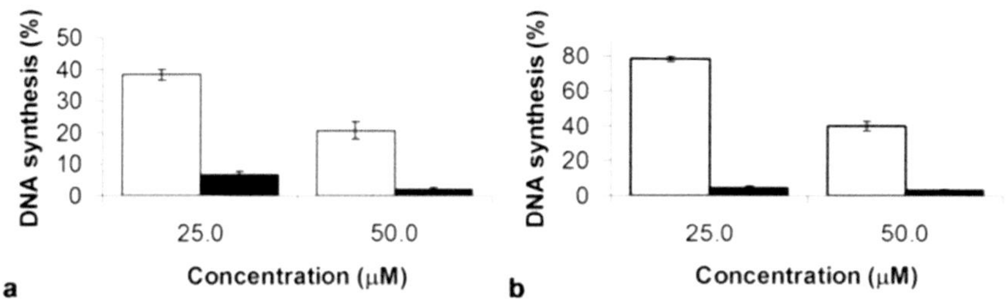

Fig. (5). Inhibition of DNA synthesis in cisplatin-sensitive (L1210, **a**) and cisplatin-resistant (L1210-R, **b**) murine leukemia cells incubated for 3 h with either cisplatin (□) or AUL12 (■) (adapted from ref. [52]).

As concerns the solution chemistry, these gold(III) complexes were proved to hydrolyze in a physiological-like environment by delivering two moles of halide per mole of starting complex, thus leading to the corresponding gold(III)-diaquo counterparts within 30-40 min. Intriguingly, the hydrolyzed species were proved to be reasonably stable in physiological solution, reduction to gold(I) occurring after 12-24 h. Since the physiological environment is generally reducing, gold(III) complexes, often characterized by high redox potentials, are likely to undergo reduction to the corresponding less active gold(I) species, a major drawback for their pharmacological development. Thus, the inherent electrochemical properties of our gold(III) compounds have been studied in a physiological-like solution by cyclic voltammetry, showing that both DMDT (AUL10 and AUL14) and ESDT (AUL12 and AUL13) derivatives undergo irreversible stepwise reduction processes, leading to the corresponding dinuclear gold(I) species $[Au^{I}(DMDT)]_2$ and $[Au^{I}(ESDT)]_2$, at *ca.* -300 mV and -180 mV (*vs* saturated calomel electrode, SCE), respectively. Remarkably, these reduction reactions occur at potentials considerably lower than the typical values for the Au(III)/Au(I) couple known for the corresponding $K[Au^{III}X_4]$ (X = Cl, Br) precursors (*ca.* +1.29 V) [54]. Therefore, coordination by dithiocarbamates induces a large stabilization of the metal ion in the +3 oxidation state, owing to the electron-donating capability and the stabilizing chelate effect of the dithiocarbamato moiety.

Given the strict structural and chemical analogy of these gold(III) complexes with cisplatin, we started from the hypothesis that their cytotoxic properties should have arisen from a direct interaction with intracellular DNA. Experimental evidences established their high affinity toward some biologically-relevant isolated macromolecules, resulting in a dramatic inhibition of both DNA and RNA synthesis in a non-dose-dependent way, whereas, as expected, cisplatin promoted a strong dose-dependent inhibition of DNA without significantly affecting RNA synthesis (Fig. **6**).

In addition, these compounds showed extremely fast DNA binding rates. With reference to Fig. (**7**), in which the binding affinity of AUL10 to calf thymus DNA is reported as an example, it is apparent that this gold(III) compound has a great affinity toward DNA with evidence of binding observable even soon after contact (time zero). Reaction with DNA appears to be extremely rapid and dependent on both r_i value and contact time, achieving 100% binding after less than 3 h compared to 51% reached by cisplatin tested under the same experimental conditions after 24 h.

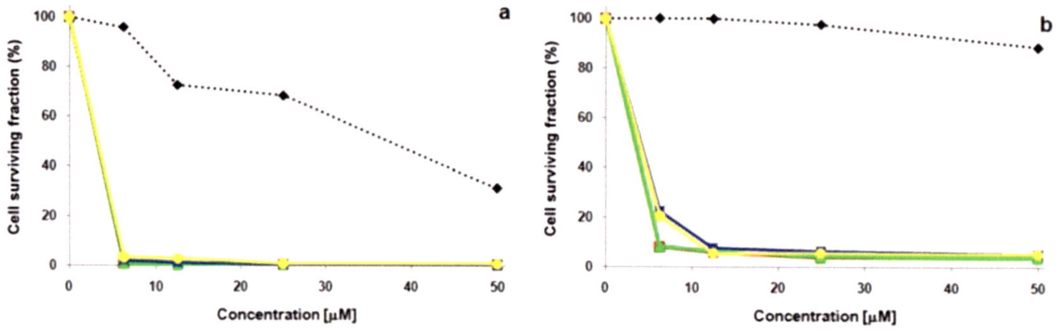

Fig. (6). Inhibition of macromolecular synthesis in HL60 cells incubated for 3 h with increasing concentrations of cisplatin (♦), AUL10 (■), AUL14 (▲), AUL13 (×) and AUL12 (●). Data expressed in terms of H^3-thymidine (**a**) and H^3-uridine (**b**) percentage uptake (adapted from ref. [52]).

These compounds were also proved to form interstrand cross-links with faster kinetics than cisplatin, whereas they were found to be totally unable to induce DNA-protein cross-links, contrary to cisplatin that may act as a bifunctional agent [29]. This behavior is, besides surprising, extremely interesting, since exposure to several agents inducing DNA-protein cross-links gives rise to genotoxic and carcinogenic effects, and the primary mutagenic effects induced by some xenobiotics are believed to be mediated through the formation of this kind of lesions [55].

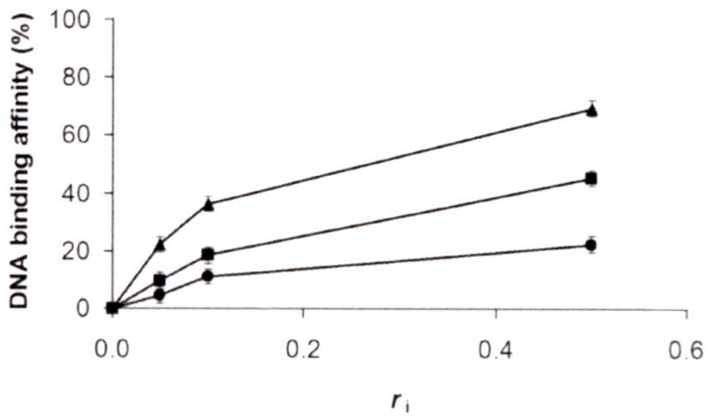

Fig. (7). Binding affinity of AUL10 to calf thymus DNA at 0 min (●), 15 min (■), and 30 min (▲). Data are expressed in terms of percentage of DNA-bound gold at the different r_i (molar ratio of tested compound to nucleotides) values (0.05, 0.1, and 0.5). (Adapted from ref. [52]).

Inhibition of the Selenoenzyme Thioredoxin Reductase

Altogether, our preliminary results showed that the mechanism of action of these gold(III)-dithiocarbamato derivatives differs from that of the classical platinum(II)-based anticancer drugs. Although they were proved to bind DNA to a greater extent than cisplatin, this evidence is more likely to be a consequence of their extremely high reactivity toward isolated biologically-relevant macromolecules rather than undoubtedly assessing DNA as their ultimate target.

In this regard, recent reports have identified the enzyme thioredoxin reductase (TrxR) as a reliable target for anticancer gold compounds [56]. The thioredoxin (Trx) system plays a key role in regulating the overall intracellular redox balance. TrxR is a large homodimeric selenoenzyme controlling the redox state of Trx. TrxR was proved to be inhibited by a number of gold derivatives, which trigger alterations of the mitochondrial functions and induce severe oxidative stress, eventually leading to cell apoptosis. In order to get insights into their mechanism of action, the four gold(III) complexes AUL10, AUL12, AUL13 and AUL14 have been studied in-depth as inhibitors of the thioredoxin system [57]. All the tested compounds were proved to induce cancer cell death through both apoptotic and non-apoptotic mechanisms, and to inhibit TrxR activity. Based on our results, we proposed a working model suggesting that deregulation of the TrxR/Trx system is a major mechanism involved in their anticancer activity (Fig. **8**).

These compounds were proved to trigger cell death, favor generation of reactive oxygen species (ROS), modify some mitochondrial functions (*i.e.* membrane potential, thus promoting mitochondrial swelling), and to inactivate both cytosolic and mitochondrial thioredoxin reductase. Trx protects cells from a variety of oxidative stresses by regulating the redox state and activity of many cellular proteins controlling cell growth. All the tested complexes inhibit TrxR by irreversibly binding to the catalytic site, thus hampering the function of TrxR that acts as mediator of electron flow from nicotinamide adenine dinucleotide phosphate (NADPH) to peroxiredoxins through Trx, eventually leading to the accumulation of ROS (especially hydrogen peroxide). Moreover, the inhibition of the Trx/TrxR redox system promotes the dissociation of the Trx-ASK-1 (apoptosis signal-regulating kinase-1) and the subsequent activation of the MAPK (mitogen-activated protein kinase) system. Both the increased level of ROS and the activation of the MAPK system induce elevated long-lasting levels of phosphorylated extracellular signal-regulated kinases-1 (phosphor-ERK-1) and -2 (phosphor-ERK-2) that may lead to cell death. Intriguingly, ERK phosphorylation, and the consequent cell death, were inhibited by the antioxidant L-NAC (itself preventing the dissociation of the complex Trx-ASK-1 by keeping Trx in the reduced state), whereas the peroxyl scavenger Trolox (6-hydroxy-2,5,7,8-tetramethylchroman-2-carboxylic acid) was proved only slightly efficient. Thus, we hypothesized that a persistent ERK-1/-2 activation triggered first by accumulation of hydrogen peroxide and then by ASK-1 pathway deregulation might be responsible for cell death through both apoptotic and non-apoptotic routes, whereas cisplatin leads to cell death only through an apoptotic pathway (as determined by the poly-(ADPribose)-polymerase (PARP) cleavage).

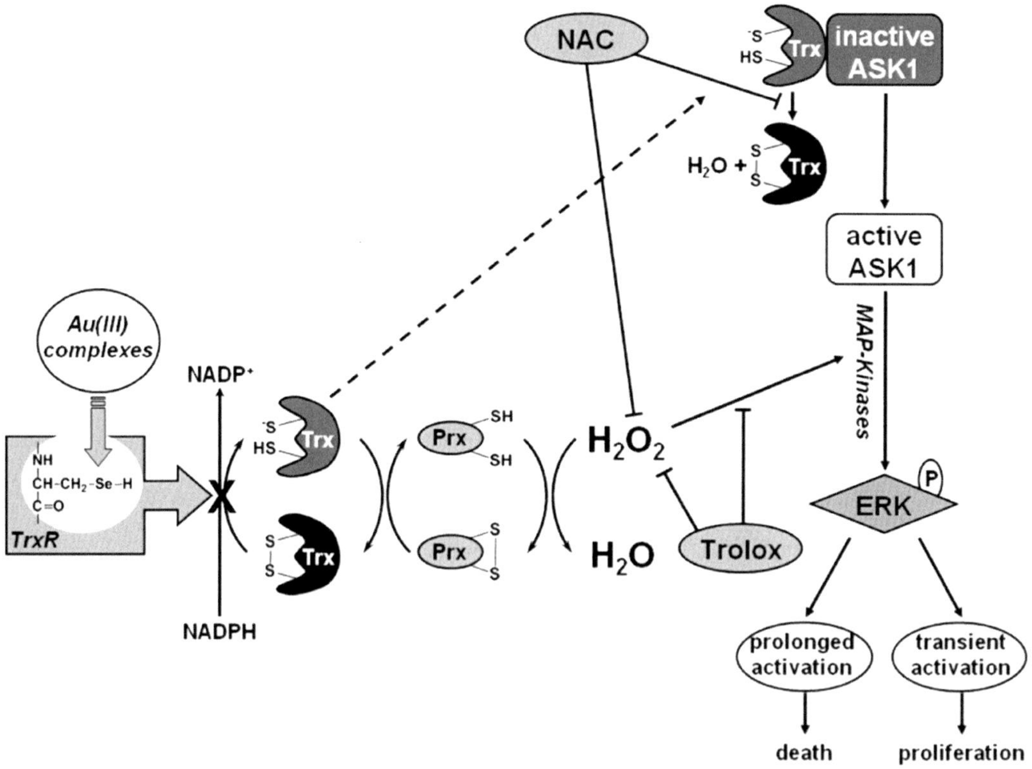

Fig. (8). Proposed model of the molecular mechanisms involved in the gold(III)-dithiocarbamato derivatives-induced cell death (adapted from ref. [57]).

Higher levels of Trx and TrxR, compared to those observed in the corresponding healthy counter-cells from the same patient, are found in many different types of tumors and transformed cell lines [58], including prostate cancer [59]. Increased levels of Trx have been also associated with resistance to several anticancer drugs currently in clinical use for the treatment of prostate cancer, including cisplatin [60] and docetaxel [61]. Therefore, the key role in regulating apoptosis and the high levels of expression detected in different cancer histotypes have prompted interest in the development of drugs that, either on their own or in combination with other chemotherapeutic agents, might target the Trx system [62]. In this regard, we have recently investigated the biological activity and molecular mechanisms of our gold(III)-dithiocarbamato derivatives toward prostate cancer [63], that is, the most common malignancy and the second cause of cancer-related death in males. Despite the benefits of androgen ablation in the early stages of the disease, many tumors recur in an androgen-independent form, with a dramatic increase in the mortality rates [64]. *In vitro* cytotoxic activity was investigated toward the androgen receptor-negative prostate cancer PC3 and DU145 cell lines. Among all, AUL10 resulted to be the best performer, with IC_{50} values about four and ten times lower than cisplatin on PC3 and DU145 cells, respectively. It was proved cytotoxic *in vitro* also against the cisplatin-resistant PC3-R cells, with activity levels comparable to those detected for the parent cisplatin-sensitive PC3 cell line, ruling out (again) the occurrence of cross-resistance phenomena. Further studies showed that the investigated gold(III) complex exerts a powerful cytotoxic effect on PC3 cells by inducing apoptosis, as assessed by Annexin-V and APO2.7 staining assays, which confirmed a strong induction of APO2.7, that is, a mitochondrial membrane protein exposed on the cell surface of cells undergoing apoptosis. Moreover, it induces mitochondrial membrane depolarization, cytochrome-c release and caspase-9 activation, indicating that its activity is exerted through the mitochondrial intrinsic apoptotic pathway. In fact, it significantly reduces the expression of the antiapoptotic protein Bcl-2 and, at the same time, increases the expression of the proapoptotic Bax protein, two regulators playing a major role in the mitochondrial apoptotic pathway [65,66]. Finally, it was proved to cause early cell damage (Fig. **9a**) and to slightly affect the cell cycle (Fig. **9b**), and, in agreement with results above discussed, strongly inhibits TrxR enzyme activity in PC3 cells and induces the production of large amounts of ROS.

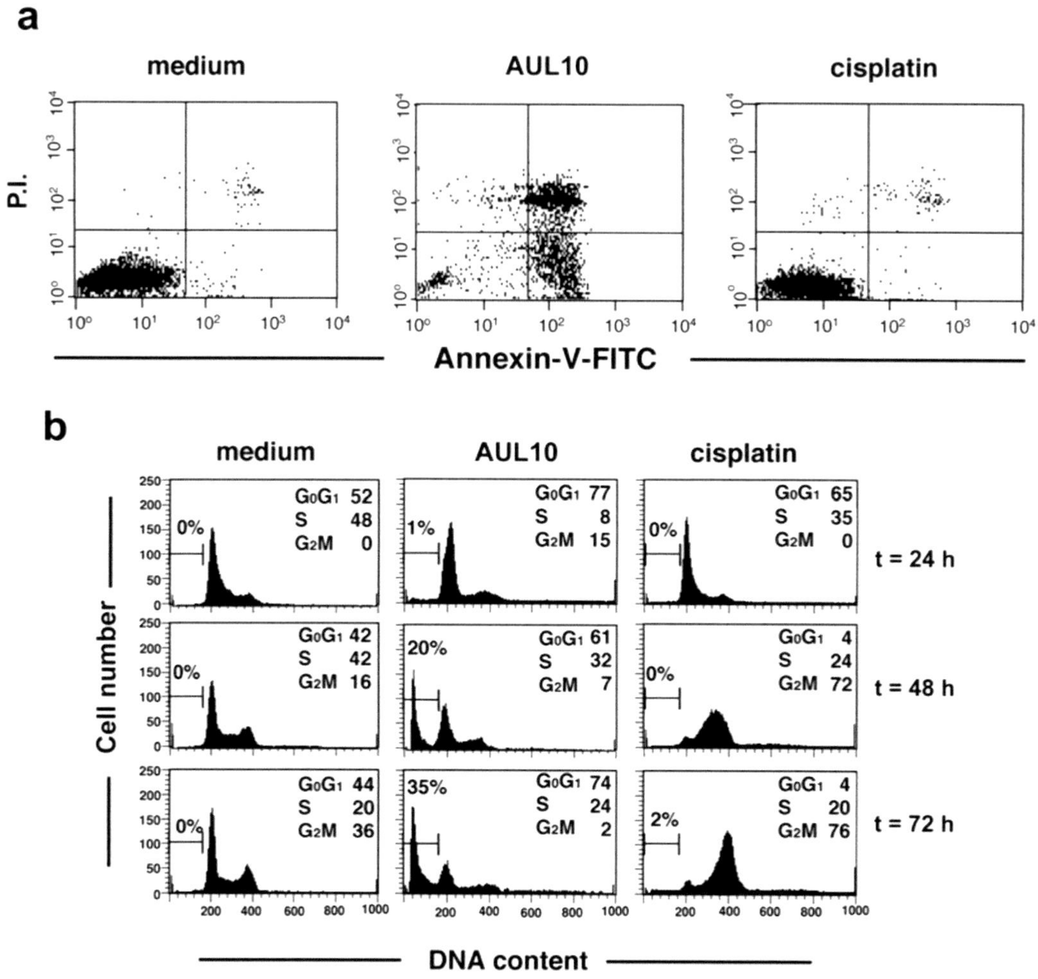

Fig. (9). Induction of apoptosis and DNA fragmentation by AUL10: (**a**) FACS analysis of prostate cancer cells in drug-free medium and after 12 incubation with either AUL10 or cisplatin (5 μM), and double-stained with Annexin-V-FITC and propidium iodide (PI), and (**b**) subsequent detection of DNA fragmentation and cell cycle progression after 24, 48 and 72 h (adapted from ref. [63]).

Androgen-independent prostate cancer is characterized by a greater invasive potential than its hormone-responsive counterpart. A successful therapeutic approach is aimed at suppressing not only cell proliferation, but also the metastatic potential of any cells escaping from the primary tumor site to colonize the bone marrow [67]. As far as we are aware of, our study shows for the first time that an antitumor agent (*i.e.* AUL10), is able to both inhibit PC3 cell migration and reduce the expression of the surface-expressed and phosphorylated forms of the epithelial growth factor receptor (EGFR), whose ligands are paracrine and autocrine growth factors for prostate cancer and are involved in prostate cancer metastasis [68,69,70].

An Intriguing Unexpected Surprise: Proteasome Inhibition

In order to further investigate the mechanism of action of our gold(III)-dithiocarbamato complexes, we have subsequently identified the proteasome as a major *in vitro* and *in vivo* target [71]. The ubiquitin-proteasome pathway (Fig. **10**) plays a major role in the degradation of oxidatively damaged and mutated proteins as well as of proteins involved in cell cycle progression, proliferation and apoptosis [72].

The 26S proteasome is a large multisubunit protease complex, localized in both the nucleus and the cytosol, that identifies and degrades damaged proteins previously tagged by a chain of ubiquitin molecules. The 20S proteasome, the proteolytic core of 26S complex, contains multiple peptidase activities (chymotrypsin-, trypsin- and caspase-like) and acts as a catalytic machine. Ubiquitinated proteins are escorted to the 26S proteasome where they undergo final degradation and the ubiquitin is released and recycled. Aberrant proteasome-dependent proteolysis seems to be associated with the pathophysiology of some malignancies, including cancer, in which some regulatory proteins are either stabilized due to decreased degradation or lost due to accelerated degradation. Therefore, the ubiquitin-proteasome pathway has become an attractive target for the development of new anticancer agents, the validation of which arises from the approval of the proteasome-inhibiting chemotherapeutic agent bortezomib for the treatment of multiple myeloma [73].

The proteasome-inhibiting properties of AUL14 have been investigated [74]. First, it was shown to inhibit cell proliferation on several breast cancer cells. In particular, it exhibited greater *in vitro* cytotoxic activity than cisplatin towards the highly metastatic and invasive estrogen receptor α-negative MDA-MB-231 breast cancer cell line (85% *vs* $<20\%$ inhibition, respectively, both at 5 μM

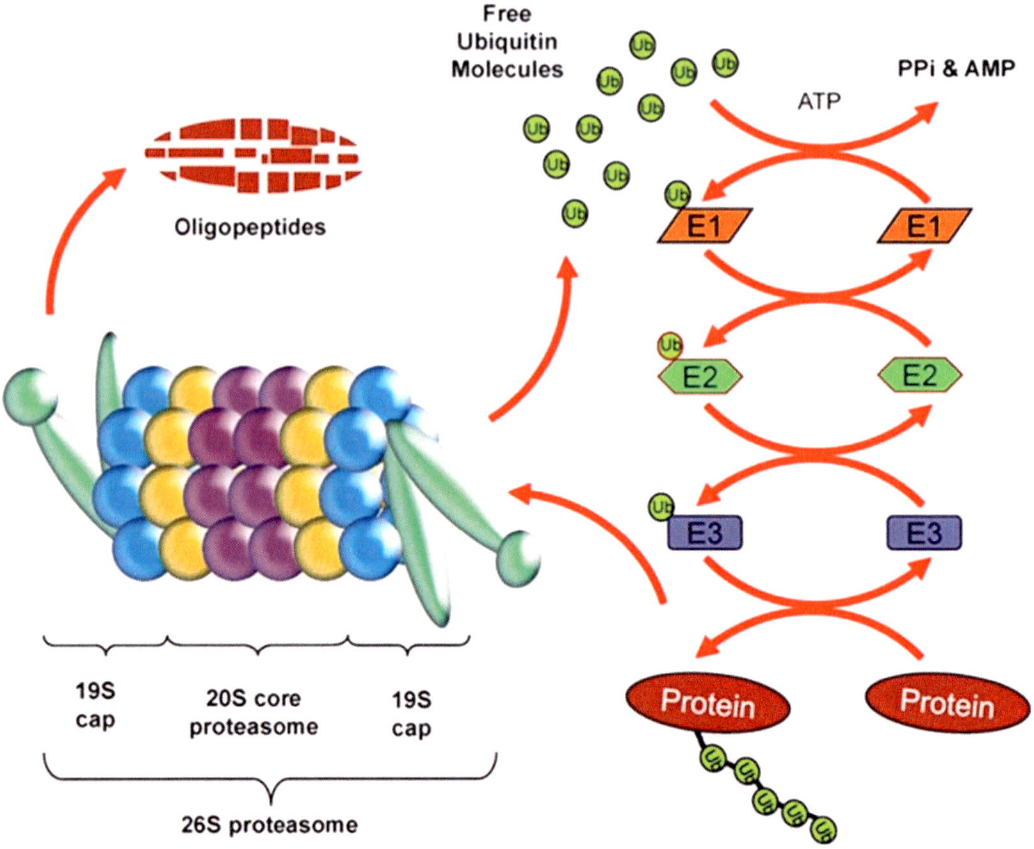

Fig. (10). The ubiquitin-proteasome pathway. A target protein degraded by the ubiquitin-proteasome pathway is first covalently modified by multiple ubiquitin (Ub) molecules in a three-step, highly regulated enzymatic process involving an Ub-activating (E1), Ub-conjugating (E2), and the Ub-ligating (E3) enzymes. The ubiquitinated protein is then escorted to the 26S proteasome, recognized by the 19S cap, de-ubiquitinated and then degraded by the catalytic 20S core into oligopeptides. The ubiquitin molecules are released and recycled (adapted from ref. [72]).

concentration over 24 h). AUL14 was also proved to strongly inhibit the proteasomal chymotrypsin-like activity in MDA-MB-231 whole-cell extract in a dose-dependent way, and this evidence is particularly important since inhibition of chymotrypsin-like activity is associated with growth arrest and/or apoptosis induction in cancer cells [75]. Proteasomal inhibition was further detected in intact MDA-MB-231 cells, confirmed by decreased proteasomal activity and increased levels of ubiquitinated proteins and the proteasome target protein p27. Induction of apoptosis by AUL14 *in vitro* has been confirmed by multiple assays identifying cellular and biochemical hallmarks, such as apoptotic morphological changes, the presence of apoptotic nuclei, and apoptosis-specific PARP cleavage (Fig. **11**).

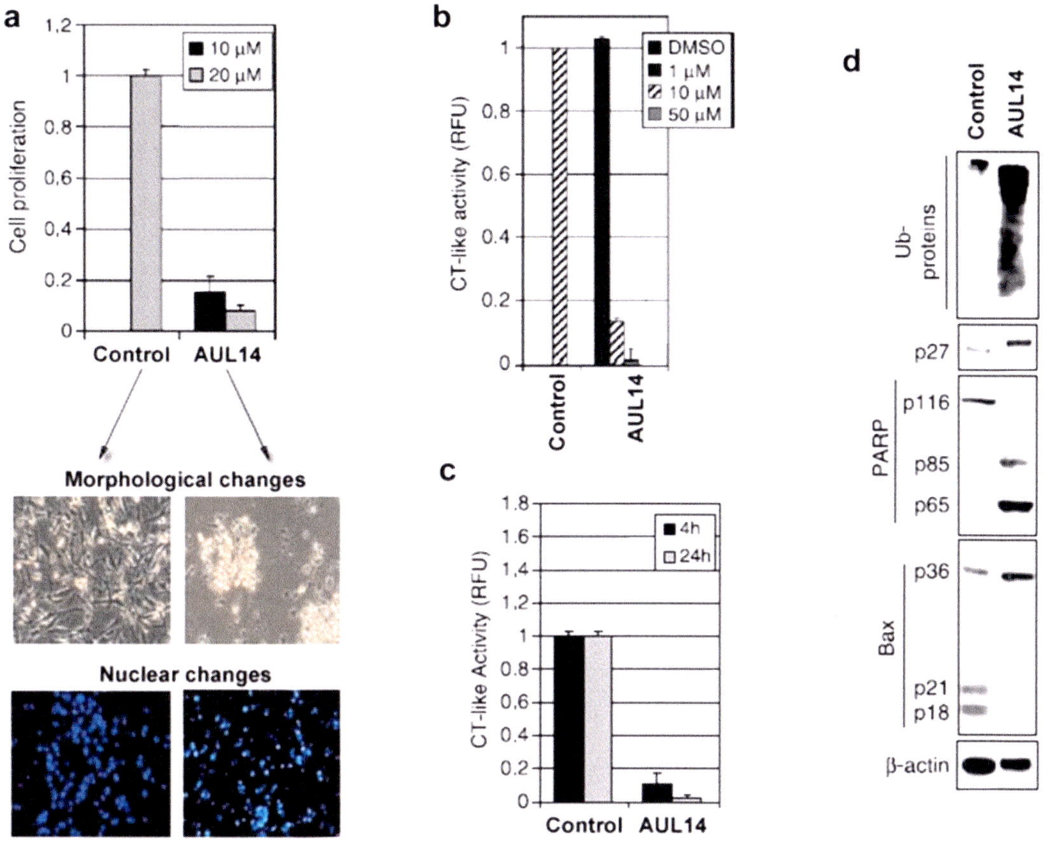

Fig. (11). Inhibition of (**a**) cell proliferation over 24 h, (**b**) chymotrypsin-like activity in cell extract, (**c**) chymotrypsin-like activity in intact cells, and (**d**) apoptosis induction upon treatment of MDA-MB-231 breast cancer cells with AUL14 (adapted from ref. [74]).

Remarkably, proteasomal inhibition and apoptosis induction were proved to be effectively reversed by the addition of a reducing agent. The reversal of AUL14-mediated proteasomal inhibition by L-NAC or dithiothreitol (DTT), was proposed to be the result of the reaction that pulls the complex away from the proteasome, thereby preventing it from binding and, thus, from inhibiting the proteasome itself. On the other hand, it is also possible that L-NAC or DTT could reduce gold(III) to gold(I), an oxidation state that does not have or has lower affinity for binding and inhibiting the proteasome. Another suggested possibility was based on the report that gold(III)-porphyrin 1a induces intracellular oxidation, altering GSH levels in the cell [76]. Therefore, a possibility that AUL14 might stimulate production of ROS that oxidize and inactivate the proteasome was proposed. This hypothesis was supported by a well-established susceptibility of the proteasome to oxidative modification and inactivation upon exposure to free radical-generating systems [77].

As previously mentioned, since gold(III) complexes are often easily reduced to the corresponding gold(I) counterparts (or even to metallic gold) under the generally reducing physiological conditions, when we started our research in the field we could not rule out beforehand that their biological activity might be triggered by the initial reduction of the gold(III) center to gold(I). For this reason, we first synthesized the gold(I) derivative $[Au^{I}(ESDT)]_2$ (AUL15, Fig. **3**) and tested for its *in vitro* cytotoxicity. Remarkably, it was proved to induce a smaller inhibitory effect toward tumor cell lines, compared to the gold(III) analogues $[Au^{III}Br_2(ESDT)]$ (AUL12) and $[Au^{III}Cl_2(ESDT)]$ (AUL13) tested under the same experimental conditions, although its antiproliferative activity was higher or, at least comparable with cisplatin [51]. Nevertheless, in order to evaluate the importance of the oxidation state of the metal center for the mechanism of action and the overall antitumor activity of our gold complexes, we have recently carried out a detailed comparative study on two gold-dithiocarbamato derivatives owning metal centers with different oxidation states, namely AUL12 and AUL15, to provide insights into their possible mechanism of action [78]. When comparing their antiproliferative activities, we found that AUL15 was less potent than AUL12 against human breast cancer MDA-MB-231 cells (IC_{50} = 13.5 and 4.5 μM, respectively; Fig. **12a**). Since both gold compounds own the same ESDT ligand, this finding suggests that the observed effect is mediated by the different oxidation states of the gold centers. In agreement with these results, both compounds were shown to inhibit the proteasomal chymotrypsin-like activity of a purified 20S proteasome (*i.e.* cell-free conditions), AUL15 being less potent then AUL12 (IC_{50} = 17.7 and 1.13 μM, respectively; Fig. **12b**).

Further studies showed that both complexes inhibit the chymotrypsin-like activity of 26S proteasome in human breast cancer MDA-MB-231 cells as well, resulting in decreased proteasomal activity, increased levels of ubiquitinated proteins, and accumulation of ubiquitinated form of the proteasomal target protein IκB-α, and induce cell death by triggering both apoptotic and non-apoptotic (calpain-dependent but DNA-damage-independent necrosis) pathways, AUL12 being (again) more effective than AUL15. The observation that the gold(I) compound displayed a lower cytotoxic profile may point to the lower affinity of gold(I) to the proteasome, since this different effect was observed under cell-free conditions and intact cells. In agreement with our previous reports concerning AUL14 [74], different reducing agents, either DTT or L-NAC, were able to reverse the effects induced by the investigated gold complexes in a cell-free system and in intact MDA-MB-231 cells.

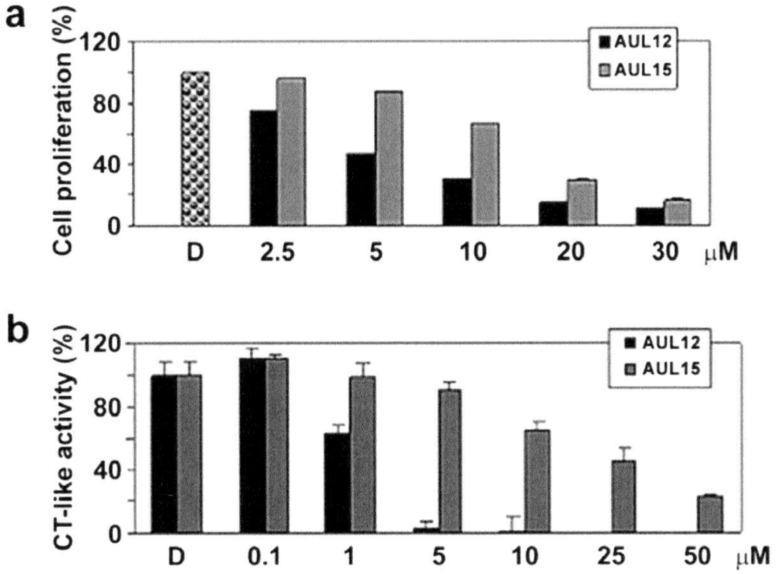

Fig. (12). (**a**) Antiproliferative effect on MDA-MB-231 cells treated for 24 h with either AUL12 or AUL15 at indicated concentrations, with DMSO as a control. (**b**) Inhibition of the chymotrypsin-like activity of purified 20S proteasome in the presence of either AUL12 or AUL15 at the indicated concentrations, with DMSO as a control (adapted from ref. [78]).

Interestingly, the gold(III) complex was able to induce production of ROS in intact breast cancer cells, whereas the gold(I) analogue was not. Furthermore, ROS induction by AUL12 could be effectively blocked by the addition of the reducing agent L-NAC. These results show that ROS induced by gold(III) but not gold(I) compound could be, at least partly, responsible for the observed different proteasome-inhibitory levels. The observation that the treatment with L-NAC and AUL12 could effectively block the production of ROS, argues that the addition of the reducing agent may increase the pool of ROS scavengers, thereby preserving cellular integrity.

In conclusion, we hypothesize that there are at least two mechanisms responsible for the biological activity of these gold compounds, including ROS production and direct interaction of the metal with the proteasome, and the reversion of gold(I/III) compounds-mediated effects by L-NAC could be due to either ROS scavenging or direct interaction with the investigated complexes. Finally, the different activity of AUL12 and AUL15 may result from the different oxidation state (+3 *vs* +1) and geometry (tetracoordinate square-planar *vs* dicoordinate linear) of the gold centers. This is not surprising since it is well-known that the activity of metal complexes is not determined only by the presence of the metal, especially when metals exist in different oxidation states and have rich coordination chemistry. In fact, in that case, even subtle changes in the charge of a metal can result in a significant change in the geometry of the complex, leading to dramatic alterations of its biological properties.

All together, these results clearly identify the proteasome as a primary target of the investigated gold(III) complexes. Anyway, it is worth pointing out that this hypothesis is not in contrast with the previously discussed model related to the TrxR/Trx system as potential target. In fact, it has been recently reported that the proteasome inhibitor bortezomib induces apoptosis through generation of ROS [79]. Since ROS are produced also in our case, the observed proteasome inhibition can favor the long-lasting persistence of phosphorylated ERK-1/2.

In Vivo Anticancer Activity

Among all, the gold(III)-dithiocarbamato derivatives, AUL12 has been selected, due to its overall favorable solubility, stability and antitumor properties, for additional *in vivo* studies.

First, we evaluated the anticancer activity *in vivo* of AUL12 on three transplantable murine tumor models (*i.e.* solid Ehrlich carcinoma, Ehrlich ascites and Lewis lung carcinoma) to confirm the promising results previously obtained *in vitro* toward several human tumor cell lines [80]. Chemotherapy with AUL12 at 10 mg kg^{-1} was proved much more effective than cisplatin toward all three tumor types. Remarkably, treatment of Ehrlich solid tumor-bearing mice with AUL12 induced up to 74% reduction of tumor mass compared to an average 50% inhibition recorded in cisplatin-treated animals (Table **2**). Similar results have been obtained for Lewis lung carcinoma, that is, AUL12 turning out to be the best performer inducing up to 80% inhibition of tumor growth (Table **2**). Analogously, when tested on Ehrlich ascites tumor-bearing mice, the gold(III) complex showed a noticeably higher capability than the reference drug in increasing the lifespan of treated animals (T/C = 157.2 *vs* 130.0%). Intriguingly, 37.5% of AUL12-treated mice survived more than 30 d after tumor implantation (LTS), showing complete tumor regression (Table **3**).

Table 2. *In vivo* anticancer activity toward Ehrlich solid carcinoma and Lewis lung carcinoma (Day 1: tumor implantation; Days 2-7: daily *i.p.* administration of the tested compounds; Day 11: mice sacrificed and tumors explanted)

Compound	Daily Dose (mg kg^{-1})	Average Tumor Weight (Mean ± S.D., g)	Inhibition of Tumor Growth (%)
control	–	0.139 ± 0.01	–
AUL12	5	0.075 ± 0.09	46.04
AUL12	10	0.036 ± 0.01	74.10
cisplatin	3.5	0.070 ± 0.02	49.64

Table 3. *In vivo* anticancer activity toward Ehrlich ascites tumor (Day 1: tumor implantation; Days 2-7: daily *i.p.* administration of the tested compounds).

Compound	Daily Dose (mg kg^{-1})	Average Surviving Time[a] (Mean ± S.D., d)	Anticancer Activity[b] (T/C, %)	LTS[c] (%)
control	–	15.01 ± 0.51	-	–
AUL12	5	18.94 ± 1.23	126.2	12.5
AUL12	10	23.60 ± 2.06	157.2	37.5
cisplatin	3.5	19.50 ± 1.70	130.0	25.0

[a]Survivors excluded. [b]Average surviving time of treated mice *vs* control untreated mice. [c]Long-term survivors 30 d after tumor implantation.

Although such *in vivo* experiments undoubtedly demonstrate the greater anticancer activity of AUL12, it might be argued that these results could have been largely predictable owing to the higher administered dose of the gold(III) compound. Actually, the anticancer activity of AUL12 was shown to be dose-dependent, and the best results were achieved when an approximately three-fold dose, compared to cisplatin, was injected. On the other hand, this choice was not accidental. In fact, for both AUL12 and cisplatin, the maximum daily dose corresponds to one-third of the median lethal dose (LD_{50} = 30 and 11.4 mg kg^{-1}, respectively) calculated under the same experimental conditions, thus allowing the safe administration of such a high amount of the gold(III)-dithiocarbamato complex. Moreover, the effectiveness of this protocol is also supported by the observation that chemotherapy with AUL12 was well tolerated. In this regard, the body weight loss of the animals was recorded daily as a sign of general toxicity. Intriguingly, although mice treated with either AUL12 or cisplatin initially showed a significant weight loss, hosts treated with the gold(III) derivative did not suffer from anorexia and rapidly recovered the lost body weight, whereas those treated with the platinum drug looked prostrate and did not recover the lost weight.

It is worth pointing out that very few toxicity data are available in the literature for gold derivatives, mainly concerning gold(I)-based antiarthritic drugs, such as solganal, myochrysine and auranofin, for which acute toxicity represents a major drawback [81]. Moreover, gold nanoparticles have attracted great attention in recent years because of their unique properties and potential applications in medicine [82]. Unfortunately, toxicity was again proved to be a severe dose-limiting factor [83] Therefore, as far as we are aware of, the LD_{50} value of 30 mg kg^{-1} recorded for AUL12 is among the higher ever reported for gold-based therapeutics, confirming its favorably low acute toxicity profile.

Gold compounds whose anticancer activity has been already reported in the literature have often shown promising *in vitro* cytotoxicity that, unfortunately, was not confirmed by *in vivo* studies afterwards [13]. On the contrary, the *in vivo* antitumor activity of our gold(III)-dithiocarbamato derivatives is fully consistent with *in vitro* results. For example, treatment of MDA-MB-231 breast tumor-bearing nude mice with AUL14 resulted in significant inhibition of tumor growth (*ca.* 50% inhibition upon daily treatment with 1.0 mg kg^{-1} for 29 d, compared to untreated control mice), associated with inhibition of chymotrypsin-like proteasomal activity, accumulation of the proteasome target protein p27, and apoptosis induction, as confirmed by a massive PARP cleavage. Remarkably, during the 29-day treatment, no toxicity was observed, and mice did not display signs of weight loss, decreased activity or anorexia [74]. According to these experimental evidences, proteasome turns out to be a major biological target for this class of gold(III) derivatives not only *in vitro* but also *in vivo*.

Analogously, administration of 1 mg kg^{-1} every other day of AUL10 caused an overall 85% reduction of PC3 prostate tumor in nude mice after a 19-day treatment (compared to control untreated mice) (Fig. **13**) [63]. Remarkably, chemotherapy was well tolerated by treated mice which suffered from minimal systemic toxicity, and histology showed no detectable damages to the main animals' organs. It is worth noting that these results are extremely important since the antitumor activity *in vivo* has been evaluated against a human tumor (xenograft) implanted on immunodepressed nude mice and not just towards a murine tumor, thus providing a more reliable outcome.

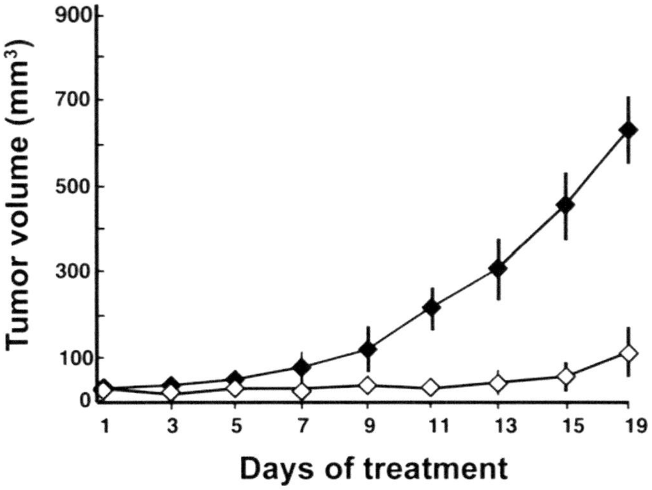

Fig. (13). *In vivo* anticancer activity of AUL10 on PC3 prostate tumor-bearing nude mice (xenografts). Tumor volume was measured in athymic nude mice after subcutaneous injection of either drug-free medium or containing 1 mg kg^{-1} of AUL10 every other day. Tumor volumes were measured three times a week using a caliper. Points (♦: drug-free medium; ◊: AUL10) represent the mean ± SD of eight animals in each group (adapted from ref. [63]).

In Vivo Nephrotoxicity Studies

As previously pointed out, the rationale of our designing strategy was to combine the anticancer activity of the gold(III) metal center with the potential chemoprotective function of coordinated dithiocarbamates so as to avoid/reduce renal failure upon treatment. Therefore, *in vivo* nephrotoxicity studies have been carried out with AUL12 or, for comparison purposes, cisplatin, by measuring some specific biomarkers ion both urines and cortical renal tissues of treated rats [80]. Increased levels of TUP (total urinary proteins), NAG (*N*-acetyl-β-D-glucosaminidase) and GS (glutamine synthetase) activity are widely recognized as signs of a general kidney injury [84]. With reference to Fig. (**14**), as expected [32], cisplatin administration induced a significant increase of TUP excretion, NAG and GS activity in urines, whereas AUL12 caused much smaller changes in the urinary profile compared to control rats, mainly observable at the higher dose (20 mg kg^{-1}).

Several xenobiotic substances damage renal proximal tubule, the portion of the nephron characterized by the greater sensitivity to nephrotoxic effects. It is subdivided into three segments, namely S_1-S_2 (*pars convoluta*) and S_3 (*pars recta*) present in the cortical labyrinth and the medullar rays [85]. It has been recently demonstrated that reduced PAH (*p*-aminohippuric acid) uptake and GS activity in the renal cortical slices of sacrificed treated rats identify specific injuries affecting S_1-S_2 and S_3 segments, respectively [86,87]. With reference to Fig. (**14e**), significant inhibition of GS activity in renal cortical slices was detected in cisplatin-treated rats due to a severe diffuse tubular necrosis of the S_3 segment of the proximal tubule in the outer stripe of the outer medulla, whereas PAH accumulation was not affected (Fig. **14d**), in agreement with data previously reported [32]. Conversely, AUL12 induced no significant changes in the renal cortical biomarkers examined, accounting for negligible nephrotoxicity. This result is extremely positive when compared to the few data reported in the literature related to the renal toxicity induced by gold derivatives. For instance, the antiarthritic drugs auranofin and myochrysine are well known to induce proteinuria and kidney dysfunction [88], and gold nanoparticles are able to penetrate renal cells causing nephrotoxicity [89].

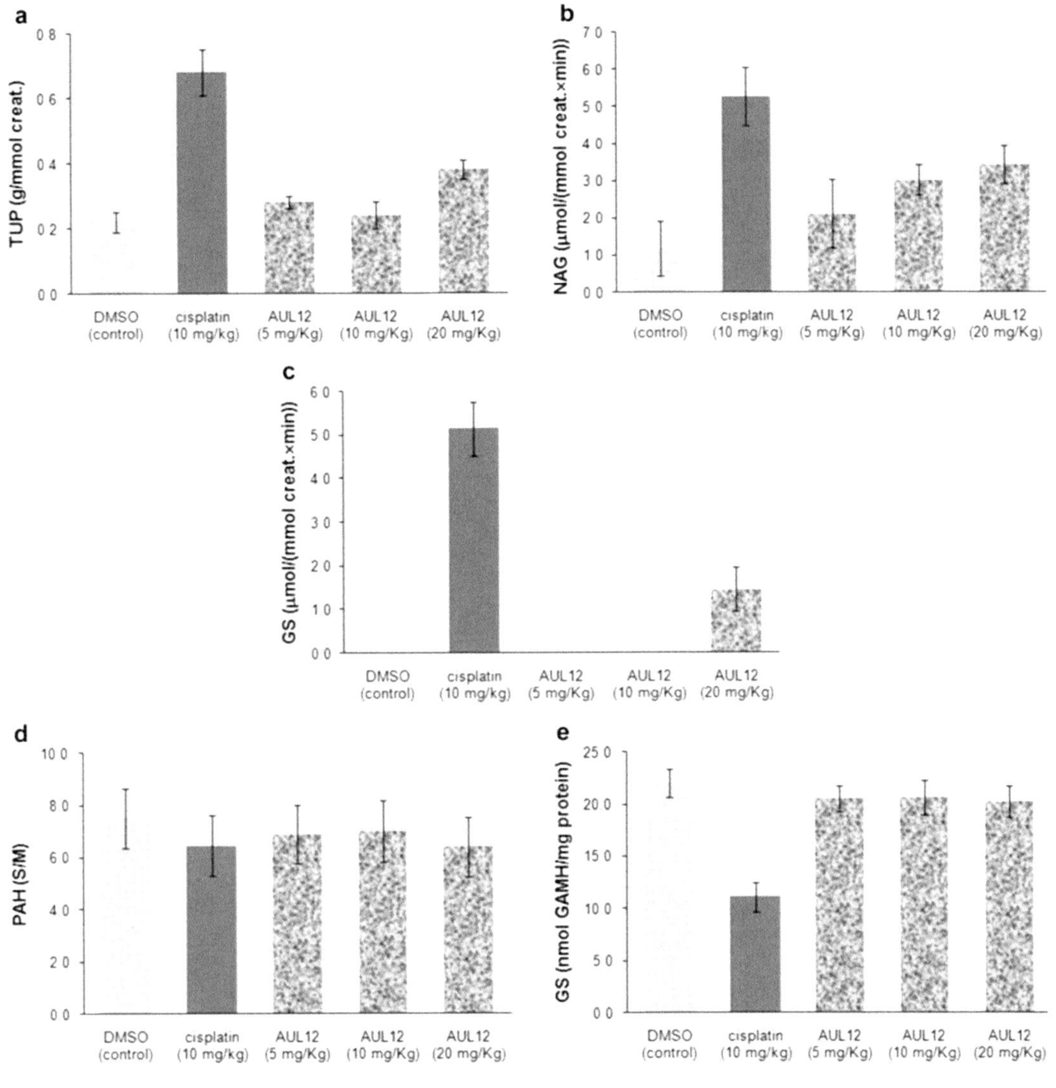

Fig. (14). Urinary and renal cortex profiles of male albino Wistar rats on a single *i.p.* injection of the tested compounds. Evaluation of (**a**) TUP excretion, (**b**) NAG activity, and (**c**) GS activity in urines collected along 24 h after administration, and evaluation of (**d**) PAH uptake and (**e**) GS activity in renal cortical slices of rats sacrificed 24 h after administration (adapted from ref. [80]).

Subsequent histopathological investigations have confirmed the favorable toxicity profile of the tested gold(III) complex. In fact, no significant histologically detectable toxicity involving treated animals' heart, liver, spleen, kidneys, testicles, pancreas, lungs and brain was observed, and SEM evaluation of the surface of all tissues examined were considered compatible with normal conditions when compared to control animals. Surprisingly, no gold was detected in the investigated tissues, thus ruling out the accumulation of the metal in any of the organs taken into account (Fig. **15**). Accumulation around the injection site (*i.e.* peritoneal area) has also been excluded, and these results are in full agreement with the fact that gold seems to be rapidly (within 48 h) cleared from the body, the large majority being excreted through the feces (>89%) and only about 10% *via* the urinary system [80].

Altogether, results reported here confirm that the idea of combining the antitumor properties of the gold(III) metal center with the potential chemoprotective function of coordinated dithiocarbamates is a somewhat winning strategy. The gold(III) compound AUL12 turned out to be extremely promising in terms of greater *in vivo* anticancer activity, reduced nephrotoxicity and acute toxicity compared to cisplatin, thus providing a solid starting point for its validation as a suitable candidate for further pharmacological testing and supporting the filing of a patent related to its use in cancer chemotherapy [90].

More recently, a group of thirteen gold(III) complexes, including AUL12, has been tested at Oncotest GmbH according to a specific comparative *in vitro* strategy for the development of new anticancer agents [91]. Among all, AUL12 turned out to be the second best performer with IC_{50} values in the low micromolar range on all the screened 36 human tumor cell lines, in particular against ovary and brain cancers, and an excellent degree of selectivity (17%). Intriguingly, from a comparative analysis toward 110 reference substances with known modes of action, AUL12 turned out to be the only gold(III) complex covered by this screening study whose mechanism of action did not resemble the mechanism of any of the reference compounds, thus supporting our previous hypotheses [92].

"SECOND GENERATION" GOLD-DITHIOCARBAMATO ANTICANCER AGENTS: TOWARD A TARGETED CHEMOTHERAPY?

Background: the "Trojan Horse"

Recently, the emphasis in cancer drug development has been shifting from cytotoxic nonspecific chemotherapies to molecularly targeted rationally designed drugs promising greater effectiveness and less side-effects [93]. The "magic

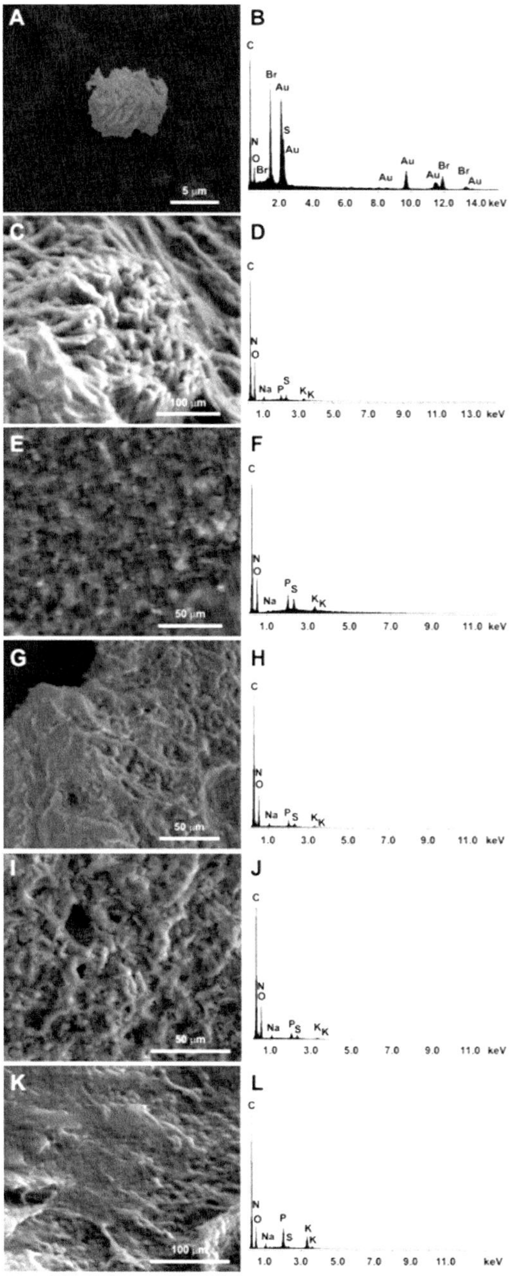

Fig. (15). Selected SEM images of (**a**) a suspension of AUL12, (**c**) heart (30 kV, ×800 magnification), (**e**) liver (30 kV, ×1,602 magnification), (**g**) spleen (20 kV, ×1,500 magnification), (**i**) kidney (20 kV, ×2,021 magnification), and (**k**) testicle (20 kV, ×1,000 magnification) taken at necropsy from male albino Wistar rats sacrificed 48 h after a single *i.p.* injection of AUL12, and associated X-ray microanalysis spectra (**b**, **d**, **f**, **h**, **j** and **l**) (adapted from ref. [80]).

bullet" concept (as first proposed by Ehrlich) [94] may be summarized in one word: targeting. Targeting and delivery are two aspects of drug design that have been receiving much attention in recent years because of the potential for improving efficacy and reducing unwanted side-effects [95]. Tumor cells express many biomarkers and receptors that can be specifically targeted by cytotoxic agents. Conjugated drugs incorporating a tumor targeting group and a cytotoxic "smart bomb" are emerging as promising therapies for cancer treatment.

A major problem of therapeutic effectiveness relies on the crossing of the cell membrane. Cellular uptake of therapeutics is still a challenging task because of the plasma membrane, which constitutes an impermeable barrier for most molecules. In order to overcome this issue, several carrier-mediated delivery strategies have been investigated. Among them, much attention has been recently given to peptide-based delivery systems. Peptide transporters are integral plasma membrane proteins that mediate the cellular uptake of di- and tripeptides and peptide-like drugs (*i.e.* peptidomimetics). Two peptide transporters, namely PEPT1 and PEPT2, have been identified in mammals. They are present predominantly in epithelial cells of the small intestine, bile duct, mammary glands, lung, choroid plexus, and kidney but are also localized in other tissues (pancreas, liver, gastrointestinal tract) and, intriguingly, seem to be overexpressed in some types of tumors [96]. In fact, cancer cells require larger amounts of peptide-bound amino acids for growth and metabolism, and consequently peptide transporters might be upregulated [97]. In this regard, it was recently reported that PEPTs are ubiquitously overexpressed in various types of tumor cells but not in the corresponding healthy tissues [98,99]. A unique feature is their capability for sequence-independent transport of most possible di- and tripeptides inside the cells. These transporters are stereoselective toward peptides containing L-enantiomers of amino acids. Intriguingly, owing to their capability to promote the cellular uptake of potentially all physiologically occurring di- and tripeptides, they can also internalize peptide-like chemotherapeutics resembling the main structural features of small peptides (*i.e.* peptidomimetics). For example, apart from degradation products of nutritional proteins, some peptidomimetic (*e.g.* bestatin, L-dopa), nonpeptidic (*e.g.* valacyclovir, AZT, 5-aminolevulinic acid) drugs and prodrugs, β-lactam antibiotics (*e.g.* cefadrine, cefadroxil, cyclacillin, cefixime, ceftibuten), and some angiotensin-converting enzyme (ACE) inhibitors, such as fosinopril, captopril and enalapril, are recognized by either PEPT1 or PEPT2 as substrates because of their resemblance to di- or tripeptides [100]. Therefore, peptide transporters represent excellent targets for the delivery of pharmacologically active compounds because their substrate binding site can accommodate a wide range of molecules with different size, hydrophobicity, and charge [101], thus acting as "Trojan horses".

Designing Strategy and Preliminary Results

Subsequent to the positive achieved outcomes previously discussed, we have extended our research toward "second generation" gold(III)-dithiocarbamato derivatives of oligopeptides as improved intracellular drug transfer and delivery systems supported by transport proteins. Therefore, during the last three years, we have been developing some gold(III)-dithiocarbamato peptidomimetics that can combine both the anticancer activity and the favorable toxicological profile of the gold(III) analogues previously studied (see above) with an improved tumor selectivity by targeting PEPT1 and/or PEPT2 *via* the oligopeptide chain. The basic idea relies on the potential recognition of the whole metal complex that, once recognized and transported by PEPTs and delivered inside the tumor cell, could exert its anticancer activity without affecting healthy tissues.

Accordingly, we have recently reported on a number of gold(III)-dithiocarbamato complexes of the type [$Au^{III}X_2$(pdtc)] (X = Cl, Br; pdtc = oligopeptidedithiocarbamate) [102] and, among all, the dipeptide derivative [$Au^{III}Br_2$(dtc-Sar-Aib-O(*t*-Bu))] (AUD8, Fig. **16**) turned out to be the best performer.

The choice of such a dipeptide chain was not accidental. We first decided to maintain the sarcosinedithiocarbamato moiety to resemble our "first generation" gold(III) analogues. Moreover, the sarcosine-containing dipeptide Gly-Sar is often used as reference substrate for peptide transport studies because of its good affinity toward both PEPT1 and PEPT2 [103]. Esterification of the C-terminus was proved again necessary; although conferring less water solubility, the bulky *t*-butyl group is unlikely to undergo easy hydrolysis (occurring only in strongly acidic conditions), thus providing stability to the final compound and, consequently, avoiding intramolecular cyclization of the dipeptide chain.

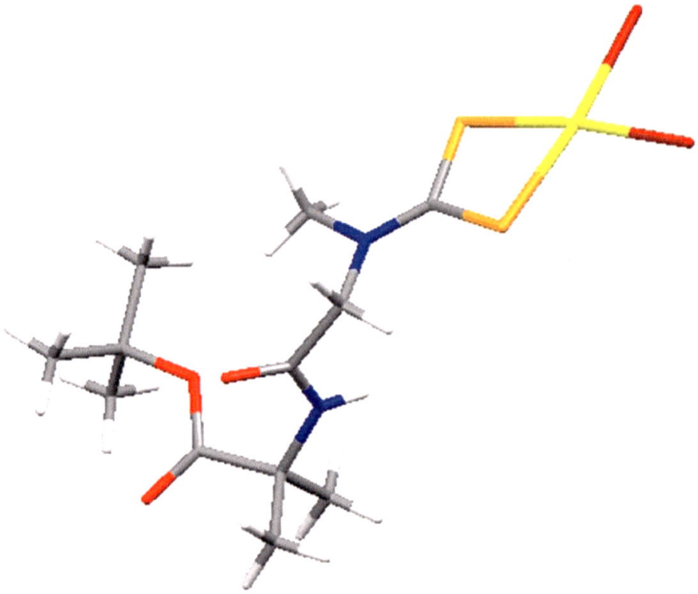

Fig. (16). X-ray crystal structures of [$Au^{III}Br_2$(dtc-Sar-Aib-O(*t*-Bu))] (AUD8).

AUD8 was tested for *in vitro* cytotoxicity toward human prostate cancer (PC3 and DU145), Hodgkin's lymphoma (L540), and ovarian adenocarcinoma cisplatin-sensitive (2008) and -resistant (C13) cell lines over 72 h. So far, the peptide transporters PEPT1 and PEPT2 have not been localized in either the normal genitourinary apparatus or healthy lymphocytes [100]. Therefore, according to our designing strategy, we first evaluated their expression in the selected tumor cells and, remarkably, both peptide transporters were shown to be expressed to a good extent in all five tumor cell lines, thus making them suitable for preliminary screening tests.

The object gold(III) complex was the most effective toward all the human tumor cell lines evaluated, reporting IC_{50} values (in the low micromolar range) up to five-fold lower than cisplatin. In particular, it was proved about 30-fold more active than cisplatin in inhibiting cell proliferation of cisplatin-resistant ovarian adenocarcinoma C13 cells, ruling out the occurrence of cross-resistance phenomena. Remarkably, apoptosis was the major mechanism involved in the growth inhibition of PC3, DU145 and cisplatin-resistant C13 cells. Conversely, it exerted its cytotoxic effect on L540 and cisplatin-sensitive 2008 cells mainly by inducing late apoptosis/necrosis. All together, these results are likely to account for a different mechanism of action compared to that of clinically-established platinum drugs.

The evidence that Aib-containing complex AUD8 showed a higher cytotoxic effect is not surprising. The α-aminoisobutyric acid (Aib) is a natural noncoded amino acid and is abundant in a class of peptide antibiotics (namely, antibiotic peptaibols) exhibiting antiviral and anticancer activity [104,105]. It was recently suggested that Aib plays a crucial role in the biological activity of peptaibols because it forces the peptide backbone to fold into helical arrangements, providing a relevant capability to cross and/or perturb cell membranes [106]. Therefore, the presence of an Aib residue in the gold(III) complex AUD8 might increase its bioavailability and, consequently, the biological activity. Remarkably, its corresponding IC_{50} values are comparable to those reported for the "first generation" analogue [$Au^{III}Br_2$(dtc-Sar-OEt)] (previously referred to as [$Au^{III}Br_2$(ESDT)], AUL12) toward the same tumor cell lines, thus confirming that the favorable anticancer properties are preserved notwithstanding the modification of the organic chain.

Complex AUD8 is currently under investigation for its *in vivo* anticancer activity as well as for the elucidation of the mechanism of action. Should it really resemble the behavior of its previous analogues, we are expecting the proteasome to be a major biological target, and preliminary outcomes seem to confirm this hypothesis. Preliminary up-to-date results are extremely promising, reporting up to 85% and 65% reduction of breast and prostate cancer, respectively, on xenografts, together with negligible acute toxicity (unpublished data), thus supporting our synthetic approach and confirming its the enormous potential. These results represent a solid starting point for the recognition of this class of gold(III) peptidomimetics as suitable candidates for further pharmacological testing and, remarkably, allowed us to file an international patent for their use in cancer chemotherapy (just extended in several countries worldwide) [107].

CONCLUDING REMARKS

Our more than decennial work on gold-dithiocarbamato derivatives as potential anticancer agents is here reported and summarized. The idea of combining the well-known antitumor properties of the gold(III) metal center with the promising chemoprotective function of dithiocarbamates was proved a somewhat winning strategy. Among all, some "first generation" gold(III) derivatives (*e.g.* AUL10, AUL12, AUL13, AUL14) turned out to be the most promising in terms of greater *in vitro* and *in vivo* antitumor activity, reduced nephrotoxic side-effects and negligible acute toxicity compared to cisplatin. The capability to overcome both acquired and intrinsic resistance showed by some types of tumors toward cisplatin confirm that they exert their antitumor activity by activating different apoptotic and non-apoptotic pathways compared to the clinically established platinum-based drugs. Although their mechanism of action has not been completely elucidated yet, some potential biological targets have been considered, and proteasome has been identified as a major *in vitro* and *in vivo* target as well as the mitochondrial selenoenzyme thioredoxin reductase. Nevertheless, further in-depth studies are still in progress.

Anyway, all that glitters is not gold! And this saying well suits our complexes. In fact, despite the positive achieved outcomes, poor water solubility and low selectivity toward tumor cells are still a challenging issue to overcome. Therefore, we are currently exploring alternative routes to improve the therapeutic efficiency of this class of complexes.

In this regard, as a further extension of our previous research on gold(III)-dithiocarbamato anticancer agents, we have been developing "second generation" gold(III) peptidomimetics that are able to maintain both the outstanding antitumor activity and the favorable nephrotoxicity and acute toxicity levels of their "first generation" analogues, together with an improved selectivity toward tumor cells by exploiting peptide transporters. The real breakthrough is not simply the use of gold compounds to treat cancer but the rational design of gold-based drugs which may be very effective, nontoxic, and potentially selective toward cancer cells, their enormous potential impact relying on the possible site-specific delivery in localized cancers, thus strongly improving the cellular uptake and minimizing unwanted side-effects. As far as we are aware of, this appears to be the first time that metal-based peptidomimetic anticancer agents are designed specifically to target peptide transporters. Eventually, this idea appears to be an original and innovative strategy in order to develop novel and more selective chemotherapeutic agents that could provide a valuable alternative to the platinum-based anticancer drugs in clinical use.

CONFLICT OF INTEREST

The authors declare that there is no conflict of interest.

ACKNOWLEDGEMENTS

Financial support from the European Union (Marie Curie European Re-Integration Grant 204828-PEPMIDAS to LR), Fondazione Cassa di Risparmio di Padova e Rovigo (CARIPARO Ph.D. grant to GB), Fondazione Ing. Aldo Gini (overseas mobility allowance to CN), and Fondazione ABO (www.fondazioneabo.org) is acknowledged. The authors are grateful to present and past members of our group and many collaborators who have made important contributions to this research work.

DISCLOSURE

This e-Book chapter is an updated version of the article entitled "Latest Insights into the Anticancer Activity of Gold(III)-Dithiocarbamato Complexes" published in *Anti-Cancer Agents in Medicinal Chemistry*, **2010**, *10*(4), 283-292.

REFERENCES

[1] Rosenberg, B. Fundamental studies with cisplatin. *Cancer*, **1985**, *55*, 2303-2316.

[2] Kelland, L. The resurgence of platinum-based cancer chemotherapy. *Nat. Rev. Cancer*, **2007**, *7*, 573-584.

[3] Sun, R.W.-Y; Ma, D.-L.; Wong, E.L.-M; Che, C-M. Some uses of transition metal complexes as anti-cancer and anti-HIV agents. *Dalton Trans.*, **2007**, 4884-4892.

[4] Bruijnincx, P.C.A.; Sadler, P.J. New trends for metal complexes with anticancer activity. *Curr. Opin. Chem. Biol.*, **2008**, *12*, 197-206.

[5] Reedijk, J. Platinum anticancer coordination compounds: study of DNA binding inspires new drug design. *Eur. J. Inorg. Chem.*, **2009**, 1303-1312.

[6] Kostova, I. Platinum complexes as anticancer agents. *Recent Pat. Anti-Cancer Drug Discovery*, **2006**, *1*, 1-22.

[7] Boulikas, T.; Pantos, A.; Bellis, E.; Christofis, P. Designing platinum compounds in cancer: structures and mechanisms. *Cancer Ther.*, **2007**, *5*, 537-583.

[8] Jakupec, M.A.; Galanski, M.; Arion, V.B.; Hartinger, C.G.; Keppler, B.K. Antitumour metal compounds: more than theme and variations. *Dalton Trans.*, **2008**, 183-194.

[9] Sanchez-Cano, C.; Hannon, M.J. Novel and emerging approaches for the delivery of metallo-drugs. *Dalton Trans.*, **2009**, 10702-10711.

[10] Nobili, S.; Mini, E.; Landini, I.; Gabbiani, C.; Casini, A.; Messori, L. Gold compounds as anticancer agents: chemistry, cellular pharmacology, and preclinical studies. *Med. Chem. Res.*, **2010**, *30*, 550-580.

[11] Kostova, I. Gold coordination complexes as anticancer agents. *Anti-Cancer Agents Med. Chem.*, **2006**, *6*, 19-32.

[12] Berners-Price, S.J.; Filipovska, A. Gold compounds as therapeutic agents for human diseases. *Metallomics*, **2011**, *3*, 863-873.

[13] Ott, I. On the medicinal chemistry of gold complexes as anticancer drugs. *Coord. Chem. Rev.*, **2009**, *253*, 1670-1681.

[14] Tiekink, E.R.T. Anti-cancer potential of gold complexes. *Inflammopharmacology*, **2008**, *16*, 138-142.

[15] Lima, J.C.; Rodriguez, L. Phosphine-gold(I) compounds as anticancer agents: general description and mechanisms of action. *Anti-Cancer Agents Med. Chem.*, **2011**, *11*, 921-928.

[16] Johnson, N.P.; Butour, J.L.; Villani, G.; Wimmer, F.L.; Defais, M.; Pierson, V.; Brabec, V. Metal antitumor compounds: the mechanism of action of platinum complexes. *Prog. Clin. Biochem. Med.*, **1989**, *10*, 1-24.

[17] Aldinucci, D.; Ronconi, L.; Fregona, D. Groundbreaking gold(III) anticancer agents. *Drug Discov. Today*, **2009**, *14*, 1075-1076.

[18] Hanigan, M.H.; Devarajan, P. Cisplatin nephrotoxicity: molecular mechanisms. *Cancer Ther.*, **2003**, *1*, 47-61.

[19] Pabla, N.; Dong, Z. Cisplatin nephrotoxicity: mechanisms and renoprotective strategies. *Kidney Int.*, **2008**, *73*, 994-1007.

[20] Wang, X; Guo, Z. The role of sulfur in platinum anticancer chemotherapy. *Anti-Cancer Agents Med. Chem.*, **2007**, *7*, 19-34.

[21] Dorr, R.T. A review of the modulation of cisplatin toxicities by chemoprotectants. In: *Platinum and Other Metal Coordination Compounds in Cancer Chemotherapy 2*, Pinedo, H.M and Schornagel, J.H., Eds.; Plenum Press: New York, 1996; pp. 131-154.

[22] Jones, M.M.; Basinger, M.A.; Holscher, M.A. Control of the nephrotoxicity of cisplatin by clinically used sulfur-containing compounds. *Fundam. Appl. Toxicol.*, **1992**, *18*, 181-188.

[23] Borch, R.F.; Dedon, P.C.; Gringeri, A.; Montine, T.J. Inhibition of platinum drugs toxicity by diethydithiocarbamate. In: *Platinum and Other Metal Coordination Compounds in Cancer Chemotherapy*, Nicolini, M., Ed.; Martinus Nijoff Publishing: Boston, 1988; pp. 216-281.

[24] Yee, S.; Fazekas-May, M.; Walker, E.M.; Montague, D.; Stern, S.; Heard, K.W. Inhibition of cisplatin toxicity without decreasing antitumor efficacy. Use of a dithiocarbamate. *Arch. Otolaryngol. Head Neck Surg.*, **1994**, *120*, 1248-1252.

[25] Segovia, N.; Crovetto, G.; Lardelli, P.; Espigares, M. *In vitro* toxicity of several dithiocarbamates and structure-activity relationships. *J. Appl. Toxicol.*, **2002**, *22*, 353-357.

[26] Scarcia, V.; Furlani, A.; Fregona, D.; Faraglia, G.; Sitran, S. Palladium and Platinum dithiocarbamato complexes containing mono and diamines. *Polyhedron*, **1999**, *18*, 2827-2837.

[27] Faraglia, G.; Fregona, D.; Sitran, S,; Giovagnini, L.; Marzano, C.; Baccichetti, F.; Casellato, U.; Graziani, R. Mixed platinum(II) and palladium(II) complexes with dithiocarbamates and amines: synthesis, characterisation and cell assay. *J. Inorg. Biochem.*, **2001**, *83*, 31-40.

[28] Marzano, C.; Trevisan, A.; Giovagnini, L.; Fregona, D. Synthesis of a new platinum(II) complex: anticancer activity and nephrotoxicity *in vitro*. *Toxicol. In Vitro*, **2002**, *16*, 413-419.

[29] Marzano, C.; Baccichetti, F.; Trevisan, A.; Giovagnini, L.; Fregona, D. Cytotoxicity and DNA damage induced by a new Pt(II) complex with pyridine and dithiocarbamate. *Chem.-Biol. Interact.*, **2002**, *140*, 215-219.

[30] Fregona, D.; Giovagnini, L.; Ronconi, L.; Marzano, C.; Trevisan, A.; Sitran, S.; Biondi, B.; Bordin, F. Pt(II) and Pd(II) derivatives of ter-butylsarcosinedithiocarbamate. Synthesis, chemical and biological characterization and *in vitro* nephrotoxicity", *J. Inorg. Biochem.*, **2003**, *93*, 181-189.

[31] Alverdi, V.; Giovagnini, L.; Marzano, C.; Seraglia, R.; Bettio, F.; Sitran, S.; Graziani, R.; Fregona, D. Characterization studies and cytotoxicity assays of Pt(II) and Pd(II) dithiocarbamate complexes by means of FT-IR, NMR spectroscopy and mass spectrometry. *J. Inorg. Biochem.*, **2004**, *98*, 1117-1128.

[32] Marzano, C.; Bettio, F.; Baccicchetti, F.; Trevisan, A.; Giovagnini, L.; Fregona, D. Antitumor activity of a new platinum(II) complex with low nephrotoxicity and genotoxicity. *Chem.- Biol. Interact.*, **2004**, *148*, 37-48.

[33] Giovagnini, L.; Ronconi, L.; Aldinucci, D.; Lorenzon, D.; Sitran, S.; Fregona, D. Synthesis, characterization and comparative *in vitro* cytotoxicity studies of platinum(II), palladium(II) and gold(III) methylsarcosinedithiocarbamate complexes. *J. Med. Chem.*, **2005**, *48* 1588-1595.

[34] Giovagnini, L.; Marzano, C.; Bettio, F.; Fregona, D. Mixed complexes of Pt(II) and Pd(II) with ethylsarcosinedithiocarbamate and 2-/3-picoline as antitumor agents. *J. Inorg. Biochem.*, **2005**, *99*, 2139-2150.

[35] Trevisan, A.; Marzano, C.; Cristofori, P.; Borella Venturini, M.; Giovagnini, L.; Fregona, D. Synthesis of a palladium-dithiocarbamate complex: biological assay and nephrotoxicity in rats. *Arch. Toxicol.*, **2002**, *76*, 262-268.

[36] Aldinucci, D.; Cattaruzza, L.; Lorenzon, D.; Giovagnini, L.; Fregona, D.; Colombatti, A. Antiproliferative and apoptotic effects of two new Pd(II)-methylsarcosinedithiocarbamate derivatives on human acute myeloid leukemia cells *in vitro*. *Oncol. Res.*, **2008**, *17*, 103-113

[37] Ronconi, L.; Fregona, D. The Midas touch in cancer chemotherapy: from platinum- to gold-dithiocarbamato complexes. *Dalton Trans.*, **2009**, 10670-10680.

[38] Ronconi, L.; Aldinucci, D.; Dou, Q.P.; Fregona, D. Latest insights into the anticancer activity of gold(III)-dithiocarbamato complexes. *Anti-Cancer Agents Med. Chem.*, **2010**, *10*, 283-292.

[39] Giovagnini, L.; Sitran, S.; Castagliuolo, I.; Brun, P.; Corsini, M.; Zanello, P.; Zoleo, A.; Maniero, A.; Biondi, B.; Fregona, D. Ru(III)-based compounds with sulfur donor ligands: synthesis, characterization, electrochemical behaviour and anticancer activity. *Dalton Trans.*, **2008**, 6699-6708.

[40] Giovagnini, L.; Mancinetti, E.; Ronconi, L.; Sitran, S.; Marchiò, L.; Castagliuolo, I.; Brun, P.; Trevisan, A.; Fregona, D. Preliminary chemico-biological studies on Ru(III) compounds with S-methyl pyrrolydine/dimethyl dithiocarbamate. *J. Inorg. Biochem.*, **2009**, *103*, 774-782.

[41] Nagy, E.M.; Nardon, C.; Giovagnini, L.; Marchiò, L.; Trevisan, A.; Fregona, D. Promising anticancer mono- and dinuclear ruthenium(III) dithiocarbamato complexes: systematic solution studies. *Dalton Trans.*, **2011**, *40*, 11885-11895.

[42] Milacic, V.; Chen, D.; Giovagnini, L.; Diez, A.; Fregona, D.; Dou, Q.P. Pyrrolidine dithiocarbamate-zinc(II) and -copper(II) complexes induce apoptosis in tumor cells by inhibiting the proteasomal activity. *Toxicol. Appl. Pharmacol.*, **2008**, *231*, 24-33.

[43] Nagy, E.M.;. Sitran, S.; Montopoli, M.; Favaro, M.; Marchiò, L.; Ronconi, L.; Caparrotta, L.; Fregona, D. Chemical and biological profiles of zinc(II) complexes containing S-donor ligands for the treatment of cancer. *Submitted.*

[44] Giovagnini, L.; Sitran, S.; Montopoli, M.; Caparrotta, L.; Corsini, M.; Rosani, C.; Zanello, P.; Dou, Q.P.; Fregona, D. Chemical and biological profiles of novel copper(II) complexes containing S-donor ligands for the treatment of cancer. *Inorg. Chem.*, **2008**, *47*, 6336-6343.

[45] Nagy, E.M.; Ronconi, L.; Nardon, C.; Fregona, D. Noble metal-dithiocarbamates: precious allies in the fight against cancer. *Mini-Rev. Med. Chem.*, **2012**, *in press*.

[46] Osswald, H.; Frank, N. Sacrosine- and prolinedithiocarbamate pretreatment increases the therapeutic efficacy of doxorubicin, methotrexate, teniposide, mitoxantrone or cyclohexylchloroethylnitrosourea in leukemia L1210. *J. Cancer Res. Clin. Oncol.*, **1990**, *116*, 448-452.

[47] Ronconi, L.; Maccato, C.; Barreca, D.; Saini, R.; Zancato, M.; Fregona, D. Gold(III) dithiocarbamate derivatives of N-methylglycine: an experimental and theoretical investigation. *Polyhedron*, **2005**, *24*, 521-531.

[48] Giovagnini, L.; Ronconi, L.; Aldinucci, D.; Lorenzon, D.; Sitran, S.; Fregona, D. Synthesis, characterization and comparative *in vitro* cytotoxicity studies of platinum(II), palladium(II) and gold(III) methylsarcosinedithiocarbamate complexes. *J. Med. Chem.*, **2005**, *48*, 1588-1595.

[49] Aldinucci, D.; Lorenzon, D.; Stefani, L.; Giovagnini, L.; Colombatti, A.; Fregona, D. Antiproliferative and apoptotic effects of two new gold(III) methylsarcosinedithiocarbamate derivatives on human acute myeloid leukemia cells *in vitro*. *Anti-Cancer Drugs*, **2007**, *18*, 323-332.

[50] Eastman, A. The mechanisms of action of cisplatin: from adducts to apoptosis. In: *Cisplatin. Chemistry and Biochemistry of a Leading Anticancer Drug*, Lippert, B., Ed.;Wiley-VCH: Weinheim, 1999; pp. 111-134.

[51] a) Ronconi, L.; Giovagnini, L.; Marzano, C.; Bettio, F.; Graziani, R.; Pilloni, G.; Fregona, D. Gold dithiocarbamate derivatives as potential antineoplastic agents: design, spectroscopic properties and *in vitro* antitumor activity. *Inorg. Chem.*, **2005**, *44*, 1867-1881; b) Boscutti, G.; Feltrin, L.; Lorenzon, D.; Sitran, S.; Aldinucci, D.; Ronconi, L.; Fregona, D. *t*-Butylsarcosinedithiocarbamato gold(III)-based anticancer agents: design, *in vitro*, biological evaluation and interaction with model biomolecules. *Inorg. Chim. Acta*, **2012**, *393*, 304-317.

[52] Ronconi, L.; Marzano, C.; Zanello, P.; Corsini, M.; Miolo, G.; Maccà, C.; Trevisan, A.; Fregona, D. Gold(III) dithiocarbamate derivatives for the treatment of cancer: solution chemistry, DNA binding, and hemolytic properties. *J. Med. Chem.*, **2006**, *49*, 1648-1657.

[53] Arnesano, F.; Natile, G. Mechanistic insight into the cellular uptake and processing of cisplatin 30 years after its approval by FDA. *Coord. Chem. Rev.*, **2009**, *253*, 2070-2081.
[54] Koelle, U.; Laguna, A. Electrochemistry of Au-complexes. *Inorg. Chim. Acta*, **1999**, *290*, 44-50.
[55] Minko, I.G.; Zou, Y.; Lloyd, R.S. Incision of DNA-protein crosslinks by UvrABC nuclease suggests a potential repair pathway involving nucleotide excision repair. *Proc. Natl. Acad. Sci. U.S.A.*, **2002**, *99*, 1905-1909.
[56] Bindoli, A.; Rigobello, M.P.; Scutari, G.; Gabbiani, C.; Casini, A.; Messori, L. Thioredoxin reductase: a target for gold compounds acting as potential anticancer drugs. *Coord. Chem. Rev.*, **2009**, *253*, 1692-1707.
[57] Saggioro, D.; Rigobello, M.P.; Paloschi, L.; Folda, A.; Moggach, S.A.; Parsons, S.; Ronconi, L.; Fregona, D.; Bindoli, A. Gold(III)-dithiocarbamato complexes induce cancer cell death triggered by thioredoxin redox system inhibition and activation of ERK pathway. *Chem. Biol.*, **2007**, *14*, 1128-1139.
[58] Lincoln, D.T.; Ali Emadi, E.M.; Tonissen, K.F.; Clarke, F.M. The thioredoxin–thioredoxin reductase system: overexpression in human cancer. *Anticancer Res.*, **2003**, *23*, 2425-2434.
[59] Singh, S.S.; Li, Y.; Ford III, O.H.; Wrzosek, C.S.; Mehedint, D.C.; Titus, M.A.; Mohler, J.L. Thioredoxin reductase 1 expression and castration-recurrent growth of prostate cancer. *Transl. Oncol.*, **2008**, *1*, 153-157.
[60] Yamada, M.; Tomida, A.; Yoshikawa, H.; Taketani, Y.; Tsuruo, T. Increased expression of thioredoxin/adult T-cell leukemia-derived factor in cisplatin-resistant human cancer cell lines. *Clin. Cancer Res.*, **1996**, *2*, 427-432.
[61] Kim, S.J.; Miyoshi, Y.; Taguchi, T.; Tamaki, Y.; Nakamura, H.; Yodoi, J.; Kato, K.; Noguchi, S. High thioredoxin expression is associated with resistance to docetaxel in primary breast cancer. *Clin. Cancer Res.*, **2005**, *11*, 8425-8430.
[62] Powis, G.; Kirkpatrick, D.L. Thioredoxin signaling as a target for cancer therapy. *Curr. Opin. Pharmacol.*, **2007**, *7*, 392-397.
[63] Cattaruzza, L.; Fregona, D.; Mongiat, M.; Ronconi, L.; Fassina, A.; Colombatti, A.; Aldinucci, D. Antitumor activity of gold(III)-dithiocarbamato derivatives on prostate cancer cells and xenografts. *Int. J. Cancer*, **2011**, *128*, 206-215.
[64] Jemal, A.; Siegel, R.; Ward, E.; Hao, Y.; Xu, J.; Thun, M.J. Cancer statistics. *CA Cancer J. Clin.*, **2009**, *59*, 225-229.
[65] Brunelle, J.K.; Letai, A. Control of mitochondrial apoptosis by the Bcl-2 family. *J. Cell. Sci.*, **2009**, *122*, 437-441.
[66] Kang, M.H.; Reynolds, C.P. Bcl-2 inhibitors: targeting mitochondrial apoptotic pathways in cancer therapy. *Clin. Cancer Res.*, **2009**, *15*, 1126-1132.
[67] Bonaccorsi, L.; Marchiani, S.; Muratori, M.; Forti, G.; Baldi, E. Gefitinib ('IRESSA', ZD1839) inhibits EGF-induced invasion in prostate cancer cells by suppressing PI3 K/AKT activation. *J. Cancer Res. Clin. Oncol.*, **2004**, *130*, 604-614.
[68] Di Lorenzo, G.; Tortora, G.; D'Armiento, F.P.; De Rosa, G.; Staibano, S.; Autorino, R.; D'Armiento, M.; De Laurentiis, M.; De Placido, S.; Catalano, G.; Bianco, A.R.; Ciardiello, F. Expression of epidermal growth factor receptor correlates with disease relapse and progression to androgen-independence in human prostate cancer. *Clin. Cancer Res.*, **2002**, *8*, 3438-3444.
[69] Schlomm, T.; Kirstein, P.; Iwers, L. Daniel, B.; Steuber, T.; Walz, J.; Chun, F.H.K.; Haese, A.; Kollermann, J.; Graefen, M.; Huland, H.; Sauter, G.; Simon, R.; Erbersdobler, A.

Clinical significance of epidermal growth factor receptor protein overexpression and gene copy number gains in prostate cancer. *Clin. Cancer Res.*, **2007**, *13*, 6579-6584.

[70] Bratland, A.; Boender, P.J.; Høifødt, H.K. Osteoblast-induced EGFR/ERBB2 signaling in androgen-sensitive prostate carcinoma cells characterized by multiplex kinase activity profiling. *Clin. Exp. Metastasis*, **2009**, *26*, 485-496.

[71] Milacic, V.; Fregona, D.; Dou, Q.P. Gold complexes as prospective metal-based anticancer drugs. *Histol. Histopathol.*, **2008**, *23*, 101-108.

[72] Milacic, V.; Dou, Q.P. The tumor proteasome as a novel target for gold(III) complexes: implications for breast cancer therapy. *Coord. Chem. Rev.*, **2009**, *253*, 1649-1660.

[73] Dalla Via, L.; Nardon, C.; Fregona, D. Targeting the ubiquitin-proteasome pathway with inorganic compounds to fight cancer: a challenge for the future. *Future Med. Chem.*, **2012**, *4*, 525-543.

[74] Milacic, V.; Chen, D.; Ronconi, L.; Landis-Piwowar, K.R.; Fregona, D.; Dou, Q.P. A novel anticancer gold(III) dithiocarbamate compound inhibits the activity of a purified 20S proteasome and 26S proteasome in human breast cancer cell cultures and xenografts. *Cancer Res.*, **2006**, *66*, 10478-10486.

[75] Lopes, U.G.; Erhard, P.; Yao, R.; Cooper, G.M. p53-dependent induction of apoptosis by proteasome inhibitors. *J. Biol. Chem.*, **1997**, *272*, 12893-12896.

[76] Wang, Y.; He, Q.Y.; Sun, R.W.; Che, C.M.; Chiu, J.F. Gold(III) porphyrin 1a induced apoptosis by mitochondrial death pathways related to reactive oxygen species. *Cancer Res.*, **2005**, *65*, 11553-11564.

[77] Szweda, P.A.; Friguet, B.; Szweda, L.I. Proteolysis, free radicals, and aging. *Free Radical Biol. Med.*, **2002**, *33*, 29-36.

[78] Zhang, X.; Frezza, M.; Milacic, V.; Ronconi, L.; Fan, Y.; Bi, C.; Fregona, D.; Dou, Q.P. Inhibition of tumor proteasome activity by gold dithiocarbamato complexes *via* both redox-dependent and -independent processes. *J. Cell. Biochem.*, **2010**, *109*, 162-172.

[79] Perez-Galan, P.; Roue, G.; Villamar, N.; Montserrat, E.; Campo, E.; Colomer, D. The proteasome inhibitor bortezomib induces apoptosis in mantle-cell lymphoma through generation of ROS and Noxa activation independent of p53 status. *Blood*, **2006**, *107*, 257-264.

[80] Marzano, C.; Ronconi, L.; Chiara, F.; Giron, M.C.; Faustinelli, I.; Cristofori, P.; Trevisan, A.; Fregona, D. Gold(III)-dithiocarbamato anticancer agents: activity, toxicology and histopathological studies in rodents. *Int. J. Cancer*, **2011**, *129*, 487-496.

[81] Bird, H.A. Drug toxicity. *Ann. Rheum. Dis.*, **1990**, *49*, 331-336.

[82] Salata, O.V. Applications of nanoparticles in biology and medicine. *J. Nanobiotechnol.*, **2004**, *2*, 3-6.

[83] Ponyala, N.R.; Pena-Mendez, E.M.; Havel, J. Gold and nano-gold medicine: overview, toxicology and perspectives. *J. Appl. Biomed.*, **2009**, *7*, 75-91.

[84] Trevisan, A.; Cristofori, P.; Fanelli, G. Glutamine synthetase activity in rat urine as sensitive marker to detect S_3 segment-specific injury of proximal tubule induced by xenobiotics. *Arch. Toxicol.*, **1999**, *73*, 255-262.

[85] Khan, K.N.M.; Alden, C.I.; Kidney. In: *Handbook of Toxicologic Pathology*, 2nd ed., Haschek, W.M.; Rousseaux, C.G. and Wallig M.A., Eds.; Academic Press: San Diego, 2002; vol. 2, pp. 2255-2330.

[86] Trevisan, A.; Giraldo, M.; Borella, M.; Bottegal, S.; Fabrello, A. Tubular segment-specific biomarkers of nephrotoxicity in the rat. *Toxicol. Lett.*, **2001**, *124*, 113-120.

[87] Cristofori, P.; Zanetti, E.; Fregona, D.; Piaia, A.; Trevisan, A. Renal proximal tubule segment-specific nephrotoxicity: an overview on biomarkers and histopathology. *Toxicol. Pathol.*, **2007**, *35*, 270-275.

[88] Cheriathundam, E.; Alvares, A.P. Species differences in the renal toxicity of the antiarthritic drug, gold sodium thiomalate. *J. Biochem. Toxicol.*, **1996**, *11*, 175-181.

[89] Sereemaspun, A. Effect of gold nanoparticle on renal cell: an implication for exposure risk. *Renal Fail.*, **2008**, *30*, 323-325.

[90] Fregona, D.; Ronconi, L.; Marzano, C. Dithiocarbamate complexes of gold(III) and their use as antitumor agents. *It. Pat.*, **2008**, IT1347835B1

[91] Oncotest GmbH. http://www.oncotest.de/drug-screening/index.php.

[92] Casini, A.; Kelter, G.; Gabbiani, C. Cinellu, M.A.; Minghetti, G.; Fregona, D.; Fiebig, H.H.; Messori, L. Chemistry, antiproliferative properties, tumor selectivity, and molecular mechanisms of novel gold(III) compounds for cancer treatment: a systematic study. *J. Biol. Inorg. Chem.*, **2009**, *14*, 1139-1149.

[93] de Bono, J. S.; Ashworth, A. Translating cancer research into targeted therapeutics. *Nature*, **2010**, *467*, 543-549.

[94] Strebhardt, K.; Ulrich, A. Paul Herlich's magic bullet concept: 100 years of progress. *Nat. Rev. Cancer*, **2008**, *8*, 473-480.

[95] Harper, B.W.; Krauser-Heuer, A.M.; Grant, M.P.; Manohar, M.; Garbutcheon-Singh, K.B.; Aldrich-Wright, J.R. Advances in platinum chemotherapeutics. *Chem. Eur. J.*, **2010**, *16*, 7064-7077.

[96] Rubio-Aliaga, I.; Daniel, H. Peptide transporters and their roles in physiological processes and drug disposition. *Xenobiotica*, **2008**, *38*, 1022-1042.

[97] Rubio-Aliaga, I.; Daniel, H. Mammalian peptide transporters as targets for drug delivery. *Trends Pharmacol. Sci.*, **2002**, *23*, 434-440.

[98] Mitsuoka, K.; Miyoshi, S.; Kato, Y.; Murakami, Y.; Utsumi, R.; Kubo, Y.; Noda, A.; Nakamura, Y.; Nishimura, S.; Tsuji, A. Cancer detection using a PET tracer, ^{11}C-glycylsarcosine, targeted to H^+/peptide transporter. *J. Nucl. Med.*, **2008**, *49*, 615-622.

[99] Landowski, C.P.; Vig, B.S.; Song, X.; Amidon, G.L. Targeted delivery to PEPT1-overexpressing cells: acidic, basic, and secondary floxuridine amino acid ester prodrugs. *Mol. Cancer Ther.*, **2005**, *4*, 659-667.

[100] Brandsch, M.; Knütter, I.; Bosse-Doenecke, E. Pharmaceutical and pharmacological importance of peptide transporters. *J. Pharm. Pharmacol.*, **2008**, *60*, 543-585.

[101] Brandsch, M. Transport of drugs by proton-coupled peptide transporters: pearls and pitfalls. *Expert Opin. Drug Metab. Toxicol.*, **2009**, *5*, 887-905.

[102] a) Negom Kouodom, M.; Ronconi, L.; Celegato, M.; Nardon, C.; Marchiò, L.; Dou, Q.P.; Aldinucci, D.; Formaggio, F.; Fregona, D. Toward the selective delivery of chemotherapeutics into tumor cells by targeting peptide transporters: tailored gold-based anticancer peptidomimetics. *J. Med. Chem.*, **2012**, *55*, 2212-2226; b) Negom Kouodom, M.; Boscutti, G.; Celegato, M.; Crisma, M.; Sitran, S.; Aldinucci, D.; Formaggio, F.; Ronconi, L.; Fregona, D. Rational design of gold(III)-dithiocarbamato peptidomimetics for the targeted anticancer chemotherapy. *J. Inorg. Biochem.*, **2012**, *117*, 248-260.

[103] Geissler, S.; Zwarg, M.; Knütter, I.; Markwardt, F.; Brandsch, M. The bioactive dipeptide anserine is transported by human proto-coupled peptide transporters. *FEBS J.*, **2010**, *277*, 790-795.

[104] Brown, K.L.; Hancock, R.E.W. Cationic host defense (antimicrobial) peptides. *Curr. Opin. Immunol.*, **2006**, *18*, 24-30.

[105] Johnstone, S.A.; Gelmon, K.; Mayer, L.D.; Hancock, R.E.; Bally, M.B. *In vitro* characterization of the anticancer activity of membrane-active cationic peptides. I. Peptide-mediated cytotoxicity and peptide-enhanced cytotoxic activity of doxorubicin against wild-type and p-glycoprotein overexpressing tumor cell lines. *Anti-Cancer Drug Des.*, **2000**, *15*, 151-160.

[106] Toniolo, C.; Brückner, H. *Peptaibiotics*; Wiley-VCD/VHCA: Weinheim/Zürich, 2009.

[107] Fregona, D.; Ronconi, L.; Formaggio, F.; Dou, Q. P.; Aldinucci, D. Gold(III) complexes with oligopeptides functionalized with sulfur donors and use thereof as antitumor agents. *PCT Int. Appl.*, **2010**, WO2010105691A1.

Send Reprints Orders on reprints@benthamscience.net

Advances in Anticancer Agents in Medicinal Chemistry, 2013, Vol. *2*, 173-253

CHAPTER 4

Toward Anticancer Therapeutics Based on Glycidic Structures

Luca Gabrielli, Alice Capitoli, Laura Russo, David Bini, Francesca Taraballi, Cristina Lupo and Laura Cipolla*

Department of Biotechnology and Biosciences, University of Milano-Bicocca, P.za della Scienza 2, 20126 Milano, Italy

Abstract: Recent efforts in the design and synthesis of potential anti-cancer vaccines based on carbohydrates are outlined, covering literature up to 2012. This approach capitalises on the fact that cancer cells often display alterations in their glycan repertoire if compared to normal cells, resulting in the accumulation of new structures, usually referred as to tumour-associated carbohydrate antigens (TACA). Several preclinical and clinical studies demonstrate that naturally acquired, passively administered, or actively induced antibodies against TACAs are able to eliminate circulating tumour cells and micro-metastases in cancer patients. TACAs can be ideal candidates to elicit an antitumor immune response, however they are often not immunogenic enough to induce protection, since many of them are of embryonic origin or expressed in normal tissue, even if at low levels, and consequently tolerated by the immune system. Approaches toward breaking self-tolerance in the design of novel glycocnjugates structures, together with new conjugation methods appeared in the last years will be considered.

Keywords: Glycopeptides, glyconanoparticles, tumour-associated carbohydrate antigens, glycoconjugates, anti-tumour vaccines.

1. HISTORICAL INTRODUCTION

As far as the late 19th century, the idea emerged that the immune system can recognise and hence react against tumours, and several decades later it was demonstrated that tumour-rejection antigens are tumour-specific [1, 2]. The concept that the immune system can recognize and destroy nascent transformed cells was initially proposed by Burnet [3] and Thomas [4], later supported by the existence of cancer immunosurveillance and evidence of a more general process

***Address correspondence to Laura Cipolla:** Department of Biotechnology and Biosciences, University of Milano-Bicocca, P.za della Scienza 2, 20126 Milano, Italy; Tel: +39 02 64483460; Fax: 39 02 64483565; E-mail: laura.cipolla@unimib.it

Michelle Prudhomme (Ed)

of cancer immunoediting [5]. Since then, research focused on the development of cancer vaccines [6], considered as specific active immunotherapy of cancer (as opposed to adaptive or passive immunotherapy) which entails immunizing patients against the antigens that are expressed in cancer cells with the goal of eradicating these cancer cells. In the design of a vaccine to treat cancer, one must first identify structural features unique to malignant transformed tumour cells, which may be exploited to prompt the immune system to recognise the cancer cells as "nonself". In this context, it is now well known that altered glycosylation patterns either on glycoproteins or glycolipids are a hallmark of the tumour phenotype. This phenomenon was first described by Meezan *et al.* in 1969 with the demonstration that healthy fibroblasts have smaller membrane glycoproteins than their transformed counterparts [7]. This finding was later corroborated with histological evidence that lectins show differential binding to healthy compared with malignant tissue [8]. More recently, cancer-associated cell-surface glycans have been directly characterized using specific monoclonal antibodies and mass spectrometry [9], have been introduced changes, very recently, advanced NMR techniques Changes in glycosylation include both the under- and overexpression of naturally-occurring glycans, as well as neo-expression of glycans normally restricted to embryonic tissues, most often arising from changes in the expression levels of glycosyltransferases in the Golgi compartment of cancerous cells. One of the most common changes is an increase in the size and branching of *N*-linked glycans, often due to an increased activity of *N*-acetylglucosaminyltransferase V (GlcNAc-TV, also known as MGAT5; the enzyme that leads to β1,6GlcNAc branching). The increased branching creates additional sites for terminal sialic acid residues, which, in conjunction with a corresponding upregulation of sialyltransferases, ultimately leads to an increase in global sialylation [10].

Tumour-Associated Carbohydrate Antigens (TACAs) can be categorized into two major groups (Fig. **1**): glycolipids such as GM2, GD2, GD3, and fucosyl GM1 (gangliosides), and Lewis y (Le^y) and globo H (neutral glycolipids); glycoproteins, such as the mucin-related epitopes Tn (GalNAcα-O-Ser/Thr), TF or T (Thomsen-Friedenreich, Galβ1→3GalNAcα-O-Ser/Thr) and sTn (NeuAcα2→6GalNAcα-O-Ser/Thr) [11].

Glycolipids such as GM2, GD2, GD3, 9-*O*-acetyl GD3, fucosyl GM1, Lewis y, and globo H are attached to the lipid bilayer at the cell surface by hydrophobic forces through the ceramide moiety. In glycoproteins, carbohydrate antigens such as Thomsen-Friedenreich, sialylated Tn, Tn, Le^y and globo H are generally attached to the hydroxyl group of serine or threonine in mucins (MUC) through a glycosidic linkage (*O*-linked), but may also be *N*-linked to other proteins through asparagine. Whether expressed as glycolipids or glycoproteins, these antigens are more abundantly expressed at the cell surface than any protein antigens, and the immune response appears to be predominantly against the carbohydrate moiety.

Many of these epitopes are observed in malignant tissues throughout the body (Table **1**), including the brain, breast, colon and prostate.

Table 1. Common TACAs Expressed on Malignant Tissues[a]

Tumour	Antigens
B cell lymphoma	GM2, GD2
Breast	GM2, Globo H, TF(c)[b], Le^y
Colon	GM2, TF(c), sTn(c), Le^y, Tn, sLe^a
Lung	GM2, Globo H, Le^y
Melanoma	GM2, GD2, GD3L, GD3
Neuro-blastoma	GM2, GD2, GD3L, PSA
Ovary	GM2, Globo H, TF(c), sTn(c), Le^y, Gb_3
Prostate	GM2, Globo H, TF(c), Tn(c), sTn(c), Le^y
Sarcoma	GM2, GD2, GD3L, GD3
Small cell Lung cancer	GM2, FucGM1, Globo H, PSA, sLe^a
Stomach	GM2, Le^y, Le^a, sLe^a

[a]Based on Ref. [99b]; [b](c) = clustered.

Another common feature of tumours is the overproduction of certain glycoproteins and glycolipids. For example, epithelial tumours often overproduce mucin glycoproteins, which are characterized by dense clusters of *O*-linked glycans. Mucins are highly *O*-glysosylated proteins (about 75% of total weight) expressed on endodermal epithelial cells. Mucins are used as diagnostic markers

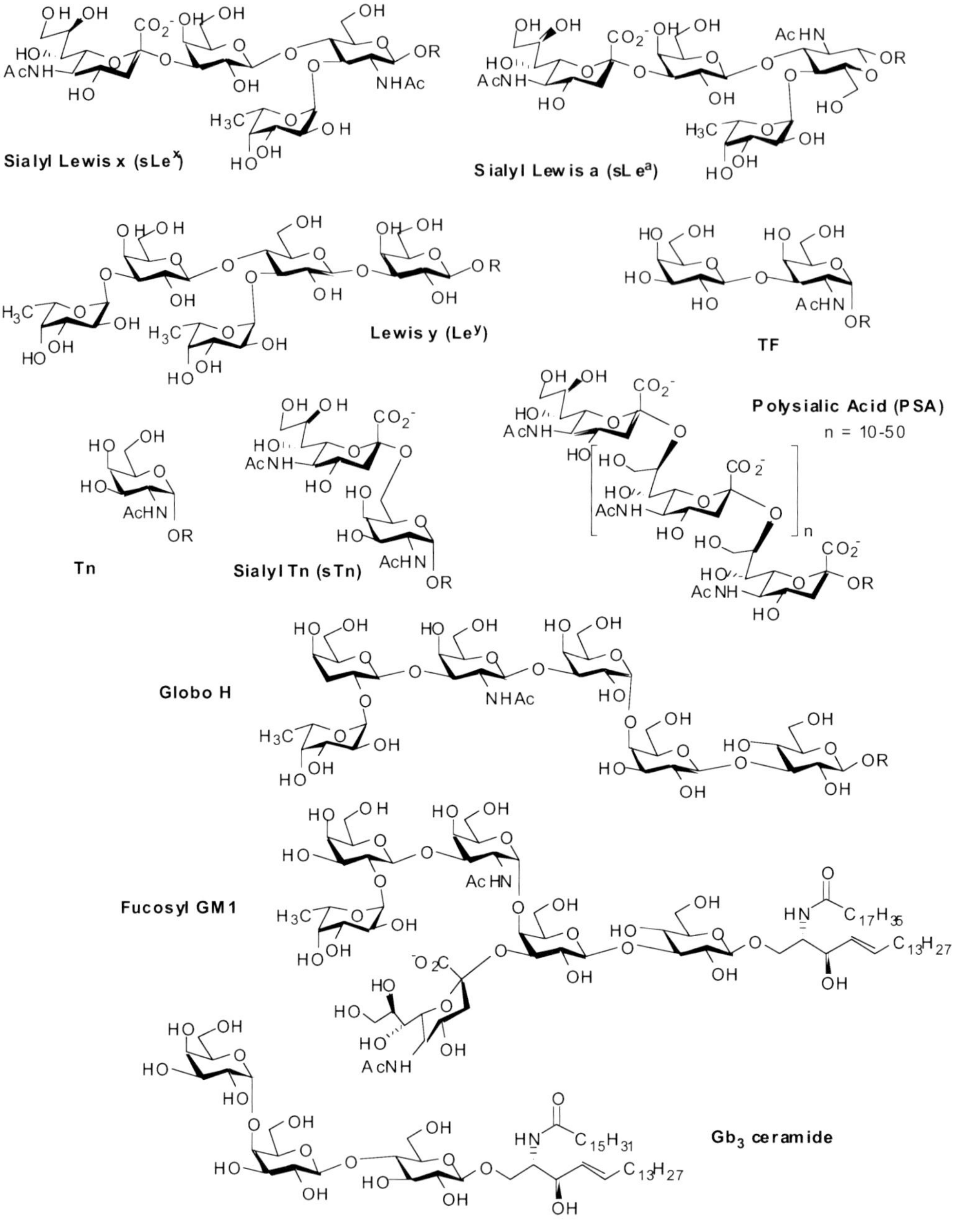

Fig. (1). Tumour-Associated Carbohydrate Antigens (TACAs).

of cancer and can also function as scaffolds for most of the above-listed cancer-associated epitopes [12]. Additionally, cancer tissues can display an increase in ganglioside expression. For example, complex gangliosides (for example, GD2,

GD3 and fucosyl GM1) are found at elevated levels in small-cell lung carcinomas, neuroblastomas and melanomas [11b]. Among cancer-associated antigens, T, Tn, sialyl-Tn (sTn) and the ganglioside GM2 are the most well known. TF, Tn, and sTn (Fig. **1**), antigens are expressed in carcinoma-associated mucins. The Tn structure in normal cells is cryptic since it is further glycosylated to construct complex *O*-linked glycans on mucin-type glycoproteins, whereas in most human carcinomas this cryptic structure is exposed at the cellular surface due to incomplete synthesis of carbohydrate chains. Increased expression of Tn and STn antigens has been correlated with tumour aggressiveness and poor prognosis in a number of epithelial tumours. In addition to Tn and sTn, T antigen (also known as the Thomsen-Friedenreich TF antigen), is often referred to as a tumour-associated blood group antigen. Although gross changes in glycosylation of tumour tissues are apparent, no single change seems to distinctly differentiate normal and malignant cells. Instead, each type of malignant tissue is characterized by a distinct set of changes in glycan expression (Table **1**).

2. CARBOHYDRATE-BASED ANTICANCER VACCINES: GENERAL CONSIDERATIONS

Because cancer cell glycans differ from those found on their healthy counterparts, it might be possible to recruit the immune system to target cancer cells on the basis of their altered glycosylation. Although atypical glycans can render cancer cells mildly antigenic, they are rarely immunogenic [13]. Many tumour-associated glycans have an embryonic origin or are expressed at low levels in normal tissue and at elevated levels on tumours, in which cases B cells expressing high-affinity antibodies for these structures would have been eliminated during development [14]. Consequently, the glycans can be perceived as 'self' by the human immune system; for this reason, many attempts at generating anticancer vaccines have focused on breaking immune self-tolerance for tumour-associated glycans [15]. Furthermore, complicating factors arise from the degree of heterogeneity of carbohydrates expressed on the tumour cell surface, even within a particular cancer type [16].

The development of a clinically active carbohydrate-based vaccine is a long-standing goal for the treatment and the prevention of cancer and metastasis. Successful tumour immunotherapy might require a T-cell-mediated immune response, in addition to B-cell response. However, till recently it has been believed that carbohydrate-based antigens raise a T-cell independent humoral response, so that the immune system, upon vaccination with tumour-associated carbohydrate-containing constructs reacts with short-lived B-cell immunoglobulins (Ig)M with poor memory and without the support typically provided by T-cells. In recent years several reports provided evidence that carbohydrate-based vaccines do result in a T-cell response [17]. Moreover, additional studies establish the feasibility of tumour-associated carbohydrate antigen-presenting glycopeptides as CD8+ T-cell-based vaccines [18, 19].

There are different strategies in order to pursue an immune responce, including mimicking the cancer cell surface by displaying vaccine glycans in a multivalent context, or chemically modifying cancer glycans to make them more 'foreign', and actively recruiting T-cell. Each of these glycan-based strategies will be discussed.

In the past two decades, research has focused on many aspects of vaccine construction: choice of antigen [15a], development of procedures for the synthesis [20] or isolation of antigens, conjugation to an appropriate immunogenic carrier [21], and selection of adjuvants for coadministration [22]. However, advances in immune system knowledge must be flanked by sound synthetic carbohydrate and glycoconjugate chemistry, which is still challenging and hard task, even if the synthesis can now rely on efficient methods. In the next section, these will be briefly outlined. It's not unreasonable to belive that, while carbohydrates themselves may not be particularly immunogenic, their conjugation to an appropriate carrier may well overcome this problem [23, 24].

3. SYNTHETIC STRATEGIES TOWARDS GLYCOCONJUGATES

The synthesis of merely the core fragments, the regions in closest proximity to the polypeptide backbone, can require complex orthogonal protection schemes to form branched oligosaccharide structures. The methods for such transformations that are currently at our disposal are not compatible with the complex functionality of the polypeptide backbone, precluding the chemical elaboration of the oligosaccharide from the polypeptide scaffold [25]. Despite these challenges, some impressive structures have been reported [26]. In addition, advances in glycosylation methods, including enzymatic methodologies [27-29] and in recombinant DNA technologies [30, 31] promise to relieve the strain of protecting-group manipulations in glycoprotein syntheses.

Typically, syntheses of glycoconjugates adopt one of three strategies. The first is the linear assembly of glycosylated amino acids using protected glycosylated amino acids as building blocks for automated solid-phase peptide synthesis (SPPS) to generate glycosylated peptide fragments [32] (Fig. **3A**). Fmoc-based peptide synthesis methods are sufficiently mild that the oligosaccharide remains intact throughout the synthesis. The linear assembly of glycosylated amino acids in particular usually provides well-defined products; following this approach, the required carbohydrate structure is attached to an amino acid residue, typically serine and threonine for *O*-linked glycopeptides and asparagine for *N*-linked glycopeptides [33-35] (Fig. **2**).

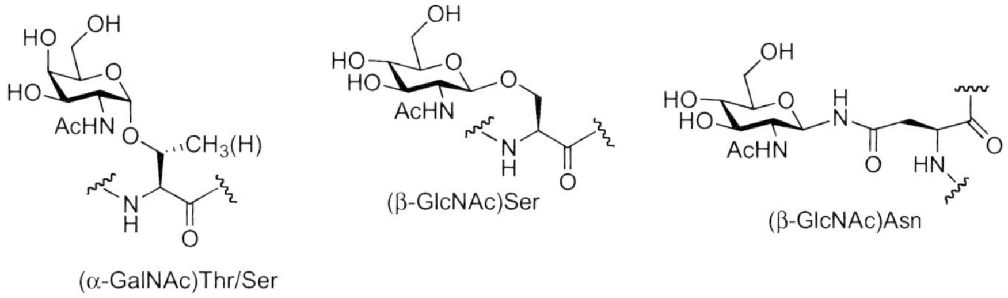

Fig. (2). Common *O*-linked serine and threonine glycosides and *N*-linked asparagine glycosides found in protein glycosylation.

Factors limiting the synthesis are the need of extensive carbohydrate and amino acid protection and the chemical lability of the glycosidic bond with the amino acid residues [32, 34, 36, 37]. In general, peptides larger than 50-60 residues are difficult to obtain due to low yields and by-products.

Convergent condensation of unprotected or partially protected peptide/ glycopeptide segments has been proposed as alternative approach to total synthesis of glycoproteins (Fig. **3B**) (see next section), and Fig. (**3C**).

3.1. Strategies for the Construction of the Oligosaccharidic Chain

Two general strategies can be used for oligosaccharide production: enzymatic (or chemoenzymatic syntheses) and chemical synthesis. In enzymatic and chemoenzymatic routes, saccharide intermediates are elaborated with enzymes, typically glycosyltransferases or glycosidases, to generate oligosaccharides (Fig. **4A**) [38-40].

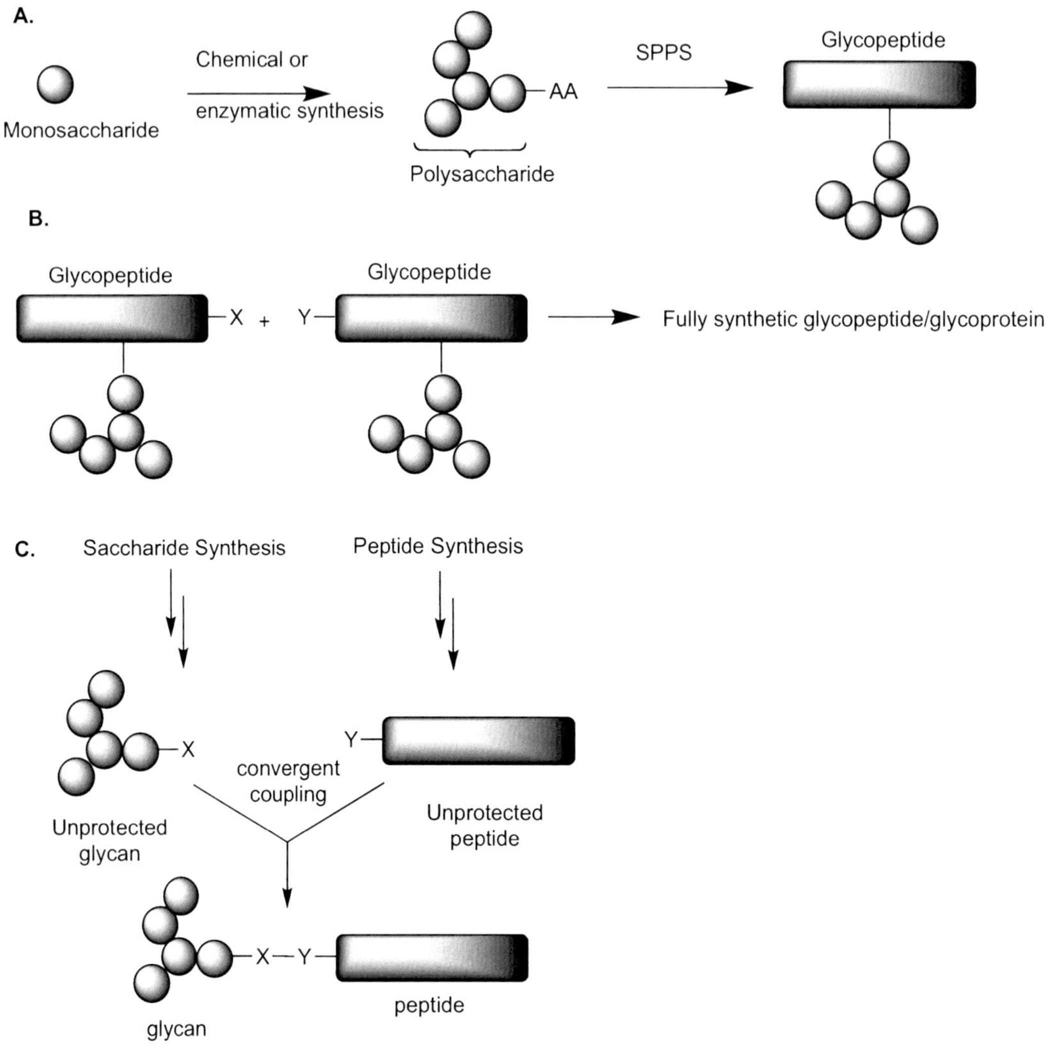

Fig. (3). General strategies for glycopeptide/glycoprotein synthesis.

In chemical synthesis [41], the appropriate building blocks are produced and assembled into oligosaccharides (Fig. **4B**). Enzymes perform glycosylation with absolute regio- and stereocontrol; enzymatic synthesis is limited by the availability of the required enzyme. On the other hand, chemical synthesis is much more flexible, since both natural and non-natural saccharide building blocks can be assembled with natural or non-natural linkages but it requires stereochemical and regiochemical control in glycosidic linkage formation. Remarkables advances in carbohydrate chemistry have been done in the last few years [29] and many complex, highly branched oligosaccharides have been prepared [23, 42], using solution- and/or solid-phase approaches [43], and automated oligosaccharide syntheses have been developed [44]. Recent advances in glycosylation methods [45] comprise, among others, the glycal assembly method proposed by Danishefsky and co-workers [20, 46], Boons [47], Kunz [48]. More recently Davis [49] described a strategy for the construction of glycoconjugate vaccines, using glycosyl disulphide donors for the oligosaccharide's synthesis. Their aglycon flexibility allows iterative assembly of complex carbohydrates and protective group freedom since the "armed" or "disarmed" disulphide status is altered through the aglycon rather than the protective groups of the sugar. Moreover the use of glycosyl disulphides delivers glycosyl thiol products that are suitable for site-specific protein ligation. Two major advances are being applied to make more efficient the chemical synthesis of oligosaccharides: one-pot reactions [29i, 50] and polymer-supported synthesis [42, 44, 51, 52]. Progress on this front has also facilitated the generation of oligosaccharide libraries containing up to 1300 compounds [53].

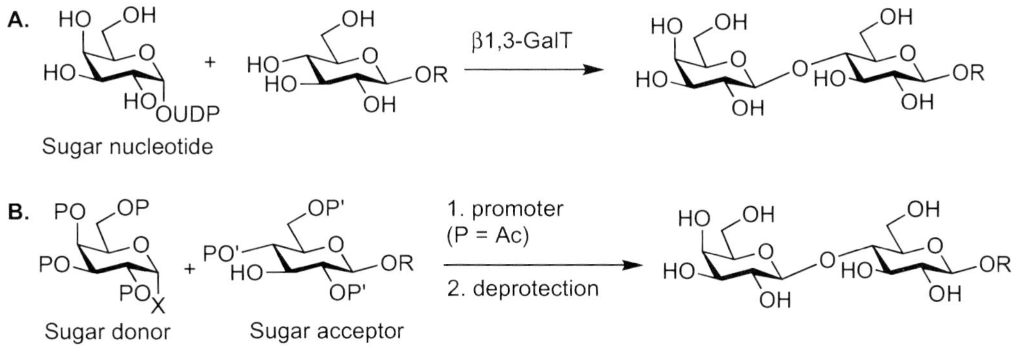

Fig. (4). General stategies for oligosaccharide productions.

3.2. Glycosidic Bond Formation Between the Oligosaccharide and the Amino Acid/Peptide Moieties

Three main strategies can be applied to the glycosidic bond formation between the glycan moiety and the peptide moiety for the formation of short glycopeptides (Fig. **5**).

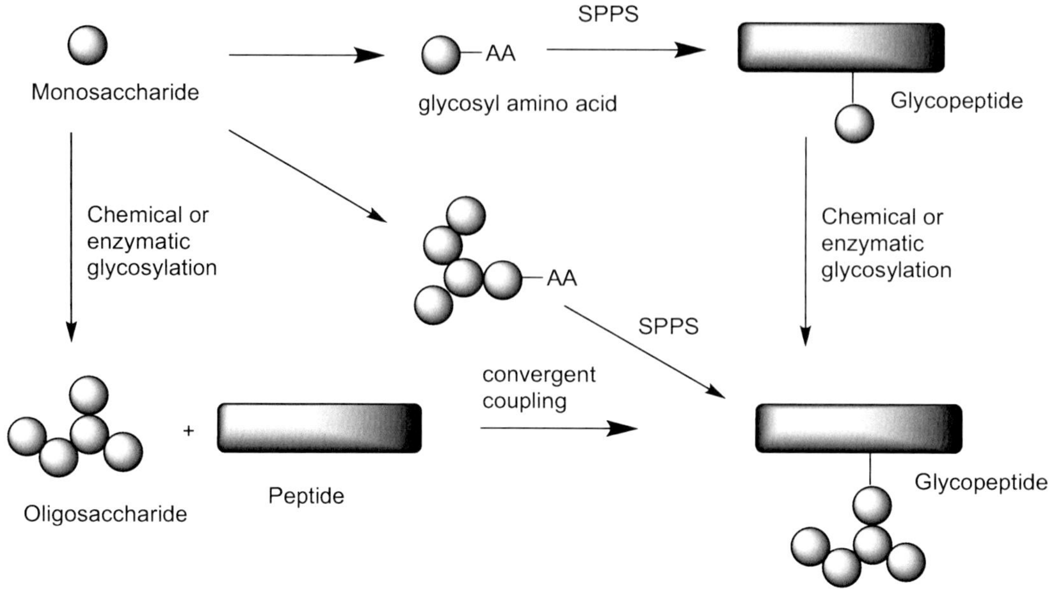

Fig. (5). General strategies for the synthesis of short glycopeptides.

Most commonly, pre-formed protected glycosylated amino acids building blocks are employed in the stepwise assembly of the peptide preferentially *via* automated solid-phase peptide synthesis (SPPS) to generate glycosylated peptide fragments [32, 37]. It is important to note that *O*-glycosidic and intersaccharidic linkages are relatively labile towards acids [54]. Under strongly basic conditions, β-elimination of the carbohydrate may also occur at the *O*-linked serine and threonine glycosides [55]. Thus, the proper selection of protecting groups, which is necessary to block the functional groups on both the glycan and the peptide part, is a matter of importance for the solid-phase as well as solution-phase synthesis of glycopeptides. It has been found that the glycosidic linkages of fully acylated carbohydrates can withstand short treatment with TFA used for removal of side-chain protecting groups of amino acids. Furthermore, β-elimination of the *O*-linked serine and threonine glycosides is usually not promoted by relatively weak bases, such as morpholine and piperidine. Modern Fmoc-based peptide synthetic methods are sufficiently mild that the oligosaccharide remains intact throughout the synthesis (Fig. **6**).

The preparation of the glycosylated building blocks rely on diferrent methodologies, depending on the glycosidic bond (*O*-linked or *N*-linked).

A majority of *O*-linked glycosyl amino acids have been synthesized by standard glycosylation techniques with glycosyl donors [34, 45c, 56].

Different valuable methods exist for the formation of the *N*-link in glycosyl asparagine amino acids. The most widely exploited is the diimide-mediated coupling of glycosylamines with an Asp side chain carboxylate [57]. This method is often plagued by the ready anomerization of the glycosylamine, and this may lead to the formation of anomeric mixtures of glycopeptides [26c, 58]. Other reported methods rely on the reaction of the isothiocyanate of the protected saccharide with the carboxylate side chain of a partially protected Asp [59]. Use of the Ritter reaction involving hydrolysis of glycosyl nitrilium intermediates by the carboxylate side chain of Asp results in direct amide formation [60]. A silylated amide asparagine side chain has been directly *N*-glycosylated with glycosyl sulfoxide donors [61]. Reaction of glycosyl azides with Asp side chain carboxylates in the presence of PPh_3 affords Asn *N*-glycosides [62].

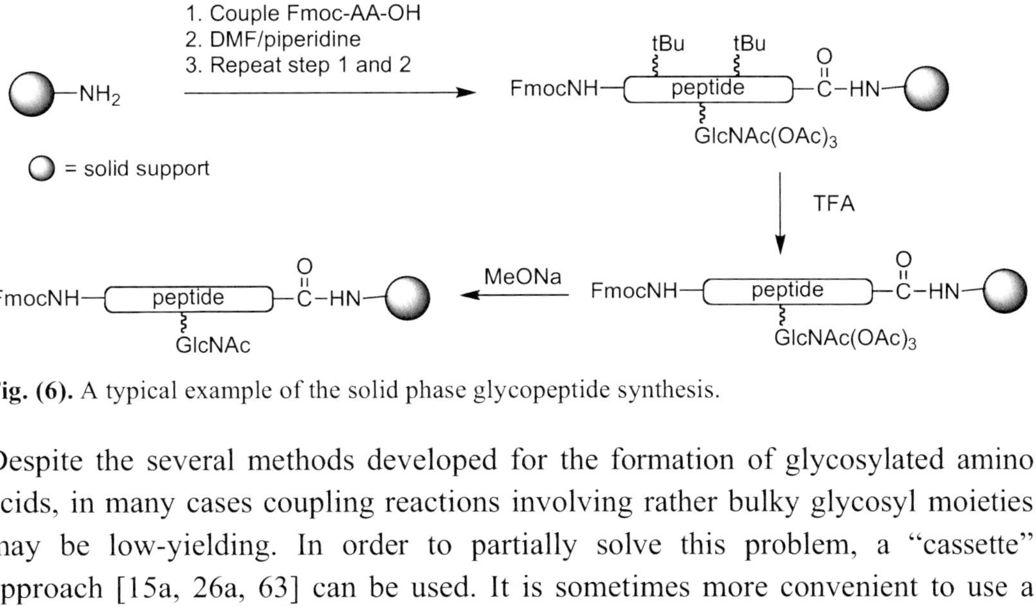

Fig. (6). A typical example of the solid phase glycopeptide synthesis.

Despite the several methods developed for the formation of glycosylated amino acids, in many cases coupling reactions involving rather bulky glycosyl moieties may be low-yielding. In order to partially solve this problem, a "cassette" approach [15a, 26a, 63] can be used. It is sometimes more convenient to use a glycosyl amino acid with a relatively simple saccharide side chain in the peptide assembly and then elaborate the glycopeptide chemically or chemoenzymatically to expand the glycan [64].

3.3. Peptide/Glycopeptide Fragments Ligation

Convergent assembly of peptide/glycopeptide fragments has been proposed to avoid by-product formation and low yields. In this approach, the *C*-terminus of the acceptor fragment must be selectively activated in the presence of a variety of proteinogenic functional groups, while at the same time a donor fragment with compatible reactivity must be available. Toward this aim, different chemistries have been developed. The native chemical ligation method [65, 66] (Fig. **7**), is based on the functionalisation of one fragment as a COOH-terminal thioester, while the other bears an NH_2-terminal cysteine residue.

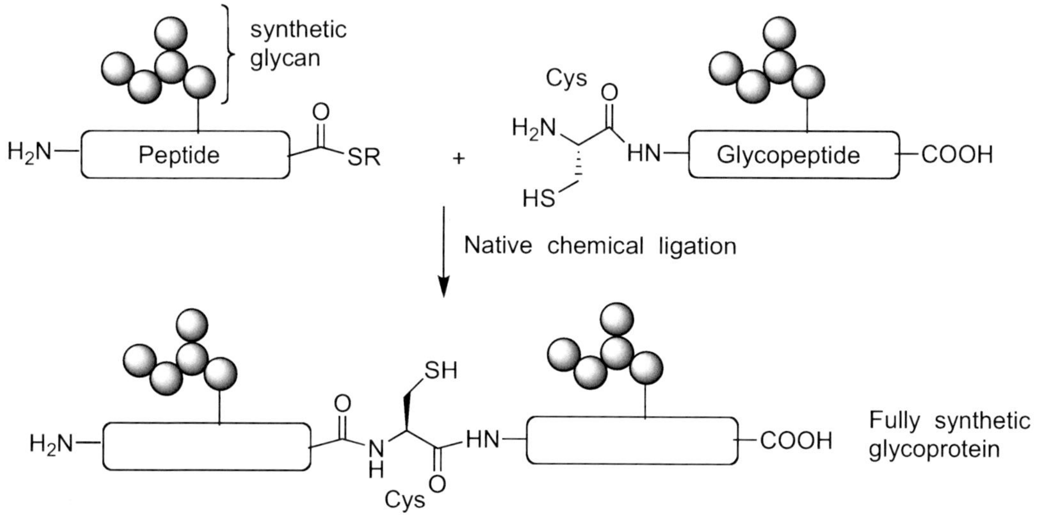

Fig. (7). The native chemical ligation method.

Hence, when an unprotected peptide thioester is mixed with a second unprotected peptide containing an *N*-terminal cysteine residue as the donor fragment, they undergo rapid transthioesterification. The resulting thioester intermediate then undergoes a spontaneous and irreversible S→N acyl transfer. In this way the two peptide fragments are linked together *via* a "native" amide bond. This process enabled the convergent condensation of unprotected glycopeptide fragments, each generated by automated SPPS, and has been widely applied to form full-length, fully functional glycoproteins [67-69]. It is important to note that native chemical ligation is effected in aqueous solution with unprotected peptides, and the reaction conditions are entirely compatible with carbohydrates and native proteins. The main drawback of native chemical ligation is the synthesis of suitable peptide/glycopeptide thioesters. Another limitation of native chemical ligation is its intrinsic reliance on having a cysteine residue at the ligation juncture. Cysteine is uncommon, comprising only 1.7% of all residues in proteins. To solve this problem an emerging strategy in protein synthesis has been the use of removable auxiliaries that act as cysteine surrogates to mediate the chemical ligation of peptide fragments [70]. The difficulty of synthesizing glycopeptide thioesters can be overcome by using the techniques proposed by Danishefsky and co-workers [71], such as the masked glycopeptide acyl donor approach [72] (Fig. **8**).

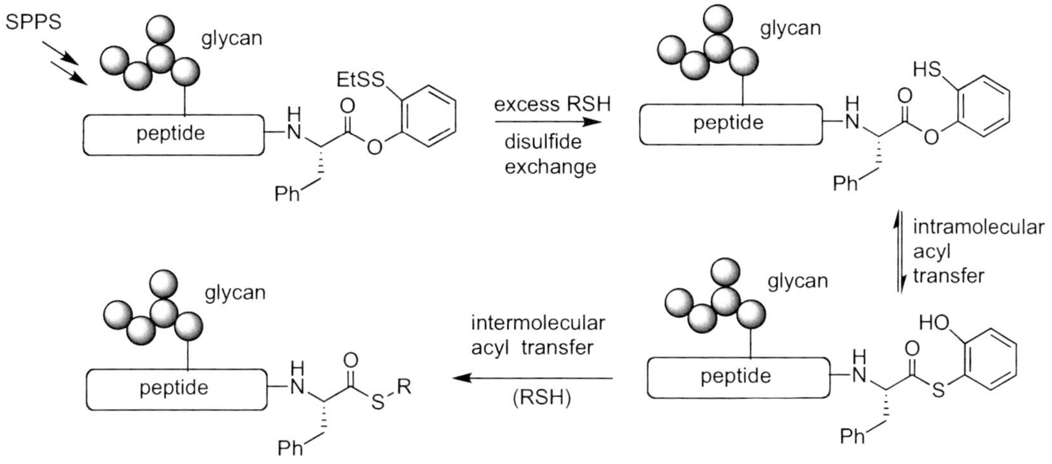

Fig. (8). Masked glycopeptide acyl donor technique as a novel solution to native chemical ligation.

In this methodology a peptide phenolic ester equipped with an ortho-disulfide moiety can be ligated to a peptide containing an *N*-terminal cysteine residue after the disulfide bond is reductively cleaved. The mechanism of this interesting ligation reaction is thought to involve a dynamic O→S acyl transfer in the reduced phenolic ester intermediate equipped with an ortho mercaptal group.

Related to "native chemical ligation" is "expressed protein ligation" [73]; this methodology permits the chemical union of recombinant protein fragments with synthetic glycopeptides, further relieving the burden of large protein synthesis. Furthermore, facile production of recombinant fragments also renders expressed protein ligation a cost efficient method.

Two additional techniques emerged as valuable tools for peptide/glycopeptide fragments ligation, the protease-catalysed ligation [74] (Fig. **9A**), and the traceless Staudinger ligation [75] (Fig. **9B**). It is well known that proteases are valuable biocatalysts for the assembly of peptide/glycopeptide fragments under kinetically controlled conditions [76].

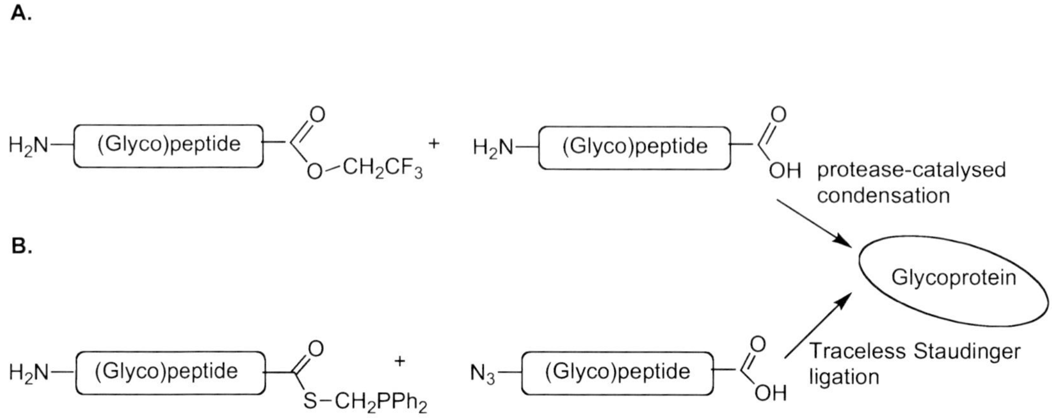

Fig. (9). Glycoprotein synthesis by **A**. protease-catalysed condensation and **B**. Staudinger ligation.

3.4. Convergent Assembly

Initially, convergent assembly of oligosaccharides and proteins was limited by a lack of suitable chemical methods. Recently, different methods have been developed for protein chemical glycosylation and post translation modification is emerging as an important method for glycoprotein synthesis. Most natural glycan-protein linkages are *N*-(Asn) and *O*-(Ser/Thr) glycosides; the most common *N*-linked motifs are GlcNAc*β*-Asn and for *O*-linked GlcNAc*β*-Ser/Thr or GalNAc*α*-Ser/Thr, although other unusual linkage forms are observed [77] such as *C*-linked Man-Trp [78].

Many indiscriminate glycosylation methods have been reported in literature, for the synthesis of *N*, *O*, C and *S*-linked glycoproteins [79, 80].

***N*-linked Glycans.** One of the most used methodology for the synthesis of N-linked glycans is the coupling between protected or unprotected glucosamine and a protected Asp derivated (Fig. **10A**). The Staudinger reaction of glycosyl azide with Asp or Asn side chains has been described for both protected and unprotected sugars (Fig. **10B**, **C**). N-glycosyl Asp have also been prepared *via* mild photochemical coupling using a photoreactive side chain amine of aspartate (Fig. **10D**). A frequently used strategies involves reductive amination (Fig. **10E**); carbohydrate-derived isothiocyanates react more selectively with amino groups alone (Fig. **10F**). Mixed-anhydride methods are well established for the activation of carboxylic acids to form carboxyl derivatives, and in this way aldonic acids may similarly be coupled to proteinaceous amines (Fig. **10G**). In a reverse sense, carbodiimide chemistry has also been employed in an attempt to activate, and therefore glycosylate, protein carboxylates (Fig. **10H**).

***O*-linked Glycans.** The *O*-glycosidic bond is normally installed through glycosylation of a suitable Ser o Thr. Trichloroacetimidate (TCA) donors have been used previously and recently this method has been improved by using $HClO_4$ silica supported as acidic catalyst (Fig. **11A**). Activation of thioglycosides by Ph_2SO/Tf_2O has been used for the preparation of Tn and Tf antigen building blocks (Fig. **11B**). Also n-pentenyl glycosides have been used as glycosyl donors, for the synthesis of glyco-peptides (Fig. **11C**). Glycosidic aromatic diazonium salts can also be used as electrophiles to functionalize a wide range of electron-rich side chains within protein structures, such as those of aromatic tyrosinyl and tryptophanyl or nucleophilic lysinyl and histidinyl residues (Fig. **11D**). Carbohydrate-derived isothiocyanates have been successfully used (Fig. **11E**). The use of highly activated acyl azides for the formation of amides from proteinaceous amines and carboxylate ester terminus spacer arm on carbohydrates (Fig. **11F**), has also been described. Diethyl squarate was also used for the coupling of carbohydrates bearing amino-terminus spacer arms to amines in BSA (Fig. **11G**).

***C*-linked Glycans.** The synthesis of a C-linked glycosyl amino acid, *via* ring opening, has been described recently. Functional group conversion and deprotection furnished a glycoamino acid suitable for peptide elongation (Fig. **12**).

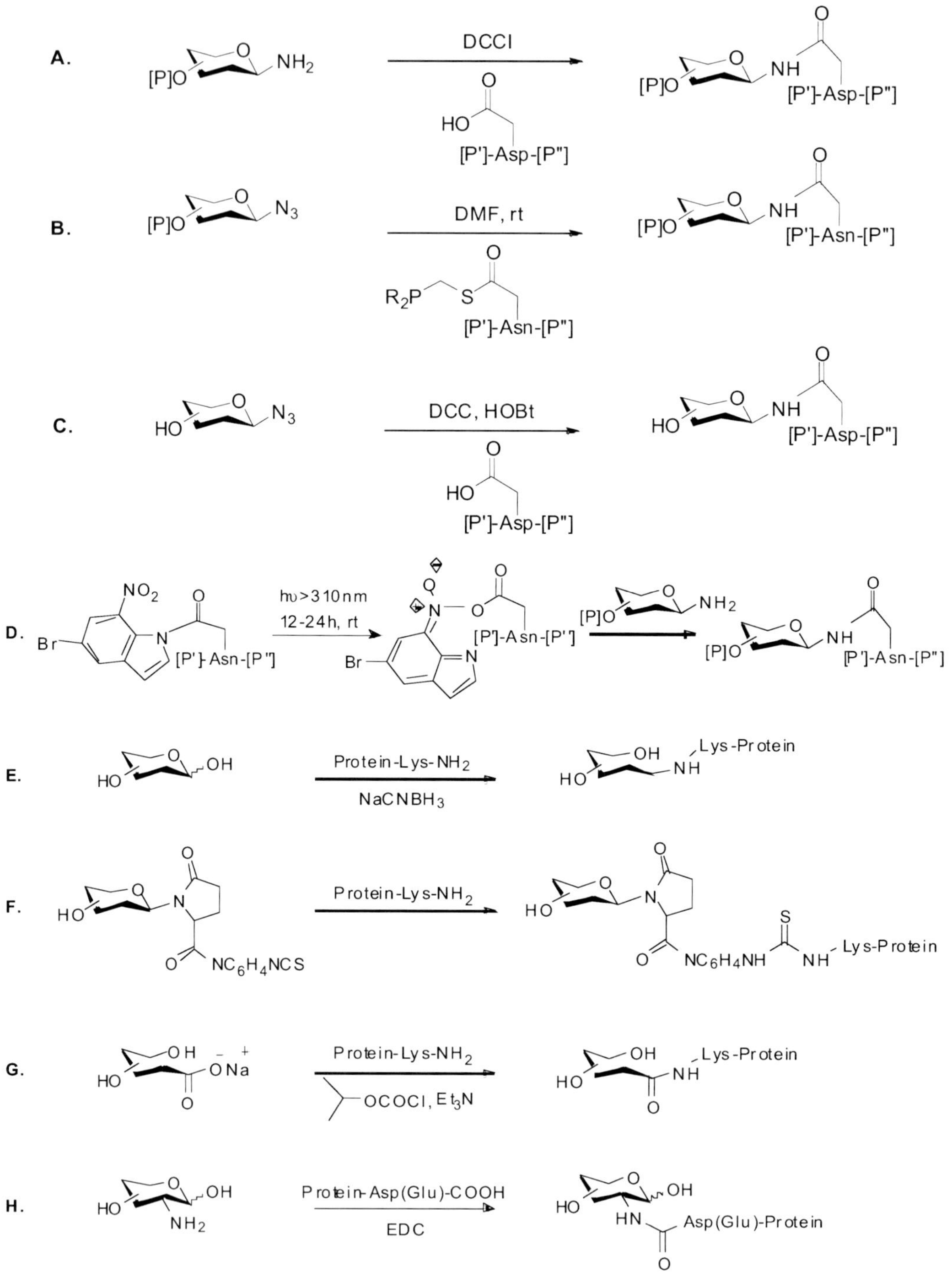

Fig. (10). Chemical methods for the conjugation of *N*-linked carbohydrates to proteins/peptides.

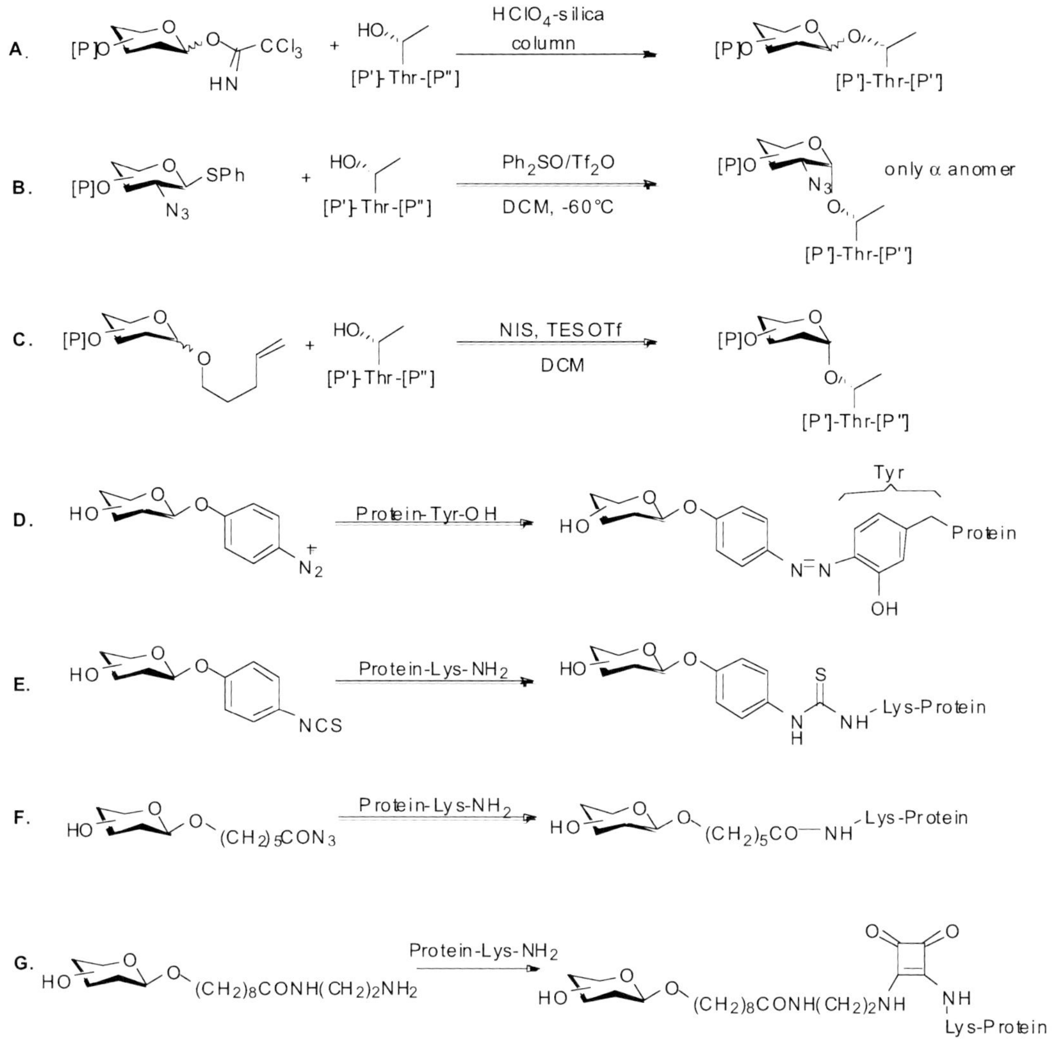

Fig. (11). Chemical methods for the conjugation of *O*-linked carbohydrates to proteins/peptides.

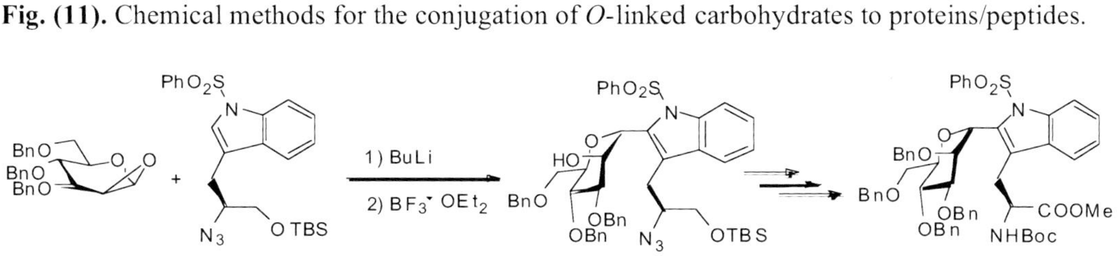

Fig. (12). Chemical methods for the conjugation of *C*-linked carbohydrates.

***S*-linked Glycans.** Different methods have been applied for the preparation of unnatural glycan-peptide system; as a primary linkage type, thioethers or variants have been explored heavily. One of the most frequently used and timed strategies for protein glycosylation, involve the use of 2-iminomethoxymethyl thioglycosides (Fig. **13A**). A serine-derived sulfamidate allows in water reaction with thioexoses to create S-linked glycoamino acids (Fig. **13B**). Aziridine-containing peptides have been used to create S-linked glycopeptides with high stereoselectivity (Fig. **13C**). Peptides containing β-bromoalanine and γ-bromohomoalanine were coupled with protected 1-thio-sugars to furnish S-linked glycopeptides in good yields (Fig. **13D**). In a reverse way, thiol containing peptides have been reacted with glycosyl bromides (Fig. **13E**). Also mesylates have been used to alkylate cysteine residues (Fig. **13F**). Reaction of glycosylthiomethyl azides with peptide-derived thioacids results in a variety of glycopeptidomimetics (Fig. **13G**). In a similar way a glycosylthiomethyl bromide have been coupled to a pepdide *via* cysteine (Fig. **13H**).

2-Chloroethyl-1-thioglycosides have also been used to indiscriminately alkylate protein amino and hydroxyl groups [81]; an essentially analogous technique using 2-bromoethylglycosides with short peptide sequences containing cysteine or homocysteine and no basic residues allowed some selectivity for *S*-alkylation [82]. A novel high-temperature method has been described for the modification of proteins that are lyophilized with reducing oligosaccharides [83], involving an Amadori rearrangement with protein lysines, which destroys the integrity of the reducing end residue.

Although high levels of functionalization are thus easily accessible using the above methods, a lack of residue selectivity is often a drawback in the synthesis of well-defined conjugates. In addition, these techniques may alter the overall charge of the protein or destroy the cyclic nature of the glycans introduced.

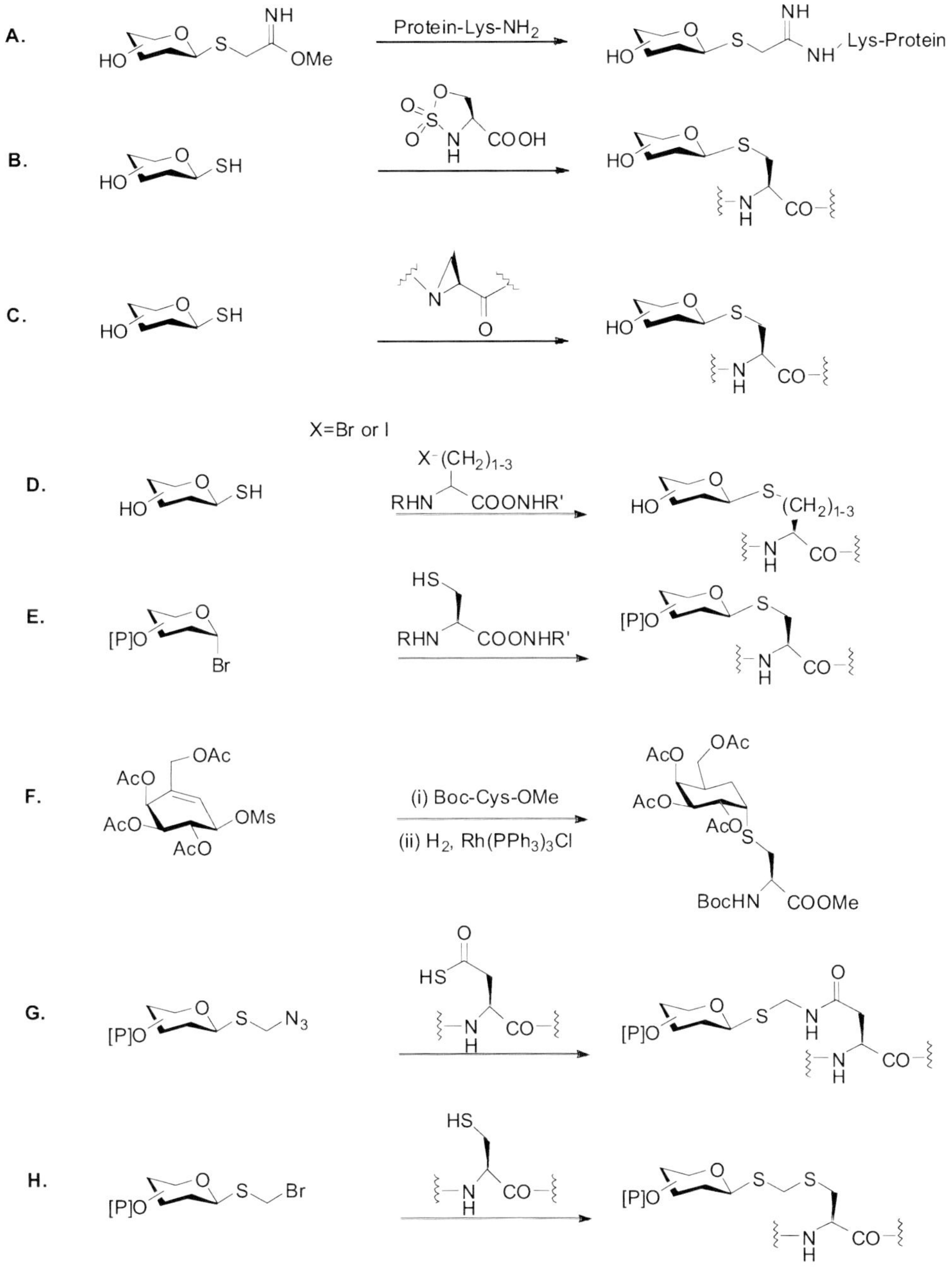

Fig. (13). Chemical methods for the conjugation of *S*-linked carbohydrates to proteins/peptides.

As already mentioned, the glycosidic linkage is a too difficult bond to be made between an oligosaccharide and a large protein. In response, chemists have begun to explore various approaches to the construction of glycopeptide/protein mimetics that have superior properties for therapeutic applications, or lend themselves to an easier convergent assembly from proteins and synthetic oligosaccharides. Hence, in an attempt to increase the selectivity and predictability of protein glycosylation, various novel approaches have been described, all of which exploit the chemoselectivities of different enzymatic and traditional methods [84]. Chemoselective ligation, first described by protein chemists as the coupling of two mutually and uniquely reactive groups in an aqueous environment, provides access to complex glycoconjugates in an elegant and convergent way. In this technique, uniquely reactive couples of functional groups (generally an elecrophile and a nucleophile) are introduced in the peptide and sugar fragments, giving rise to a selective covalent bond formation even in the presence of an array of other unprotected functional groups.

Different chemoselective techniques have been developed for neoglycoconjugate synthesis using reactions between a ketone or an aldehyde with strong nucleophiles (Fig. **14**), or adding sulfur nucleophiles to a variety of electrophiles (Fig. **15**) [79].

By mixing a thiol and a cysteine-tagged protein it's possible to generate a mixed disulfide after air oxidation. However, under such conditions unwanted symmetrical disulfides can form. In contrast, reagents that bear methanethiosulfonate (MTS) [85, 86], phenylthiosulfonate (PTS) [87], or phenylselenenylsulfide (SeS) [88], react rapidly and specifically with cysteine to provide mixed disulfides. These transformations are nearly instantaneous, allow kinetic control of product formation, and do not require large excesses of reagents. Moreover the selensulfide method allowed the coniugation of an heptasaccaride, one of the larged synthetic glycans to be atteached to a protein [88].

Disulphides are often stable *in vivo*, but they may be labile under reducing conditions; disulphide glycoconjugates may be transformed in the more stable thioethers, by reaction with electron-rich phosphines, such as hexamethylphosphorus triamide (HMPT) [89].

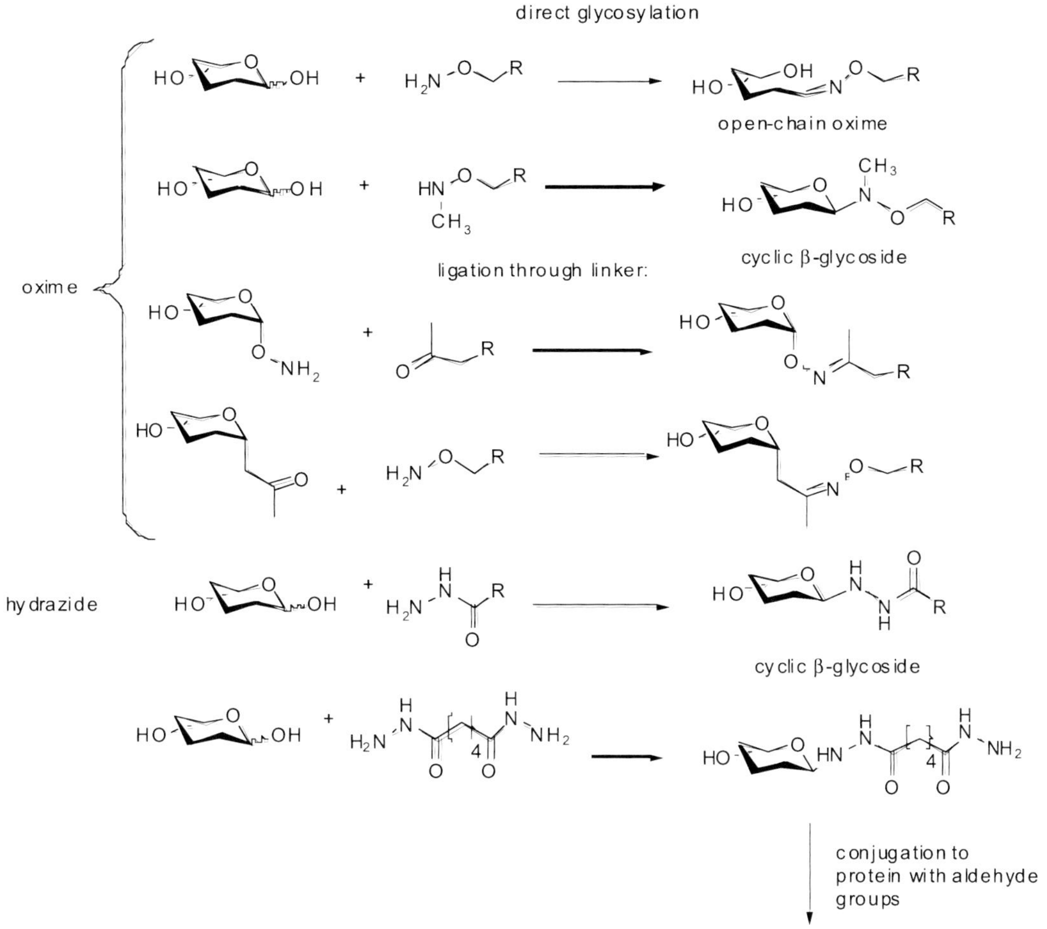

Fig. (14). Chemoselective glycosylation methods based on carbonyl chemistry.

Recently the free-radical thiol-ene coupling (TEC) emerged as an important click process proceeding with the assistance of the greenest catalyst such as visible light, without damaging any delicate biomolecules (*e.g.* proteins) [90].

After the applications of TEC in functionalization, also the sister reaction consisting of the hydrothiolation of alkynes, referred to as thiol-yne coupling (TYC), is receiving increased attention. Also the TYC reaction can be photoinitiated in the UV-visible range and it has been used for the preparation of dually glycosylated peptides, between glycosyl thiols and alkynyl peptides [91].

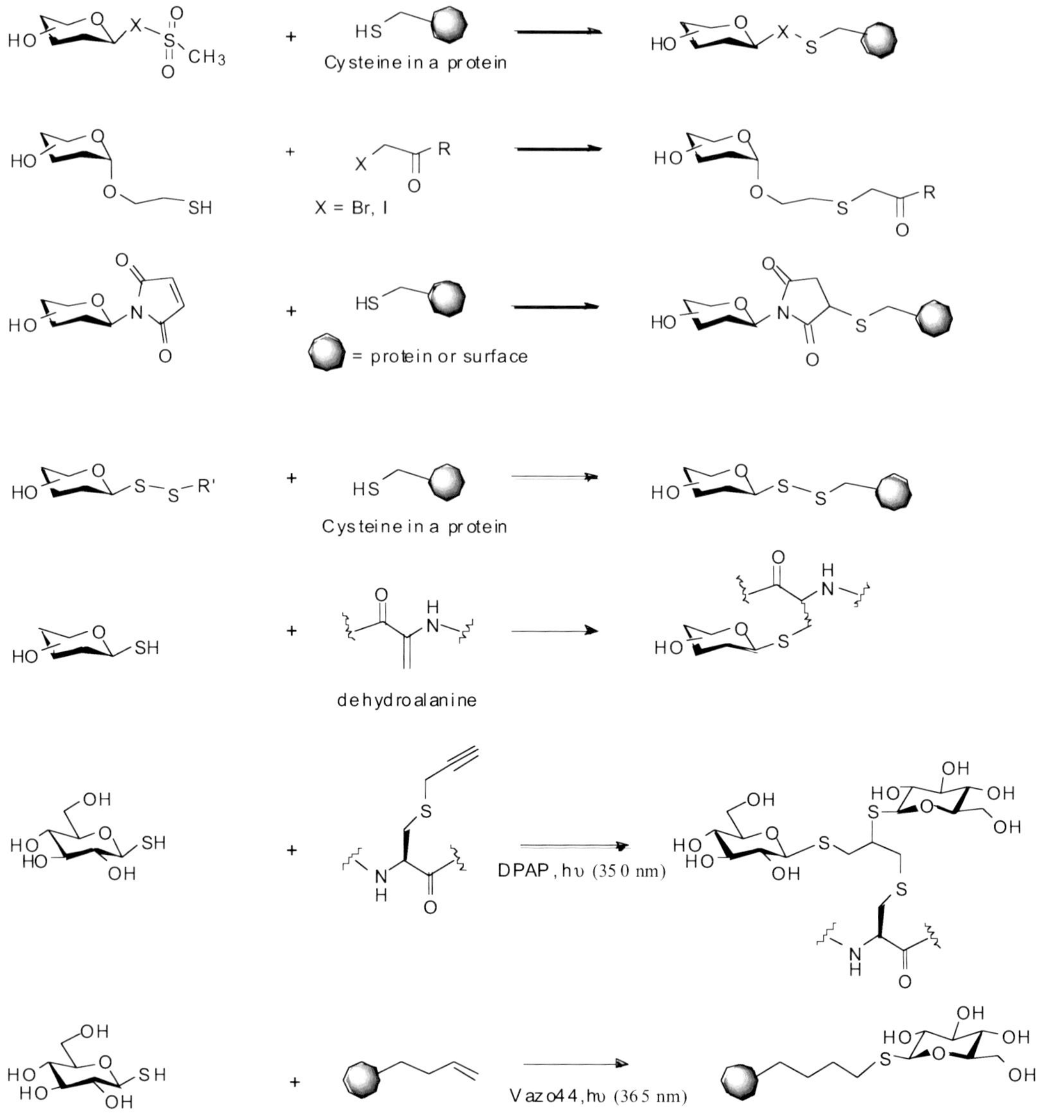

Fig. (15). Sulfur-based chemoselective glycosylation methods.

For full control of glycosylation both choice of site (site selectivity) and glycan are needed. A combined site-directed mutagenesis and chemical modification approach has solved this problem [47d, 92]. This "tag and modify" approach provides a general method that allows both regio- and glycan-specific glycosylation of proteins. Using different synthetic aminoacids it's possible to tag the biosynthesized proteins and later modify it by disulphide, thioether, cross-metathesis and triazole modification [89] (Fig. **16**).

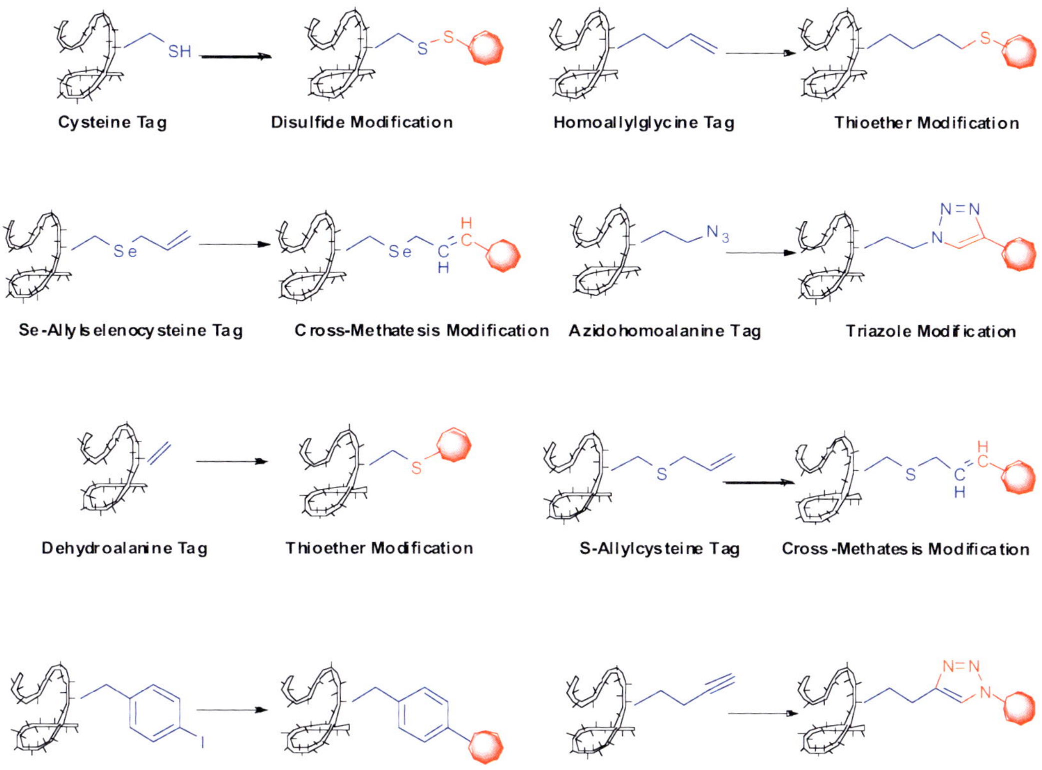

Fig. (16). Proteins tag and modify methods.

The chemical mutagenesis, defined as a chemical modification on an expressed and folded protein, in order to install a desired side chain at a desired site, it's becoming an important tool for the "tag and modify" approach [93]. As we previously showed, cysteine and dehydroalanine (Dha) rapresent useful amino acids for proteins modifications by chemoselective methods. Interconversion from serine to cysteine has been reported [94-96]. Cystein was also used as a common precursor to multiple amino acids: formylglycine, glycine and serine [97, 98]. Koshland showed that the sulfonylated serine can be eliminated under basic conditions to give dehydroalanine [99]. Davis reported a novel chemical method to oxidatively eliminate cysteine directly to Dha, using O-mesitylenesulfonylhydroxylamine (MSH) [100]. Dehydroalanine can be considered as a general chemical mutagenesis handle; aryl and aliphatic nucleophiles may allow access to a diverse functional set of amino acid side chains. Moreover Dha is a useful precursor to cysteine derivatives, including natural residues such as glycosyl-, phosphoryl-, and farnesyl cysteine.

3.5. Recombinant Methods

Recombinant methods [30, 101] are emerging for creating artificial post-translational modification of proteins. Among these, glycoprotein remodelling and tRNA technology should be mentioned (Fig. **17**).

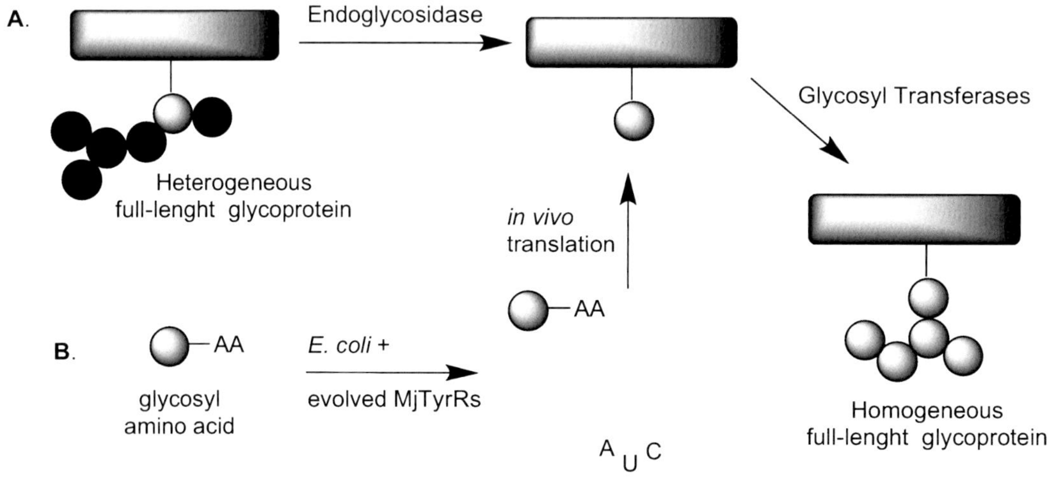

Fig. (17). **A**. Glycoprotein remodelling. **B**. *In vivo* suppressor tRNA technology: homogeneous neoglycoproteins and glycoproteins can be produced by *in vivo* suppressor tRNA technology. An orthogonal tRNA synthetase and tRNA pair can be evolved to accept and to supply the glycosyl amino acids during protein biosynthesis *in vivo* (MjTyrRS: *Methanococcus jannaschii* tyrosine-tRNA synthetase).

Glycoprotein remodelling techniques [102] involve the use of enzymes to transform a heterogeneous population of protein glycoforms into a single homogeneous glycoprotein. In the initial step in this process endoglycosidase treatment affords a glycoprotein containing a single GlcNAc attached to an Asn residue. As different endoglycosidases recognize different glycan chains, it is possible, through proper choice of the enzyme, to selectively trim different glycans. The resulting GlcNAc residue can then be modified using glycosyltransferases and sugar nucleotides to build up a complex glycan.

Although the use of glycosyltransferases allows for the rapid production of highly complex glycans, it suffers from a limitation in that sometimes the reactions do not proceed to completion. An alternative approach relies on the use of the endoglycosidases Endo A and Endo M to transfer a fully elaborated glycan chain to the GlcNAc-Asn residue through a transglycosylation reaction [103].

In vivo suppressor tRNA technology (Fig. **13**), has been exploited for the recombinant production of neoglycoproteins and glycoproteins [104]. An orthogonal tRNA synthetase and tRNA pair can be evolved to accept and supply different unnatural [105] or glycosylated [31, 106] amino acids in response to the stop codon TAG during protein biosynthesis *in vivo*, affording a homogeneous glycoprotein population. The glycoproteins were easily isolated and the incorporated monosaccharide can serve as a primary glycosylation site to which saccharides can be added sequentially with glycosyltransferases *in vitro*.

A related approach, the bioorthogonal chemical reporter strategy, using unnatural substrates has been proposed by Bertozzi and co-workers [107]. In this strategy a chemical reporter linked to a suitable substrate, such as a monosaccharide, is introduced into a target biomolecule through cellular metabolism. In a second step, the reporter is further manipulated through chemistry to function as probes, markers, or points for elaboration for oligosaccharide chemoselective ligation.

In general, the genetic incorporation of saccharide-modified amino acids directly into proteins should considerably enhance the ability to analyze and manipulate glycoprotein structure and function.

4. GLYCOCONJUGATES AS ANTICANCER THERAPY

As previously described, the synthetic tumour associated carbohydrate antigen (TACA) must be conjugated to an appropriate carrier protein to transform the epitope into a fully functional vaccine. The main role of the carrier proteins is to increase the immunogenicity of the carbohydrate antigen, that is the titer of anti-carbohydrate antibodies produced in terms of IgG and IgM. In particular, the long term immunological response and tumour cell killing by complement-dependent cytotoxicity or by ADCC is dependent on the IgG production. To obtain high titer

IgG production, the co-administration of substances called adjuvants is always needed, and their use is widely diffused in immunology. However, most adjuvants have undesirable side effects: the induction of arthritis in rats and uveitis in rabbits caused by the use of Freund's complete adjuvant (FCA), have been described [108]. FCA is derived from the extraction of mycobacteria cell wall and is universally used for immunization of animals. The only adjuvants acceptable for use on humans are the class of calcium and aluminium salts such as alum (aluminium hydroxide); the stronger but more toxic adjuvant QS-21, a saponin fraction purified from the bark of the tree *Quillaja saponaria,* and GPI-0100 have been used both for mice immunization and for clinical tests on humans at the Sloan-Kettering Institute [15a]. Because adjuvants have an undefined chemical structure (they are generally complex mixtures of compounds) they can in principle interfere with a series of physiological processes causing undesired side effects. The use of these substances introduces irrelevant determinants and ambiguity in composition and structure and for these reasons has been defined the "dirty trick" of immunology. To eliminate the side effects, extensive structure-activity relationship on FCA have been done and significant progress has been made to identify the minimal active structure derived from the mycobacterial cell wall essential for adjuvant effects. Noteworthy examples include muramyl dipeptide analogues which represent the minimal active structure of FCA. Similarly, the lipopeptide tripalmitoyl-S-glyceryl-cysteinylserine (Pam_3CS) derived from the *N*-terminal portion of Braun's lipoprotein of *Escherichia coli* has been found as a potent adjuvant for vaccines [109]. The use of Pam_3CS as an internal, built-in adjuvant has been reviewed [110]. With such a molecular system high-titer antibodies against HIV protein gp120 were obtained without the use of external adjuvants. As outlined in Fig. (**18**), the upgrading of a synthetic carbohydrate epitope to functional vaccine that elicits a therapeutically useful immunological response can be accomplished in two alternative ways: by conjugation with a carrier protein or through the design of a totally synthetic vaccine, in which a T-helper cell peptide epitope and an adjuvant are covalently linked to the sugar epitope. These two strategies lead respectively to semi-synthetic (with a carrier protein) or fully synthetic vaccines.

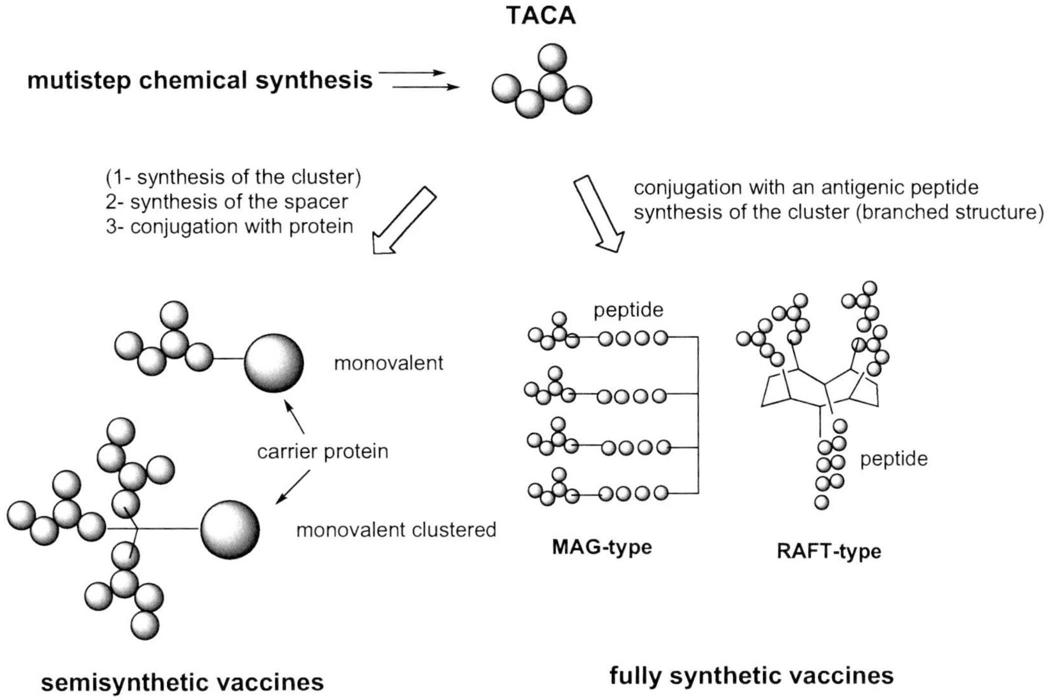

Fig. (18). General strategies for the preparation of semi-synthetic and fully synthetic vaccines.

The use of fully synthetic vaccines has several advantages:

1. These vaccines have chemically defined structures, while in semi-synthetic vaccines a mixture of compounds is obtained composed of different conjugates, each having a different carbohydrate epitope density.

2. No antibodies are produced that recognize specifically the chemical scaffold (generally a dendrimeric structure) on which the sugar epitopes are assembled. On the contrary, the immune response to the carrier proteins is much more superior to the one directed against the carbohydrate antigen, and this may lead to carrier-induced epitopic suppression. The epitopic suppression was first observed in the case of peptide epitopes conjugated to tetanus toxoid (TT) as the carrier [111]. It was shown that immunization of mice with TT strongly inhibited the subsequent antibody response to synthetic peptides conjugated to the same carrier. The problem of epitopic suppression has nowadays been partially addressed by the use of

immunostimulants. However, the existence of this phenomenon limits the number of proteins that can be used as carriers thus limiting the efficacy of these glycoconjugates.

3. In principle, in fully synthetic vaccines, the adjuvant function can be incorporated directly in the molecule; this would avoid the use of external adjuvants.

For these reasons, totally synthetic vaccines still remain a very interesting and challenging therapeutic target.

In the following sections, different approaches towards the design of anti-tumour carbohydrate-containing constructs will be outlined. For the sake of clarity throughout the following sections, glycoconjugate constructs will be classified based on their valency, that is on the number and type of carbohydrate antigens; they will not be differentiated upon their carrier construct (peptide, protein, lipid, nanoparticle, *etc*…). Hence, we can distinguish mainly three types of conjugates:

- **Monovalent constructs**: only one type of carbohydrate antigen is conjugated to the carrier construct;
- **Monovalent clustered constructs**: one type of carbohydrate antigen presented in clusters of two to several units, conjugated to the molecular construct;
- **Multivalent constructs**: several different carbohydrate antigens displayed on a single carrier structure.

4.1. Monovalent Constructs

A great deal of work on monovalent constructs as potential vaccines, defined also as first-generation vaccines, has been proposed by Danishefsky and co-workers [112]. The first carbohydrate vaccines investigated were monomeric, containing a single carbohydrate antigen conjugated, through an appropriate linker, to an immunogenic carrier protein, such as keyhole-limpet hemocyanine (KLH). Different TACAs were hence synthesised and then conjugated to the carrier.

Among these, Globo H (Fig. **1**), is a hexasaccharide first isolated from the human breast cancer cell line MCF-7 [113], and then shown to be overexpressed on the surfaces of a number of other cancer cell lines [114] (see Table **1**), as a glycolipid and possibly as a glycoprotein, identified and defined by murine MoAb MBr1 generated by immunization of mice with human breast cancer cell MCF-7. Globo H has been synthesised and then conjugated to the carrier by the highly convergent glycal protocol and investigated in a number of different cancers [115].

Pre-clinical studies in mice were conducted using the vaccine prepared with Globo H ceramide alone or with adjuvants such as *Salmonella minnesota* mutant R595 or Globo H allyl glycoside covalently conjugated to KLH or BSA by reductive amination, plus QS-21 as adjuvant. The Globo H-KLH conjugate plus QS-21 was proven to be the optimal vaccine, inducing high titer IgM and IgG responses to the Globo H antigen [116]. It is worthy of note that the antibodies thus obtained were found to be reactive with Globo H-positive MCF-7 cancer cells, but not with Globo H-negative B78.2 melanoma cells. On the basis of these results, Globo H monovalent KLH-conjugate vaccine was advanced to Phase I clinical trial against prostate cancer [123c] and breast cancer [123a], and Phase II/III clinical trials should also commence.

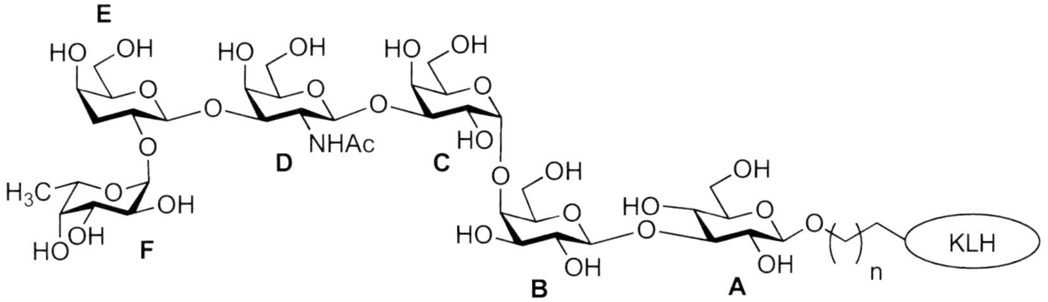

Fig. (19). Monovalent Globo H containing vaccine proposed by Danishefsky and co-workers.

The vaccines resulted safe, no significant toxicity was detected, and they induced specific high titer IgM antibodies against Globo H. This was the first demonstration of a complex synthetic carbohydrate antigen inducing an immune response in humans [123b]. In most patients, after immunization, both IgM and IgG antibodies were detected against synthetic Globo H. In prevaccinated patients no serological reactivity against synthetic Globo H was detected. In some patients the antibody titers were present 2 years after the last vaccination. A trial compared the Globo H-KLH vaccine prepared by direct reductive amination or by using a bifunctional cross-linker 4-(4-*N*-maleimidomethyl) cyclohexane-1-carboxyl hydrazide (MMCCH). The antibody response in all groups was similar to that described above.

Truncated, synthetic versions of the Globo H antigen were also prepared and investigated for their ability to bind the MBr1 MoAb. The terminal fucosyl residue (ring F) was shown to be critical for antibody recognition, whereas the A and B rings were found to be less significant. This suggests that the binding domain is localized in the CDEF ring system. This phenomenon was also seen for vaccines containing the KH-1 antigen [46, 117], a nonasaccharide comprising both the Lewis y tetrasaccharide and the Lewis x trisaccharide epitopes (Fig. **1**). The antibodies elicited by the KH-1 vaccine constructs recognized the KH-1 antigen in addition to the Lewis y antigen, which is similar to the four saccharides found at the non-reducing end of the KH-1 nonasaccharide. The Globo H-KLH conjugate vaccine was the first semi-synthetic vaccine to enter in clinical trials, and since then a variety of monovalent constructs have been prepared by Danishefsky and co-workers and tested to complete phase I clinical trial (Table **2**).

Table 2. Completed Phase I Clinical Trials with Monovalent KLH-Conjugates with QS-21 Adjuvant[a]

Antigen	Immune Response	Tumour
FucGM1	IgM[b], IgG	Small cell lung cancer
FucGM2	IgM, IgG	Small cell lung cancer
Lewis y	IgM, some IgG	Ovarian cancer
Globo H	IgM, IgG	Breast cancer, Prostate cancer

[a]Based on Ref. [99a]; [b]Ig = Immunoglobulin.

The immunogenicity of TF and sTn antigens has been studied in a series of small clinical trials in colon, breast and ovarian cancer patients by immunization with TF-KLH and STn-KLH conjugate vaccines plus different adjuvants [118].

Fully synthetic anticancer vaccines, composed by the tetrasaccharide Le^y coupled to the protein carrier KLH using several different linkers were also proposed by

Boons and co-workers [119]. The objective was to investigate the influence of the linker on the immunogenicity of the tetrasaccharide. It was found that a highly immunogenic linker such as 4-(maleimidomethyl)-cyclohexane-1-carboxylate (Fig. **20**), dramatically reduced titers of antibodies against the weakly immunogenic Le^y tetrasaccharide antigen. The use of a less immunogenic linker such as 3-(bromoacetamido)-propionate improved the immunological response considerably.

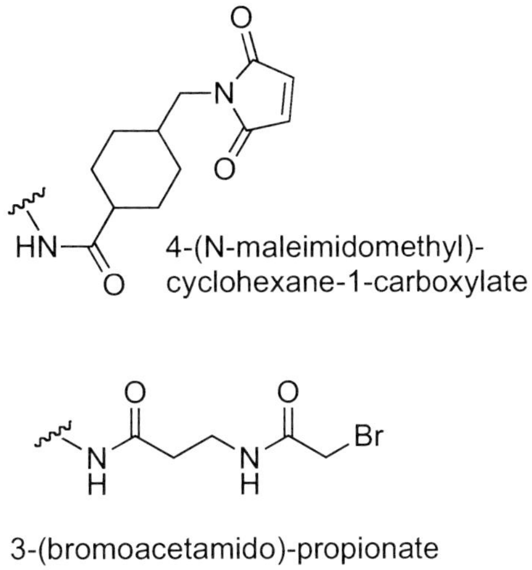

Fig. (20). Linkers used for the conjugations to proteins.

To further investigate the ideal presentation of the Le^y antigen, the presentation of Le^y in a dimeric form was also pursued [42b]. Naturally occurring Lewis antigens exist not only as positional isomers in monomeric forms, but also as homo and heterodimers. For example, the Le^y-Le^x heterodimer (Fig. **21**), is part of the KH-1 antigen that was isolated from human colonic adenocarcinoma cells [120]. This antigen has only been found on the surface of adenocarcinomas cells, and has never been isolated from normal colonic tissue, thus, providing a highly specific marker for colon malignancies [121]. The Le^y-Le^x heptasaccharide, modified by an artificial aminopropyl spacer, was synthesized by a highly convergent approach that employed two orthogonally protected lactosamine building blocks. The artificial aminopropyl moiety was modified by a thioacetyl group, which allowed an efficient conjugation to keyhole limpet hemocyanin (KLH) that had been activated with electrophilic 3-(bromoacetamido)-propionyl groups.

Mice were immunized with the Le^y-Le^x-BrAc-KLH antigen. Analysis of the sera by ELISA established that a helper T-cell immune response was raised against the Le^y-Le^x saccharide. Further ELISA analysis showed that the titer for monomeric Le^y tetrasaccharide was ten fold lower whereas recognition of the Le^x trisaccharide was negligible. This data demonstrated that the raised antibodies have high specificity for the Le^y-Le^x heptasaccharide, indicating that the recognized epitope is spanning the two Lewis antigen monomers; it was also determined that the antibody recognition of the internal Lewis x trisaccharide was very low.

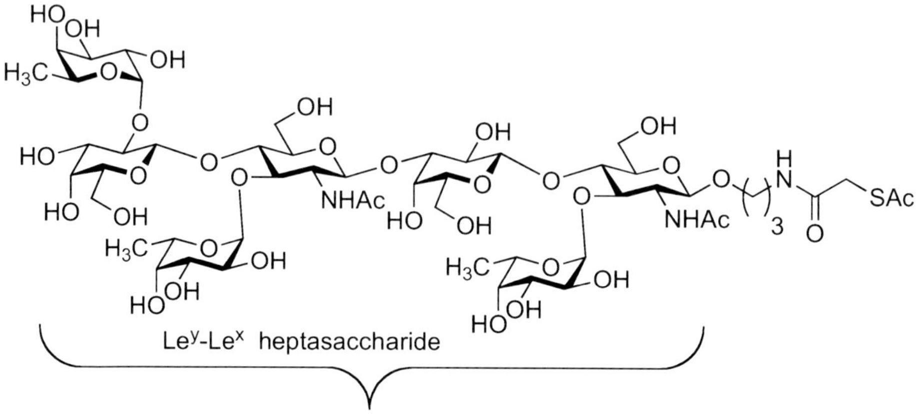

Fig. (21). Structure of the Le^y-Le^x heptasaccharide, modified by an artificial spacer for conjugation to KLH.

The synthesis and immunological evaluation of a lipidated glycopeptide containing the tumour-associated Tn antigen was also proposed [122], since the Tn antigen is an excellent target for immunotherapy [123]. The structurally well-defined, fully synthetic anticancer vaccine candidate (Fig. **22**), constitutes the minimal structural features required for a focused and effective T cell dependent immune response; the vaccine is composed of the tumour-associated Tn antigen, the peptide T epitope YAFKYARHANVGRNAFELFL (YAF), and the lipo-peptide *S*-[(*R*)-2,3-dipalmitoyloxy-propyl]-*N*-palmitoyl-*R*-cysteine (Pam_3Cys).

To overcome the T cell independent properties of the carbohydrate antigen, the YAF peptide was incorporated. This 20-amino acid peptide sequence is derived from an outer-membrane protein of *Neisseria meningitidis* and has been identified as an MHC class II restricted site for human T cells [124]. It was envisaged that this helper T cell epitope would induce a T cell dependent immune response that results in the production of IgG antibodies against the Tn antigen. The combined B cell and helper T cell epitope lacks the ability to provide appropriate "danger signals" [125] for dendritic cell maturation. Therefore, the lipopeptide Pam_3Cys, which is derived from the immunologically active *N*-terminal sequence of the principal lipoprotein of *Escherichia coli* [126], was incorporated.

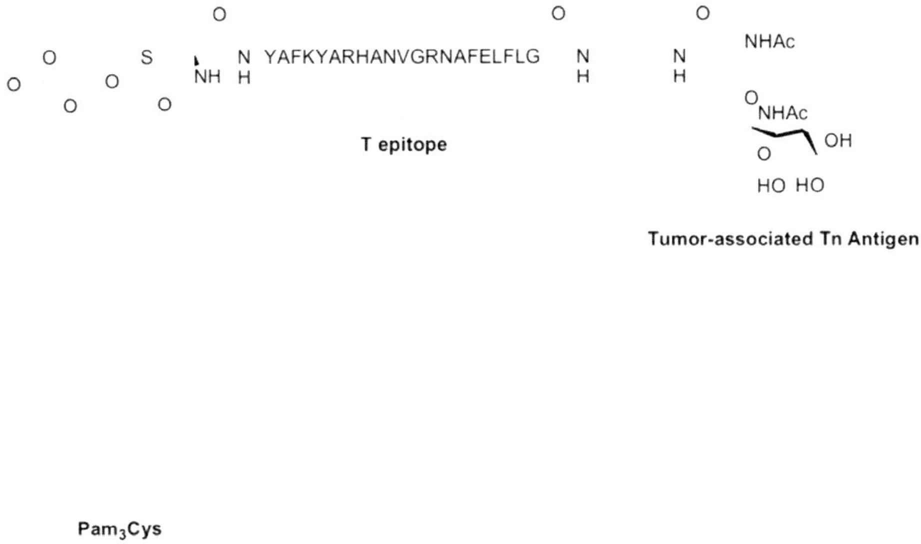

Fig (22). Structure of lipidated vaccine containing the tumour-associated Tn antigen.

Vaccine was included into phospholipid-based liposomes prior to administration; the mice that were immunized with the liposome preparations elicited IgM and IgG antibodies against the Tn antigen.

Kunz and co-workers [48] synthesised the linear glycopeptide shown in Fig. (**23**), containing the sialyl-Tn glycododecapeptide epitope linked through a spacer to a T cell peptide type (YSYFPSV) tetanus toxoid (TT), as the T cell epitope, while the peptide motif PDTRPAP was incorporated as the immunodominant peptide domain [127]. The two portions were conjugated using a flexible oligoethylene glycol spacer. In addition, glycopeptides have been synthesised which contain tumour-associated saccharide antigens, such as the Thomsen-Friedenreich (T), Tn or sTn antigen, in combination with peptide sequences of the tandem repeat region of MUC1. MUC1 is a heavily glycosylated membrane glycoprotein containing a domain of numerous tandem repeats of the 20 amino acid sequence TAPPAHGVTSAPDTRPAPGS in its extracellular part. Most of the *O*-glycosylation sites are located within the tandem repeat region. This glycopeptide was administered to cultured peripheral blood lymphocytes (PBL) and induced proliferation of CD3+ cells. Interestingly, antibodies against a sTn-MUC1 tandem-repeat glycopeptide conjugate specifically recognize not only the glycan but also the peptide backbone [128]. Recently Payne and co-workers have described an efficient method for the convergent assembly of MUC1-lipopeptide vaccine candidates; these chimeras consisting of MUC1 glycopeptides (bearing multiple couple of Tn or T tumor-associated antigens) tetherd to the lipopeptide immunoadjuvant Pam3CysSer were synthesized in high yields using a fragment-based condensation strategy [129].

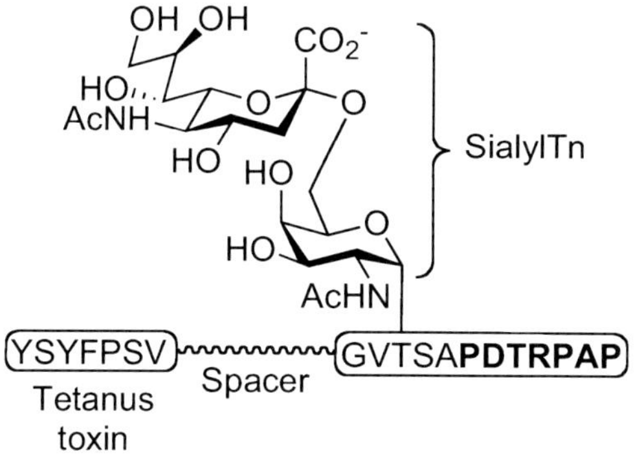

Fig. (23). Sialyl-Tn glycopeptide as anticancer vaccine.

Recently Gendler and co-workers [130] have identified the minimum requirements to consistently induce CTLs and ADCC-mediating antibodies specific for the tumor form of MUC1 resulting in a therapeutic response in a mouse model of mammary cancer. The vaccine is composed of the immunoadjuvant Pam_3CysSK_4, a peptide T-helper epitope and an aberrantly glycosylated MUC1 peptide. Covalent linkage of the three components was essential for maximum efficacy. The vaccine produced CTLs, which recognized both glycosylated and nonglycosylated peptides, whereas a similar nonglycosylated vaccine gave CTLs which recognized only nonglycosylated peptide. Antibodies elicited by the glycosylated tripartite vaccine were significantly more lytic compared with the unglycosylated control. As a result, immunization with the glycosylated tripartite vaccine was superior in tumor prevention.

Covalent Conjugate Ganglioside Vaccines

On the basis of exciting progress made with bacterial polysaccharide conjugate vaccines, several laboratories explored the use of gangliosides and related carbohydrates conjugated to BSA or tetanus toxoid for the production of antibodies and monoclonal antibodies [131]. The effect of the covalent conjugation of protein carriers on ganglioside GD3 and their immunogenicity was systematically established by Helling *et al.* [132]. Of the many methods of conjugation, and diverse carriers and adjuvants studied, covalent attachment of GD3 with KLH by reductive amination and immunological adjuvant QS-21 proved optimal [133]. High-titer IgM and IgG responses against GD3, which could mediate complement lysis of human melanoma cells expressing GD3, were seen in most mice. Striking findings in these studies were the absolute necessity of conjugation of ganglioside to the immunogenic carrier KLH, the importance of the method of conjugation, and the need for a potent immunological adjuvant such as QS-21. The same GD3-KLH conjugate with other immunological adjuvants, other conjugation procedures, or immunization with ganglioside alone or covalently attached to other carriers plus QS-21, resulted in a minimal response. The demonstration of immunogenicity of GM2 in man was documented in a series of clinical trials conducted with the GM2-KLH conjugate alone or GM2-KLH mixed with the immunological adjuvants BCG, Detox (containing BCG cell wall skeletons and monophosphoryl lipid A) or QS-21 in patients with melanoma [134]. The covalently conjugated GM2- KLH without adjuvant or with BCG or Detox was moderately immunogenic. GM2-KLH plus QS-21 not only induced the highest IgM titers, but also induced durable IgG antibodies in most patients.

Based on the findings of studies on the GM2-KLH conjugate vaccine, various clinical trials have been conducted with other gangliosides. Small groups of melanoma patients were vaccinated with GD2-KLH or GD3-KLH conjugate plus QS-21, GD2, GD3, GD3-lactone or fucosyl GM1 conjugated with KLH plus QS-21 vaccines. The GD2-KLH vaccine induced a moderate anti-GD2 IgM antibody titer in all patients vaccinated [135]. As seen with purified GD3, the GD3-KLH conjugate vaccine was unable to induce antibodies against GD3. Other attempts have been made to induce anti-GD3 antibodies with a GD3-lactone [136].

A neoglycopeptide immunogen displaying one or two copies of the GM2 tetrasaccharidic moiety has been synthesized. These glycopeptides were prepared using the Huisgen cycloaddition, which enables the efficient ligation of the alkyne-functionalized biosynthesized GM2 with an azido CD4+ T cell epitope peptide. Interestingly, the monovalent but not the divalent form of GM2 peptide construct, induced antimelanoma antibodies [137].

4.1.1. Chemically Modified Glycan Structure in Glycoconjugates

Successful tumour immunotherapy might require the induction of cytotoxic T lymphocytes (CTLs) in addition to antibodies. There are strategies currently being pursued to recruit T-cell help, including mimicking the cancer cell surface by displaying vaccine glycans in a multivalent context (see next section), or by chemically modifying cancer glycans to make them more 'foreign'; hence, chemical modification of monosaccharide structures can augment the immunogenicity of glycan based vaccines [138]. In addition, any approach to the synthesis TACA analogues might clarify the structure-antigenic relationship of key carbohydrate epitopes. The concise preparation of complex oligosaccharides in the laboratory still remains a significant challenge for synthetic organic chemists. The demands of regio- and stereoselectivity in glycosylation reactions often lead to lengthy synthetic schemes and extensive protecting group manipulations. Analogues might somehow simplify the chemical synthesis.

Lewis y (Le^y) and KH-1 are carbohydrate tumour-associated antigens that are often overexpressed on the surfaces of breast and prostate cancer cells as membrane glycolipids [11b]. Recent preclinical [139] and clinical trials [22, 140] with mixtures of individual KLH-conjugates and multivalent KLH-conjugate vaccines with the same antigens revealed the strong immunogenic properties of KH-1; in addition, antibodies generated in response to the KH-1-KLH construct recognized not only KH-1 antigen but also the Lewis y antigen as well, with antibody titer levels much higher than those observed after immunization with individual Le^y-KLH vaccine constructs. In order to explore the structure-antigenic relationship of these carbohydrate epitopes, several analogues of KH-1 were synthesized by Danishefsky and co-workers [46]. Having established the potency of KH-1 as an antigen to induce Le^y antibodies, the syntheses of a series of truncated analogues, each containing the crucial Le^y tetrasaccharide fragment in the context of a more elaborate construct, which is not normally encountered, was proposed. Since KH-1 contains within it the Le^y tetrasaccharide motif (Fig. **24**), this substructure was "conserved". As the "variable" part of the molecules different oligosaccharide linkers, attached to the *core* tetrasaccharide structure through a β-1,3-glycosidic bond, were chosen: lactose (Fig. **24**, V-1); a tetrasaccharide consisting of acetyl lactosamine attached to lactose (Fig. **24**, V-2); and α-fucosylated lactose (Fig. **24**, V-3). The main consideration in the selection of analogues was that of including compounds with more rigid conformations, of the type likely to enhance immunogenicity. The presence of both fucose and acetylaminosugars in oligosaccharides are known to impart structural rigidity to the molecular framework [141].

The three analogues have been prepared with high stereoselectivity and in reasonable yields using five common building blocks. Conjugation of these analogues to carrier protein by previously applied sequences has been accomplished and immunological tests are currently being completed.

GM3 is one of the most abundant TACAs on several types of tumours, such as malignant melanoma and neuroectodermal tumours [142]. Consequently, an effective vaccine based on GM3 can be widely useful. Unfortunately, GM3 is poorly immunogenic, and the problem of immunotolerance to GM3 seriously hinders its usage in cancer vaccine development. To solve this problem a new strategy based upon metabolic engineering of cell surface *N*-acetylneuraminic acid (Neu5Ac) was proposed: the keyhole limpet hemocyanin (KLH) conjugates of a series of GM3 derivatives containing chemically modified sialic acid residues with unnatural *N*-acyl side chains, such as *N*-propanoyl, *N*-butanoyl, *N*-phenylacetyl and *N*-levulinoyl were synthesized and screened as therapeutic cancer vaccines [143]. Neu5Ac is a natural sialic acid and is significantly overexpressed by many tumours [144]. The underlining concept of this strategy is to first immunize cancer patients with a synthetic vaccine consisting of an artificial derivative or analogue of a natural TACA that has its sialic acid residues chemically modified. After an immune response specific to the artificial antigen is established, the patients are treated with correspondingly modified mannosamine, which serves as a biosynthetic precursor of modified sialic acid, to initiate the expression of the artificial antigen in place of the natural TACA on tumours. The activated immune system will thereby eliminate the marked tumour cells. The concept is further supported by recent results from Jennings' group [145]. In principle, this strategy should be applicable to various TACAs.

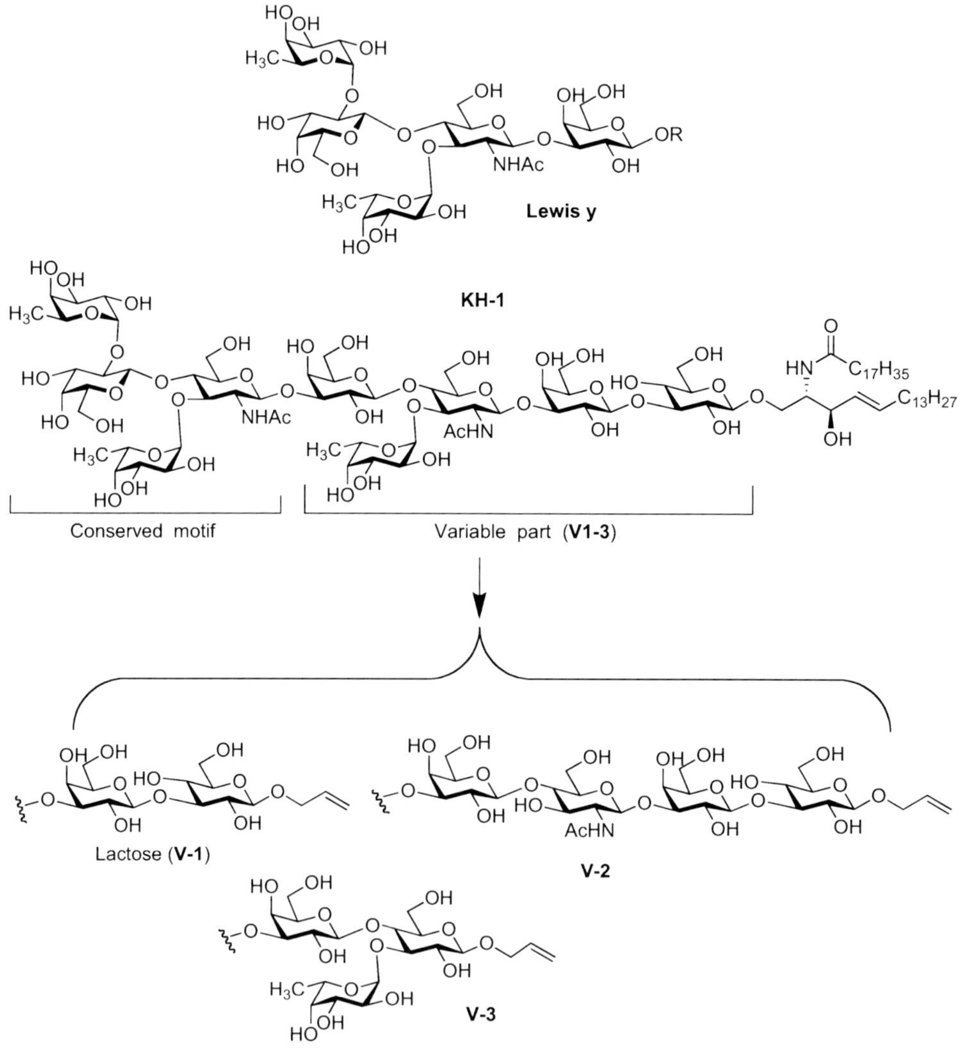

Fig. (24). Structure of KH-1, Le^y and their analogues.

Modification of the sialic acid residue of GM3 is particularly interesting because previous studies suggest that chemically modified sialic acids and sialo-carbohydrates are significantly more immunogenic than their natural counterparts [146]. More importantly, Bertozzi [115a, 147], Reutter [148], and Varki [149] have demonstrated that a variety of cells, including tumour cells, can uptake unnatural *N*-acyl mannosamines to biosynthesize artificial sialic acids and sialoglycoconjugates and present them onto cell surfaces. Thus, metabolic engineering of GM3 on tumour cells may be conveniently achieved by incorporating unnatural sialic acids.

Four unnatural *N*-acyl derivatives of GM3 (Fig. **25**), including *N*-propionyl GM3 (GM3NPr), *N*-butanoyl GM3 (GM3NBu), *N*-*iso*-butanoyl GM3 (GM3N*i*Bu), and *N*-phenylacetyl GM3 (GM3NPhAc), which comprise a range of structural variations were synthesised and studied. KLH was employed to form glycoconjugate vaccines, because KLH conjugates are often highly immunogenic and induce IgG antibody responses that are desirable for cancer immunotherapy. Alternatively, human serum albumin (HSA) conjugates were prepared as capture reagents for ELISA assays in immunological studies, which would avoid detection of antibodies specific for KLH.

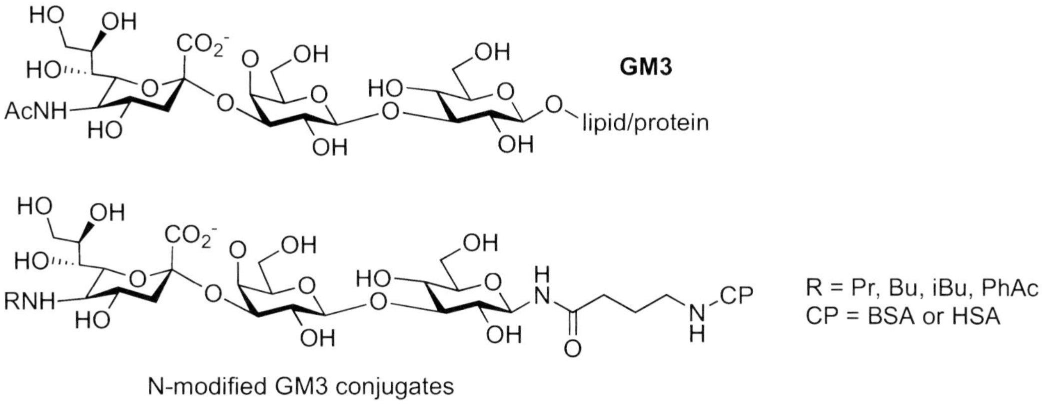

Fig. (25). Structure of vaccines containing GM3 analogues.

The properties of these glycoconjugates were studied to explore the impact of structural changes of GM3 on its immunogenicity. It was revealed that derivatized GM3 antigens are generally more immunogenic than GM3 itself. Moreover, whereas GM3 induces mainly IgM responses, derivatized GM3 antigens induce both IgM and IgG responses. GM3NPhAc proved to be the most immunogenic among the GM3 derivatives investigated, and its antisera were the least cross reactive with the natural GM3. These results indicate that GM3NPhAc is an excellent candidate as an antitumour vaccine.

Similarly, Livingston and co-workers conducted a preliminary clinical trial in which small-cell lung carcinoma patients were vaccinated with polysialic acid (PSA)-KLH or *N*-propionylated PSA-KLH (PrPSA-KLH) conjugates. The modified PrPSA-KLH conjugate elicited specific antibodies that crossreacted with PSA, whereas the natural PSA conjugate did not [147].

Jennings and co-workers demonstrated that administration of a monoclonal antibody raised against a synthetic PrPSA-KLH conjugate prevented metastasis of a leukaemic cell line when the mice were treated with *N*-propanoylmannosamine, a biosynthetic precursor of *N*-propionylated PSA [150].

The sTF antigen is present on breast tumours, thus, glycopeptide fragments containing this structure are of interest in the preparation of anticancer vaccines [15a]. A glycosyl amino acid in which a protected thiol substitutes the hydroxyl group (Fig. **26**), was used for the synthesis of glycopeptide analogues by thiol alkylation [151, 152].

The building block used for SPPS contains an unnatural 3-thio-GalNAc residue that can undergo chemoselective condensation with *N*-bromoacetamido sugars, following its incorporation into a peptide by Fmoc-based solid-phase peptide synthesis (SPPS). The thiol group can be alkylated selectively over all natural amino acids except cysteine. The resulting product contains an unnatural thioether linkage at the C-3 position, a common branch point of mucin-type oligosaccharides, but retains the native sugar peptide linkage. In this manner, carbohydrate ligands have been appended to native mucin-like scaffolds in a chemoselective fashion. This methodology was applied to the synthesis of thioether-linked analogues of the mucin-related 2,3-sialyl-TF (STF) (Fig. **27**).

Finally, the anti-MUC1 antibody, called CTM01, has been chosen to target the potently cytotoxic calicheamicin anti-tumour antibiotics to solid tumours of epithelial origin that express this antigen [153]. The calicheamicins are highly potent anti-tumour antibiotics of the enediyne family, while the murine monoclonal antibody CTM01 [154] is an internalizing IgG1 that recognizes the MUC1 antigen present on a broad spectrum of solid tumours of epithelial origin.

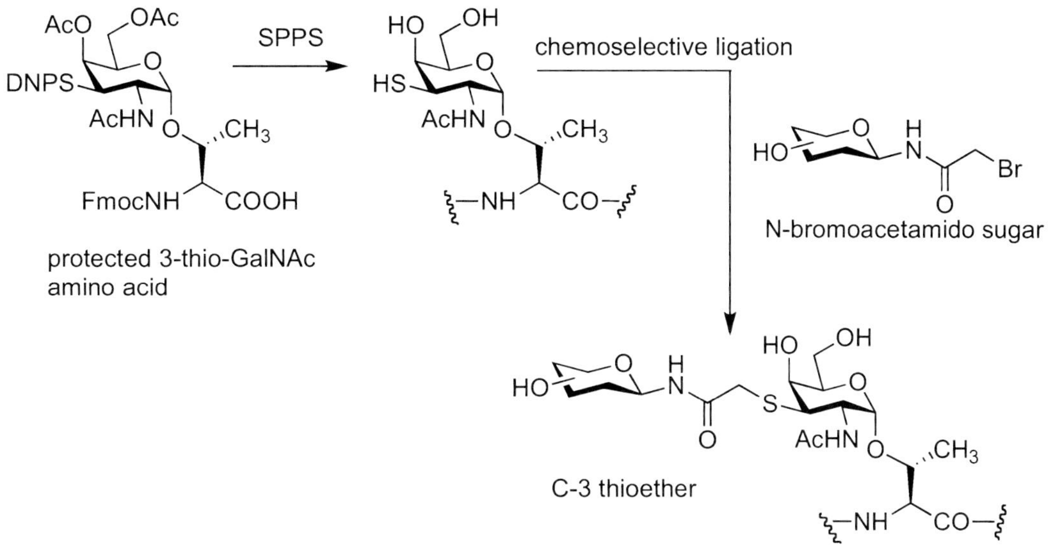

Fig. (26). Synthesis of glycopeptide analogues by thioalkylation.

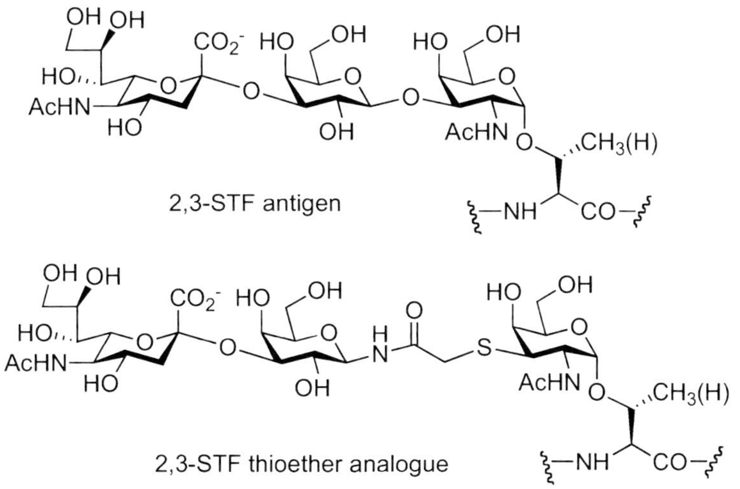

Fig. (27). Structure of 2,3-STF and their thioether analogues.

Calicheamicin was conjugated to the carbohydrates that occur naturally on antibodies: this produced a "carbohydrate conjugate" capable of releasing active drug by hydrolysis in the lysosomes where the pH is low. Both *in vitro* and *in vivo* data showed that the efficacy of the calicheamicins toward such tumours is unexpectedly enhanced by antibody conjugation.

4.2. Monovalent Clustered Constructs

Further improvement of the "first generation" monovalent vaccines comes from the possibility of mimicking more closely the complex carbohydrate structures found in glycoprotein arrangements often found on the tumour cell surface. It is known that in the mucin family of glycoproteins, carbohydrate epitopes are carried on adjacent serine and threonine residues in clusters of two to five. Since such carbohydrate clusters are apparently the preferred targets of monoclonal antibodies, it can be postulated that it would be possible to improve the immunogenity of the vaccine constructs by "clustering" groups of antigens upon a single polypeptide backbone, which would then be conjugated to a carrier molecule. Moreover glycodendrimers of certain sizes (generation) may be, on their own, capable of cross-linking immunoglobulin receptors on B-cells and thus trigger signalization leading ultimately to B-cell proliferations [155]. Monovalent clustered constructs hence constitute the "second generation" vaccines.

4.2.1. Tn-Pam$_3$CS Conjugates

The Jung adjuvant system based on the use of the lipopeptide tripalmitoyl-S-glyceryl-cysteinylserine (Pam$_3$CS) was inserted in a series of synthetic vaccines. After the pioneering example of Tam's synthetic vaccines with a built-in adjuvant directed against HIV, Toyokuni and Singhal reported the synthesis and the biological properties of an anti-cancer fully synthetic vaccine with the carbohydrate epitope Tn linked to Pam$_3$CS as the internal adjuvant [136b, 156]. Pam$_3$CS is non-immunogenic and has no toxic side effects nor does it cause tissue damage in animals. In addition, its adjuvancy is comparable to the classical Freund's adjuvant. It is speculated that lipopeptide Pam$_3$CS acts as a lipid anchor to mediate direct binding of the antigen to Ig molecules which then leads to T helper cell activation [157]. The asialylated ovine submaxillary mucin (A-OSM) which contains a high superficial density of the Tn epitope has been used to immunize mice and provided protection against the highly invasive mouse mammary carcinoma TA3-Ha that expresses Tn antigen [158]. These findings demonstrated that the Tn antigen presented on a protein backbone is capable of providing cellular immunity and protection against tumours in mice.

The essential structure recognized by antibodies directed against the Tn epitope was elucidated in the case of monoclonal antibody MLS 128 [159]. The A-OSM protein was digested with various proteases and, from the tryptic digest glycopeptides that retained high immunoreactivity were isolated. The common motif present in the highly reactive glycopeptide fragments called GP-I and GP-II is Ser*-Thr*-Thr* (the asterisks indicate glycosylation with GalNAc). Other anti-Tn monoclonal antibodies, NCC-LU-35 and CA 3239, showed essentially the same reactivity to these peptides as MLS 128 did. The α-GalNAc STT cluster is therefore an essential part of the epitope recognized by anti-Tn antibodies. Further systematic studies on the nature of Tn epitope have been done by Lo-Man and co-workers and will be described in the next section.

In Toyokuni-Singhal's fully synthetic vaccine a dimeric Tn epitope was associated to the Pam_3CS lipopetide, as shown in Fig. (**28**).

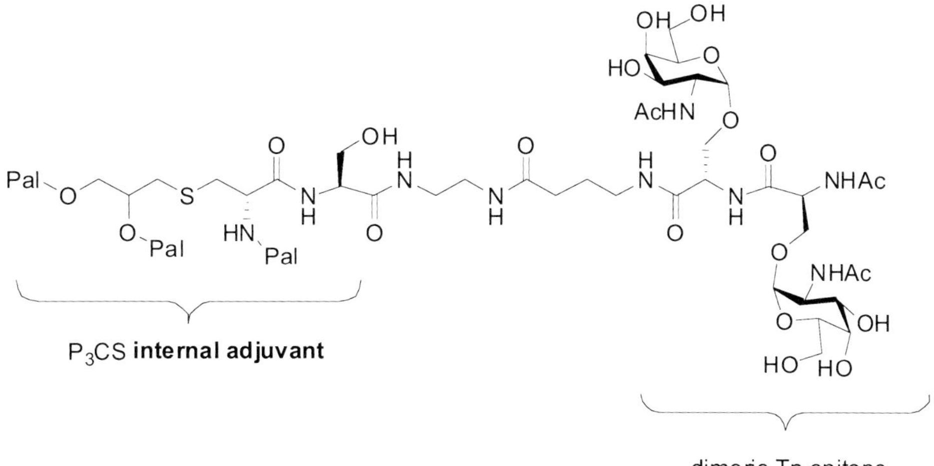

Fig. (28). Chemical structure of the di-Tn-P_3CS construct.

The di-Tn-Pam_3CS vaccine was the first example demonstrating that a synthetic, small carbohydrate antigen can generate an immune response against a TACA without the use of a macromolecular carrier or adjuvant. In this case, the Ser*-Ser* dimer was linked to the lipopeptide Pam_3CS through a nine-atom spacer constituted by an ethylendiamine coupled to a 4-aminobutyric acid. Mice immunized with this compound showed high anti-Tn antibody titers (determined as binding against A-OSM). Interestingly, this immunisation generated not only a high IgM antibody response but also a measurable IgG anti-Tn response. The production of IgG is fundamental for long term immunization and antibody-dependent cellular cytotoxicity (ADCC) against cancer cells. IgG are produced in this case, thus indicating helper T cell enlistment in the absence of external adjuvants.

More recently, Danishefsky and co-workers [15a] compared the efficiency of a very similar tri-Tn-Pam_3CS construct with the same Tn trimeric (clustered) epitope linked to KLH, namely Tn(c)-KLH (Fig. **29**).

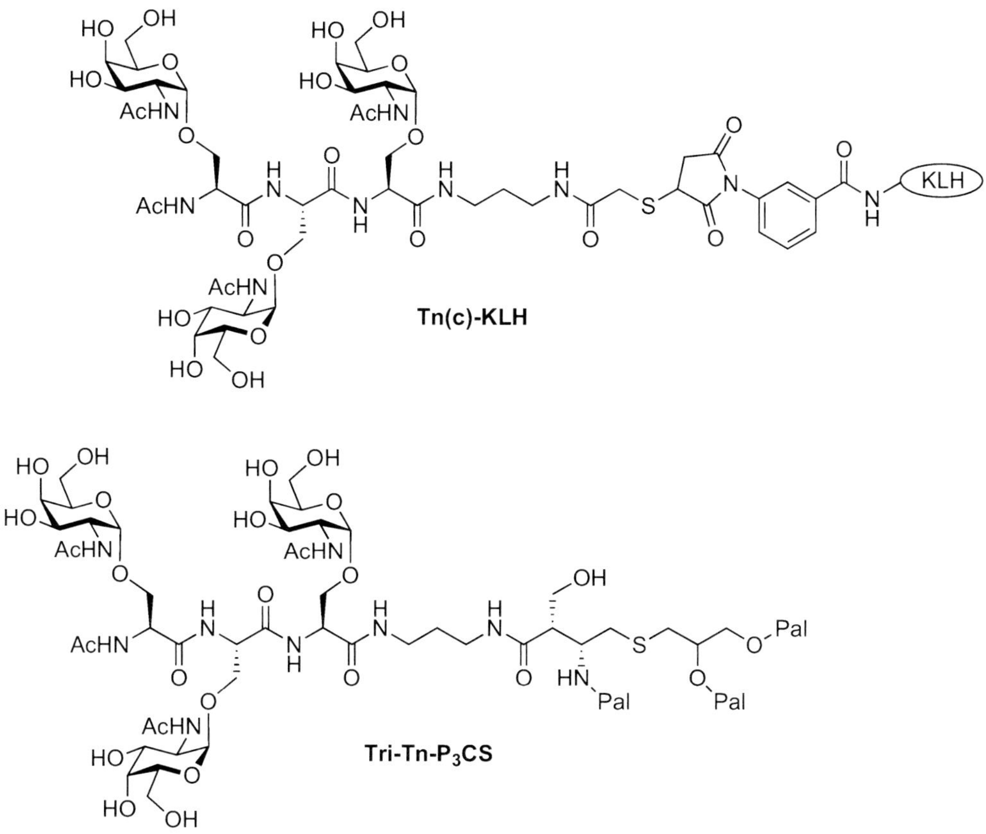

Fig. (29). Structure of the tri-Tn-Pam$_3$CS construct and Tn trimeric epitope linked to KLH (Tn(c)-KLH).

The totally synthetic vaccine tri-Tn-Pam$_3$CS in conjunction with QS-21 failed to show strong immunological reaction in mice, while a higher titer of both IgG and IgM was found in sera of animal immunised with KLH-containing vaccines. These data support, in the author's opinion, the superior immunogenicity of KLH conjugates compared to the fully synthetic constructs.

Several trimeric clustered vaccine constructs, including Tn(c), TF(c), sTn(c), 2,6-sTF(c) and Le^y(c) were synthesised by Danishefsky and co-workers [121a, 160] (Fig. **30**).

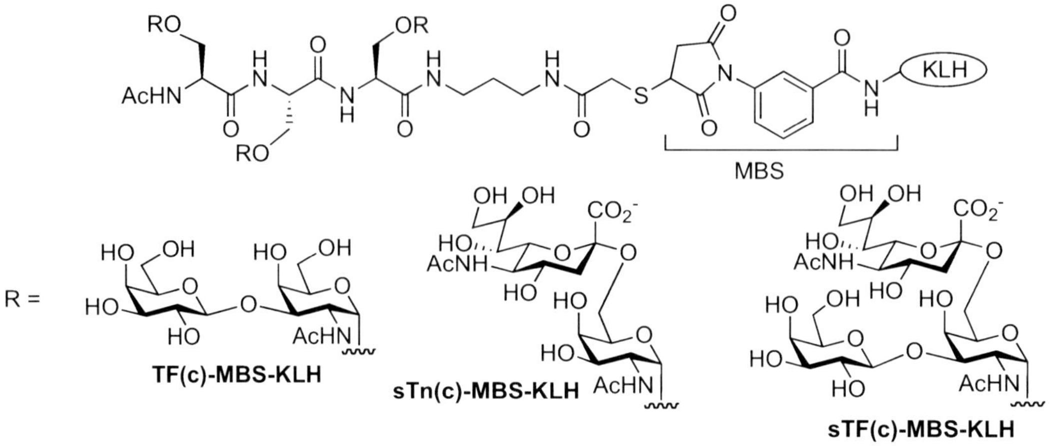

Fig. (30). Several trimeric clustered vaccine constructs proposed by Danishefsky and co-workers.

TF(c) doses of 1, 3, 10 and 30 μg were conjugated to KLH and administered with QS-21 to patients with biochemically relapsed prostate cancer. All doses induced high-titer IgM and IgG antibodies against TF. There did not appear to be increased antibody production with increasing doses of vaccine; higher titers of IgM and IgG antibodies developed at the lowest dose level (1 μg). In general such clustered vaccines exhibited enhanced levels of antibody induction compared to their non-clustered congeners, and are being evaluated in preclinical and clinical trials.

4.2.2. Multiple Antigen Glycopeptides (MAG) Presenting the Tn Epitope

Lo-Man and co-workers [161] ideated a synthetic vaccine named Multiple Antigen Glycopeptide (MAG) presenting in an efficient manner the Tn epitope to the immune system. The concept underlying this type of carbohydrate-based vaccines was inspired by the MAP (Multiple Antigen Peptide) introduced by Tam in 1988 [162].

The MAG molecules were first formed by a non immunogenic tri-lysine core providing four points of attachment that were linked to a T cell epitope and to the Tn antigen. As shown in Fig. (**31**), a second generation of MAG molecules with superior immunological properties presented a trimeric cluster as Tn epitope instead of the GalNAc-α-*O*-Ser monomeric epitope.

The T-helper peptide was the PV peptide in experiments on mice [161a] while for human vaccination [163] a TT or PADRE peptide was used as "universal" CD4+ T-cell epitopes known to stimulate effective T-helper cell responses in human populations with many HLA diversity. In these experiments, sera recognized Tn when located in the middle of the MUC1 peptide, although less efficiently than Tn located at the edge of the peptide chain. Initial encouraging results were obtained with the molecule containing four copies of monomeric Tn epitopes. This MAG, called B4-T4 MAG system was tested *in vitro* and was recognized by anti-Tn monoclonal antibodies MLS 128 (IgG) and 83 D4 (IgM). Surprisingly enough, in the same ELISA test, B4-MAG without the T cell peptide (PV peptide) did not show any interaction with antibodies. The fact that the presence of the PV peptide facilitated the recognition of the B cell Tn epitope by antibodies is not trivial to understand, because antibody specificity is directed exclusively towards the sugar moiety. The PV peptide probably acts as a spacer between the lysine core and the sugar residues in B4-T4 MAG thus facilitating sugar recognition.

In subsequent studies, MAG with trimeric Tn epitopes were used. In particular, the S*T*T* sequence of MAG:Tn_3-PV was designed (Fig. **31**), as optimal mimetic of the natural Tn epitope found on A-OSM. The immunogenicity of MAG:Tn_3-PV was compared to that of the MAG:Tn-PV (previously called B4-T4 MAG by the same authors). When BALB/c mice were immunized with these compounds with alum adjuvant, Tn-specific IgM and IgG were produced with higher titer when using MAG:Tn_3-PV [164]. To ensure that Tn-specific antibodies induced by this molecule can recognize native Tn structures, the binding of sera from immunised mice to tumour cells was analyzed by flow cytometry. Titration of sera from MAG:Tn_3-PV-immunised mice on murine adenocarcinoma TA3-Ha cells demonstrated positive binding of both IgM and IgG antibodies. Likewise, the human Jurkat cell was well recognized by antibodies induced after immunisation with MAG:Tn_3-PV. The capacity of MAG:Tn_3-PV to induce antibodies that reject the highly tumourigenic TA3-Ha adenocarcinoma *in vivo* was also verified. Mice were vaccinated three times with MAG:Tn_3-PV and alum, then, 10 days after the boost, were challenged with TA_3-Ha cells, and survival of animals was followed for 100 days. All untreated mice died within 30 days following tumour challenge, while 80% of mice vaccinated three times with MAG:Tn_3-PV and alum survived the tumour challenge. In contrast, MAG:Tn_3-PV vaccination did not protect mice against the Tn-negative carcinoma CT26 cell line, showing the Tn specificity of the protection provided by MAG.

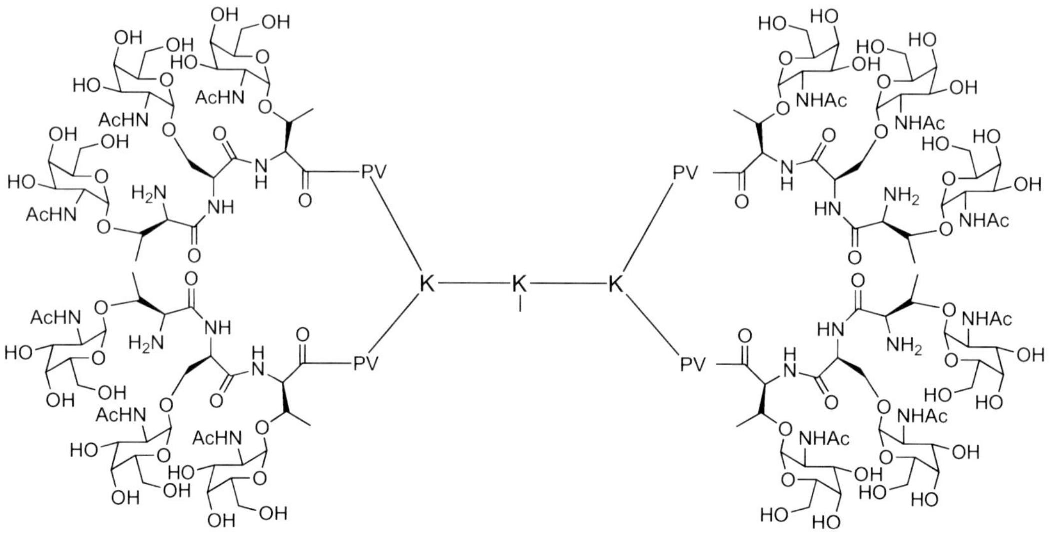

Fig. (31). Chemical structure of MAG:Tn3-PV.

Interestingly, the percentage of survival of mice treated with a linear glycopeptide containing a T cell epitope associated with a double tri-Tn glycotope (Tn_6-PV) was lower than for mice treated with MAG:Tn_3-PV. This result was somehow surprising because the same microgram doses of Tn_6-PV and MAG:Tn_3-PV corresponds to a 1.5-fold greater amount of tri-Tn in the case of Tn_6-PV. There is probably much more rigidity in the double tri-Tn cluster structure of the Tn_6-PV, whereas MAG can display a large variety of Tn glycotopes through its four flexible peptidic arms that can better mimic the diversity of natural Tn clusters.

In a recent study with the goal of optimizing the development of MAG:Tn immunogens, the influence of the amino acid carrying the GalNAc was investigated [184]. MAG were synthesized displaying different trimeric glycopeptides to mimic the Tn epitope: the S*T*T* (used in the immunological studies discussed so far), S*S*S*, hS*hS*hS* (hS = homoserine) sequences. The S*T*T* backbone was found to be the most permissive in generating antibodies that recognise also the other glycotope. On the contrary, IgG generated by MAG containing S*S*S* and hS*hS*hS* backbones were scarcely cross-reactive against the other epitopes. The capacity of the antibodies induced by the different MAG immunogens to recognise the "native form" of Tn on tumour cells was also investigated by flow cytometry. No significant difference was found for the recognition of the Tn-positive Jurkat cell by antibodies elicited by MAG displaying S*T*T* and S*S*S* sequences, while hS*hS*hS* non-natural glycotope induced antibodies that displayed reduced reactivity for native Tn on Jurkat. These data indicate that the nature of the amino acid linked to the GalNAc and the sequence of the glycotope somehow influence the specificity and immunological efficiency of produced antibodies. A further conclusion, in partial contrast with data presented in the next section, is that the Tn epitope would include part of the amino acid structure and the use of Ser of Thr backbones is not equivalent from an immunological point of view.

In the same study a second important point was highlighted: full synthetic MAG:Tn is able to induce anti-Tn IgG antibodies with a mild adjuvant setting (alum), whereas the KLH-Tn conjugate requires the use of a much more powerful adjuvant, such as QS-21. Finally, two MAG were designed and synthesized for human therapy, containing the two different CD4 T-cell peptides, namely TT and PADRE, and were able to provide help for anti-Tn antibody production in all immunized primates. Importantly, in all of the experimental settings, no adverse reaction was observed in any animal such as local inflammation or weight loss assessing the safety of the MAG. Tn-specific antibodies elicited in these nonhuman primates were able to recognize glycosylated human mucin sequences as well as Tn-positive human tumour cells. Antibodies specific for TACA are able to mediate tumour cell killing by complement-dependent cytotoxicity or by ADCC.

Dumy and Lo-Man [165] presented the synthesis and the immunological properties of a novel multiepitopic glycopeptide in which four copies of monomeric Tn antigen analogue are presented on Mutter's Regioselectively Addressable Functionalized Templates (RAFT) [166].

RAFT (Fig. **32**), are topological templates composed of a cyclic decapeptide containing two Pro-Gly β-turns that induce conformational rigidity in solution

[167]. The six lysine residues composing the β-strand provide six attachment points through their side chains in two independent functional faces (four in the upper face and two in the lower, as shown in Fig. **32**). This allowed the construction of a molecule presenting four Tn epitopes on one face of the scaffold and T cell peptides (PV peptides) on the opposite RAFT side.

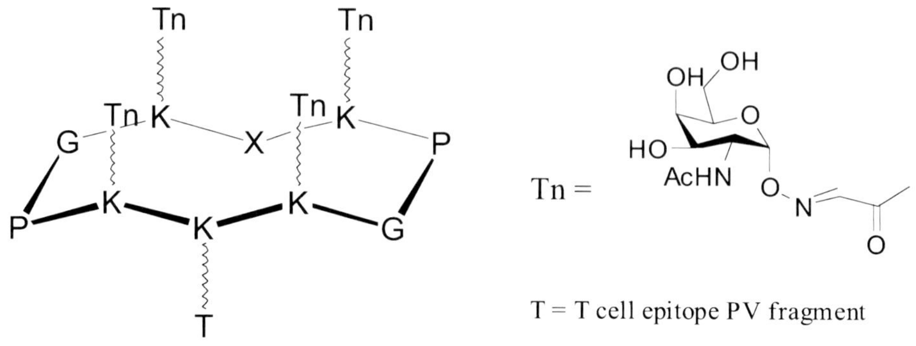

X = Ala: RAFT (4GalNAc, 1PV)
X = Lys-T cell epitope: RAFT(4GalNAc, 2PV)

Fig. (32). Chemical structure of RAFT(4GalNAc, 1PV) and RAFT(4GalNAc, 2PV).

The synthetic vaccines RAFT(4GalNAc, 2PV) and RAFT(4GalNAc, 1PV) were assembled *via* a convergent synthetic way based on the chemoselective ligation of sugar and peptide fragments to the cyclic scaffold. The RAFT intermediate with four serine residues in the upper face and two hydroxylamine groups was first chemoselectively linked to one or two PV peptide fragments with a *C*-terminal aldehyde group. Then the serines were oxidized to aldehydes and condensed with four units of α-GalNAc hydroxylamine. As a consequence of the chemoselective assembly, sugars and peptides were linked to the RAFT through non-natural oxime bonds. Despite the presence of oxime "non native" bonds between GalNAc monosaccharides and lysine side chains, the biotinylated variant RAFT(4GalNAc, Biotin) was recognised in ELISA tests by anti-Tn monoclonal antibodies 6E11 (IgG) and 83D4 (IgM). In contrast with previous observations on MAG:Tn systems, these data indicate that the recognition of antibodies is specifically directed toward the carbohydrate moiety of the RAFT vaccine. Recently RAFT peptides have been successfully glycosylated by alkyne-azide cycloaddition, instead of the oximation procedure [168].

Concerning the T cell PV peptide part, experiments were performed on dendritic cells (DC) in the presence of a population of CTLL cells. The activities RAFT(4GalNAc, 1PV) and the non-glycosylated synthetic precursor RAFT(4Ser, 1PV) were tested. Upon recognition of PV peptide, DC present this peptide in MHCII complexes on their surface, the complex interacts with T-cell receptor (TCR) leading to IL-2 secretion by activated T-cell hybridoma. The IL-2 production was then measured by tritiated- thymidine incorporation by the IL-2 dependent CTLL cell line. Both the unglycosylated and the glycosylated RAFT stimulated the PV-specific T cell hybridoma. This indicates that the presence of a non native oxime bond at the *C*-terminal does not interfere negatively with the T cell determinant presentation by DC to CD4+ T cells. Interestingly enough, the response (IL-2 production) induced by RAFT(4GalNAc, 1PV) was dramatically enhanced at significantly lower doses compared to the response obtained with the non-glycosylated RAFT(4Ser, 1PV). This surprising result would indicated that the presence of the sugar antigens somehow facilitate the presentation of the PV peptide by MHC class II molecules.

BALB/c mice were immunized with RAFT(4GalNAc, 1PV) and alum and a high titer of IgG was found by analyzing sera from immunized mice with ELISA tests. These antibodies were found to be able to bind to human tumour Jurkat cell line expressing the Tn antigen in flow cytometry experiments. It can be concluded that, like MAG systems, also RAFT constructs bearing Tn and PV epitopes with non natural oxime bonds are able to elicit an immune response specifically directed against the native form of Tn displayed by cancer cells.

The use of a single chemoselective ligation for the functionalization of RAFT peptides limits the design complexity of the macromolecule. Dumy proposed that the way [169] to achive the preparation of more sophisticated compounds is to use one-pot triple orthogonal chemoselective ligations, through the combination of a CuAAC reaction, oxime ligation and thioether bond formation.

In a recent work [170] different RAFT constructs have been covalently linked to different sugar headgroups (βGal, βLac and αTF). The relative inhibitory activities of glycocluster with the three ligands reflected the affinity of the free carbohydrates. Headgroup tailoring is thus one route to optimize activity and selectivity of RAFT glycocluster. They studied also the effect of different ligands density and the increase of ligand density from tetra- to hexadecavalency added a second route.

The ligand density effect has been further investigated: a new series of molecularly-defined glycoclusters (Fig. **33**), were synthesized in a controlled manner [171]. Starting from a RAFT carrier, either a polylysine dendritic framework or a second RAFT, then 16 copies of *b*Gal, *a*Man, *b*Lac or cancer-related *a*TF antigen were successively conjugated within the same molecule using oxime chemistry. These macromolecules rapresent a new generation of dendri-RAFTs glycoclusters with high glycosidic density and variable spatial organizations. Further biological assays between a model lectin from *Canavalia ensiformis* (ConA) and mannosylated glycoclusters revealed a higher inhibition potency than the tetravalent counterpart, in particular for the hexadecavalent polylysine skeleton. This result clearly confirms that not only the carbohydrate copy number, but also the tridimensional structure of the glycocluster affects its

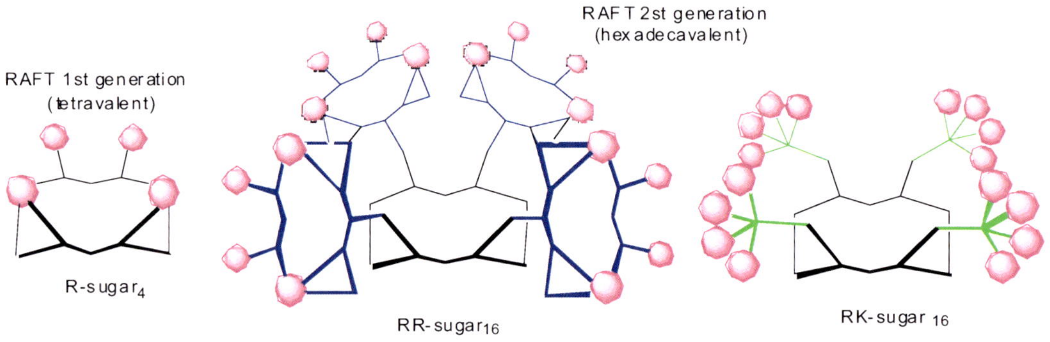

Fig. (33). Chemical structure of different RAFT constructs.

recognition properties. Although these hexadecavalent compounds only differ in their peptide skeleton, the higher inhibition potency might be explained by the higher degree of freedom of carbohydrates and a suitable distribution for multivalent interaction.

Very recently Dumy and co-workers [172] investigated a RAFT construct conteining Tn analogues and a CD8+ CTL peptide, a transmembrane receptor-like glycoprotein with tyrosine kinase activity. They positioned the TLR-2 palmitic acid agonist in different positions of the peptide sequences (Fig. **34**), and they concluded that the attachment at the peptide N-terminal afforded most advantageous results. After challenge inoculation with cancerous MO5 cells, vaccinated mice showed 100% survival after 90 days. The position of the TLR-2 ligand palmitic acid appeared to influence the cross presentation pathway of GLP vaccines constructs within DCs, and this might be a consequence of a difference in binding/internalization process *via* TLR-2. Recently it has been reported that peptides linked to Pam(3)Cys of R-configuration lead to better activation of DCs compared to those with S-configuration [173, 174].

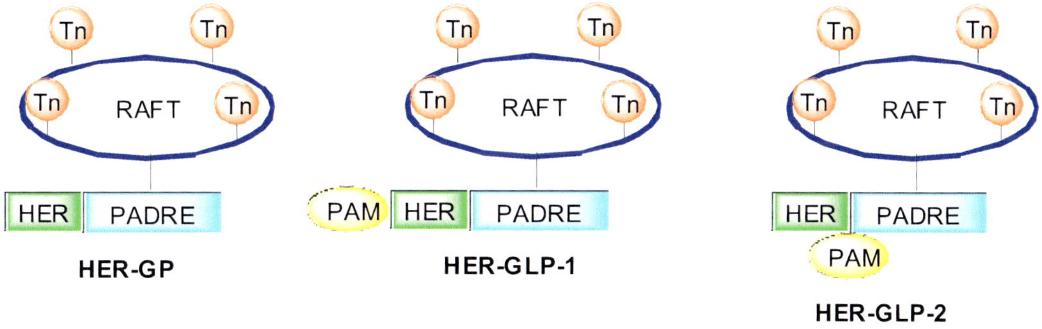

Fig. (34). RAFT constructs with the TLR-2 palmitic acid agonist in different positions.

4.2.3. Other Tn Epitope Containing Constructs

The same chemoselective technique used for RAFT assembly was used for the synthesis of linear glycopeptides formed by the *C*-glycoside analogue of α-GalNAc. As shown in Fig. (**35**), linear molecular constructs were obtained by chemoselective coupling of one or two units of the α-*C*-glycosyl analogue of GalNAc to an *N*-terminal appendage of T cell peptide epitope bearing one or two hydroxylamino groups. In this case too, the final glycoconjugates contain an unnatural oxime bond between the sugar and the peptide unit, through an aminoxyacetic acid spacer (AOA). The T cell epitope of choice was the short peptide fragment 327-339 from chicken ovalbumin (OVA).

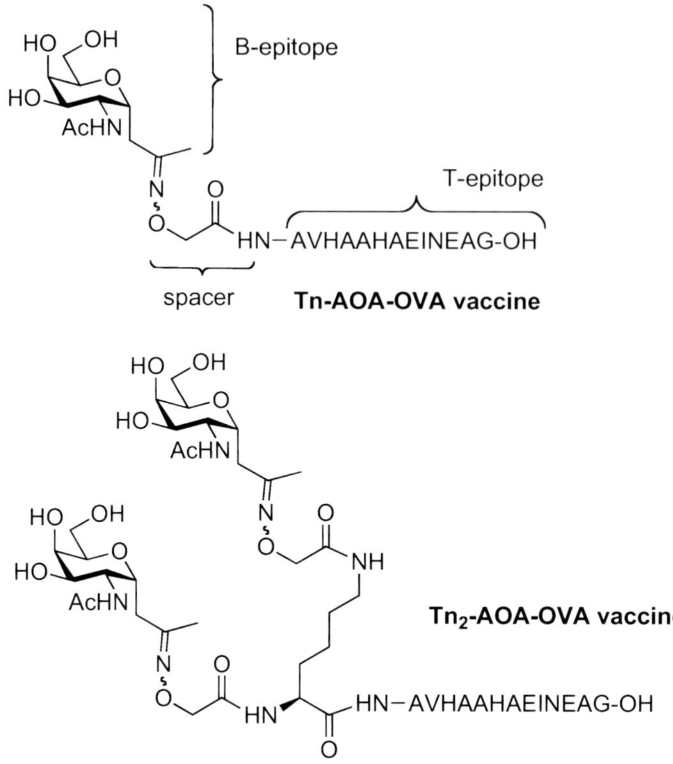

Fig. (35). Structure of unnatural Tn-containing glycoconjugates.

As described in the previous section, the ability of dendritic cells to present the OVA peptide as MHC type II complex to the T cell receptor was analyzed by measuring the incorporation of [^{3}H]-thymidine by the IL-2 dependent T-cell clone CTLL. The glycopeptide containing two sugar units was presented more efficiently than that with just one sugar. In accordance with experiments on MAG:Tn, these data indicate that the non natural oxime bond does not hamper the OVA peptide presentation by DC. Moreover, as observed by Lo-Man, the presence of the sugar units facilitate the T cell epitope presentation.

Kunz and co-workers [48] synthesised also the *N*-terminal glycotripeptide of M blood group asialoglycophorin A (Fig. **36**); the deprotected *N*-acetylated glycotripeptide of exactly specified structure carrying two tumour-associated T-antigen side chains was coupled to bovine serum albumin (BSA) to give the T antigen glycopeptide BSA conjugate as a synthetic vaccine.

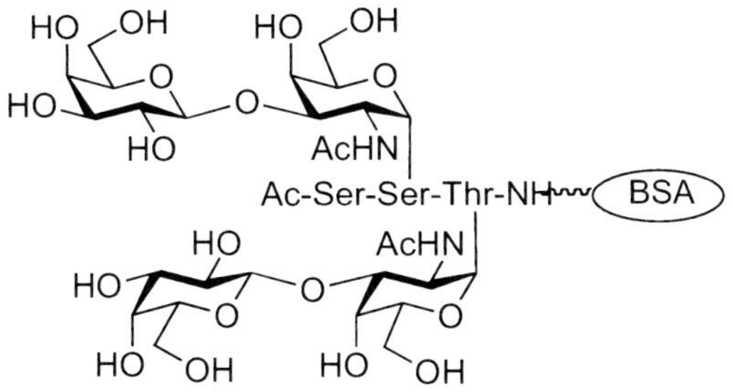

Fig. (36). Structure of the *N*-terminal glycotripeptide conjugated to BSA.

A vaccine consisting of sialyl Tn carbohydrate epitopes coupled to a highly immunogenic carrier molecule, mAb17-1A, adsorbed on alhydrogel and co-formulated with a strong adjuvant, QS-21 was also synthesised [175]. It has been shown by the authors that the sialyl Tn carbohydrate conjugate vaccine, coformulated with QS-21 adjuvant, can induce an IgG response against the sTn moiety [176]. The proposed strategy consisted of coupling tumour-associated carbohydrate epitopes to a highly immunogenic murine antibody with intrinsic antitumour activity [177], in order to use an immunogenic carrier protein to increase the immunogenicity of the carbohydrate antigen and to benefit from the antitumour immune response induced by the carrier molecule itself. Different types of presentation of sialyl Tn (Fig. **37**), (monomeric *vs* trimers *vs* clustered *via* a branched polyethylenimine linker) were studied.

The sialyl Tn-mAb17-1A conjugate vaccine was administered in Rhesus monkeys, and the immune responses against mAb17-1A, sialyl Tn, ovine submaxillary mucin, and tumour cells were analyzed. The data demonstrated that the density of carbohydrate epitopes on the carrier is an essential parameter for induction of anti-carbohydrate specific memory IgG immune responses. Furthermore, the influence of different types of presentation of sialyl Tn

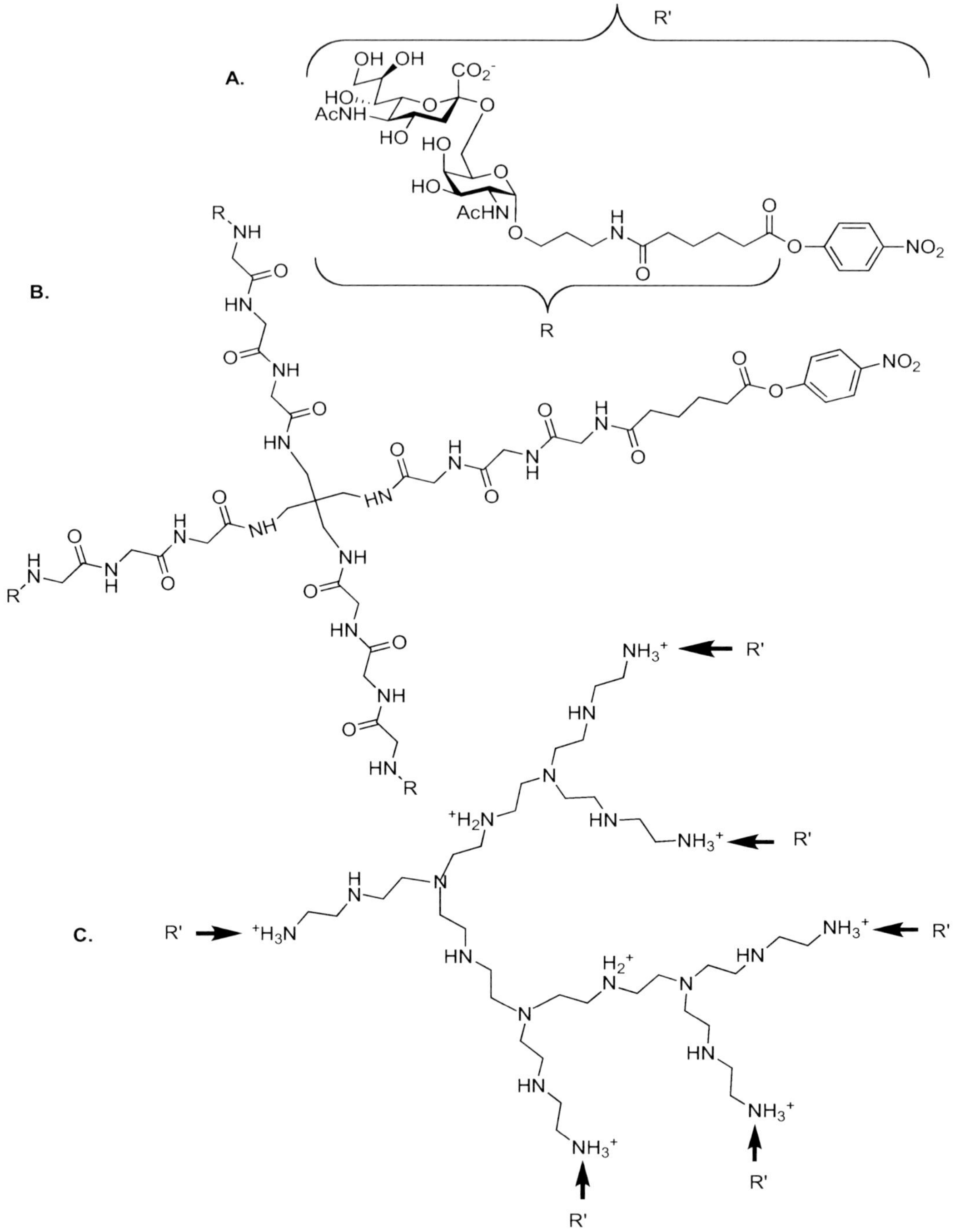

Fig. (37). Different presentation of sialyl Tn epitope: **A**. monomeric; **B**. trimers; **C**. clustered *via* branched linker.

(monomeric *vs* trimers *vs* clustered *via* a branched polyethylenimine linker) on antibody titers and specificity was studied. High density coupling of sialyl Tn epitopes to mAb17-1A induced the strongest immune response against synthetic sialyl Tn and showed also the highest reactivity against natural targets, such as OSM and tumour cells.

Immunization using peptides that mimic carbohydrate Ags has resulted in both Ab and T-cell responses; a fifteen-mer peptide mimic (Fig. **38**), of the TF-Ag (H-I-H-G-W-K-S-P-L-S-S-LG- G-G) was selected by phage display biopanning using

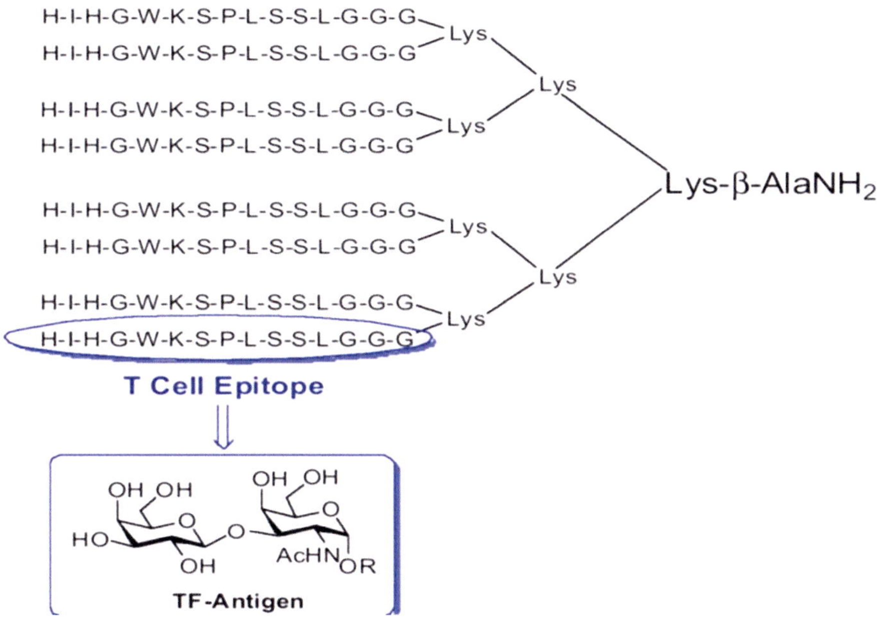

Fig. (38). Dendritic glycomimetic of a carbohydrate related antigen.

IgG3 antibody (JAA-F11) and rabbit anti-TF-Ab and was analyzed *in vitro* to confirm TF-Ag peptide mimicry [178]. *In vivo*, the immunization with TF-Ag-mimicking multiple antigenic peptides induced TF-Ag reactive Ab production. This novel active immunotherapy approach will hopefully decrease tumor burden in cancer patients by specifically targeting TF-Ag positive cancer cells and blocking metastasis. This represented, to the best of our knowledge, the first case of a dendritic glycomimetics of a carbohydrate related antigen.

According to the principle of multiple antigen presentation (MAP), a di-lysyl lysine core was used for the synthesis of tetramers of a glycododecapeptide antigen from the tandem-repeat sequence of the tumor-associated mucin, MUC1, which carries a sialyl- TN-antigen saccharide side chain (Fig. **39**) [179]. The NMR spectra of these dendrimeric compounds in water showed only one set of signals indicating structural equivalency as well as very similar flexibility of the glycopeptide portions of these dendrimers. This result was considered promising for the use of such constructs in immunological treatment of epithelial tumors. In particular, not only a B cell, but also a T cell immune response should be inducible with these multimeric antigens.

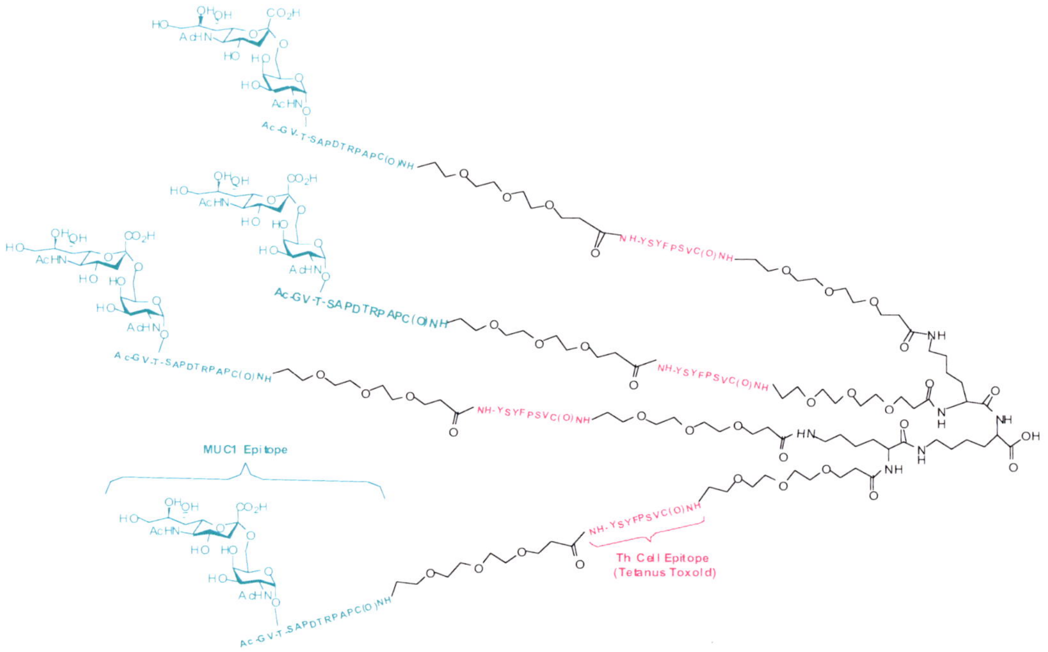

Fig. (39). Sialyl-TN MUC1 Lys2-Lys dendrimer vaccines.

Taking advantage of the overexpression of Gb_3 antigen [180] and the MUC5AC-based peptide marker on ovarian cancer [181], Danishefsky and co-workers designed and synthesized a vaccine construct targeting ovarian carcinoma [182]. The efficient synthesis was enabled by the preparation of a Gb3-MUC5AC thioester cassette as a key building block for constructing three alternating repeats of Gb3 and MUC5AC (Fig. **40**). Both nonconjugate and KLH-conjugate vaccine

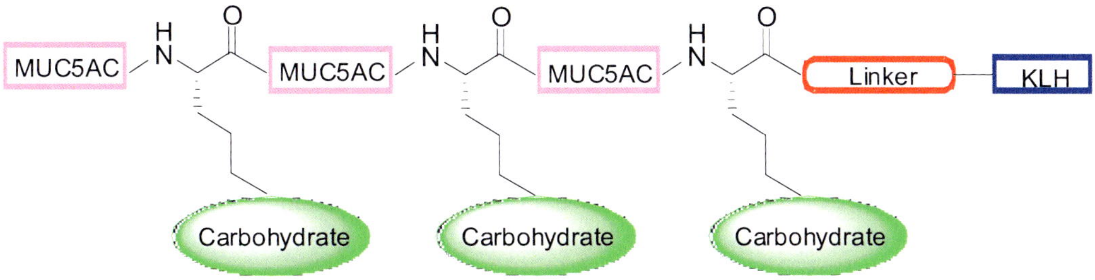

Fig. (40). New model of antitumor vaccine based on carbohydrate-peptide conjugated system.

candidates have been prepared and the results of immunological evaluations will be forthcoming. Due to the fact that Gb3 exists as a ceramide form, the authors prepared Gb3 glycosylamino acid using non-natural extended hydroxynorleucine linker in the hopes of mimicking the ceramide chain.

4.3. Multivalent Constructs

As outlined previously, each type of malignant tissue is characterized by a distinct set of changes in glycan expression. The design of the first generation carbohydrate vaccines, displaying only multiple copies of one TACA did not take into account the degree of heterogeneity of carbohydrates expressed on transformed cell surfaces. Even within a particular cancer type, there is a considerable amount of variation in the level and nature of cell-surface carbohydrates expressed [16]. In principle, a vaccine that targets several cancer-associated glycans should lead to a stronger and more specific immune response than one that targets a single cancer glycan [183].

In an effort to mirror the heterogeneous nature of cancer-cell surface glycans, Danishefsky and co-workers prepared multiantigenic vaccines that contain several different glycan structures [184], closely associated with a specific cancer on a single molecule (unimolecular multivalent construct).

Inspired by the way of presentation in natural mucins, multiple tumour antigens were included into a single polypeptide construct. Non-natural amino acids have been used for the conjugation of the glycans, supposing that such unnatural linkages might result in an enhanced immune response. Furthermore, the use of amino acids containing long, aliphatic side chains may serve to distance the glycosides from the peptide backbone and facilitate glycopeptide synthesis.

A unimolecular trivalent (Fig. **41**), and a pentavalent vaccine (Fig. **42**), employing non-natural amino acids as linkers to carbohydrate domains have been prepared. The trivalent construct containing carbohydrate epitopes Tn, Lewis y, and Globo H has undergone preliminary investigation; preclinical evaluation has shown promising levels of immunogenicity, with antibody responses observed against each individual carbohydrate antigen, demonstrating proof of principle for a unimolecular multivalent vaccine construct with a non-natural amino acid linker.

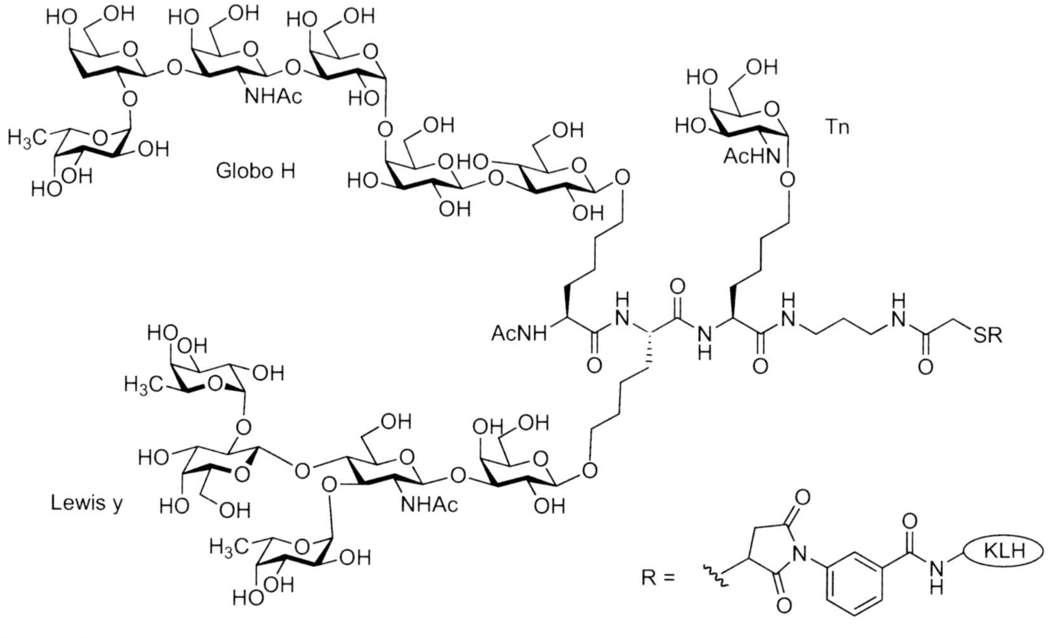

Fig. (41). Unimolecular trivalent vaccine.

In order to target prostate cancer the pentavalent vaccine conjugate containing five carbohydrate antigens known to be expressed in high levels on prostate cancer cell surfaces, Tn, TF, sTn, Lewis y, and Globo H (Fig. **42**), was also prepared.

The vaccine was conjugated separately to two different carrier proteins, KLH and Pam_3Cys (P_3CS) (Fig. **42**). *In vivo* preclinical serological results of these pentavalent constructs, including ELISA assays and FACS analysis, were conducted [185]. The cumulative data suggest that the immunological properties of the individual antigens are preserved in these highly elaborate vaccines and constitute a strong case for evaluating the central concept of the unimolecular multiantigenic fully synthetic vaccine in the setting of clinical trials. Also a hexavalent vaccine containing the Tn, TF, sTn, Le^y, Globo H and GM2 TACAs was synthesised.

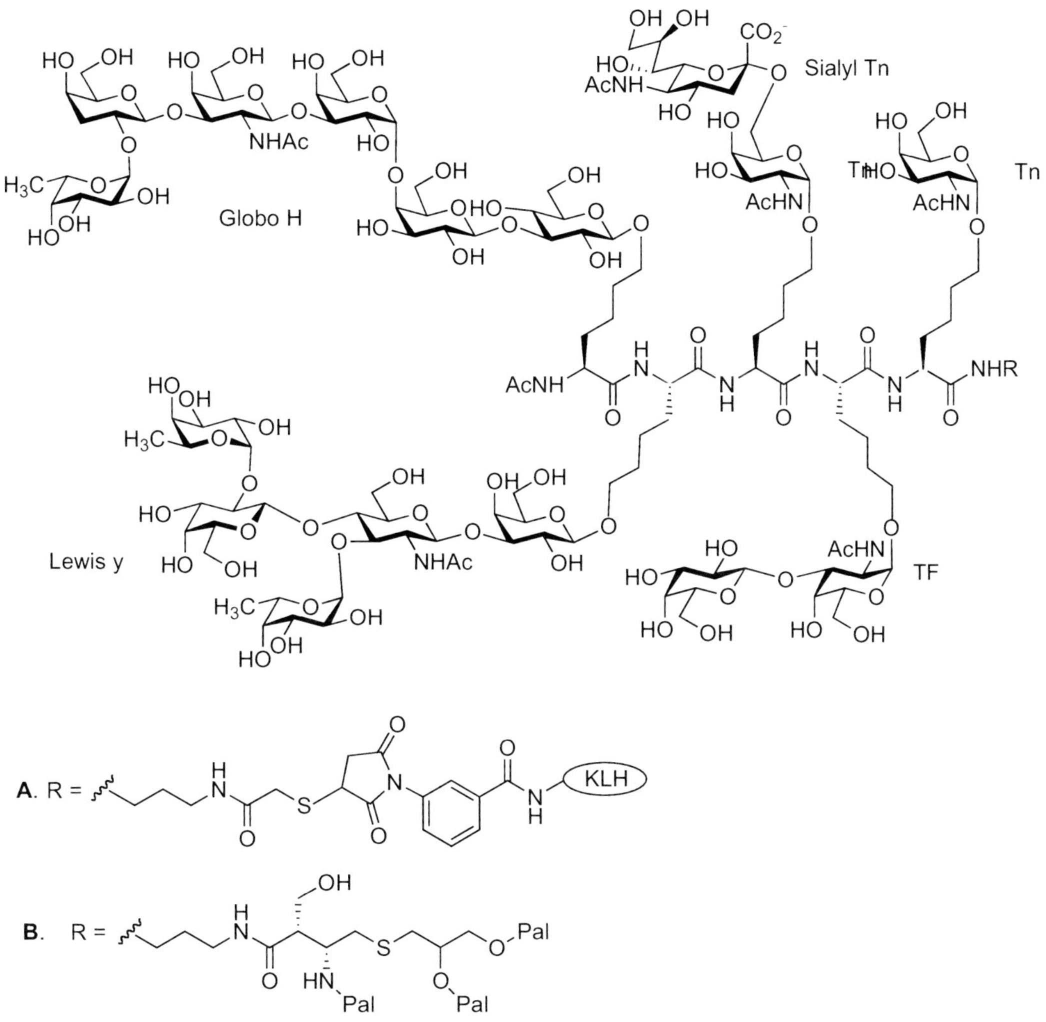

Fig. (42). Pentavalent vaccine conjugated to two different carrier proteins, **A**. KLH and **B**. Pam_3Cys (Pal = palmitoyl).

The over-expression of MUC1, a human tumor-associated epithelial mucin, is correlated with the progression of breast, ovarian, and colon cancer [186]. Based on these observations and the promising biological properties of the unimolecular pentavalent vaccine, Danishefsky's group prepared a hybrid vaccine construct containing a unimolecular pentavalent glycopeptide domain covalently linked to the MUC1 peptide (Fig. **43**) [187]. The preparation of the KLH conjugate of this construct is currently underway.

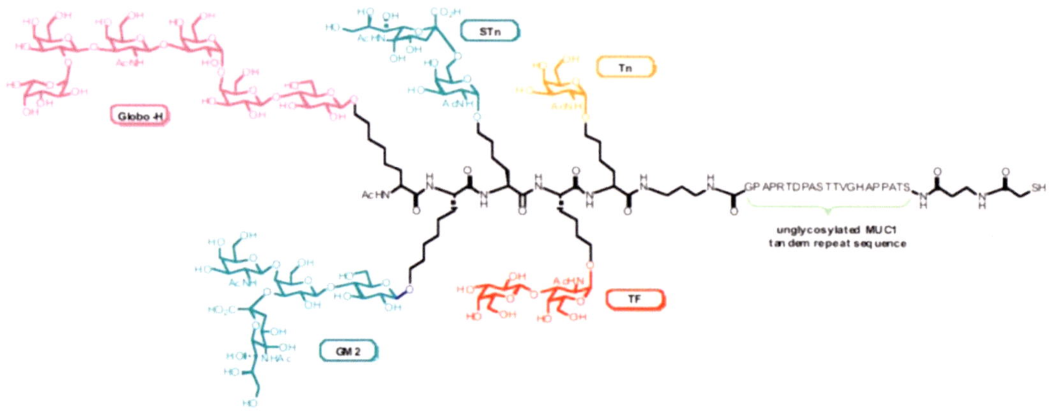

Fig. (43). A complex unimolecular pentavalent MUC1 glycopeptide construct for prostate and breast cancer.

Recently Danishefsky and co-workers [188] prepared multiantigenic vaccines using a cyclic peptide scaffold, as reported in Fig. (**44**). Positions A and F may contain handles for glycan attachments, whereas position G is a cysteine suitable for linkage to a carrier protein or biological marker. They synthesized a multiantigenic construct incorporating both Tn and STn antigens. This type of multivalent construct is intended to reflect the degree of carbohydrate heterogeneity associated with most cancer. Morover the authors used also a cross-linking methatesis between the carbohydrates in order to ridify the construct and prevent undesired spreading of glycan units. Immunological investigation of these new macromolecules are not yet reported.

4.4. Nanotechnology for Cancer Therapy

Nanosciences and nanotechnologies are widely seen as having huge potential to bring advantages and innovations in different areas such as new drug development, information and communication technologies and the production of stronger, lighter materials. Bio-nanotechnologies, in particular, are concerned with

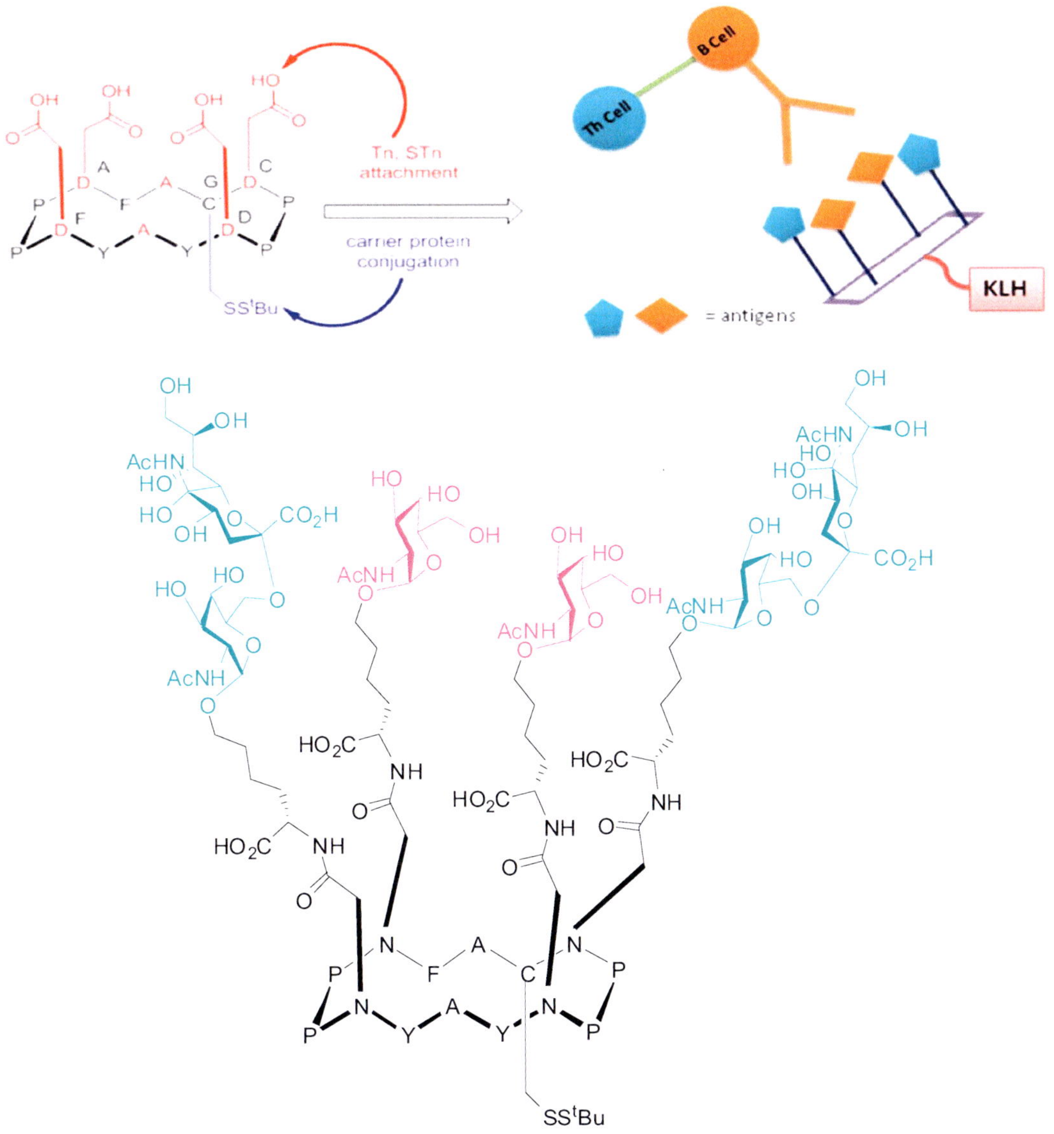

Fig. (44). Multivalent RAFT glycoconjugate.

molecular scale properties and applications of biological nanostructures and work at the interface between chemical, biological and physical sciences.

Bio-nanotechnologies can be used for the development of new anti-cancer therapies; construction of carbohydrate clustered systems on gold nanoparticles affords nano-glycoconjugates presenting anti-tumour activity. Gold glyconanoparticles can be considered as a bio-mimetic model of carbohydrate presentation at the cell surface. This represents a very important feature because of the carbohydrate key role in cell-adhesion and cell-recognition events regarding many physiological but also pathological processes, such as infection [189], inflammation [190] and metastasis development [191]. Their employment allows us to achieve systems that present some peculiar characteristics: high degree of multiple antigen presentation, high storage and biological stability against enzymatic degradation, easy control of ligand number and nanoparticle size [192].

In recent years Penades and co-workers developed a one step versatile methodology to prepare gold GNPs based on Brust's procedure [193]. In particular, the *in situ* reduction of a gold salt in the presence of an excess of the appropriate thiol-derivatized glycan leads to the GNPs (Fig. **45**) [194].

The influence of ligand density and presentation on the recognition by protein receptors has been evaluated by examining the interaction of lactose-functionalized GNPs with two different galactose-specific carbohydrate-binding proteins: an enzyme, *E. coli* β-galactosidase, and a lectin, Viscum album agglutinin [195]. The results suggest that the proper selection of ligand densities and spacers in GNP functionalization is an important requisite to match the topological requirements of the target receptor while escaping glycosidase degradation. The authors observed that ligand clustering is not necessarily correlated with improved binding affinity and a higher valence of GNP does not imply a superior inhibitory potential. In this regard, the use of flexible spacers may facilitate matching the geometrical requirements of the receptor.

Glyco-nanoparticles were employed as anti-adhesion devices against metastasis progression [196]. In fact, one of the most critical steps in metastasis is the adhesion of tumour cells to the vascular endothelium, followed by their transmigration and generation of new tumour *foci*. Tumour cell metastasis is promoted by interactions between tumour-associated antigens and selectins of epithelial cells, but also carbohydrate-carbohydrate interactions between glycosphingolipids expressed on the tumour and endothelial cell surfaces seem to

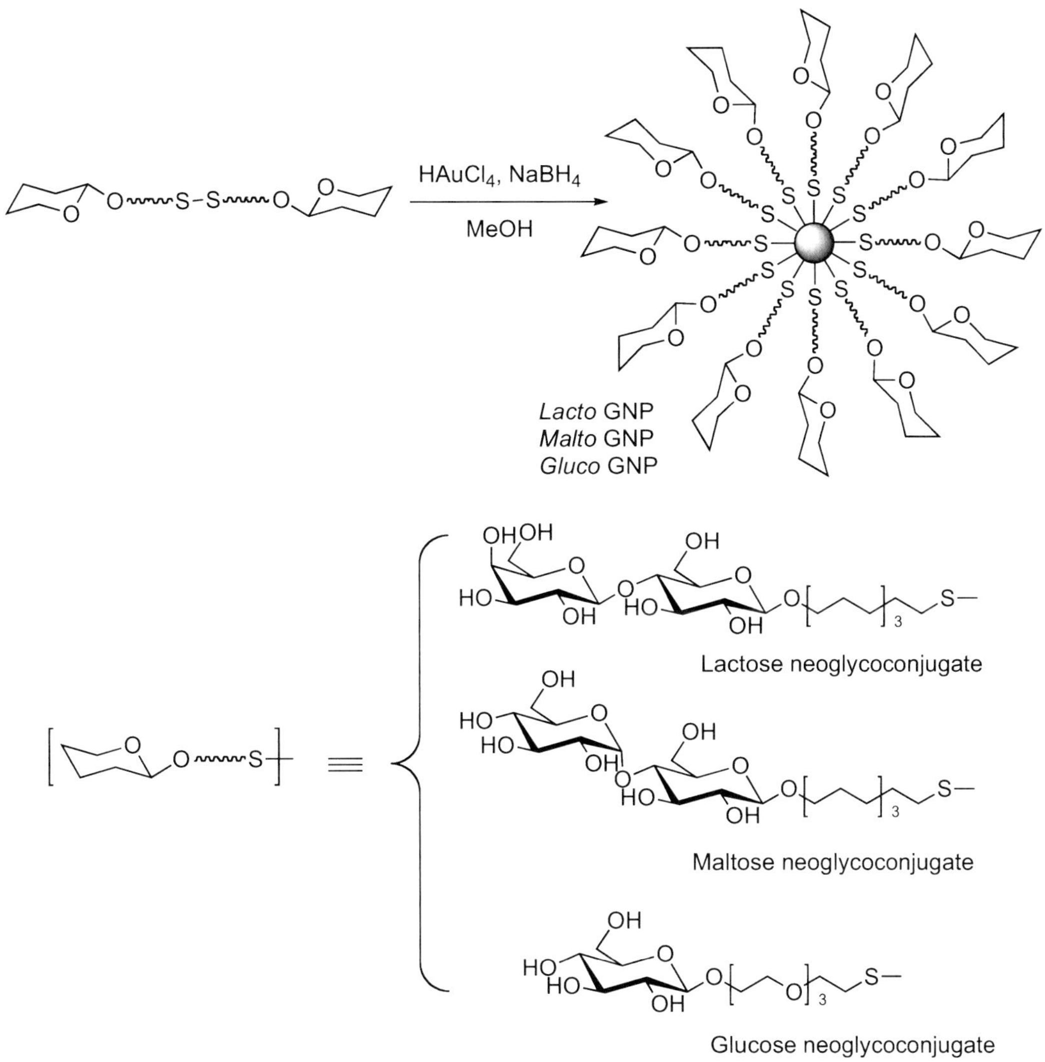

Fig. (45). Procedure for the preparation of gold glyconanoparticles.

be involved in the critical adhesion step. It has been proposed that a carbohydrate-carbohydrate interaction between GM3 expressed in a murine melanoma cell line (B16), that generates aggressive metastasis in lung [197] and Gg3 or lactosylceramide of endothelium cells is crucial for this process [198]. As a consequence, inhibition of this event by glyco-nanoparticles presenting carbohydrate antigens expressed either in the tumour or the endothelium cells could represent an effective anti-adhesion therapy. In particular, as the antigen lactosylceramide is involved in cell adhesion, lactose gold glyco-nanoparticles (*lacto*-GNPs) were tested as potential inhibitor of the interaction between melanoma cells and endothelium cells. According to the author's results, a 70% tumour inhibition was obtained when mice injected with melanoma cells pre-incubated with lactose-gold glyconanoparticles were sacrificed after three weeks and both lungs evaluated under the microscope for analysis of tumour *foci*. Glyco-nanoparticles functionalised with the disaccharide maltose (Glcα1→4Glc, *malto*-GNPs) and the monosaccharide glucose (*gluco*-GNPs), which are not involved in this adhesion process, have also been prepared and tested as negative control systems (Fig. **45**).

An additional application of gold glyco-nanoparticles was illustrated by Svarovsky and co-workers [199]. They proposed the synthesis of gold nanoparticles bearing the Thomsen-Friedenreich (TF) disaccharide. Applying the method previously described, they prepared 3-dimensional self assembled monolayers (3D-SAMs) of gold particles functionalized with the TF moiety (Fig. **46**).

According to preliminary data, *in vitro* and *in vivo* anti-tumour and anti-metastatic bioassays revealed the TF-gold nanoparticle ability to inhibit tumour growth and lung metastasis formation against an implanted metastatic breast cancer cell line.

Barchi *et al.* prepared gold nanoparticles bearing the TF antigen at different densities and in different context [200]. GNPs containing a range of densities 'diluted' with copies of the PEG-thiol spacer unit showed that lower antigen density affords more uniform particles. The authors also studied the constitution of the actual antigen by synthesizing nanoparticles not only with the linker-extended disaccharide, but also within the context of the surrounding peptide sequence where it may be presented *in vivo*. The synthesis of TFag-containing glycopeptide thiols based on a mucin peptide repeating unit were prepared, assembled into gold nanoparticles and their physical properties evaluated. Sizing data showed that certain sugar presentations result in the assembly of particles that may have reasonable uniformity in their gold core diameters by TEM analysis, but they can be polydispersed and 'non-uniform' in solution. Glycopeptide-coated nanoparticles result in more uniform particles as seen by

TEM analysis, however, GNP's and GPNP's contain some larger size elements that could be a consequence of either aberrations in the self-assembly process or aggregation events. An important conclusion gleaned from this work is that nanoconstructions with various surface chemistries may display very different behavior when comparing microscopy to sizing measurements in solution.

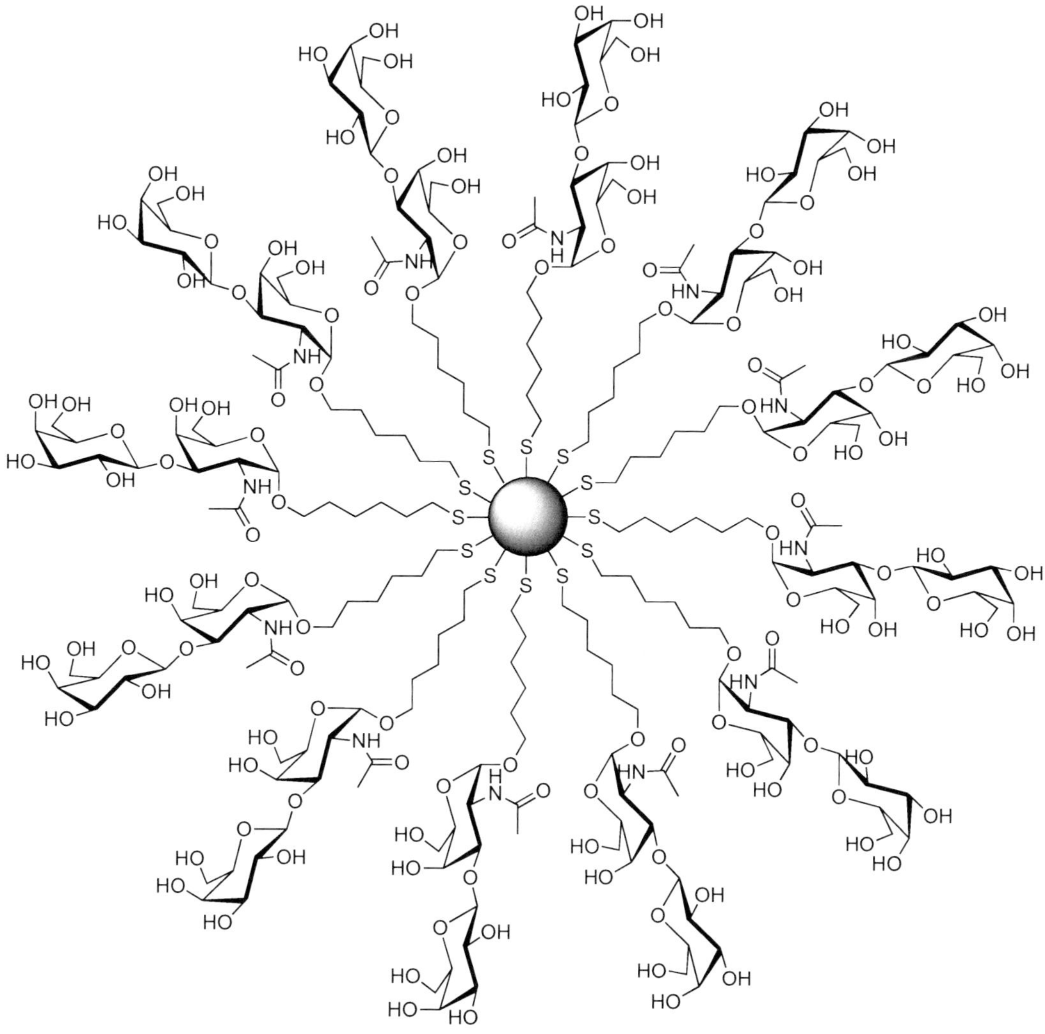

Fig. (46). Gold nanoparticles bearing the Thomsen-Friedenreich disaccharide.

Surprisingly, in 2005 P. Mukherjee *et al.* [201] demonstrated that gold nanoparticles present a particular intrinsic property: they are capable of binding to heparin-binding growth factors like VEGF165 and bFGF, and inhibiting these growth factor-mediated signalling. VEGF165 and bFGF are two endothelial cell mitogens and mediators of angiogenesis. Gold nanoparticle ability to selectively inhibit VEGF165- and bFGF-induced proliferation of HUVECs and fibroblasts means that they present an intrinsic anti-angiogenic activity.

It is known that highly patterned displays of antigens can lead to earlier B cell amplification for potent IgM responses as well as efficient switching to IgG. Antigen organization has a great influence on B cell tolerance, with B cells unresponsive to poorly organized antigens while responding promptly to the same antigen presented in a highly organized manner. Recently, viral capsids have emerged as a promising platform for antigen presentation. Peptide epitopes presented on the surface of viral capsids can stimulate an adaptive immune response by effective activation of antigen presenting cells as well as stimulation of B-cell mediated response by direct cross-linking of B cell receptors ([202, 203]). Huang and co-workers [204] selected the cowpea mosaic virus capsid (CPMV), which is high immunogenic yet non-infectious to humans; in particular the authors used a mutant capsid bearing reactive cysteines on the exterior surface, used for the selective conjugation with Tn antigens. The glycoconjugate was then injected into mice and pre- and post-immune antibody levels in the mice sera were measured by enzyme-linked immunosorbant assays. High total antibody titers and, more importantly, high IgG titers specific for Tn were obtained in the post-immune day 35 serum, suggesting the induction of T cell-dependent antibody isotype switching by the glycoconjugate. The antibodies generated were able to recognize Tn antigens presented in their native conformations on the surfaces of both MCF-7 breast cancer cells and the multidrug resistant breast cancer cell line NCIADR RES. These results suggest that the CPMV capsid can greatly enhance the immunogenicity of weak antigens such as Tn and this can provide a promising tool for the development of carbohydrate based anti-cancer vaccines.

Low production cost, the ease with which they can be functionalized with bioconjugates presenting anti-tumour activity, associated with their intrinsic anti-angiogenic properties, make nanoparticles a viable tool for the development of new anti-cancer drugs.

Moreover magnetic glyconanoparticles (*glyco*-ferrites) rapresents a usefull tool for selective immunolabeling and imaging of cells [205, 206]. Antibody-MGNPs conjugates are excellent candidates to accomplish sensitive and highly specific detection of cells. The presence of the outer gold layer ensures possibilities for easy chemical conjugation of diverse molecules in varying ratios. The hybrid nature of these nanoparticles is a great advantage, as the carbohydrate molecules provide resistance to nonspecific adsorption and lack of immunogenicity, while allowing specific targeting and keeping the size of the nanoparticles smaller than other stabilizers. This feature represents an advantage for *in vivo* applications, as it facilitates longer blood half-life, avoiding RES clearance. The possibility of conjugating different vectors (peptides, DNA, small molecules, and others) to these sugar/carboxyl hybrid magnetic nanoparticles (MGNPs) makes them excellent candidates for the production of high-quality contrast agents, capable of detecting targets at the cellular and molecular level.

5. CONCLUSION AND PERSPECTIVES

The ensemble of results presented in this review on the immunological activity of Tn-containing artificial vaccines suggests some general remarks. The advantages in the use of fully synthetic vaccines instead of carrier protein glycoconjugates presented in the introductory section have been only partially attained. While some of Danishefsky's vaccines based on KLH conjugates are in an advanced phase of clinical trials, the experimentation on humans of fully synthetic is still at a less advanced stage. However, the efficiency of MAG:Tn or RAFT:Tn or Tn-P_3CS constructs in eliciting antibody response both in mice and non-human primates is a matter of fact documented by elegant and exhaustive studies. The greater potency of synthetic vaccines over carrier-protein glycoconjugates is still controversial. According to Lo-Man, the MAG:Tn vaccines would be superior to KLH-Tn conjugates and would induce higher titer of IgG requiring for this less potent and safer adjuvants such as alum. In this perspective, MAG derivatives would be more suitable molecules than KLH glycoconjugates for the clinical development of an anti-cancer vaccine for humans. On the contrary, Danishefsky showed that KLH conjugates are more efficient than Toyokuni's Tn-P_3CS molecules in inducing anti-Tn IgG response.

The use of virus capsid as carrier for the development of carbohydrate based antitumor vaccines, seems to be promising: Huang observed a statistically significant increase in binding to MCF-7 cells by IgG, which was similar to those obtained from a trivalent vaccine construct. This suggests the IgG antibodies generated were able to recognize Tn in its native configurations on the tumor cell surface.

Some interest arises from structure-activity relationship (SAR) in synthetic vaccines. The investigation of SAR in these molecular constructs is particularly difficult because the complex molecular events responsible for antibody production have been only partially clarified. Penadès observed that ligand clustering in gold glyconanoparticles is not necessarily correlated with improved binding affinity.

The fact that both sugar Tn antigen and peptide T cell antigen must be present in the same molecule does not indicate that these antigens are processed and recognized simultaneously. On the contrary, the sugar epitope recognition by B-cells and the peptide presentation as MHC complex to TCR for T cells activation, are events that occur in different phases of the antibody generation process. In the design of RAFT molecules it has also been shown that the presentation of sugar and peptide epitopes on different sides of a rigid scaffold could facilitate the recognition of both epitopes thus making the vaccine more efficient. In this sense, the MAG:Tn constructs tested so far which present the peptide and the sugar as directly linked could be improved by presenting the sugars and the peptides in different spatial regions.

However, experimental data on linear Tn-T peptide and MAG:Tn also indicate that the presence of sugar units (clusters) facilitate the presentation of the T epitope peptide on MHC molecules, and, on the other hand, the peptide helps the sugar to be recognized by Tn-specific antibodies.

This unexpected synergy between the sugar Tn and peptide epitopes is an important element to take into account in the design of novel anticancer vaccines.

Glyconanoparticles rapresent a usefull tool for the development of new synthetic vaccines. Moreover *lacto*-nanoparticles have proved to be a poor substrate for *E.*

Coli β galactosidase. The observed stability toward degradation, togheter with the lack of toxicity against severall cell lines, makes the GNP technology a promising strategy for the development of new potential drugs.

CONFLICT OF INTEREST

The authors declare that there is no conflict of interest.

ACKNOWLEDGEMENT

Declared none.

DISCLOSURE

This chapter is an update of the previously published review Glycoconjugates in cancer therapy appeared in *Anti-Cancer Agents Med. Chem.*, **2008**, *8*, 92-121.

REFERENCES

[1] Prehn, R.T.; Main, J.M. *J. Natl. Cancer Inst.*, **1957**, *18*, 769.
[2] Klein, G.; Sogren, H.O.; Klein, H.; Hellstrom, K.E. *Cancer Res.*, **1960**, *20*, 1561.
[3] a) Burnet, F.M. *Brit. Med. J.*, **1957**, *1*, 841; b) Burnet, F.M. *Prog. Exp. Tumor Res.*, **1970**, *13*, 1.
[4] Thomas, L. In *Cellular and Humoral Aspects of the Hypersensitive States;* Lawrence, H.S. Ed.; Hoeber-Harper, New York, **1959**; pp. 529–532.
[5] Dunn, G.P.; Bruce, A.T.; Ikeda, H.; Old, L.J.; Schreiber, R.D. *Nature Immunol.*, **2002**, *3*, 991.
[6] a) Gilboa, E. *Nature Rev. Cancer*, **2004**, *4*, 401; b) Astronomo, R.D.; Burton, D.R. Nature Rev. Drug Discov. **2010**, *9*, 308; c) Slovin, S.F.; Keding, S.J.; Ragupathi, G. *Immunol. Cell Biol.* **2005**, 83, 418; d) Keding, S.J.; Danishefsky, S.J. PNAS, **2004**, *101*, 11937; e) Jäger, E.; Jäger, D.; Knuth, A. *Curr. Opin. Immunol.*, **2002**, *14*:178.
[7] Meezan, E.; Wu, H.C.; Black, P.H.; Robbins, P.W. *Biochemistry*, **1969**, *8*, 2518; b) Dube, D.H.; Bertozzi, C.R. *Nature Rev. Drug Discov.* **2005**, *4*, 477.
[8] Rabinovich, G.A.; Croci, D.O. *Cell*, **2012**, *36*, 322; b) Turner, G.A. *Clin. Chim. Acta*, **1992**, *208*, 149; c) Saussez, S.; Marchant, H.; Nagy, N.; Decaestecker, C.; Hassid, S.; Jortay, A.; Schüring, M.-P.; Gabius, H.-J.; Danguy, A.; Salmon, I.; Kiss, R. *Cancer*, **1998**, *82*, 252.
[9] Shriver, Z.; Raguram, S.; Sasisekharan, R. *Nature. Rev. Drug Discov.*, **2004**, *3*, 863.
[10] a) Matsumoto, A.; Cabral, H.; Sato, N.; Kataoka, K.; Miyahara, Y. *Angew. Chem. Int. Ed.* **2010**, *49*, 5494; b) Ohtsubo, K.; Marth, J.D. *Cell* **2006**, *126*, 855; c) Kim, Y.J.; Varki, A. *Glycoconj. J.*, **1997**, *14*, 569.
[11] Sell, S. *Human Path.*, **1990**, *21*, 1003;b) Hakomori, S.; Zhang, Y. *Chem. Biol.*, **1997**, *4*, 97; c) Taylor Papadimitriou, J.; Epenetos, A.A. *Trends Biotechnol.*, **1994**, *12*, 227; d) Gabius,

H.J. *Angew. Chem. Int. Ed.,* **1988**, *27*, 1267; e) Ju, T.; Otto, V.I.; Cummings, R.D. *Angew. Chem. Int. Ed.* **2011**, *50*, 1770.

[12] Hollingsworth, M.A.; Swanson, B.J. *Nature Rev. Cancer,* **2004**, *4*, 45.

[13] Fukuda, M. *Cancer Res.,* **1996**, *56*, 2237.

[14] a) Jurianz, K.; Ziegler, S; Garcia-Schuler, H.; Kraus, S.; Bohana-Kashtan, O.; Fishelson, Z.; Kirschfink, M. *Mol. Immunol.,* **1999**, *36*, 929; b) Speiser, D.E.; Miranda, R.; Zakarian, A.; Bachmann, M.F.; McKall-Faienza, K.; Odermatt, B.; Hanahan, D.; Zinkernagel, R.M.; Ohashi, P.S. *J. Exp. Med.,* **1997**, *186*, 645.

[15] Danishefsky, S.J.; Allen, J.R. *Angew. Chem. Int. Ed.,* **2000**, *39*, 836; b) Livingston, P.O. *Immunol. Rev.,* **1995**, *145*, 147; c) Freire, T.; Bay, S.; Vichier-Guerre, S.; Lo-Man, R.; Leclerc, C. *MiniRev. Med. Chem.,* **2006**, *6*, 1357.

[16] Zhang, S.; CordonCardo, C.; Zhang, H.S.; Reuter, V.E.; Adluri, S.; Hamilton, W.B.; Lloyd, K.O.; Livingston, P.O. *Int. J. Cancer,* **1997**, *73*, 42; b) Zhang, S.; Zhang, H.S.; CordonCardo, C.; Reuter, V.E.; Singhal, A.K.; Lloyd, K.O.; Livingston, P.O. *Int. J. Cancer*, **1997**, *73*, 50.

[17] Dzhambazov, B.; Holmdahl, M.; Yamada, H.; Lu, S.; Vestberg, M.; Holm, B.; Johnell, O.; Kihlberg, J.; Holmdahl, R. *Eur. J. Immunol.*, **2005**, *35*, 357.

[18] Xu, Y.; Sette, A.; Sidney, J.; Gendler, S.J.; Franco, A. *Immunol. Cell Biol.*, **2005**, *83*, 440.

[19] Bettahi, I.; Dasgupta, G.; Renaudet, O.; Chentou, A.A.; Zhang, X.; Carpenter, D.; Yoon, S.; Dumy, P.; BenMohamed, L. *Cancer. Immunol. Immun.*, **2009**; *58*, 187-200.

[20] Danishefsky, S.J.; Bilodeau, M.T. *Angew. Chem. Int. Ed.,* **1996**, *35*, 1380.

[21] a) Keding, S.J.;Danishefsky, S. J. In *Carbohydrate-Based Drug Discovery*, Wong, C.-H. Ed.; Wiley-VCH, Weinheim, Germany, **2003** Vol. *1*, pp. 381-406; b) Bundle, D.R. *Vaccine Design* **2011**, 69.

[22] Ragupathi, G.; Koide, F.; Kagan, E.; Spassova, M.; Bornmann, W.; Gregor, P.; Reis, C.; Clausen, H.; Danishefsky, S.J.; Livingston, P.O. *Cancer Immunol. Immunother.,* **2003**, *52*, 608.

[23] Ingale, S.; Wolfert, M.A.; Buskas, T.; Boons, G.J. *Chembiochem.*, **2009**, *10*, 455-463.

[24] Zhu, J.; Warren, D.; Danishefsky, S.J. *Expert Rev Vaccines.*, **2009**, *8(10)*, 1399-1413.

[25] For a comprehensive review on glycopeptide/glycoprotein synthesis see for example: Davis, B.J. *Chem. Rev.,* **2002**, *102,* 579.

[26] a) Mathieux, N.; Paulsen, H.; Meldal, M.; Bock, K. *J. Chem. Soc., Perkin Trans. 1*, **1997**, 2359; b) Sames, D.; Chen, X.-T.; Danishefsky, S.J. *Nature*, **1997**, *389*, 587; c) Danishefsky, S.J.; Hu, S.; Cirillo, P.F.; Eckhardt, M.; Seeberger, P.H. *Chem. Eur. J.,* **1997**, *3*, 1617; d) Wang, Z.-G.; Zhang, X.-F.; Ito, Y.; Nakahara, Y.; Ogawa, T. *Carbohydr. Res.*, **1996**, *295*, 25; e) Seifert, J.; Unverzagt, C. *Tetrahedron Lett.*, **1996**, *37*, 6527; f) Meinjohanns, E.; Meldal, M.; Paulsen, H.; Dwek, R.A.; Bock, K. *J. Chem. Soc., Perkin Trans. 1*, **1998**, 549. g) Dudkin, V.Y.; Miller, J.S.; Danishefsky, S.J. *J. Am. Chem. Soc.,* **2004**, *126*, 736; h) Mandal, M.; Dudkin, V.Y.; Geng, X.; Danishefsky, S.J. *Angew. Chem., Int. Ed.,* **2004**, *43*, 2557; i) Geng, X.; Dudkin, V.Y.; Mandal, M.; Danishefsky, S.J. *Angew. Chem., Int. Ed.,* **2004**, *43*, 2562; j) Pratt, M.R; Bertozzi, C.R. *Org. Lett.*, **2004**, *6*, 2345.

[27] Zhu, X.; Schmidt, R.R. *Angew. Chem. Int. Ed.* **2009**, *48*, 1900; b) Unverzagt, C. *Carbohydr. Res.*, **1998**, *305*, 423.

[28] Seitz, O.; Wong, C.-H. *J. Am. Chem. Soc.*, **1997**, *119*, 8766.

[29] a) Khan, S.H.; O'Neill, R.A. Eds., Modern Methods in Carbohydrate Synthesis; Frontiers in Natural Product Research (Harwood Academic, Australia, 1996), Vol. 1; Preparative

Carbohydrate Chemistry Dekker, New York, **1997**; b) Davis, B.G. *J. Chem. Soc. Perkin Trans.* I, **2000**, 2137; c) Paulsen, H. *Angew. Chem., Int. Ed.*, **1982**, 21, 155; d) Boons, G.-J. *Contemp. Org. Synth.*, **1996**, 3, 173; e) Boons, G.-J. *Tetrahedron*, **1996**, 52, 1095; f) Toshima, K.; Tatsuta, K. *Chem. Rev.*, **1993**, 93, 1503; g) Whitfield, D.M.; Douglas, S.P. *Glycoconj. J.*, **1996**, 13, 5; h) Sears, P.; Wong, C.-H. Science, **2001**, 291, 2344; i) Koeller, K.M.; Wong, C.-H. *Chem. Rev.*, **2000**, 100, 4465; j) Danishefsky, S.J.; Bilodeau, M.T. *Angew. Chem., Int. Ed.*, **1996**, 35, 1381; l) Paulsen, H.; Brockhausen, I. Glycoconj. J., **2003**, 18, 867; m) Lopez, J.C.; Agocs, A.; Uriel, C.; Gomez, A.M.; Fraser-Reid, B. *Chem. Commun.*, **2005**, 5088; n) Uriel, C.; Gomez, A.M.; Lopez, J.C.; Fraser-Reid, B. *J. Carbohydr. Chem.*, **2005**, 24, 665; m) Lu, J.; Fraser-Reid, B.; Gowda, C. *Org. Lett.*, **2005**, 7, 3841; n) Voglmeir, J.; Sardzik, R.; Weissenborn, M.J.; Flitsch, S.L. *Omics: J. Integr. Biol.* **2010**, *14*, 437.

[30] Davis, B.G. *Science*, **2004**, *303*, 480; b) Zhang, Z.; Gildersleeve, J.; Yang, Y.-Y.; Xu, R.; Loo, J.A.; Urya, S.; Wong, C.-H.; Schultz, P.G. *Science*, **2004**, *303*, 371.

[31] Herzner, H.; Reipen, T.; Schultz, M.; Kunz, H. *Chem. Rev.*, **2000**, *100*, 4495.

[32] Taylor, C.M. *Tetrahedron,* **1998**, *54*, 11317.

[33] Arsequell, G.; Valencia, G. *Tetrahedron: Asymmetry,* **1997**, *8*, 2839.

[34] Arsequell, G.; Valencia, G. *Tetrahedron: Asymmetry,* **1999**, *10*, 3045.

[35] Kunz, H. *Angew. Chem., Int. Ed.*, **1987**, *26*, 294.

[36] See for example a) Mizuno, M. *Trends Glycosci. Glycotechnol.,* **2001**, *13*, 11; b) St Hilaire, P. M.; Meldal, M. *Angew. Chem., Int. Ed.,* **2000**, *39*, 1162; c) Seitz, O. *ChemBioChem,* **2000**, *1*, 214.

[37] a) Schmaltz, R.M.; Hanson, S.R.; Wong, C.-H. *Chem. Rev.* **2011**, *111*, 4259; b) Matsushita, T.; Nishimura, S.-I. *Methods Enzymol.* **2010**, *478*, 485; c) Mahajan, R.; Khare, N.K. *Trends Carbohydr. Res.* **2010**, *2*, 28; d) Kittl, R.; Withers, S.G. *Carbohydr. Res.*, **2010**, *345*, 1272; e) Monsan, P.; Remaud-Simeon, M.; Andre, I. *Curr. Opin. Microbiol.* **2010**, *13*, 293; f) Seibel, J.; Buchholz, K. *Adv. Carbohydr. Chem. Biochem.* **2010**, *63*, 101.

[38] Flitsch, S.L. *Curr. Opin. Chem. Biol.,* **2000**, *4*, 619; b)Palcic, M.M. *Curr. Opin. Biotechnol.,* **1999**, *10*, 616; c) David, S.; Auge, C.; Gautheron, C. *Adv. Carbohydr. Chem. Biochem.,* **1991**, *49*, 175

[39] Hanson, S.; Best, M.; Bryan, M.C.; Wong, C.-H. Trends Biochem. Sci. **2004**, *29*, 656; b) Muthana, S.; Cao, H.; Chen, X. Curr. Opinion Chem. Biol. **2009**, *13*, 573; c) Karst, N.A.; Linhardt, R.J. Curr. Med. Chem. **2003**, *10*, 1993.

[40] Galan, M.C.; Benito-Alifonso, D.; Watt, G.M. *Org. & Biomol. Chem.* **2011**, *9*, 3598; b) Kajihara, Y.; Yamamoto, N.; Okamoto, R.; Hirano, K.; Murase, T. *Chem. Record* **2010**, *10*, 80.

[41] See for example a) Nicolaou, K.C.; Winssinger, N.; Pastor, J.; DeRoose, F. *J. Am. Chem. Soc.,* **1997**, *119*, 449; b) Buskas, T.; Li, Y.; Boons, G.-J. *Chem. Eur. J.,* **2005**, *11*, 5457; c) Wu, B.; Hua, Z.; Warren, J.D.; Ranganathan, K.; Wan, Q.; Chen, G.; Tan, Z.; Chen, J.; Endo, A.; Danishefsky, S.J. *Tetrahedron Lett.*, **2006**, *47*, 5577; d) Wang, Z.-G.; Warren, J.D.; Dudkin, V.Y.; Zhang, X.; Iserloh, U.; Visser, M.; Eckhardt, M.; Seeberger, P.H.; Danishefsky, S.J. *Tetrahedron*, **2006**, *62*, 4954; e) Geiger, J.; Barroca, N.; Schmidt, R.R. *Synlett*, **2004**, 836; f) Jayaprakash, K.N.; Lu, J.; Fraser-Reid, B. *Angew. Chem., Int. Ed.*, **2005**, *44*, 5894.

[42] a) Hölemann, A.; Seeberger, P.H. *Curr. Opin. Biotechnol.*, **2004**, *15*, 615; b) Palmacci, E.R.; Plante, O.J.; Seeberger, P.H. *Eur. J. Org. Chem.*, **2002**, 595; c) Marcaurelle, L.A.;

Seeberger, P.H. *Curr. Opin. Chem. Biol.*, **2002**, *6*, 289; d) Stallforth, P.; Lepenies, B.; Adibekian, A.; Seeberger, P.H. *J. Med. Chem.* **2009**, *52*, 5561; e) Seeberger, P.H.; Werz, D.B. *Nature* **2007**, *446*, 1046; f) Weishaupt, M.; Eller, S.; Seeberger, P.H. Methods Enzymol. 2010, 478(Glycomics), 463.

[43] a) Seeberger, P.H.; Werz, D.B. *Nature Rev. Drug Discov.*, **2005**, *4*, 751; b) Kroeck, L.; Esposito, D.; Castagner, B.; Wang, C.-C.; Bindschaedler, P.; Seeberger, P.H. *Chem. Sci.* **2012**, *3*, 1617.

[44] a) Paulsen, H.; Brockhausen, I. *Glycoconj. J.*, **2003**, *18*, 867; b) Davis, B.G.; Chambers, D.; Cumpstey, I.; France, R.; Gamblin, D. In *Carbohydrates*; Osborn, H.M.I. Ed.; Elsevier Science Ltd.: Oxford, **2003**; pp. 69-120; c) Grayson, E.J.; Ward, S.J.; Hall, A.L.; Rendle, P.M.; Gamblin, D.P.; Batsanov, A.S.; Davis, B.G. *J. Org. Chem.*, **2005**, *70*, 9740.

[45] Spassova, M.K.; Bornmann, W.G.; Ragupathi, G.; Sukenick, G.; Livingston, P.O.; Danishefsky, S.J. *J. Org. Chem.*, **2005**, *70*, 3383.

[46] a) Majumdar, D.; Zhu, T.; Boons, G.-J. *Org. Lett.*, **2003**, *5*, 3591; b) Geurtsen, R.; Boons, G.-J. *Eur. J. Org. Chem.*, **2002**, 1473; c) Geurtsen, R.; Boons, G.-J. *Tetrahedron Lett.*, **2002**, *43*, 9429; d) Watt, G.M.; Boons, G.-J. *Carbohydr. Res.*, **2004**, *339*, 181; e) Kim, J.-H.; Yang, H.; Park, J.; Boons, G.-J. *J. Am. Chem. Soc.*, **2005**, *127*, 12090; f) Kim, J.-H.; Yang, H.; Boons, G.-J. *Angew. Chem., Int. Ed.*, **2005**, *44*, 947.

[47] Kunz, H. *J. Peptide Sci.*, **2003**, *9*, 563.

[48] Grayson, E.J.; Bernardes, G.J.L.; Chalker, J.M.; Boutureira, O.; Koeppe, J.R.; Davis, B.J. *Angew. Chem., Int. Ed.*, **2011**, *50*, 4127-4132.

[49] Douglas, N.L.; Ley, S.V. ; Lücking, U.; Warriner, S.L. *J. Chem. Soc., Perkin Trans. 1*, **1998**, 51.

[50] a) Seeberger, P.H.; Haase, W.-C. *Chem. Rev.*, **2000**, *100*, 4549;b) Seeberger, P.H. *J. Carbohydr. Chem.*, **2002**, *21*, 613.

[51] Kahne, D. *Curr. Opin. Chem. Biol.*, **1997**, *1*, 130.

[52] a) Liang, R. Yan, L.; Loebach, J.; Ge, M.; Uozumi, Y.; Sekanina, K.; Horan, N.; Gildersleeve, J.; Thompson, C.; Smith, A.; Biswas, K.; Still, W.C.; Kahne, D. *Science*, **1996**, *274*, 1520; b) Sofia, M.J. Allanson, N.; Hatzenbuhler, N.T.; Jain, R.; Kakarla, R.; Kogan, N.; Liang, R.; Liu, D.; Silva, D.J.; Wang, H.; Gange, D.; Anderson, J.; Chen, A.; Chi, F.; Dulina, R.; Huang, B.; Kamau, M.; Wang, C.; Baizman, E.; Branstrom, A.; Bristol, N.; Goldman, R.; Han, K.; Longley, C.; Midha, S.; Axelrod, H.R. *J. Med. Chem.*, **1999**, *42*, 3193.

[53] Kunz, H.; Unverzagt, C. *Angew. Chem., Int. Ed.*, **1988**, *27*, 1697.

[54] Sjolin, P.; Elofsson, M.; Kihlberg, J. *J. Org. Chem.*, **1996**, *61*, 560.

[55] a) Burger, K.; Kluge, M.; Fehn, S.; Koksch, B.; Hennig, L.; Müller, G. *Angew. Chem., Int. Ed.*, **1999**, *38*, 1414; b) George, S.K.; Schwientek, T.; Holm, B.; Reis, C.A.; Clausen, H.; Kihlberg, J. *J. Am. Chem. Soc.*, **2001**, *123*, 11117; c) Cato, D.; Buskas, T.; Boons, G.-J. *J. Carbohydr. Chem.*, **2005**, *24*, 503; d) Cudic, M.; Burstein, G.D. *Methods Mol. Biol.* **2008**, *494*, 187; e) Haase, C.; Seitz, O. *Top. Curr. Chem.* **2007**, 267, 1; f) Mogemark, M.; Kihlberg, J. Eds. Levy, D. E.; Fuegedi, P. in Organic Chemistry of Sugars **2006**, 755; g) Nakahara, Y. *Trends Glycosci. Glycotechnol.* **2003**, *15*, 257.

[56] Marks, G. S.; Neuberger, A. *J. Chem. Soc.* **1961**, 4872.

[57] Teshima, T.; Nakajima, K.; Takahashi, M.; Shiba, T. *Tetrahedron Lett.*, **1992**, *33*, 363.

[58] Günther, W.; Kunz, H. *Angew. Chem., Int. Ed. Engl.*, **1990**, *29*, 1050.

[59] a) Handlon, A.L.; Fraser-Reid, B. *J. Am. Chem. Soc.,* **1993**, *115*, 3796; b) Ratcliffe, A. J.; Konradsson, P.; Fraser-Reid, B. *J. Am. Chem. Soc.,* **1990**, *112*, 5665; c) Nair, L.G.; Fraser-Reid, B.; Szardenings, A.K. *Org. Lett.,* **2001**, *3*, 317.

[60] Kahne, D.; Walker, S.; Cheng, Y.; van Engen, D. *J. Am. Chem. Soc.,* **1989**, *111*, 6881.

[61] a) Inazu, T.; Kobayashi, K. *Synlett,* **1993**, 869; b) Mizuno, M.; Muramoto, I.; Kobayashi, K.; Yaginuma, H.; Inazu, T. *Synthesis,* **1999**, 162.

[62] Tsuda, T.; Nithimura, S. *Chem. Commun.*, **1996**, 2779; b) Meinjohanns, E.; Meldal, M.; Paulsen, H.; Schleyer, A.; Bock, K. *J. Chem. Soc., Perkin. Trans. 1*, **1996**, 985; c) Nakahara, Y.; Iijima, H.; Ogawa, T. *Tetrahedron Lett.*, **1994**, *35*, 3321; d) Liebe, B.; Kunz, H. *Tetrahedron Lett.,* **1994**, *35*, 8777.

[63] Koeller, K.M.; Smith, M.E.; Wong, C.-H. *Bioorg. Med. Chem.*, **2000**, *8*, 1017; b) Koeller, K.M.; Smith, M.E.; Huang, R.-F.; Wong, C.-H. *J. Am. Chem. Soc.*, **2000**, *122*, 4241; c) Leppanen, A.; White, S.P.; Helin, J.; McEver, R.P.; Cummings, P.D. *J. Biol. Chem.*, **2000**, *275*, 39569.

[64] Goody, R.S.; Alexandrov, K.; Engelhard, M. *ChemBioChem*, **2002**, *3*, 399; b) McGrath, N.A.; Raines, R. T. *Acc. Chem. Res.* **2011**, *44*, 752; c) Wu, C.-Y.; Wong, C.-H. *Chem. Commun.* **2011**, *47*, 6201; d) Hojo, H.; Katayama, H.; Nakahara, Y. *Trends Glycosci. Glycotechnol.* **2010**, *22*, 269; e) Kumar, K. S. A.; Brik, A. *J. Pept. Sci.* **2010**, *16*, 524; f) Rohde, H.; Seitz, O. *Biopolymers* **2010**, *94*, 551.

[65] Dawson, P.E.; Muir, T.W.; Clark-Lewis, I.; Kent, S.B.H. *Science,* **1994**, *266*, 776; b) Cotton, G.J.; Muir, T.W. *Chem. Biol.,* **1999**, *6*, R247; c) Dawson, P.E.; Kent, S.B. *Annu. Rev. Biochem.*, **2000**, *69*, 923.

[66] Robertson, N.; Ramage, R. *J. Chem. Soc., Perkin Trans.,* **1999**, *1*, 1015.

[67] Shin, Y.; Winans, K.A.; Backes, B.J.; Kent, S.B.H.; Ellman, J.A.; Bertozzi, C.R. *J. Am. Chem. Soc.*, **1999**, *121*, 11684.

[68] a) Marcauelle, L.A.; Mizoue, L.S.; Wilken, J.; Oldham, L.; Kent, S.B.; Handel, T.M.; Bertozzi, C.R. *Chem. Eur. J.,* **2001**, *7*, 1129; b) Mezzato, S.; Schaffrath, M.; Unverzagt, C. *Angew. Chem., Int. Ed.,* **2005**, *41*, 1650.

[69] Offer, J.; Boddy, C.N.C.; Dawson, P.E. *J. Am. Chem. Soc.*, **2002**, *124*, 4642; b) Marinzi, C.; Offer, J.; Longhi, R.; Dawson, P.E. *Bioorg. Med. Chem.*, **2002**, *12*, 2749.

[70] a) Wan, Q.; Chen, J.; Chen, G.; Danishefsky, S.J. *J. Org. Chem.*, **2006**, *71*, 8244; b) Wu, B.; Chen, J.; Warren, J.D.; Chen, G.; Hua, Z.; Danishefsky, S.J. *Angew. Chem., Int. Ed.,* **2006**, *45*, 4116.

[71] Warren, J.D.; Miller, J.S.; Keding, S.J.; Danishefsky, S.J. *J. Am. Chem. Soc.*, **2004**, *126*, 6576.

[72] Muir, T.W.; Sondhi, D.; Cole, P.A. *Proc. Natl. Acad. Sci. U.S.A.,* **1998**, *95*, 6705.

[73] a) Zhong, Z.; Bibbs, J.; Yuan, W.; Wong, C.-H. *J. Am. Chem. Soc.*, **1991**, *113*, 2259; b) Wong, C.-H.; Schuster, M.; Wang, P.; Sears, P. *J. Am. Chem. Soc.*, **1993**, *115*, 5893; c) Witte, K.; Seitz, O.; Wong, C.-H. *J. Am. Chem. Soc.*, **1998**, *120*, 1979.

[74] Saxon, E.; Armstrong, J.I.; Bertozzi, C.R. *Org. Lett.*, **2000**, *2*, 2141.

[75] Bordusa, F. *Chem. Rev.*, **2002**, *102*, 4817.

[76] Vliegenthart, J.F.G.; Casset, F. *Curr. Opin. Struct. Biol.,* **1998**, *8*, 565.

[77] Bolsinger, S.S.; Gentzsch, M.M.; Tanner, W.W. *Biochim. Biophys. Acta,* **1999**, *1426*, 297.

[78] Davis, B.G. *Chem. Rev.*, **2002**, *102*, No. 2.

[79] Gamblin, G.P.; Scanlan, E.M.; Davis, B.G. *Chem. Rev.,* **2009**, *109*, No. 1

[80] Ticha, M.; Cerny, M.; Trnka, T. *Glycoconjugate J.,* **1996**, *13*, 681.

[81] Bengtsson, M.; Broddefalk, J.; Dahmén, J.; Henriksson, K.; Kihlberg, J.; Lönn, H.; Srinivasa, B.R.; Stenvall, K. *Glycoconj. J.*, **1998**, *15*, 223.
[82] Boratynski, J.; Roy, R. *Glycoconj. J.*, **1998**, *15*, 131.
[83] a) Marcaurelle, L.A.; Bertozzi, C.R. *Chem. Eur. J.*, **1999**, *5*, 1384; b) Lemieux, G.A.; Bertozzi, C.R. *Trends Biotechnol.*, **1998**, *16*, 506; c) Hang, H.C.; Bertozzi, C.R. *Acc. Chem. Res.*, **2001**, *34*, 727; d) Peri, F. *MiniRev. Med. Chem.*, **2003**, *3*, 658.
[84] Davis, B.G.; Lloyd, R.C.; Jones, J.B. *J. Org. Chem.*, **1998**, *63*, 9614-9615.
[85] Davis, B.G.; Maughan, M.A.T.; Green, M.P.; Ullman, A.; Jones, J.B. *Tetrahedron-Asymmetr.*, **2000**, *11*, 245-262.
[86] Gamblin, D.P.; Garnier, P.; Ward, S.J.; Oldham, N. J.; Fairbanks, A. J.; Davis, B.G. *Org. Biomol. Chem.*, **2003**, *1*, 3642-3644.
[87] Gamblin, D.P.; Garnier, P.; Van Kasteren, S.; Oldham, N.J.; Fairbanks, A.J.; Davis, B.G. *Angew. Chem. Int. Ed.*, **2004**, *43*, 828-833.
[88] Chalker, J.M.; Bernardes, G.J.L.; Davis, B.G. *Accounts Chem. Res.*, **2011**, *44*, 730-741.
[89] Dondoni, A.; Marra, A. *Chem. Soc. Rev.*, **2012**, *41*, 573-586.
[90] Lo Conte, M.; Pacifico, S.; Chambery, A.; Marra, A.; Dondoni A. *J. Org. Chem.*, **2010**, *75*, 4644-4647.
[91] a) Davis, B.G.; Jones, J.B. *Synlett*, **1999**, 1495; b) Lloyd, R.C.; Davis, B.G.; Jones, J.B. *Bioorg. Med. Chem.*, **2000**, *8*, 1537; c) Davis, B.G.; Lloyd, R.C.; Jones, J.B. *J. Org. Chem.*, **1998**, *63*, 9614; d) Davis, B.G.; Maughan, M.A.T.; Green, M.P.; Ullman, A. *Tetrahedron: Asymm.*, **2000**, *11*, 245; e) Macmillan, D.; Bill, R.M.; Sage, K.A.; Fern, D.; Flitsch, S. *Chem. Biol.*, **2001**, *8*, 125; f) Davis, B.G. *Chem. Commun.*, **2001**, 351; g) Watt, G.M.; Lund, J.; Levens, M.; Kolli, V.S.K.; Jefferis, R.; Boons, G.-J. *Chem. Biol.*, **2003**, *10*, 807.
[92] Chalker, J.M.; Davis, B.G. *Curr. Opin. Chem. Biol.*, **2010**, *14*, 781-789.
[93] Neet, K.E.; Koshland, D.E Jr. *Proc. Natl. Acad. Sci. USA*, **1966**, *56*, 1606-1611.
[94] Polga, L.; Bender, M.L. *J. Am. Chem. Soc.*, **1966**, *88*, 3153-3154.
[95] Gamblin, D.P.; Van Kasteren, S.; Bernardes, G.J.L.; Chalker, J.M.; Oldham, N.J.; Fairbanks, A.J.; Davis, B.G. *Mol. BioSyst.*, **2008**, *4*, 558-561.
[96] Clark, P.I.; Lowe, G. *J. Chem. Soc. Chem. Commun.*, **1977**, 923-924.
[97] Clark, P.I.; Lowe, G. *Eur. J. Biochem.*, **1978**, *84*, 293-299.
[98] Strumeyer, D.H.; White, W.N.; Koshland, D.E Jr. *Proc. Natl. Acad. Sci. USA*, **1963**, *50*, 931-935.
[99] Bernardes, G.J.L.; Chalker, J.M.; Errey J.C.; Davis, B.G: *J. Am. Chem. Soc.*, **2008**, *130*, 5052-5053.
[100] Wong, C.-H. *Chem. Commun.*, **2006**, 21.
[101] a) Martin, R.; Witte, K.L.; Wong, C.-H. *Bioorg. Med. Chem.*, **1998**, *6*, 1283; b) Witte, K.; Sears, P.; Martin, R. Wong, C.-H. *J. Am. Chem. Soc.*, **1997**, *119*, 2114.
[102] a) Li, B.; Zeng, Y.; Hauser, S.; Song, H.; Wang, L.-X. *J. Am. Chem. Soc.*, **2005**, *127*, 9692; b) Fujita, M.; Shoda, S.; Haneda, K.; Inazu, T.; Takegawa, K.; Yamamoto, K. *Biochem. Biophys. Acta*, **2001**, *270*, 17723; c) Yamamoto, K.; Kadowaki, S.; Fujisaki, M.; Kumagai, H.; Tochikura, T. *Biosci. Biotechnol. Biochem.* **1994**, *58*, 72.
[103] Wang, L.; Schultz, P.G. *Angew. Chem. Int. Ed.*, **2005**, *44*, 34.
[104] a) Liu, H.; Wang, L.; Brock, A.; Wong, C.-H.; Schultz, P.G. *J. Am. Chem. Soc.*, **2003**, *125*, 1702; b) Wang, L.; Brock, A.; Herberich, B.; Schultz, P.G. *Science*, **2001**, *292*, 498.
[105] Xu, R.; Hanson, S.R.; Zhang, Z.; Yang, Y.-Y.; Schultz, P.G.; Wong, C.-H. *J. Am. Chem. Soc.*, **2004**, *126*, 15654.

[106] a) Saxon, E.; Bertozzi, C.R. *Science*, **2000**, *287*, 2007; b) Lemieux, G.A.; Bertozzi, C.R. *Chem. Biol.*, **2001**, *8*, 265; c) Vocadlo, D.J.; Hang, H.C.; Kim, E.J.; Hanover, J.A.; Bertozzi, C.R. *Proc. Natl. Acad. Sci. U.S.A.*, **2003**, *100*, 9116.

[107] Adam, A. *Synthetic adjuvants: modern concepts in immunology* C.A. Bona Ed., John Wiley and Sons, New York. **1984**.

[108] a) Deres, K.; Schild, H.; Wiesmuller, K.-H.; Jung, G.; Rammensee, H. *Nature,* **1989**, *342*, 561; b) Wiesmuller, K.-H.; Jung, G.; Gillessen, D.; Loffl, C.; Bessler, W.; Boltz, T. *Immunology,* **1991**, *72*, 109.

[109] Toyokuni, T.; Singhal, A.K. *Chem. Soc. Rev.,* **1995**, 231.

[110] Schutze, M.-P.; Leclerc, C.; Jolivet, M.; Audibert, F.; Chedid, L. *J. Immunol.,* **1985**, *135*, 2319.

[111] For recent reviews on Danishefsky and co-workers research on carbohydrate-based vaccines see: a) Ouerfelli, O.; Warren, J.D.; Wilson, R.M., Danishefsky, S.J. *Exp. Rev. Vaccines*, **2005**, *4*, 677;

[112] Slovin, S.F.; Keding, S.J.; Ragupathi, G. *Immunol. Cell Biol.,* **2005**, *83*, 418.

[113] a) Kannagi, R.; Levery, S.B.; Ishigami, F.; Hakomori, S.; Shevinsky, L.H.; Knowles, B.B.; Solter, D. *J. Biol. Chem.*, **1983**, *258*, 8934; b) Bremer, E.G.; Levery, S.B.; Sonnino, S.; Ghidoni, R.; Canevari, S.; Kannagi, R.; Hakomori, S. *J. Biol. Chem.*, **1984**, *259*, 14773.

[114] Livingston, P.O. *Semin. Cancer Biol.*, **1995**, *6*, 357.

[115] a) Gilewski, T.; Ragupathi, G.; Bhuta, S.; Williams, L.J.; Musselli, C.; Zhang, X.-F.; Bencsath, K.P.; Panageas, K.S.; Chin, J.; Hudis, C.A.; Norton, L.; Houghton, A.N.; Livingston, P.O.; Danishefsky, S.J. *Proc. Natl. Acad. Sci. USA*, **2001**, *98*, 3270; b) Ragupathi, G.; Slovin, S.F.; Adluri, S.; Sames, D.; Kim, I.J.; Kim, H.M.; Spassova, M.; Bornmann, W.G.; Lloyd, K.O.; Scher, H.I.; Livingston, P.O.; Danishefsky, S.J. *Angew. Chem. Int. Ed.*, **1999**, *38*, 563; c) Slovin, S.F.; Ragupathi, G.; Adluri, S.; Ungers, G.; Terry, K.; Kim, S.; Spassova, M.; Bornmann, W.G.; Fazzari, M.; Dantis, L.; Olkiewicz, K.; Lloyd, K.O.; Livingston, P.O.; Danishefsky, S.J.; Scher, H.I. *Proc. Natl. Acad. Sci. USA*, **1999**, *96*, 5710.

[116] Ragupathi, G.; Park, T.K.; Zhang, S.; Kim, I.J.; Graber, L.; Adluri, S.; Lloyd, K.O.; Danishefsky, S.J.; Livingston, P.O.; *Angew. Chem. Int. Ed. Engl.*, **1997**, *36*, 125.

[117] Ragupathi, G.; Deshpande, P.P.; Coltart, D.M.; Kim, H.M.; Williams, L.J.; Danishefsky, S.J.; Livingston, P.O. *Int. J. Cancer,* **2002**, *99*, 207.

[118] a) Adluri, S.; Helling, F.; Ogata, S.; Zhang, S.; Itzkowitz, S.H.; Lloyd, K.O.; Livingston, P.O. *Cancer Immunol. Immunother.,* **1995**, *41*, 185; b) Miles, D.W.; Towlson, K.E.; Graham, R.; Reddish, M.; Longenecker, B.M.; Taylor-Papadimitriou, J.; Rubens, R.D. *Br. J. Cancer,* **1996**, *74,* 1292.

[119] Buskas, T.; Li, Y.; Boons, G.-J. *Chem. Eur. J.*, **2004**, *10*, 3517.

[120] Nudelman, E.; Levery, S.B.; Kaizu, T.; Hakomori, S. *J. Biol. Chem.*, **1986**, *261*, 11247.

[121] a) Kaizu, T.; Levery, S.B.; Nudelman, E.; Stenkamp, R.E.; Hakomori, S. *J. Biol. Chem.*, **1986**, *261*, 11254; b) Kim, S.Y.; Yuan, M.; Itzkowitz, S.H.; Sun, Q.; Kaizu, T.; Palekar, A.; Trump, B.F.; Hakomori, S.-I. *Cancer Res.*, **1986**, *46*, 5985.

[122] Buskas, T.; Ingale, S.; Boons, G.-J. *Angew. Chem. Int. Ed.*, **2005**, *44*, 5985.

[123] a) Springer, G.F. *J. Mol. Med.,* **1997**, *75*, 594; b) Toyokuni, T.; Hakomori, S.; Singhal, A.K. *Bioorg. Med. Chem.*, **1994**, *2*, 1119; c) Kagan, E.; Ragupathi, G.; Yi, S.; Reis, C.A.; Gildersleeve, J.; Kahne, D.; Clausen, H.; Danishefsky, S.J.; Livingston, P.O. *Cancer Immunol. Immunother.*, **2005**, *54*, 424.

[124] Wiertz, E.J.H.J.J.; van Gaans-van den Brink, A.M.; Gausepohl, H.; Prochnicka-Chalufour, A.; Hoogerhout, P.; Poolman, J.T. *J. Exp.Med.*, **1992**, *176*, 79.
[125] Medzhitov, R.; Janeway, Jr., C.A. *Science,* **2002**, *296*, 298.
[126] Braun, V. *Biochim.Biophys. Acta*, **1975**, *415*, 335.
[127] Burchell, J.; Taylor-Papadimitriou, J.; Boshell, M.; Gendler, S.; Duhig, T. *Int J. Cancer.,* **1989**, *44*, 691.
[128] Kaiser, A.; Gaidzik, N.; Westerlind, U.; Kowalczyk, D.; Hobel, A.; Schmitt, E.; Kunz, H. *Angew. Chem. Int. Ed. Engl.,* **2009**, *48*, 7551-7555.
[129] Wilkinson, B.L.; Malins, L.R.; Chun, C.K.Y.; Payne, R.J. *Chem. Commun.,* **2010**, *46*, 6249-6251.
[130] Lakshminarayanan, V.; Thompson, P.; Wolfert, M.A.; Buskas, T.; Bradley, J.M.; Pathangey, L.B.; Madsen, C.S.; Cohen, P.A.; Gendler, S.J.; Boons, J. *PNAS*, **2012**, *109* (1), 261-266.
[131] a) Wang Z.-G.; Wiliams, L.J.; Zhang, X.-F.; Zatorski, A.; Kudryashov, V.; Ragupathi, G.; Spassova, M.; Bornmann, W.; Slovin, S.F.; Scher, H.I.; Livingston, P.O.; Lloyd, K.O.; Danishefsky, S.J. *Proc. Natl. Acad. Sci. U.S.A.*, **2000**, *97*, 2719; b) Kudryashov, V.; Ragupathi, G.; Kim, I.J.; Breimer, M.E.; Danishefsky, S.J.; Livingston, P.O.; Lloyd, K.O. *Glycoconj. J.,* **1998**, *15*, 243.
[132] Helling, F.; Shang, A.; Calves, M.; Zhang, S.; Ren, S.; Yu, R.K.; Oettgen, H.F.; Livingston, P.O. *Cancer Res.,* **1994**, *54*, 197.
[133] Kensil, C.R.; Patel, U.; Lennick, M.; Marciani, D. *J. Immunol.,* **1991**, *146*, 431.
[134] Helling, F.; Zhang, S.; Shang, A.; Adluri, S.; Calves, M.; Koganty, R.; Longenecker, B.M.; Yao, T.J.; Oettgen, H.F.; Livingston, P.O. *Cancer Res.,* **1995**, *55*, 2783.
[135] Livingston, P.O.; Ritter, G.; Srivastava, P.; Padavan, M.; Calves, M.J.; Oettgen, H.F.; Old, L.J. *Cancer Res.,* **1989**, *49*, 7045.
[136] a) Ragupathi, G.; Meyers, M.; Adluri, S.; Ritter, G.; Livingston, P.O. *Proc. Am. Assoc. Cancer Res.,* **1997**, *38*, 3981a; b) Ragupathi, G.; Meyers, M.; Adluri, S.; Howard, L.; Musselli, C.; Livingston P.O. *Int. J. Cancer,* **2000**, *85*, 659.
[137] Bay, S.; Fort, S.; Birikaki, L.; Ganneau, C.; Samain, E.; Coic, Y-M.; Bonhomme, F.; Dériaud, E.; Leclerc, C.; Lo-Man, R. *Chem. Med. Chem.*, **2009**, *4*, 582-587.
[138] Krug, L.M.; Ragupathi, G.; Ng, K.K.; Hood, C.; Jennings, H.J.; Guo, Z.; Kris, M.G.; Miller, V.; Pizzo, B.; Tyson, L.; Baez, V.; Livingston, P.O. *Clin. Cancer Res.,* **2004**, *10*, 916.
[139] Kudryashov, V.; Kim, H. A.; Ragupathi, G.; Danishefsky, S.J.; Livingston, P.O.; Lloyd, K.O. *Cancer Immunol. Immunother.*, **1997**, *45*, 281.
[140] a) Sabbatini, P.; Kudryashov, V.; Ragupathi, G.; Danishefsky, S.J.; Livingston, P.O.; Bornmann, W.G.; Spassova, M.; Spriggs, D.; Aghajanian, C.; Soignet, S.; Peyton, M.; O'Flaherty, C.; Curtin, J.; Lloyd, K. *Int. J. Cancer,* **2000**, *87*, 79; b) Ragupathi, G.; Cappello, S.; Yi, S.S.; Spassova, M.; Bornmann, W.; Danishefsky, S.J.; Livingston, P.O. *Vaccine,* **2002**, *20*, 1030.
[141] Hakomori, S. In *Gangliosides and Cancer*; Oettgen, H.F., Ed.; VCH: Weinheim, Germany, **1989**; p. 59.
[142] Bitton, R.J.; Guthmann, M.D.; Babri, M.R.; Carnero, A.J.L.; Alonso, D.F.; Fainboim, L.; Gomez, D.E. *Oncol. Rep.,* **2002**, *9*, 267.
[143] Pan, Y.; Chefalo, P.; Nagy, N.; Harding, C.; Guo, Z. *J. Med. Chem.*, **2005**, *48*, 875.
[144] Takano, R.; Muchmore, E.; Dennis, J.W. *Glycobiol.,* **1994**, *4*, 665.

[145] Zou, W.; Borrelli, S.; Gilbert, M.; Liu, T.; Pon, R.A.; Jennings, H.J. *J. Biol. Chem.,* **2004**, *279*, 25390.

[146] a) Jennings, H.J. *Int. J. Infect. Dis.,* **1997**, *1*, 158; b) Ritter, G.; Boosfeld, E.; Calves, M.J.; Oettgen, H.F.; Old, L.J.; Livingston, P.O. *Immunobiol.,* **1990**, *182*, 32; c) Ritter, G.; Boosfeld, E.; Asluri, S.; Calves, M.J.; Oettgen, H.F.; Old, L.J.; Livingston, P.O. *Int. J. Cancer,* **1991**, *48*, 379.

[147] Bertozzi, C.R.; Kiessling, L.L. *Science,* **2001**, *291*, 2357; b) Mahal, L.K.; Bertozzi, C.R. *Chem. Biol.,* **1997**, *4*, 415; c) Yarema, K.J.; Mahal, L.K.; Bruehl, R.E.; Rodriguez, E.C.; Bertozzi, C.R. *J. Biol. Chem.,* **1998**, *273*, 31168; d) Mahal, K.L.; Yarema, K.J.; Bertozzi, C.R. *Science,* **1997**, *276*, 1125.

[148] Kayser, H.; Geile, C.C.; Paul, C.; Zeitler, R.; Reutter, W. *FEBS Lett.,* **1992**, *301*, 137; b) Schmidt, C.; Stehling, P.; Schnitzer, J.; Reutter, W.; Horskorte, R. *J. Biol. Chem.,* **1998**, *273*, 19146.

[149] Tangvoranuntakul, P.; Gagneux, P.; Diaz, S.; Bardor, M.; Varki, N.; Varki, A.; Muchmore, E. *Proc. Natl. Acad. Sci. U.S.A.,* **2003**, *100*, 12045.

[150] Liu, T.M.; Guo, Z.W.; Yang, Q.L.; Sad, S.; Jennings, H.J. *J. Biol. Chem.,* **2000**, *275*, 32832.

[151] Marcaurelle, L.A.; Pratt, M.R.; Bertozzi, C.R. *ChemBioChem,* **2003**, *2-3*, 224.

[152] Marcaurelle, L.A.; Bertozzi, C.R. *J. Am. Chem. Soc.,* **2001**, *123*, 1587.

[153] Hamann, P.R.; Hinman, L.M.; Beyer, C.F.; Greenberger, L.M.; Lin, C.; Lindh, D.; Menendez, A.T.; Wallace, R.; Durr, F.E.; Upeslacis, J. *Bioconj. Chem*., **2005**, *16*, 346.

[154] Aboud-Pirak, E.; Sergent, T.; Otte-Slachmuylder, C.; Abarca, J.; Trouet, A.; Schneider, Y.J. *Cancer Res.,* **1988**, *48*, 3188.

[155] Shiao, C.T.; Roy, R. *New J. Chem*., **2012**, *36*, 324-339.

[156] a) Toyokuni, T.; Dean, B.; Cai, S.; Boivin, D.; Hakomori, S.-I.; Singhal, A.K. *J. Am. Chem. Soc.,* **1994**, *116*, 395.

[157] Bessler, W.G.; Jung, G. *Res. Immunol.,* **1992**, *143*, 548; b) Wiesmuller, K.-H.; Bessler, W.G.; Jung, G. *Int. J. Pept. Protein Res.,* **1992**, *40*, 255.

[158] Singhal, A.; Fohn, M.; Hakomori, S. *Cancer Res.,* **1991**, *51*, 1406.

[159] Nakada, H.; Numata, Y.; Inoue, M.; Tanaka, N.; Kitagawa, H.; Funakoshi, I.; Fukui, S.; Yamashina, I. *J. Biol. Chem.,* **1991**, *266*, 12402.

[160] Slovin, S.F.; Ragupathi, G.; Musselli, C.; Fernandez, C.; Diani, M.; Verbel, D.; Danishefsky, S.J.; Livingston, P.; Scher, H.I. *Cancer Immunol. Immunother.*, **2005**, *54*, 694.

[161] a) Bay, S.; Lo-Man, R.; Osinaga, E.; Nakada, H.; Leclerc, C.; Cantacuzène, D. *J. Peptide Res.,* **1997**, *49*, 620; b) Lo-Man, R.; Bay, S.; Vichier-Guerre, S.; Dériaud, E.; Cantacuzène, D.; Leclerc, C. *Cancer Res.* **1999**, *59*, 1520.

[162] Posnett, D.N.; McGrath, H.; Tam, J.P. *J. Biol. Chem.,* **1988**, *263*, 1719; b) Tam, J.P. *Proc. Natl. Acad. Sci. USA,* **1988**, *85*, 5409.

[163] Lo-Man, R.; Vichier-Guerre, S.; Perraut, R.; Dériaud, E.; Huteau, V.; BenMohamed, L.; Diop, O.M.; Livingston, P.O.; Bay, S.; Leclerc, C. *Cancer Res.,* **2004**, *64*, 4987.

[164] Lo-Man, R.; Bay, S.; Vichier-Guerre, S.; Dériaud, E.; Cantacuzène, D.; Leclerc, C. *J. Immunol.,* **2001**, 2849.

[165] Grigalevicius, S.; Chierici, S.; Renaudet, O.; Lo-Man, R.; Dériaud, E.; Leclerc, C.; Dumy, P. *Bioconj. Chem.,* **2005**, *16*, 1149.

[166] Dumy, P.; Eggleston, I.M.; Cervigni, S.; Sila, U.; Sun, X.; Mutter, M. *Tetrahedron Lett.,* **1995**, *36,* 1255.

[167] Peluso, S.; Rückle, T.; Lehmann, C.; Mutter, M.; Peggion, C.; Crisma, M. *ChemBioChem,* **2001**, *2*, 432.

[168] Bossu, I.; Berthet, N.; Dumy, P.; Renaude, O. *J. Carbohydr. Chem.*, **2011**, *30*, 458-468.

[169] Galibert Galibert, M.; Renaudet, O.; Dumy, P.; Boturyn, D. *Angew. Chem.*, **2011**, *123*, 1941-1944.

[170] André, S.; Renaudet, O.; Bossu, I.; Dumy, P.; Gabius, H-J. *J. Pept. Sci.,* **2011**, *17*, 427-437.

[171] Bossu, I.; Šulc, M.; Křenek, K.; Dufour, E.; Garcia, J.; Berthet, N.; Dumy, P.; Křen, V.; Renaudet, O. *Org. Biomol. Chem.*, **2011**, *9*, 1948-1959.

[172] Renaudet, O.; Dasgupta, G.; Bettahi, I.; Shi, A.; Nesburn, A.B.; Dumy, P.; BenMohamed, L. *PLoS One*, **2010**, *5*, 1-16.

[173] Khan, K.N.; Kitajima, M.; Hiraki, K.; Fujishita, A.; Sekine, I.; Ishimaru, T.; Masuzaki, H. *Gynecol. Obstet. Invest.*, **2009**, *68*, 40-52.

[174] Khan, S.; Weterings, J.J.; Britten, C.M.; de Jong, A.R.; Graafland, D.; Melief, C.J.M.; van der Burg, S.H.; van der Marel, G.; Overkleeft, H.S.; Filippov, D.M.; Ossendorp, F. *Mol. Immunol.*, **2009**, *46*, 1084-1091.

[175] Kircheis, R.; Vondru, P.; Nechansky, A.; Ohler, R.; Loibner, H.; Himmler, G.; Mudde, G.C. *Bioconj. Chem.*, **2005**, *16*, 1519.

[176] Kircheis, R.; Vondru, P.; Zinöcker, I.; Häring, D.; Nechansky, A.; Loibner, H.; Himmler, G.; Mudde, G.C. *Vaccine*, **2006**, *24*, 2349.

[177] Riethmuller, G.; Schneider-Gadicke, E.; Schlimok, G.; Schmiegel, W.; Raab, R.; Hoffken, K.; Gruber, R.; Pichlmaier, H.; Hirsche, H.; Pichlmayr, R.; *Lancet,* **1994**, *343*, 1172.

[178] Heimburg-Molinaro, J.; Almogren, A.; Morey, S.;Glinskii, O.V.; Roy, R.; Wilding, G.E.; Cheng, R.P.; Glinsky, V.V.; Rittenhouse-Olson K. *Neoplasia*, **2009**, *11*, 780-792.

[179] Keil, S.; Kaiser, A.; Syed, F.; Kunz, H. *Synthesis,* **2009**, *8*, 1355-1369.

[180] a) Kiguchi, K.; Iwamori, Y.; Suzuki, N.; Kobayashi, Y.; Ishizuka, B.; Ishiwata, I.; Kita, T.; Kikuchi, Y.; Iwamori, M. *Cancer Sci,* **2006**, *97*, 1321-1326. b) Lingwood, C. A.; Khine, A. A.; Arab, S. *Acta Biochim. Pol.* **1998**, *45*, 351-359. c) Arab, S.; Russel, E.; Chapman, W. B.; Rosen, B.; Lingwood, C. A. *Oncol. Res.* **1997**, *9*, 553-563.

[181] Giuntoli, R. L. II; Rodriguez, G. C.; Whitaker, R. S.; Dodge, R.; Voynow, J. A. *Cancer Res.,* **1998**, *58*, 5546-5550.

[182] Zhu, J.; Wan, Q.; Ragupathi, G.; George, C.M.; Livingston, P.O.; Danishefsky, S.J. J. *Am. Chem. Soc.*, **2009**, *131*, 4151-4158.

[183] a) Livingston, P.O. *Clin. Cancer Res.,* **2001**, *7*, 1837; b) Ragupathi, G.; Coltart, D.M.; Williams, L.J.; Koide, F.; Kagan, E.; Allen, J.; Harris, C.; Glunz, P.W.; Livingston, P.O.; Danishefsky, S.J. *Proc. Natl. Acad. Sci. U. S. A.,* **2002**, *99*, 13699.

[184] Cho, Y.S.; Wana, Q.; Danishefsky, S.J. *Bioorg. Med. Chem.*, **2005**, *13*, 5259 and refs. cited therein.

[185] Ragupathi, G.; Koide, F.; Livingston, P.O.; Cho, Y.S.; Endo, A.; Wan, Q.; Spassova, M.K.; Keding, S.J.; Allen, J.; Ouerfelli, O.; Wilson, R.M.; Danishefsky, S.J. *J. Am. Chem. Soc.*, **2006**, *128*, 2715.

[186] Zhu, J.; Warren, J.D.; Danishefsky, S.J. *Expert. Rev. Vaccines.*, **2009**, *8*, 1399-1413.

[187] Lee, D.; Danishefsky, S.J. *Tetrahedron Lett.*, **2009**; *50*, 2167.

[188] Jeon, I.; Lee, D.; Krauss, I.J.; Danishefsky, S.J. *J. Am. Chem. Soc.*, **2009**; *131*, 14337.

[189] Karlsson, K.A. *Curr. Opin. Struct. Biol.*, **1995**, *5*, 622.

[190] Varki, A. *Proc. Natl. Acad. Sci.* USA, **1994**, *91*, 7390.
[191] a) Varki, A. *Glycobiology*, **1993**, *3*, 97; b) Glinsky, G.V. *Cancer Metastasis Rev.*, **1998**, *17*, 177.
[192] De la Fuente J.M., Penades, S. *Glycoconj. J.*, **2004**, *21*, 149.
[193] Brust, M.; Walker, M.; Bethell, D.; Schiffrin, D.J.; Whyman, R. *J. Chem. Soc. Chem. Commun.*, **1994**, 801.
[194] Barrientos, A.G., De la Fuente, J.M.; Rojas, T.C.; Fernandez, A.; Penades, S. *Chem. Eur. J.*, **2003**, *9*, 1909.
[195] Barrientos, A.G.; de la Fuente, J.M.; Jiménez, M.; Solís, D.; Cañada, F.J.;Martín-Lomas, M.; Penadés, S. *Carbohyd. Res.*, **2009**, *344*, 1474-1478.
[196] a) Rojo, J.; Diaz, V.; de la Fuente, J.M.; Segura, I.; Barrientos, A.G.; Riese, H.H.; Bernad, A.; Penades, S. *ChemBioChem*, **2004**, *5*, 291; b) Rafael Ojeda, Jose Luis de Paz, Africa G. Barrientos, Manuel Martin-Lomas and Soledad Penades, Carbohydrate Research, **2007**, 26;342(3-4):448-59
[197] Fidler, I.J. *Cancer Res.*, **1975**, *35*, 218; b) Fidler, I.J.; Kripke, M.L. *Science,* **1977**, *197*, 893; c) Otsuji, E.; Park, Y.S.; Tashiro, K.; Koyima, N.; Toyokuni, T.; Hakomori, S. *Int. J. Oncol.,* **1995**, *6*, 319.
[198] Oguchi, H.; Toyokuni, T.; Dean, B.; Ito, H.; Otsuji, E.; Jones, V.L.; Sadozai, K.K.; Hakomori, S. *Cancer Commun.*, **1990**, *2*, 311.
[199] Svarovsky, S.A.; Szekely, Z.; Barchi, J.J. *Tetrahedron: Asymm.,* **2005**, *16*, 587.
[200] a) Sundgren, J. J. Barchi Jr. *Carbohyd. Res.*, **2008**, *343*, 1594-1604.
[201] Mukherjee, P.; Bhattacharya, R.; Wang, P.; Wang, L.; Basu, S.; Nagy, J.A.; Atala, A.; Mukhopadhyay, D.; Soker, S. *Clin. Cancer Res.*, **2005**, *11*, 3530.
[202] J. Denis, N. Majeau, E. Acosta-Ramirez, C. Savard, M.-C. Bedard, S. Simard, K. Lecours, M. Bolduc, C. Pare, B. Willems, N. Shoukry, P. Tessier, P. Lacasse, A. Lamarre, R. Lapointe, C. Lopez Macias, D. Leclerc, *Virology*, **2007**, *363*, 59-68.
[203] a) Jegerlehner, T. Storni, G. Lipowsky, M. Schmid, P. Pumpens, M. F. Bachmann, *Eur. J. Immunol.*, **2002**, *32*, 3305-3314.
[204] Miermont, A.; Barnhill, H.; Strable, E.; Lu, X.; Wall, K.A.; Wang, Q.; Finn, M.G.; Huang, X. *Chem. Eur. J.*, **2008**, *14*, 4939-4947.
[205] García, I.; Gallo, J.; Genicio, N.; Padro, D.; Penadés, S. *Bioconjugate Chem.*, **2011**, *22*, 264-273.
[206] Gallo, J.; García, I.; Genicio, N.; Padro, D.; Penadés, S., *Biomaterials*, **2011**, 32, 9818-9825.

CHAPTER 5

Recent Highlights in the Development of Isatin-Based Anticancer Agents

Kara L. Vine[*,1,2,3,§], Lidia Matesic[*,4,5,§], Julie M. Locke[6,7] and Danielle Skropeta[5,7]

[1]School of Biological Sciences, University of Wollongong, Wollongong, NSW, 2522, Australia; [2]Centre for Medical Bioscience, University of Wollongong, Wollongong, NSW, 2522, Australia; [3]Illawarra Health and Medical Research Institute, University of Wollongong, Wollongong, NSW, 2522, Australia; [4]Life Sciences Division, Australian Nuclear Science and Technology Organisation, Lucas Heights, NSW, 2234, Australia; [5]School of Chemistry, University of Wollongong, Wollongong, NSW, 2522, Australia; [6]Intelligent Polymer Research Institute, University of Wollongong, Wollongong, NSW, 2522, Australia; [7]Centre for Medicinal Chemistry, University of Wollongong, Wollongong, NSW, 2522, Australia

Abstract: Isatin (1*H*-indole-2,3-dione) and its derivatives are responsible for a broad spectrum of biological activities. Among these the cytotoxic and antineoplastic properties have been the most widely reported. The synthetic versatility of the isatin, due to its privileged scaffold, has led to the generation of a large number of structurally diverse derivatives which include analogues derived from either mono-, di-, and tri-substitution of the aryl ring A, and/or those obtained by derivatisation of the isatin nitrogen and C2/C3 carbonyl moieties. These compounds inhibit cancer cell proliferation and tumour growth *via* interaction with a variety of intracellular targets such as DNA, telomerase, tubulin, P-glycoprotein, protein kinases and phosphatases. Herein we review recent highlights in the development of isatin-based compounds as anticancer agents with a particular focus on the cytotoxicity and structure activity relationships.

Keywords: Isatin, indolinone, cytotoxicity, anticancer, kinase, drug conjugates, enzyme inhibitor, structure-activity relationships.

***Address correspondence to Kara L. Vine:** Illawarra Health and Medical Research Institute, University of Wollongong, Wollongong, NSW, 2522, Australia; Tel: +61-2-42214256; Fax: +61-2-42214135;
E-mail: kara@uow.edu.au
Lidia Matesic: Life Sciences Division, Australian Nuclear Science and Technology Organisation, Lucas Heights, NSW, 2234, Australia; Tel: +61-2-97177337; Fax: +61-2-97179262; E-mail: lidia.matesic@ansto.gov.au

[§]These authors contributed equally to this work.

Michelle Prudhomme (Ed)

1. INTRODUCTION

Isatin (1*H*-indole-2,3-dione) (**1**), an oxidised derivative of indole, was first discovered by Erdmann and Laurent in 1840 as a product arising from the oxidation of indigo (**2**) using nitric and chromic acids [1, 2] (Fig. **1**). The compound was considered synthetic for almost 140 years until it was found to be present in plants from the *Isatis* genus [3], in fruits of the cannon ball tree, *Couroupita guianensis* Aubl. [4] and in secretions from the parotid gland of the *Bufo* frog [5]. Various substituted isatins have also been identified in plants [6-8], fungi [9], symbiotic bacteria [10] and marine molluscs [11-14], where they are postulated to play a defensive role against pathogenic organisms (Fig. **1**).

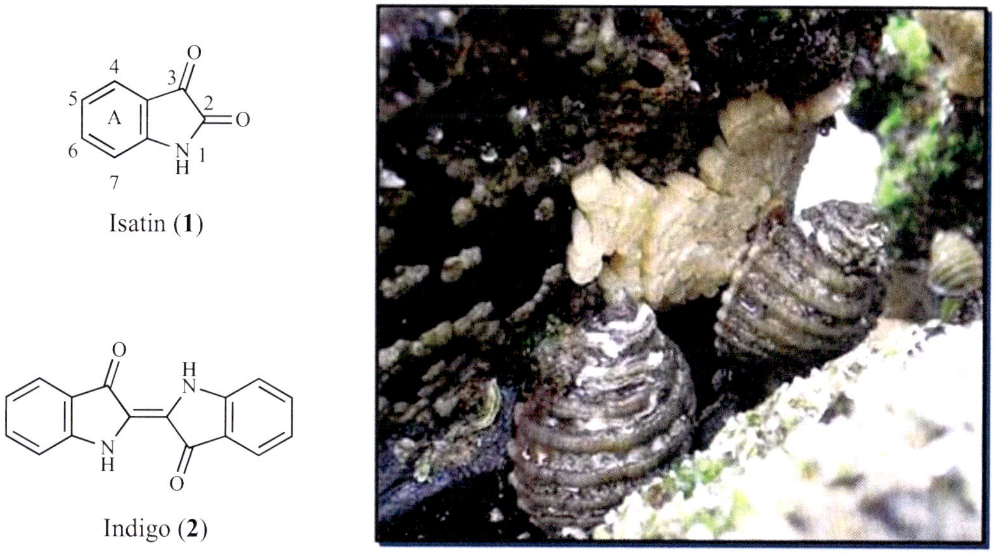

Fig. (1). The chemical structures of isatin (**1**) and indigo (**2**). The photograph shows adult Australian Muricid molluscs (*Dicathais orbita*) amongst freshly laid egg capsules, a rich source of the cytotoxic isatin derivative tyrindoleninone (6-bromo-2-methylthio-3*H*-indol-3-one) [15].

In humans and other mammals, isatin (**1**) is found as an endogenous molecule. Although the metabolic pathways of isatin (**1**) have not yet been fully elucidated, it has been proposed that it is synthesised *in vivo* from tryptophan-rich foods such as meat, dairy and whole grains. In this pathway, tryptophan is converted to indole by bacteria from the gastrointestinal tract and then transported to the liver where it is oxidized [16, 17]. Isatin (**1**) also plays a role in many physiological pathways, which are beyond the scope of this chapter (for further information see refs. [18-20]).

Isatin (**1**) contains a relatively large number of functionalisable groups and this together with its long term use in the synthetic dye industry has led to its widespread exploitation as a substrate/intermediate for organic synthesis. A number of review articles, including a comprehensive survey by da Silva *et al.* [21] describing the synthesis and chemistry of isatin have been published [22-24]. Reviews that discuss the utility of isatin as a precursor for the synthesis of other heterocyclic compounds are also available [25-27]. More recently, reviews have focused on the biological role of endogenous isatin [19, 20, 28] and the diverse range of biological activities displayed by assorted isatins and isatin derivatives [18, 29-34] including oxindoles and their copper complexes [35, 36]. Most recently, isatin derivatives have received considerable attention due to their potent anticancer activities [31]. Herein, we review the current literature describing the cytotoxic and anticancer activities of isatin analogues derived from either mono-, di-, and tri-substitution of the aryl ring A, and/or those obtained by derivatisation of the isatin nitrogen and C2/C3 carbonyl moieties (Fig. **2**). Advances in the development of more sophisticated isatin-based chemotherapeutics, including dual action drugs and selectively deliverable conjugates, and the potential utility of isatin anticancer drugs in combination therapies is also discussed.

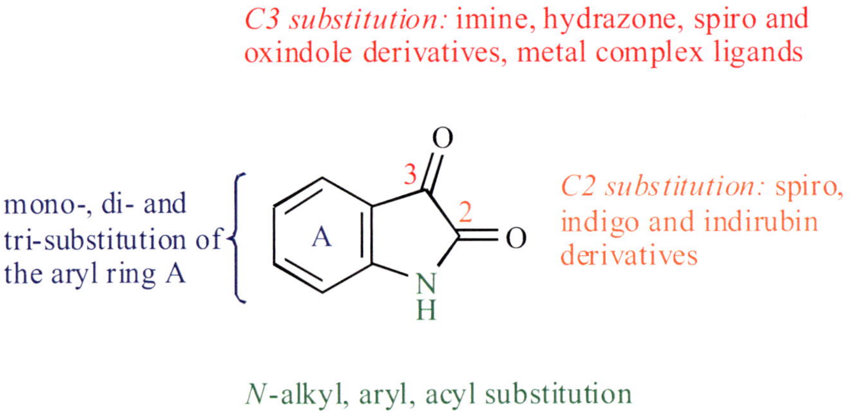

Fig. (2). The various substitution types and patterns possible for the isatin scaffold.

Finally, the cancer cell killing ability, or cytotoxicity, of a particular compound is typically defined as the concentration required to inhibit the growth of (and ultimately kill) 50% of a cell population *in vitro*, and is reported as an IC_{50}, EC_{50}, LD_{50} or GI_{50} value. It is important to note, however, that whilst this standard nomenclature allows for greater comparison of compounds across different structural classes, the use of diverse cell lines, assays (*e.g.* MTS, MTT, lactate dehydrogenase, Sulforhodamine B/Kiton Red, WST-1 and clonogenic), incubation times and concentration units (*i.e.* moles *vs* grams per litre) always need to be taken into consideration when comparing the potency of the compounds discussed in this chapter.

2. CYTOTOXIC AND ANTICANCER ACTIVITIES OF ISATIN DERIVATIVES

2.1. Mono-, Di- and Tri-Substituted Aromatic Isatin Derivatives

The isatin scaffold is a versatile moiety and its success as a new class of antineoplastic agents is supported by the approval of the oxindole, sunitinib maleate (Sutent®) by the Food and Drug Administration for the treatment of advanced renal carcinoma [37], gastrointestinal stromal tumours [38] and, more recently for neuroendocrine tumours of the pancreas (see section 2.4.1). Of importance to its activity is the fluorine atom at C5, which is not surprising, as substitution at the 5-position has previously been associated with increased biological activity for a range of isatin-based compounds. For example, in 2007 Vine *et al.* reported the *in vitro* cytotoxicity of a range of mono-substituted isatins (**3a-g**, Fig. **3**) on a human monocyte-like, histiocytic lymphoma (U937) cell line [39]. Structure activity relationship (SAR) studies revealed that substitution at position 5 was favoured over positions 4, 6 or 7, leading to greater cancer cell killing ability. Nitration at C5 (**3f**) improved the anticancer activity by a factor of 4, while the addition of a methoxy group (**3g**) only mildly improved cytotoxicity (*i.e.* decreasing the IC_{50} by 145 μM) over a 24 h period. Furthermore, halogenation yielded the most active compounds, with 5-bromo-, 5-iodo-, and 5-fluoroisatin (**3a**, **3e** and **3d** respectively) being 5-10 times more active than the unsubstituted parent compound [39]. Increasing the number of electron-withdrawing groups on the ring to make combinations of dibromo-, tribromo-, iodo- and nitroisatin derivatives (**3h-n**) also enhanced the overall activity against a panel of human cancer cell lines, by up to 100-fold from that of the parent molecule (**1**). Despite this trend, 6,7-dimethylisatin was deemed inactive in a brine shrimp lethality assay (LD_{50} 96 ppm) compared to other substituted heterocyclic isatins [40], suggesting that together with substitution on the aromatic ring A, substitution at N1, C2 and/or C3, may also significantly enhance the molecule's cytotoxic effect (see sections 2.2 - 2.4).

In terms of its mode of action, isatin itself is proposed to inhibit cancer cell proliferation *via* interaction with extracellular signal-related protein kinases (ERKs), thereby promoting apoptosis. In 2000, Cane *et al.* [41] reported that isatin inhibited the proliferation of a human promyelocytic leukemia (HL60) cancer cell line by 80% at a concentration of 0.1 mM, and consequently induced DNA fragmentation and chromatin condensation. Moreover, treatment of N1E-115 neuroblastoma cells with isatin at the same concentration inhibited the phosphorylation of ERK-2, but not ERK-1, by 35% compared to untreated control cells. A subsequent study using human neuroblastoma SH-SY5Y cells confirmed that the effect of isatin on cell proliferation was dose- and time-dependent [42]. For example, after 24 h of exposure, isatin caused 35% detachment (or cell death) of SH-SY5Y cells treated with high concentrations (400 μM) of the compound. Following a 48 h exposure, the percentage of detached cells significantly increased to 82%. Apoptosis was observed in cells exposed to lower concentrations of isatin (50 μM), as indicated by morphological changes (including cell shrinkage and nuclear condensation), internucleosomal DNA fragmentation and externalisation of plasma membrane phosphatidylserine. At higher concentrations, (greater than 200 μM) cell death increased even further, however evaluation of membrane permeability by fluorescence-activated cell sorting revealed that isatin had significantly damaged the plasma membrane, consistent with necrotic cell death [42]. Such a time- and dose-dependent switch from apoptosis to necrosis was also observed by Vine *et al.* whereby 5,6,7-tribromoisatin (**3n**) was found to be antiproliferative (and induce apoptosis) at low concentrations (4 μM), but cytotoxic (and induce necrosis) at high concentrations (130 μM) in U937 cells [39]. ERK activation was not tested in this study.

	R^1	R^2	R^3
3a	Br	H	H
3b	H	Br	H
3c	H	H	Br
3d	F	H	H
3e	I	H	H
3f	NO_2	H	H
3g	OMe	H	H

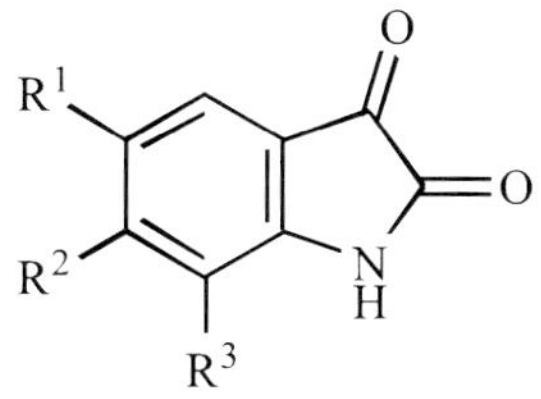

3

	R^1	R^2	R^3
3h	Br	H	Br
3i	Br	Br	H
3j	I	H	I
3k	Br	H	NO_2
3l	NO_2	Br	H
3m	NO_2	H	Br
3n	Br	Br	Br

Fig. (3). Selected isatin derivatives with mono-, di- and tri- substitution on ring A.

2.2. *N*-Alkyl Substituted Isatin Derivatives

N-Alkylated indoles are well known to exhibit anticancer activity [43-45]. However, until recently, little had been reported on the antineoplastic activity of *N*-alkyl and *N*-aryl isatins. In 2003, compound **4** (Fig. **4**), was the first *N*-alkylisatin described to induce apoptosis in a panel of human cancer cell lines, but not normal cells, at micromolar concentrations [43]. Generally it was found that normal cell lines such as peripheral blood lymphocytes and human mammary epithelial cells were resistant to *N*-(3,4-dichlorobenzyl)-1*H*-indole-2,3-dione (**4**) induced apoptosis, while cancer cell lines of lymphoid origin were the most sensitive. Further screening by the National Cancer Institute (NCI) found that the dichlorinated compound exerted a cytostatic effect (inhibiting cell growth by 50-100%) on 40 out of the 48 cell lines tested, at a concentration of 10 μM. At 10 times this concentration however, the compound exhibited 100% cytotoxicity on virtually all cell lines, suggesting that this effect may be due to non-specific toxicity [43]. Later in 2003, Liu *et al.* [44], identified a class of isatin *O*-acyl oximes (*e.g.* compound **5**) that selectivity inhibited neuronal ubiquitin *C*-terminal hydrolase (UCH-L1) at sub-micromolar concentrations in the H1299 lung cancer cell line (Fig. **4**). Despite being linked to Parkinson's disease, UCH-L1 is also expressed in many primary lung tumours and lung cancer cell lines, but not normal lung tissue [46, 47], where it is proposed to be linked to tumour progression upon upregulation [44]. Expression of UCH-L1 also correlates with tumour progression in colorectal cancer [48]. Hence, its inhibition by small molecules like compound **5**, may be of great therapeutic benefit to lung and colorectal cancer patients in the future.

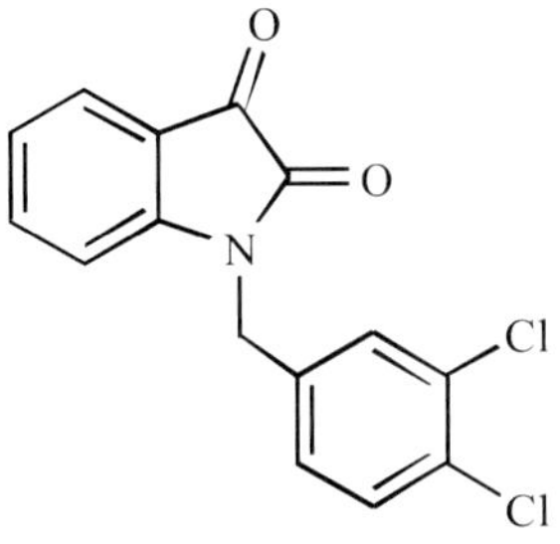

4

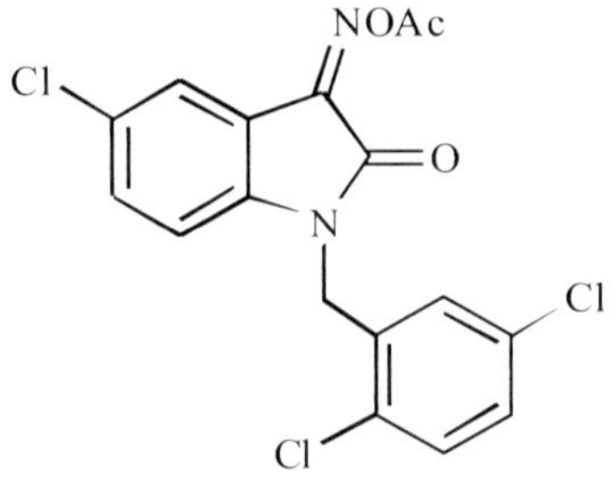

5

Fig. (4). Examples of the first synthetic cytotoxic *N*-substituted isatin-based molecules.

In 2007, Vine *et al.* [49] synthesised a series of dibrominated *N*-substituted isatins (*e.g.* **6a-d** and **7a-n**, Fig. **5**). Given the increased potency of the halogenated isatins (see section 2.1) and the fact that *N*-methylation significantly enhanced the cytotoxicity of the parent compound (**1**) [39], these compounds were evaluated for their cytotoxicity against a panel cancer cell lines *in vitro* [49]. SAR studies indicated that the introduction of an aromatic ring with a one or three carbon atom linker at N1 increased the activity relative to that of the allyl (**6a**), 2′-methoxyethyl (**6b**) and 3′-methylbutyl (**6c**) *N*-substituted isatins. Furthermore, electron-withdrawing groups substituted at the *meta* or *para* position of the substituent phenyl ring were favoured over the *ortho* orientation. Of the 24 compounds screened, nine displayed sub-micromolar IC_{50} values and in general demonstrated greater selectivity toward leukemia and lymphoma cell lines over other carcinoma cell lines tested. 5,7-Dibromo-*N*-(*p*-methylbenzyl)isatin (**7f**) was the most active compound, inhibiting the metabolic activity of two haematopoietic cancer cell lines by 50% at 0.49 μM. This effect was further enhanced by at least a factor of two when the incubation time was increased from 24 h to 72 h, making this class of compounds >10 times more active than the conventional chemotherapeutic agents 5-fluorouracil (5-FU), paclitaxel and vinblastine against U937 cells [31].

Continuing this work, in 2008 Matesic *et al.* synthesised a family of *N*-phenethyl derivatives (**8a-e**, Fig. **5**) [50]. All five *N*-phenethyl derivatives (**8a-e**) exhibited low to sub-micromolar cytotoxic activity against a panel of human leukemic, lymphoma and carcinoma cell lines where introduction of a hydrophobic bromo

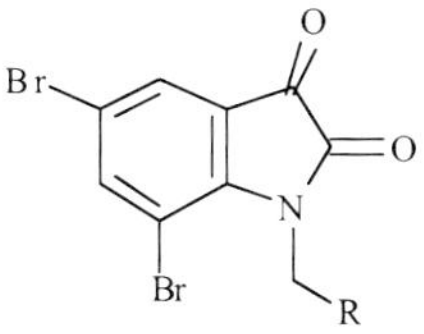

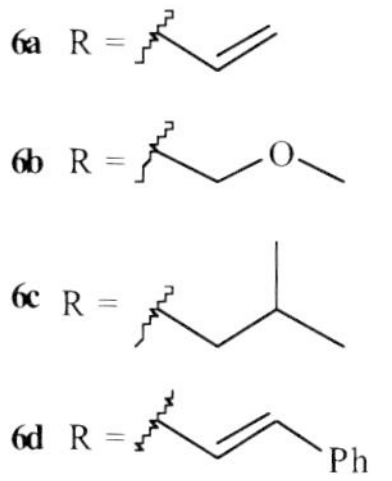

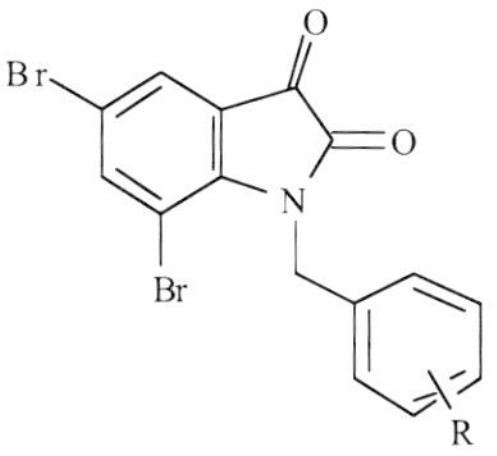

7a R = H	**7h** R = *p*-CO_2Me
7b R = *p*-I	**7i** R = *p*-(*t*-Bu)
7c R = *p*-Br	**7j** R = *p*-Ph
7d R = *p*-Cl	**7k** R = *p*-OMe
7e R = *p*-CF_3	**7l** R = *m*-OMe
7f R = *p*-Me	**7m** R = *p*-NO_2
7g R = *p*-CO_2H	**7n** R = *o*-NO_2

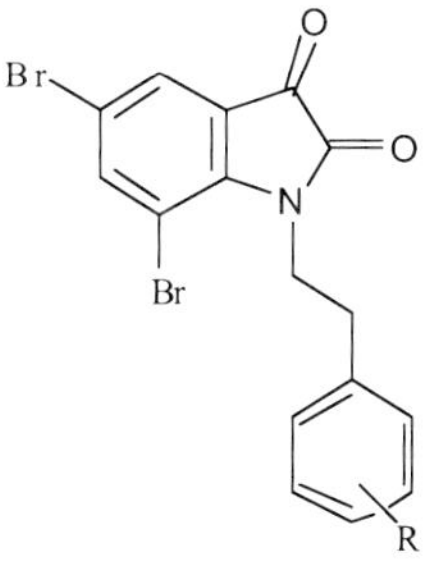

8a R = H
8b R = *m*-Br
8c R = *p*-Br
8d R = *m*-OMe
8e R = *p*-OMe

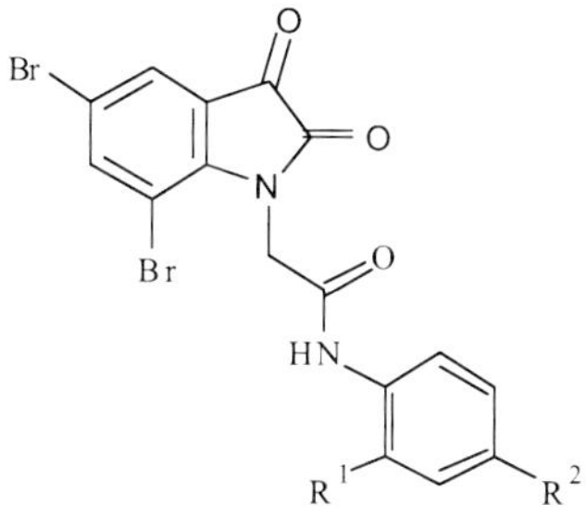

	R^1	R^2
9a	H	H
9b	NO_2	H
9c	CH_3	H
9d	H	NO_2
9e	H	CH_3

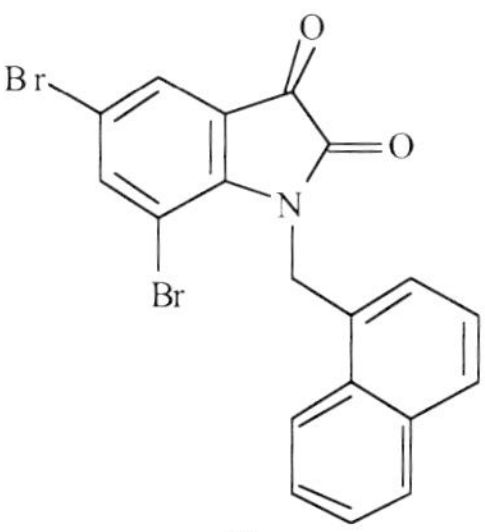

10

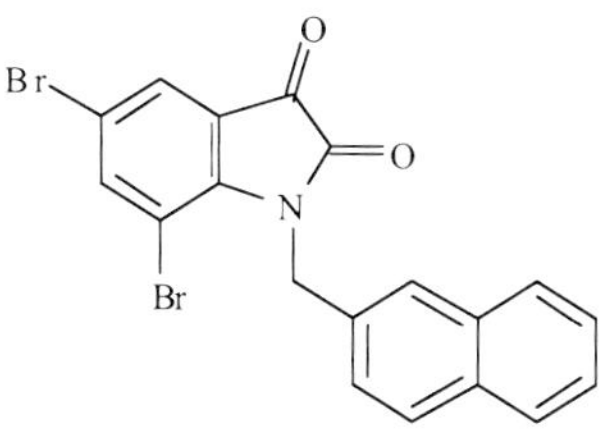

11

Fig. (5). Examples of cytotoxic *N*-substituted 5,7-dibromoisatins including the *N*-naphthyl isatin derivatives (**10** and **11**).

substituent in the *meta* (**8b**) or *para* (**8c**) position yielded the most active compounds [50]. Interestingly, the corresponding phenacyl derivatives (not shown) were at least 3-5 times less active against the U937 cells [50]. Related *N*-phenylacetamide derivatives (**9a-e**) prepared by Modi *et al.* [51] were also active against a MCF-7 human mammary adenocarcinoma cell line with IC_{50} values ranging from 1.09 - 3.91 μM and exhibiting up to 20-fold selectivity for cancer cells over non-cancerous cells.

In 2009, further examples of new *N*-alkylisatin derivatives were synthesised and evaluated for their cytotoxic activity, including Singh *et al.* [52], who described five *N*-alkylbromo and five *N*-alkylphthalimido isatin derivatives of which the most active compound gave IC_{50} values of 4.57, 10.90, 11.75, 12.40 and 54.20 μM after 48 hour incubation against HeLa, PC-3, HCT-15, THP-1 and Colo-205 cell lines respectively. Solomon *et al.* [53] prepared a series of 15 dialkyl/diaryl amino methyl, morpholinyl and piperidinyl *N*-alkylisatins bearing either an unsubstituted aromatic ring or halogenation (Cl or Br) solely at position 4 of the aromatic ring. All 15 compounds, along with their analogous 3-substituted benzothiazole derivatives (see section 2.5), were screened against three breast cancer cell lines (MDA-MB-231, MDA-MB-468 and MCF-7) and two non-cancer cell lines (184B5 and MCF10A). The derivatives were found to be active in the mid-micromolar range (>10-100 μM) after a 48 h incubation, with the most active compound, 4-bromo-1-diethylaminomethyl-1*H*-indole-2,3-dione (IC_{50} 11.68 μM; MDA-MB-468), displaying 10-15 fold greater selectivity for cancer over non-cancer cells. It is interesting to note that the derivatives in the above two studies lacked substitution at the 5- and/or 7-position of the aromatic moiety known to be important for cytotoxic activity, which may be reflected in their activities being in the mid-micromolar rather than sub-micromolar range.

Other examples of *N*-substituted isatins that display potent cytotoxic activity include the dibrominated 1- and 2-naphthyl derivatives **10** and **11** (Fig. **5**). The *N*-naphthyl isatins were found to display sub-micromolar cytotoxicity against U937 and human leukemic T-cell (Jurkat) cell lines (*e.g.* IC_{50} for the 1-naphthyl derivative (**10**) of 0.19 and 0.91 μM, respectively), along with low micromolar cytotoxicity towards a panel of human carcinoma cell lines, including those derived from breast (MDA-MB-231 and MCF-7), colon (HCT-116) and prostate

(PC-3) [50]. Interestingly, compound **10** represents one of the most cytotoxic dibrominated *N*-alkylisatin reported to date, when compared with other *N*-alkylisatins tested over a 24 h time period. This suggests that increasing the hydrophobicity of the *N*-substituent through site specific placement of an additional aromatic ring is important for activity.

In 2010, Sabet *et al.* [54] reported a QSAR study that utilised biological data from 47 of the isatin derivatives reported previously by Vine [39, 49] and Matesic [50] to reveal that positive effects to anticancer activity were related to the number of halogen atoms and secondary carbons, while negative effects were related to the number of secondary amides and ketones. Their study also further confirmed the importance of lipophilic substituents at position 5 and 7 on the aromatic ring to the anticancer activity of isatin derivatives. These findings were further supported by another QSAR study in 2011, where Modi *et al.* [51] found that electron-withdrawing substituents at the *para*-position of the phenyl ring, substitution at the 5,7-positions of the isatin ring and increasing lipophilicity of the compound enhanced the cytotoxic activity.

In addition to their potent cell killing ability, various *N*-alkylisatins were also found to induce G2/M cell cycle arrest and dramatically alter lymphocyte morphology [49, 50, 53]. As these morphological alterations were also seen in vinblastine and paclitaxel-treated cells, Vine *et al.* suggested that *N*-alkylisatins may either disrupt or stabilise microtubules in a similar fashion [49]. Various *N*-alkylbenzylisatins including representative phenethyl and naphthyl derivatives were therefore screened for their ability to interfere with microtubule dynamics and were found to strongly inhibit the rate of microtubule polymerisation. This effect was shown to be dose-dependent, and appeared to be independent of the nature of the *p*-substituent and size of the benzene carbon linker, as compounds **6d**, **7e**, **7f**, and **7j** all inhibited microtubule polymerisation at a similar rate [49]. All *N*-alkylbenzylisatins tested, including the phenethyl and naphthyl compounds were found to be potent microtubule destabilisers, which is consistent with reports that structurally similar indole [45, 55] and indolinone [56, 57] compounds inhibit tubulin polymerisation.

In 2009, Romagnoli *et al.* [58] combined the α-bromoacrylamido found in a number of natural cytotoxic alkaloids such as discorhabdin A and G with the *N*-alkylisatin type structures described earlier [49] to generate a new series of 20 α-bromoacrylamido *N*-substituted isatin derivatives (**12a-t**, Fig. **6**). The majority of the compounds exhibited sub-micromolar cytotoxicity when incubated for 72 h with IC_{50} values ranging from 0.15 - 8.53 μM against human myeloid leukemia HL60, U937, and human lymphoid leukemia MOLT-3 cells. In addition, the authors used morphological changes, flow cytometry and western blot analyses to show that the antiproliferative activity of the compounds in human leukemia cells is likely to be mediated by apoptosis caused by cytochrome c release and caspase activation.

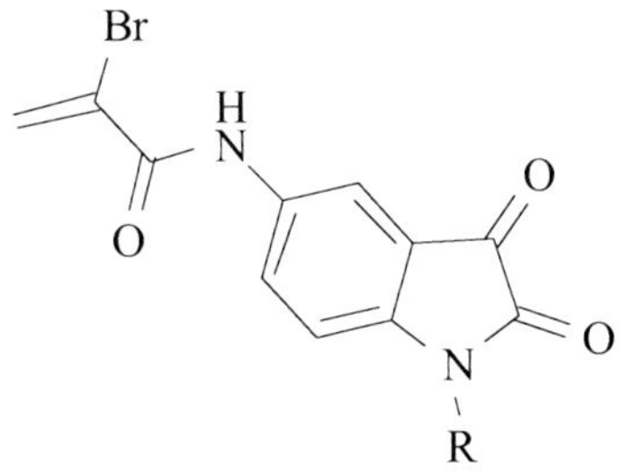

12

12a	R = H	**12k**	R = C_6H_5
12b	R = CH_3	**12l**	R = 4-Me-C_6H_4
12c	R = CH_2CH_3	**12m**	R = 4-OMe-C_6H_4
12d	R = $(CH_2)_2CH_3$	**12n**	R = 4-F-C_6H_4
12e	R = $CH_2CH{=}CH_2$	**12o**	R = $C_6H_5CH_2$
12f	R = CH_2CCH	**12p**	R = 4-Me-C_6H_4
12g	R = $CH_2CH(CH_2)_2$	**12q**	R = 4-*t*-Bu-C_6H_4
12h	R = $(CH_2)_3CH_3$	**12r**	R = 4-F-C_6H_4
12i	R = $(CH_2)_4CH_3$	**12s**	R = 4-Cl-C_6H_4
12j	R = $(CH_2)_5CH_3$	**12t**	R = 4-CF_3-C_6H_4

Fig. (6). Cytotoxic α-bromoacrylamido *N*-substituted isatin derivatives.

2.3. C2-Substituted Isatin Derivatives

The most famous of the C2-substituted isatins are the widely employed indigo pigments used since ancient times. This class includes indigo carmine (5,5'-indigodisulfonic acid sodium salt), an extensively used non-toxic, inexpensive stain for chromo-colonoscopic diagnosis and management of early colorectal cancer [59-62]. The best known cytotoxic C2-substituted isatin derivative is indirubin (**13**, Fig. **7**), the red component of indigo pigments. This compound is found in plants belonging to the genii *Indigofera*, *Isastis* and *Polygonum*, and in marine molluscs of the *Murex* genus [63]. Indirubin is the active component in the traditional Chinese antileukemia medicine Danggui Longhui Wan, and the synthesis and biological activities of indirubin and its derivatives have been well studied and reviewed [64-67]. The indirubins are thought to have great potential for pharmaceutical use however, they are plagued by extremely poor aqueous solubility. As a consequence, investigations focus on developing indirubins with improved water solubility and recent studies have often explored the more soluble 3'-oxime substituted derivatives and/or side chains designed to enhance aqueous solubility. A number of these derivatives with various substitution patterns exhibit sub-micromolar and/or high-nanomolar IC_{50} values against human cancer cell lines *in vitro* (Fig. **7**, compounds **14-16**) [68-72].

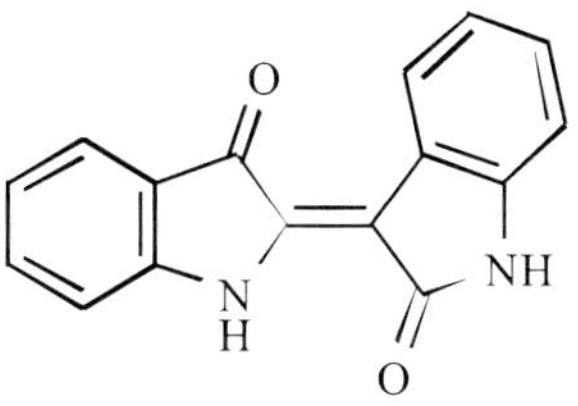

indirubin, **13**

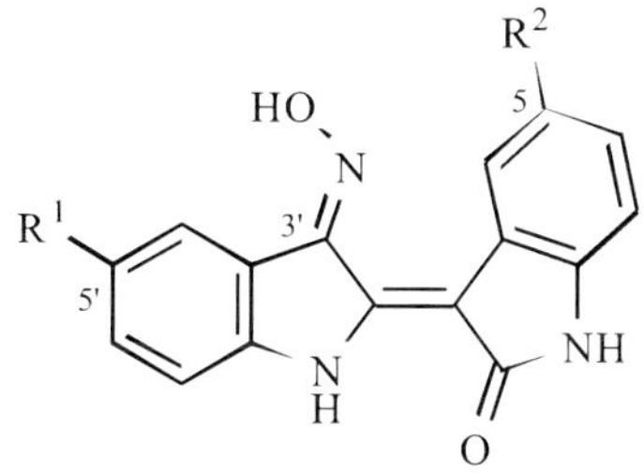

14

	R^1	R^2
14a	H	H
14b	H	NO_2
14c	OH	NO_2
14d	OH	F
14e	Cl	NO_2
14f	F	NO_2

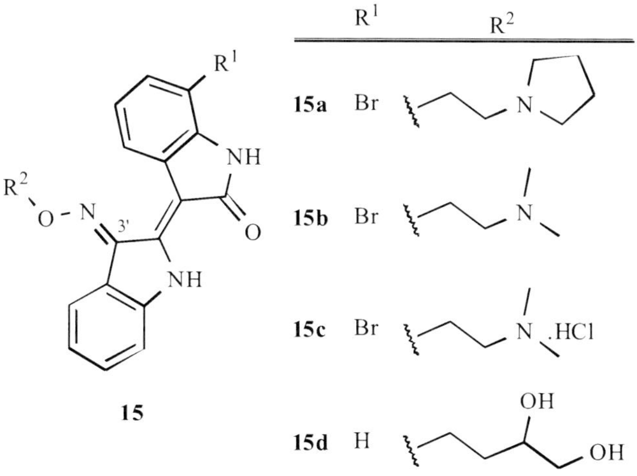

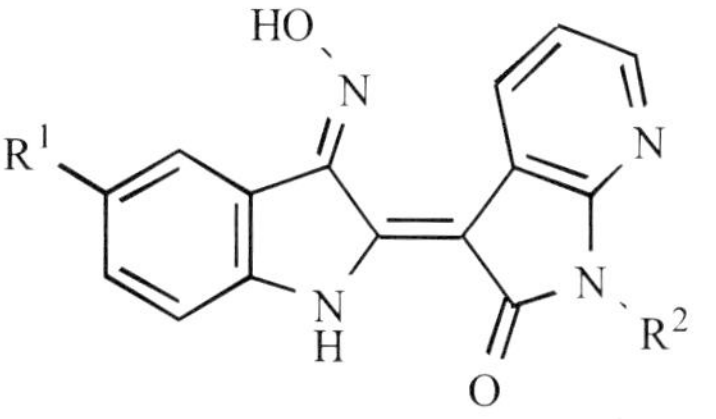

16

	R^1	R^2
16a	Cl	CH_3
16b	Cl	C_2H_5
16c	Cl	i-C_3H_7
16d	Br	i-C_3H_7

Fig. (7). The structure of indirubin (**13**) and some indirubin-3'-oxime derivatives (**14a-f**), E804 (**15d**) and a number of recently disclosed soluble indirubin-3'-oximes (**15a-c**) [68, 69] and azaindirubins (**16a-d**) [70] that exhibit low micromolar/high nanomolar IC_{50} values ($\leq$ 3.8 μM) against a variety of different human cancer cell lines *in vitro*.

Indirubins exert their cytotoxic action *via* a number of modes [73] and they are recognised for their ATP-competitive inhibition of both CDK1 and CDK2 [74-76] and induction of apoptosis through cell cycle arrest at G2/M, as a result of inhibition of GSK3 [77], c-Src kinase and NF-κB activation and expression [78, 79] as well as the activation of the aryl hydrocarbon receptor [80, 81]. Based on a range of mechanistic and crystallographic studies of indirubins with GSK3 and CDK2, a vast number of indirubin derivatives have been synthesised and their biological activity and specificity evaluated [75, 82, 83]. A number of recent studies have identified numerous alternative modes for the cytotoxic and antiangiogenic actions displayed by indirubin and some of its derivatives. Other actions of the indirubins include suppression of the VEGFR-2-mediated JAK/STAT3 signaling pathway by indirubin (**13**) [84]; inhibition of alternative kinases such as fms-like tyrosine kinase 3 by indirubin-3'-oxime (**14a**) and its 6-bromo analogue [85]; and inhibition of polo-like kinase 1 [86] as well as downregulation of Notch-1 and inhibition of Integrin β1/FAK/Akt signaling by 5-nitroindirubin-3'-oxime (**14b**) [85, 87-89].

In addition to increased solubility relative to 3'-keto compounds, the 3'-oxime substituted derivatives often exhibit either equivalent or greater cytotoxicity against cancer cell lines *in vitro* [70, 85, 90, 91]. The 3'-oxime indirubin derivative 3'-(3,4-dihydroxybutoxy)iminoindirubin or E804, (**15d**, Fig. **7**) has also recently shown potent antiangiogenic activity [92]. E804 is known to block the Src-STAT3 signaling pathway [93] and demonstrated strong inhibition of STAT5 and subsequently induced apoptosis in K562 chronic myelogenous leukemia (CML), imatinib resistant KCL-22M and primary CML cells [94]. A recent study that combined the indirubin moiety with amide-linked side chains terminating in assorted amine groups (**17a-d**, Fig. **8**) to produce derivatives with structural similarities to sunitinib (see section 2.4.1). A series of these compounds were tested against a panel of cell lines and were particularly active against SK-BR-3 breast carcinoma cells with compound **17a** showing sub-nanomolar activity (IC_{50} = 0.8 nM), significantly higher potency than that observed for the sunitinib control (3.55 μM) in this cell line [95].

In addition to indirubin derivatives, the marine environment has yielded an array of other novel C2-substituted indolinones including the alkaloid matemone (**18**, Fig. **9**)

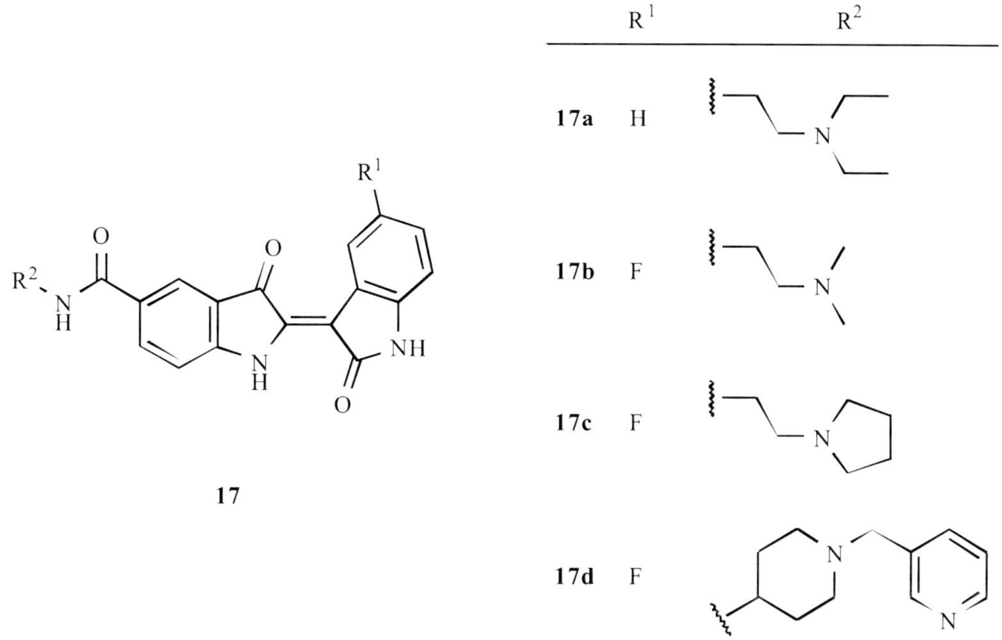

Fig. (8). Structure of indirubin derivatives whose design was based on the structure of sunitinib.

[96]. Isolated from the Indian Ocean sponge Iotrochota purpurea, matemone (**18**) was found to intercalate DNA, to inhibit the division of sea-urchin eggs and exhibited mild cytotoxicity towards a range of human carcinoma cell lines. More recent examples of marine-based isatins have been provided by the sea cucumber-associated fungus *Aspergillus fumigatus*, which was found to produce several novel prenylated indole diketopiperazine alkaloids, including compound 19 and the three spirotryprostatins C-E (**20a-c**, Fig. **9**). The prenylated indoles were evaluated for their cytotoxicity with derivative 20c exhibiting the most potent activity with IC50 values of 2-3 μM against the human non-small cell lung carcinoma (A549), the human acute lymphoblastic leukemic (MOLT-4) and HL60 cell lines [97].

Based on previous studies of the aurones, a range of 2-arylidenedihydroindole-3-ones (**21a-f**, Fig. **10**), or azaaurones, have been synthesised and evaluated for their antiproliferative and apoptotic abilities against bladder tumours. Azaaurone (**21c**), the most active compound, inhibited proliferation and induced apoptosis *via* a fibroblast growth factor receptor-3 (FGFR) dependent pathway in DAG-1 and RT112 bladder tumour cell lines [98].

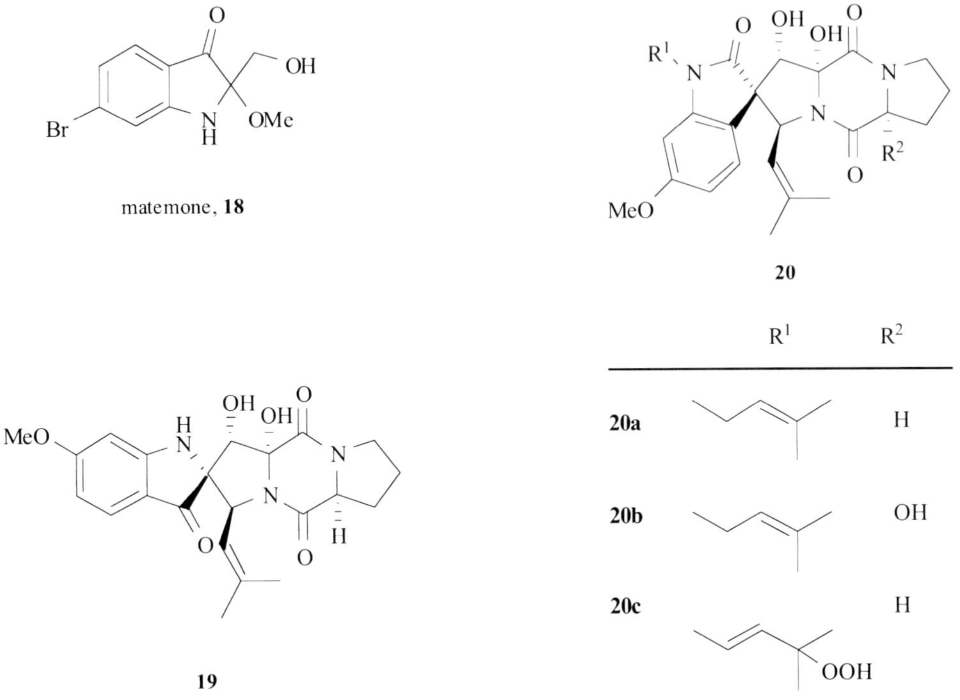

Fig. (9). Cytotoxic, marine-derived C2-substituted isatin derivatives.

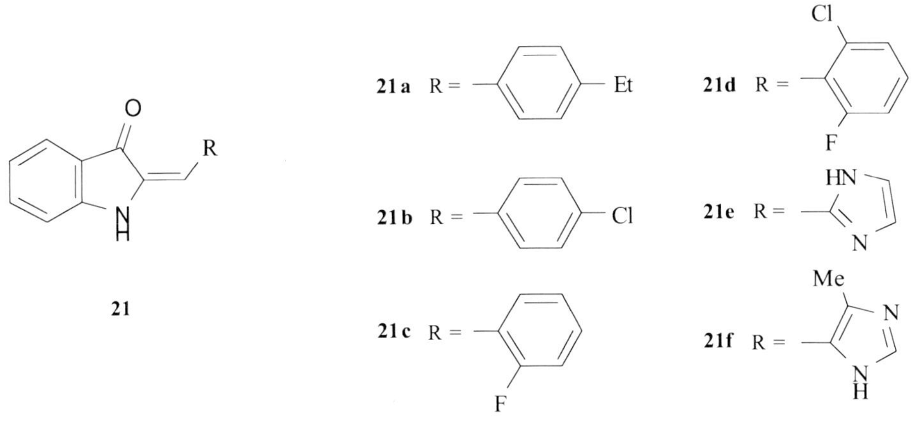

Fig. (10). Structures of some bioactive azaaurones reported by Gerby *et al.* [98].

2.4. C3-Substituted Isatin Derivatives

A plethora of C3-substituted isatins (also known as indolinones or oxindole derivatives) have been generated due to the susceptibility of isatin to be attacked by nucleophiles at the C3 position. This is reflected by the vastly greater proportion of biologically active 3-substituted isatins reported in the literature relative to the other substitution patterns. This section will highlight the recent progress of C3-substituted isatins containing arylidene, hydrazone/imine and metal functionalities, together with isoindigo and other miscellaneous isatin analogues.

2.4.1. 3-Arylidene Derivatives

Indolinones such as SU5416 (semaxanib, **22**) have been discontinued in clinical trials due to dangerous side effects [99], although the compound is extremely potent with GI_{50} values of < 10 nM against 46 out of 53 NCI cell lines [100]. In contrast, SU11248, (sunitinib, Sutent®, **23**), is now the standard first-line treatment for the treatment of gastrointestinal stromal cancers and renal cell carcinoma [101]. The drug is a multiple receptor tyrosine kinase (RTK) inhibitor, targeting VEGFR-2, platelet-derived growth receptor-β (PDGFR-β), stem cell factor receptor, fetal liver tyrosine kinase receptor-3 [99], colony-stimulating factor type 1 and glial cell-line derived neurotrophic factor receptor [102]. 3-Substituted indolinones possessing the *Z* configuration are potent inhibitors of the FGFR, while compounds adopting the *E* configuration inhibit epidermal growth factor receptor (EGFR) [55].

SU9516 (**24**) is capable of causing mitochondrial damage, caspase activation and inducing apoptosis in a dose- and time-dependent manner in U937 cells [103]. Pyrrolyllactone and pyrrolyllactam derivatives of **24** have been synthesised and described as potent CDK2 inhibitors, particularly compounds exhibiting a polar substituent in the 4-position [104].

The indolinone SU5402 (**25**), encompasses a *Z* configuration about the alkenyl bond. Twenty analogues of **25** bearing the *E* configuration were synthesised and subsequently assessed for cytotoxicity [105]. The lead compound, containing a methyl ester on the pyrrole group displayed IC_{50} values of 98 nM and 65 nM against A549 lung and MDA-MB-468 breast carcinoma cell lines after a 72 h exposure.

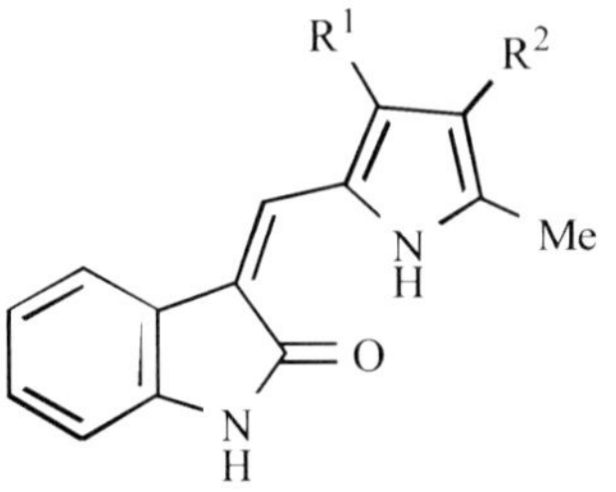

	R^1	R^2
22	Me	H
25	$(CH_2)_2COOH$	Me
26	Me	$(CH_2)_2COOH$

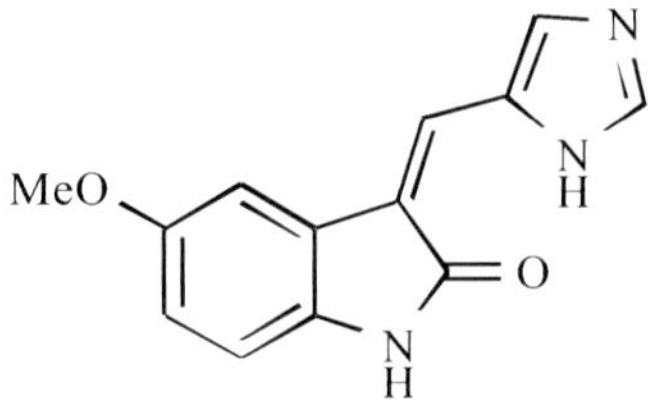

24

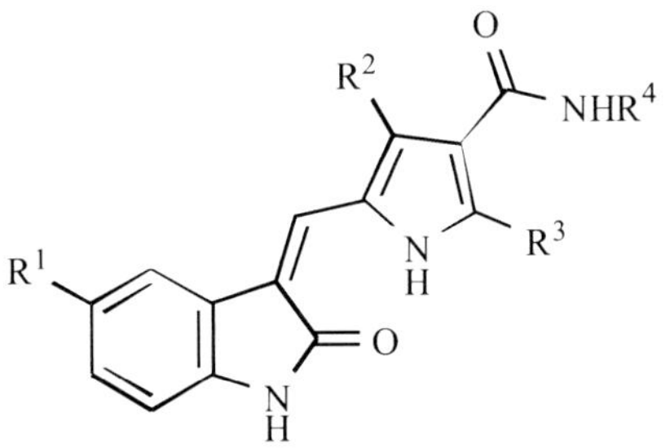

	R^1	R^2	R^3	R^4
23	F	Me	Me	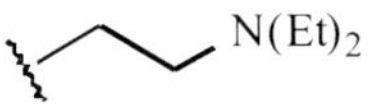
27	F	Me	Me	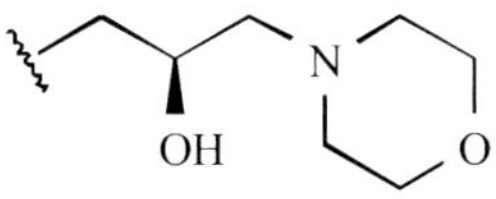
28	F	Cl	Me	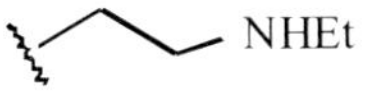
29	Cl	Cl	Me	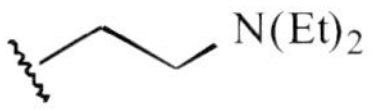
30	F	C_2H_5	Cl	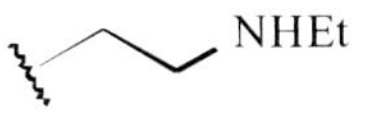

Fig. (11). Examples of 3-pyrroloarylidene isatin derivatives including the clinically used sunitinib (**23**).

SU6668 (**26**) significantly suppresses tumour angiogenesis [106], and is capable of inducing substantial tumour regression, regardless of initial tumour size. The drug was evaluated in four separate Phase I trials, but was discontinued due to the superior activity of sunitinib (**23**). SU14813 (**27**) has also emerged as a multiple RTK inhibitor with strong antiangiogenic and antitumour activity. It expresses dose-dependent antitumour efficacy and assists in the regression of human renal (786-O), human acute myelogenous leukemia (MV4;11), human colon (Colo-205 and MV522) and rat glioma (C6) tumours [107]. Additionally, the compound displays moderate systemic clearance and inhibition of tumour growth can be improved when **27** is combined with the anti-mitotic chemotherapeutic, docetaxel.

An extension of this scaffold included 18 novel 3-substituted indolinones incorporating chloropyrroles [108]. The most bioactive compounds in the series, as determined by evaluating the analogues against four tumour cell lines, were **28-30** (Fig. **11**). Indolinone **28** displayed 3-4 fold greater cytotoxicity than sunitinib (**23**) against KB oral epithelial and K111 melanoma cells, while analogues **29** and **30** were highly cytotoxic against A549 cells, with compound **29** being up to 10-fold more cytotoxic than **30** in this cell line. Furthermore, a derivative of sunitinib (**23**) containing a *N*-(dimethylamino)propyl group has been found to be up to twice as cytotoxic as **23** against HL60, K562 leukemia and MDA-MB-231 breast cancer cells [109].

Luo *et al.* have also prepared a series of 3-pyrrolo-substituted indolinones and compared their cytotoxicity to sunitinib (**23**) [110]. 5-Vinylsulfonyl indolinones such as **31a-c** (Fig. **12**) were found to exhibit IC_{50} values < 10 μM against A549, SQC-7901, ECA-109 and HCT-116 cells. Compound **31b** was more active than sunitinib (**23**) against all four cell lines. Additionally, 5-sulfonyl indolinones **32a** and **32b** were also found to possess potent cytotoxicity and compound **32b** was also more active than **23** against the four cell lines.

Indolinones incorporating a cycloalkanone fused onto the pyrrole ring have also been prepared [111]. The most cytotoxic analogue (**33**, Fig. **15**) displayed an IC_{50} value of 1.62 μM against HeLa cells after a 72 h exposure and sub-micromolar IC_{50} values against colonic HCT-116 and HT-29 cells. Additionally, the compound was efficacious as an Aurora kinase inhibitor, particularly towards Aurora kinase B. Pyrrolo-fused heterocyclic analogues have been investigated and compound **34** has been evaluated in human HT-29 colon tumour xenografts assay in BALB/cA-nude mice [112]. After 14 days of once daily administration, the compound led to antitumour efficacy in a dose-dependent manner and the tumour growth was inhibited by 74.2% at the maximum dose of 30 mg/kg.

Indolinones possessing a pyrrole ring, similar to the above mentioned compounds, have additionally been identified as inhibitors of the cAkt2 protein kinase, which is activated by phosphoinositide-dependent kinase-1 through the support of phosphoinositide 3-kinase activity in cells [113]. Activity towards the cAkt2 kinase was increased almost 400-fold through the addition of a urea group at C5 on the isatin core and a methyl group on the alkene bond at C3. The novel compound named BX-517, was optimised by exploring the C4′ position on the pyrrole ring and led to potent phosphoinositide-dependent kinase-1 inhibitors with superior pharmacokinetic properties compared to BX-517 [114].

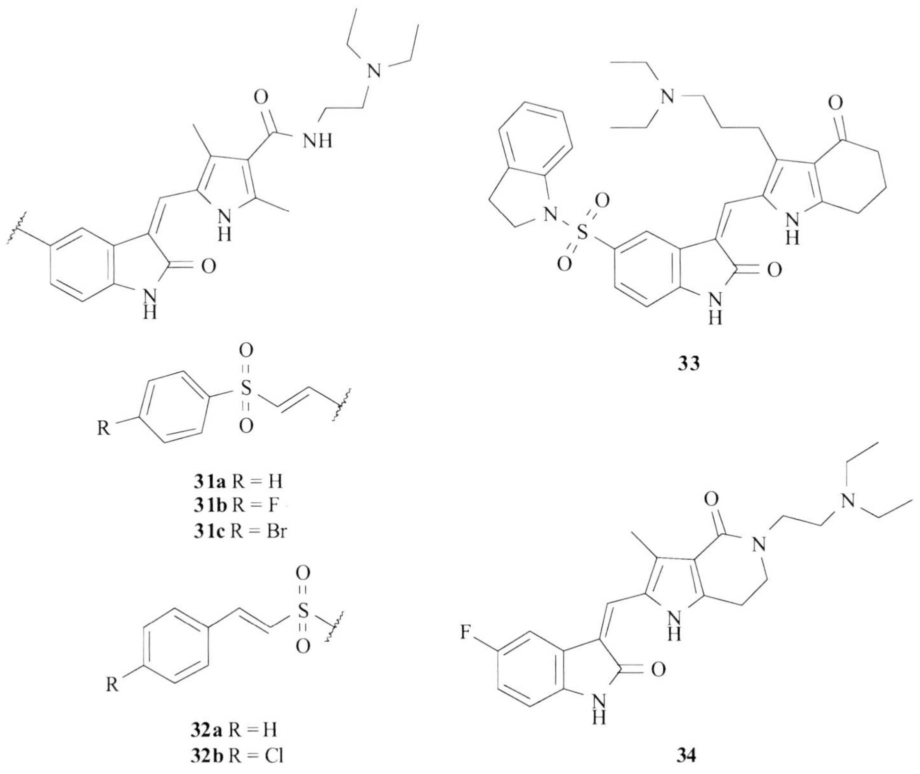

Fig. (12). Examples of 3-pyrroloarylidene isatins containing a sulfonyl functionality at C5 of isatin (**31** and **32**) and 3-pyrrolo-fused heterocyclic isatins (**33** and **34**).

Indolinones containing a dihydropyridine instead of a pyrrole ring such as **35** (Fig. **13**), have been found to be cytotoxic and exhibit 3-fold greater activity than sunitinib (**23**) against HCT-116 colon, A549 lung and HepG2 liver cells [115]. When **35** was modified to include a 4- or 7-azaindolinone core, the biological activity diminished and the analogues were less cytotoxic than sunitinib (**23**) in most of the cell lines evaluated.

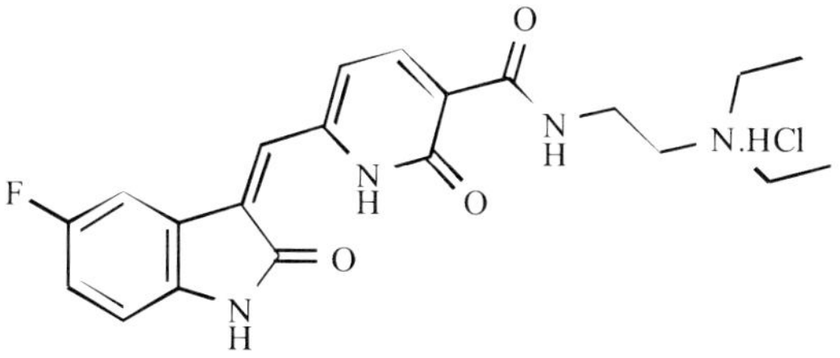

35

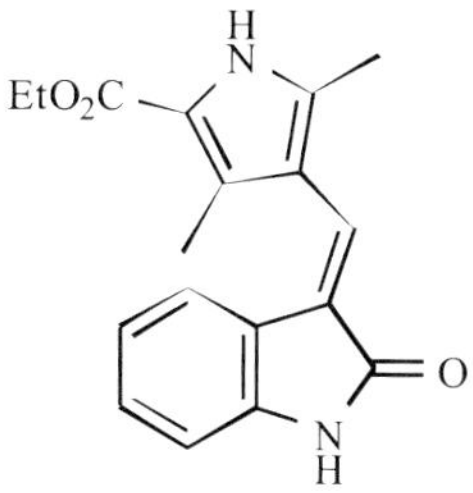

B5, **36**

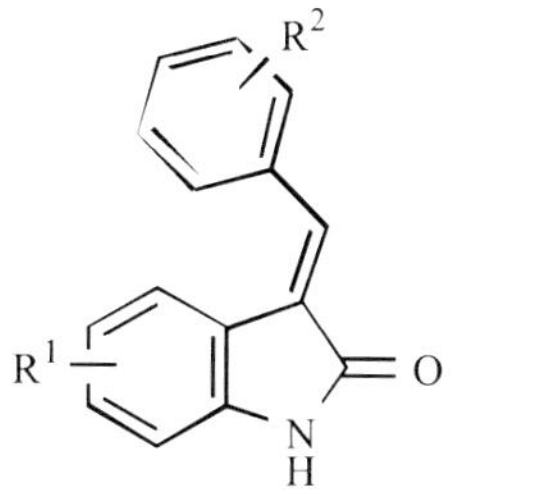

37a R^1 = 6-OCH_3, R^2 = 3-OCH_3
37b R^1 = H, R^2 = 2,5-$(OMe)_2$

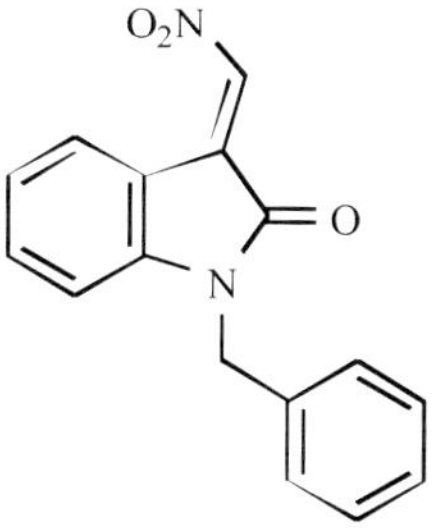

38

Fig. (13). An indolinone containing a dihydropyridine at the C3 position of isatin (**35**) and examples of (E)-3-arylidene indolinone derivatives (**36-38**).

B5 (**36**, Fig. **13**), a pyrrole-substituted indolinone possessing an *E*-isomeric configuration, has been identified as an extremely active cytotoxin against a panel of lung, breast and gastric cancer cell lines [116]. Other potent *E*-isomeric indolinones include the methoxy-substituted indolinones (**37a**) and (**37b**), which display IC_{50} values < 10 μM against MCF-7 and HCT-116 cells, together with selectivity over normal human diploid embryonic lung fibroblast (CCL-186) cells [117]. Moreover, (*E*)-3-substituted indolinones incorporating alkyl-nitromethylene units such as **38** have shown excellent inhibitory activity against P388 leukemia and A549 lung cancer cells [118].

The indolinones BIBF1000 (**39**) and BIBF1120 (**40**) induce apoptosis and both compounds have an IC_{50} value of 8 nM against the leukemic Kasumi-1 cell line, along with similar activity against the leukemic Mono-Mac-1 cell line [119]. BIBF1120 (**40**, Fig. **14**), inhibits VEGF, FGF and PDGF receptors, displays efficacy *in vivo* amongst multiple animal models and is currently in Phase III trials for the treatment of a variety of cancers [120].

RPI-1 (**41**, Fig. **14**), a 3-benzylidene-indolinone, has been shown to exhibit antiproliferative activity particularly towards a modified mouse embryonic fibroblast cell line NIH3T3 (NIH3T3^{MEN2A}) (IC_{50} 3.6 μM after 72 h) [121]. Derivatives containing a diphenyl urea functionality were introduced to the 5,6-dimethoxyindolinone core of RPI-1. This led to *N*-methyl-3-arylureidobenzylidene-indolin-2-one (**42**) being identified as the lead compound due to its increased activity against 3 modified NIH3T3 cell lines [121].

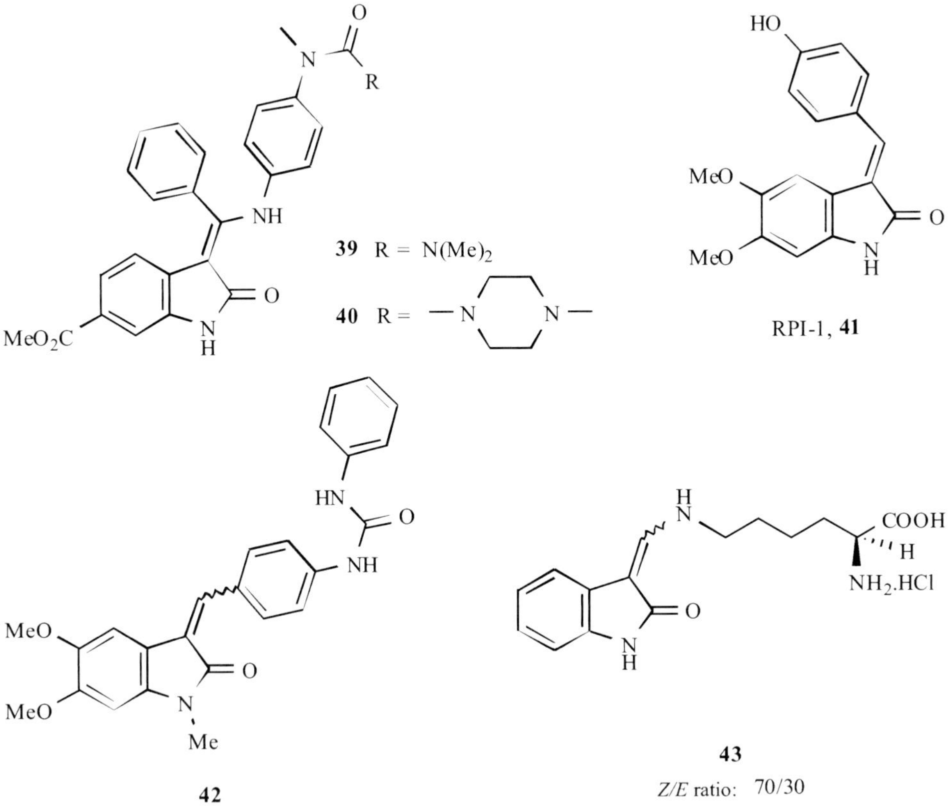

Fig. (14). Structures of the indolinones BIBF1000 (**39**), BIBF1120 (**40**), RPI-1 (**41**) and a potent derivative (**42**) as well as an example of an aminomethylene-lysine indolinone (**43**).

A C3-substituted aminomethylene-lysine indolinone (**43**, Fig. **14**) was found to exhibit cytotoxicity after 48 h towards human colon (DLD-1) and ovarian (PA-1) carcinoma cell lines (IC_{50} values ranged from 10-17 μM) [122]. Compounds containing more rigid side chains derived from D-phenylalanine and L-phenylglycine were found to be inactive.

2.4.2. Hydrazones and Imines

Isatin-based hydrazones (**44a-c**, Fig. **15**) have been identified as inhibitors of the protein tyrosine phosphatase Shp2, which plays an important role in cell signaling, cell proliferation, differentiation and migration [123]. Compounds containing a carboxylic acid group on the hydrazone aromatic ring and a *p*-halosulfonamide at the C5 position (*i.e.* **44a** and **44b**) selectively inhibit Shp2 in the low micromolar region. Analogue **44c** was the most active in the series, exhibiting an IC_{50} value of 0.8 μM against Shp2.

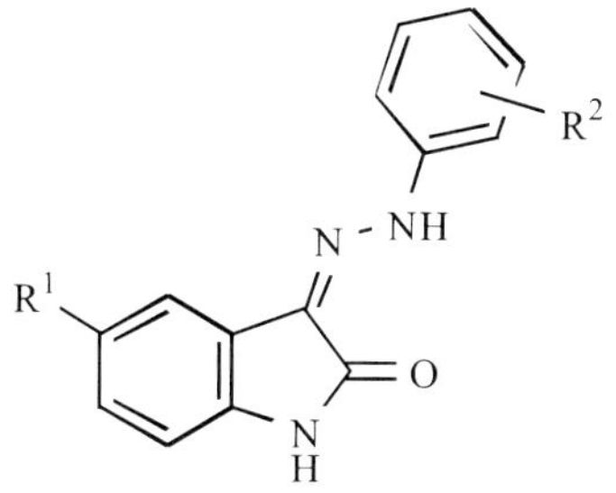

44

	R^1	R^2
44a	$SO_2NHCH_2(4\text{-}ClC_6H_4)$	$3\text{-}CO_2H$
44b	$SO_2NHCH_2(4\text{-}FC_6H_4)$	$3\text{-}CO_2H$
44c	CO_2H	$2\text{-}CO_2H$

Fig. (15). Isatin-based inhibitors of Shp2.

In recent years, Pervez and co-workers have reported the cytotoxic activity of isatin derivatives containing a thiosemicarbazone moiety (a hydrazone derivative containing a sulfur atom) [124-127]. Initially, 15 N^4-substituted isatin-3-thiosemicarbazones were screened for cytotoxicity against brine shrimp (*Artemia salina)* [124]. Only the 2-methylphenyl (**45a**), 2-methoxyphenyl (**45b**) and 3-nitrophenyl (**45c**) derivatives displayed significant cytotoxic activity (Fig. **16**). The most active analogue was **45b** with a LD_{50} value of 11 μM against *Artemia salina.* Subsequent studies assessed N^4-substituted isatin-3-thiosemicarbazones including one, two or three phenyl substituents [125]. Eleven of the 12 derivatives contained at least one fluorine atom although intriguingly, the most active compound was the trichloro-substituted analogue **45d** with a LD_{50} value of 11 μM against *Artemia salina.* Other novel N^4-substituted isatin-3-thiosemicarbazones have been synthesised and it was determined that the 3,5-dichloro-substituted derivative **45e** possessed a LD_{50} value of 17.5 μM in the brine shrimp assay [126]. Other chlorinated analogues with substituents at the 2,3-, 2,4- and 2,5- positions were far less potent, with LD_{50} values > 100 μM. To further expand the SAR of N^4-substituted isatin-3-thiosemicarbazones, the authors have also investigated the effects of an electron-withdrawing group (in this case, the trifluoromethoxy group) at the C5 position of isatin, together with mainly halogenated phenyl substituents on the thiosemicarbazone functionality [127]. Ten of the 21 compounds tested were considered to exhibit promising cytotoxicity with LD_{50} values between 11.1 and 180 μM. The 4-trifluoromethyl derivative **45f** was the most potent analogue (LD_{50} = 11.1 μM) in the series and was more active than the clinically used anticancer agent etoposide (LD_{50} = 12.7 μM) against *Artemia salina* [127].

Isatin thiosemicarbazones **45g** and **45h** (Fig. **16**) have been found to display cytotoxicity against the KB-3-1 cell line (a HeLa derivative) after a 72 h exposure (IC_{50} = 14.2 and 28.4 μM, respectively) [128]. More importantly, these compounds exhibit MDR1 selectivity (multidrug resistance that includes the P-glycoprotein (P-gp) family), which is calculated as a ratio between a compound's IC_{50} value against P-gp negative KB-3-1 cells divided by its IC_{50} value against P-gp positive KB-V1 cervical adenocarcinoma cells. A value of > 1 denotes that the compound kills P-gp-expressing cells more effectively than parental cells. Further research by this group has led to the discovery of thiosemicarbazones **45i** and **45j** which display similar cytotoxicity to **45g** and **45h** against KB-3-1 cells (IC_{50} values of 17.15 and 15.90 μM respectively), however, the MDR1 selectivity increased to 8.3 and 14.8 respectively [129].

3-Imino-substituted indolinones comprising amino acids have been assessed as kinase inhibitors and cytotoxins. Imino groups incorporating valine (**46a** and **46b**, Fig. **16**) and threonine (**47a** and **47b**) residues proved to be inactive against the CDK1/cyclin B, CDK5/p25 and GSK3α/β protein kinases [130]. Conversely, histidine imino groups (**48a** and **48b**) increased kinase activity and subsequent halogenation at C5 on the isatin nucleus yielded highly potent kinase inhibitors, with the lead compound, a 5-bromo derivative (**48b**), displaying an IC_{50} value of

0.37 μM against the CDK5/p25 kinase. Interestingly, none of the analogues synthesised displayed cytotoxicity towards human breast, lung or glioblastoma cell lines, although this may be attributed to the presence of the carboxylic acid functionality which may inhibit the entry of the compound into tumour cells.

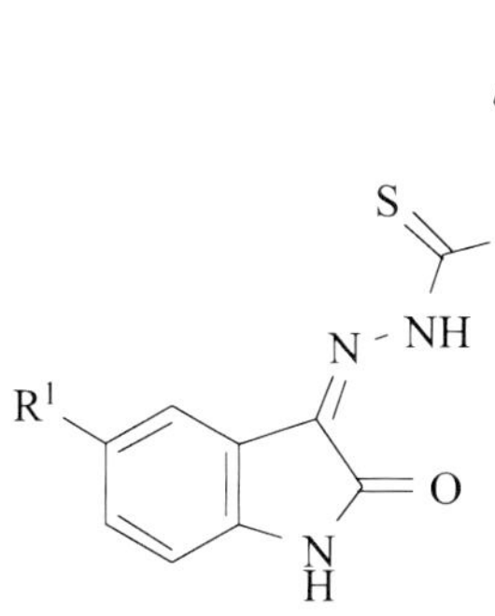

45

	R^1	R^2
45a	H	2-Me
45b	H	2-OMe
45c	H	3-NO_2
45d	H	2,4,6-Cl_3
45e	H	3,5-Cl_2
45f	OCF_3	4-F_3C
45g	H	4-OMe
45h	Br	4-NO_2
45i	H	4-NO_2
45j	H	4-*t*-Bu

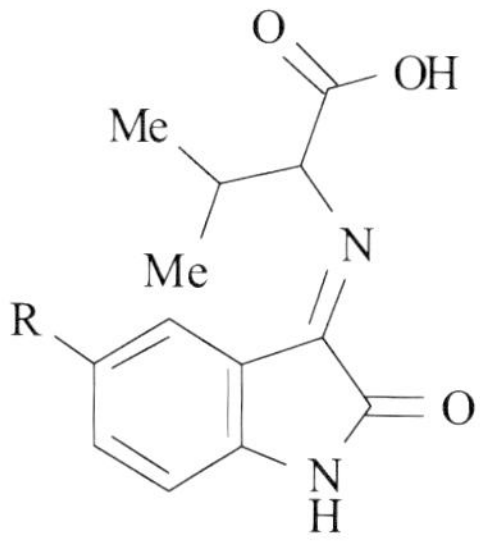

46a R = H
46b R = Br

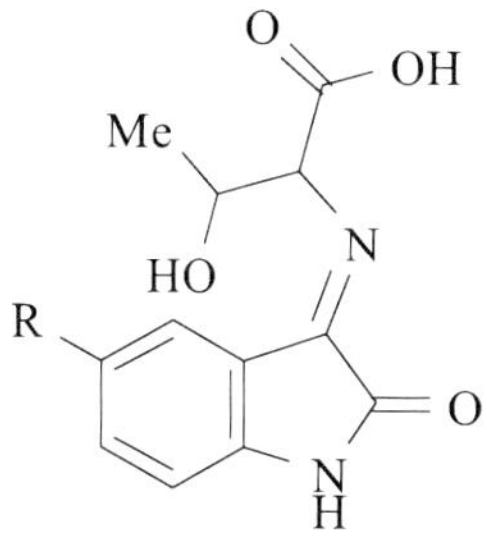

47a R = H
47b R = Br

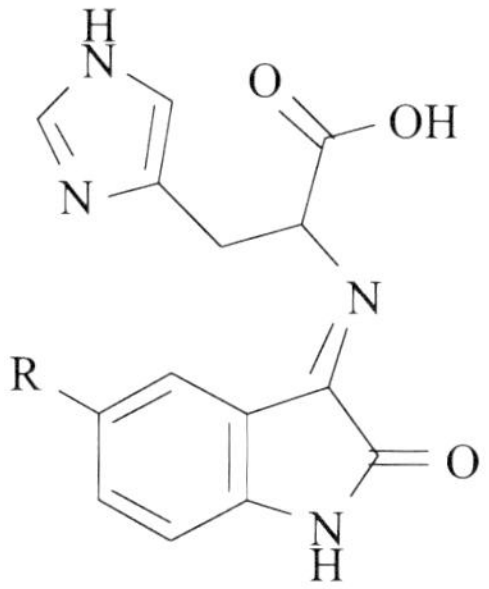

48a R = H
48b R = Br

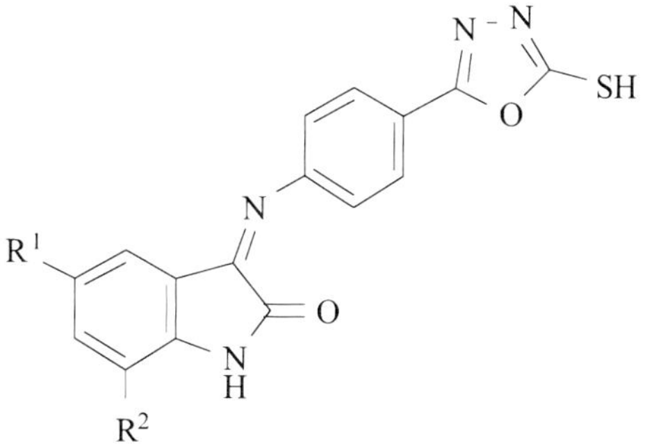

49a R^1 = F, Cl, Br; R^2 = H
49b R^1 = H; R^2 = NO_2, COOH

Fig. (16). Examples of cytotoxic isatin-3-thiosemicarbazones, iminoisatins incorporating the amino acids valine (**46**), threonine (**47**) and histidine (**48**), and examples of 3-iminoisatins monosubstituted on the isatin ring (**49**).

Gudipati *et al.* have also investigated twelve 3-iminoisatins monosubstituted at the C5 or C7 positions of the isatin ring system [131]. The compounds were tested for cytotoxic activity against HeLa, IMR-32 (neuroblastoma) and MCF-7 cells and all compounds exhibited IC_{50} values between 10.6-33.6 μM against the three cell lines, which were comparable to the IC_{50} values of cisplatin. Once again, halogen atoms at the C5 position yielded the most potent compounds (*e.g.* **49a**, Fig. **16**), while analogues bearing a C7 substituent were less active (*e.g.* **49b**).

Previously reported *N*-alkylated 3-iminoisatins [132] (**50a-e**, Fig. **17**) have been found to be extremely cytotoxic, with two derivatives (**50c** and **50e**) displaying nanomolar activity towards U937 lymphoma cells after a 24 h exposure [133]. Lysine derivatives of these 3-iminoisatins (**51a-e**) also exhibited potent cytotoxic effects, with all five analogues possessing nanomolar activity and being more cytotoxic than their corresponding imino derivatives (a 19-fold increase in the case of **50d** *vs* **51d**). Within the 3-iminoisatin series, the increase in chain length correlated with an increase in cytotoxicity (*i.e.* **50a** < **50c** and **50d** < **50e**), however, this trend was not observed within the isatin-lysine series (**51a-e**). Generally, *meta*-substituted compounds were more cytotoxic than their corresponding *para*-substituted analogues. The enhanced cytotoxicity of the isatin-lysine series (**51a-e**) when compared to the 3-iminoisatins (**50a-e**), suggests that increasing the alkyl chain length of 3-iminoisatins leads to a change in intracellular target.

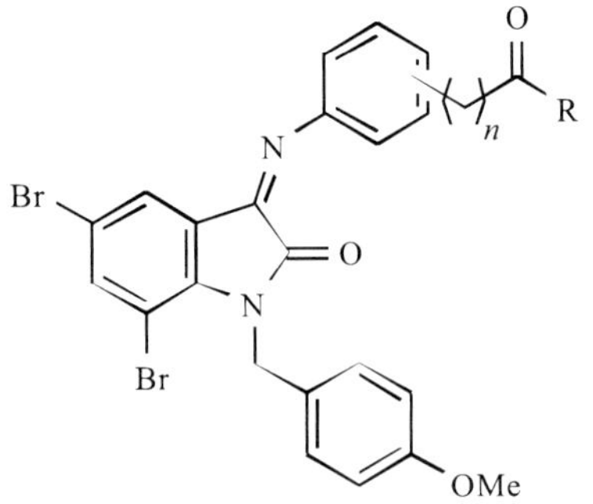

Imine	*n*	Substitution	IC_{50} (uM)
R = OH			
50a	0	*para-*	1.95 (± 0.69)
50b	1	*para-*	2.13 (± 0.51)
50c	2	*para-*	0.422 (± 0.09)
50d	0	*meta-*	3.14 (± 0.39)
50e	1	*meta-*	0.463 (± 0.08)
R = $(CH_2)_4CH(NHAc)CO_2Me$			
51a	0	*para-*	0.575 (± 0.37)
51b	1	*para-*	0.642 (± 0.03)
51c	2	*para-*	0.399 (± 0.11)
51d	0	*meta-*	0.165 (± 0.06)
51e	1	*meta-*	0.391 (± 0.13)

Fig. (17). Cytotoxic 5,7-dibrominated-*N*-alkylated 3-iminoisatins.

Furthermore, bis-Schiff bases of 5-fluoroisatin (**3d**) such as 3,3'-[oxybis(4,1-phenylenenitrilo)]bis(1,3-dihydro)-5-fluoro-2*H*-indol-2-one have been identified to be cytotoxic towards the human embryonic cell line (HEL) while a dichlorinated derivative, 3,3'-[methylenebis(2-chloro-3,5-diethyl-4,1-phenylenenitrilo)]bis(1,3-dihydro)-2*H*-indol-2-one, displayed cytotoxicity at 16 μg/mL against African green monkey kidney (Vero) and HeLa cell lines [134].

2.4.3. Metal Complexes

Isatin-diimine copper complexes, Cu(isapn) (**52**, Fig. **18**) and Cu(isaepy)$_2$ (**53**), have been evaluated against SH-SY5Y, M14 (melanoma) and U937 cell lines and were found to induce apoptosis through the mitochondrial pathway and/or copper-dependent oxidative stress [135]. Apoptosis of these copper complexes was also caspase-dependent, which appears to be the principal mechanism of cell death.

Bis-isatin thiocarbohydrazones have been coordinated to Cu(II), Ni(II), Co(II) and Zn(II) ions (**54a-d**, Fig. **18**) [136]. All of the compounds displayed cytotoxic activity after 24 h in the brine shrimp assay and produced 50% cell death at or below a concentration of 19.1 μg/mL against Ehrlich ascitic carcinoma (EAC) cells. *In vivo* studies involving female Swiss Albino mice inoculated with EAC cells revealed that the compounds reduced weight gain, prolonged the mean survival times and reversed the tumour-induced increase in white blood cell counts compared to the control [136].

Karki *et al.* synthesised the isatin thiosemicarbazone ligand, itsz, (**55**, Fig. **18**) and subsequently chelated it to ruthenium-1,10-phenathroline and 2,2'-bipyridine derivatives [137]. The compounds were tested *in vitro* against leukemic human (MOLT 4/C8 and CEM) and murine (L1210) cell lines. The ruthenium complexes displayed greater activity than their ligands and the 1,10-phenathroline derivative was the more active of the two with an IC_{50} value of 3.9 μM against the CEM cell line. These compounds were once again evaluated *in vivo* against EAC bearing mice and found to increase life span and mean survival time compared to the control.

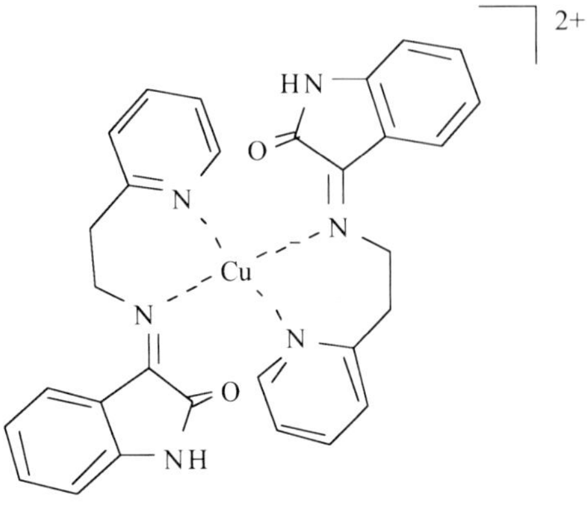

$[Cu(isapn)]^{2+}$, **52**

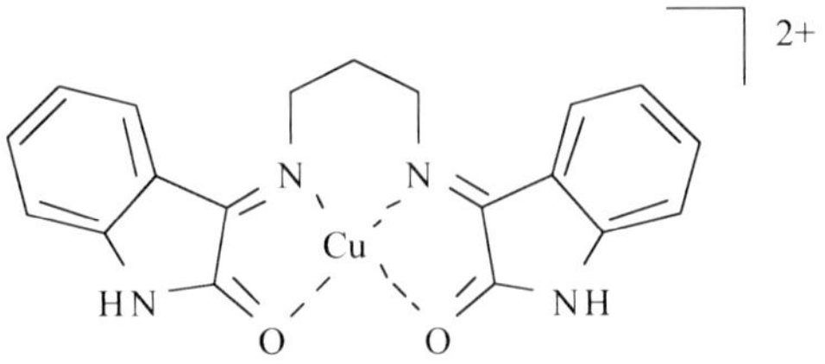

$[Cu(isaepy)_2]^{2+}$, **53**

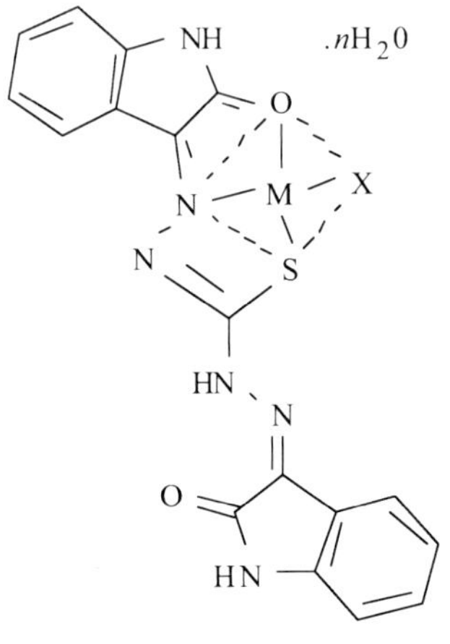

54a M = Cu(II) X = Cl, OAc n = 2
54b M = Ni(II) X = Cl, OAc n = 0

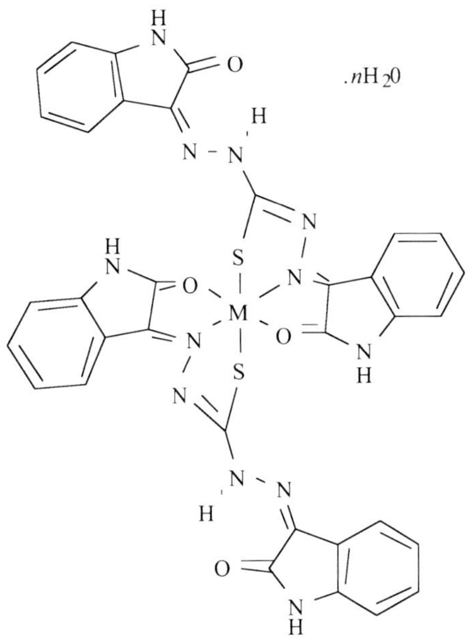

54 c M = Co(II) n = 0
54 b M = Zn(II) n = 2

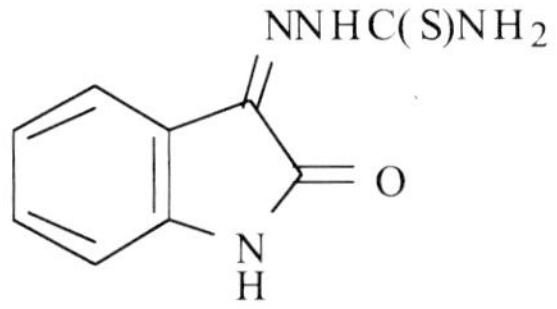

itsz, **55**

Fig. (18). The structures of some Isatin diimine complexes (**52**, **53**), bis-isatin thiocarbohydrazone metal complexes (**54a-d**) and an isatin thiosemicarbazone ligand (**55**).

Isatins containing sulfonamides through an imine or hydrazone linkage have been complexed with Co(II), Ni(II), Zn(II) and Cu(II) ions (**56a-d**, Fig. **19**) [138]. Evaluation of the complexes in the brine shrimp bioassay revealed one Ni(II) and

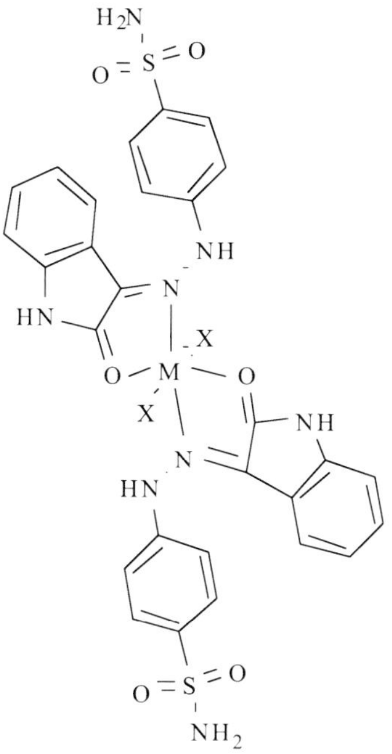

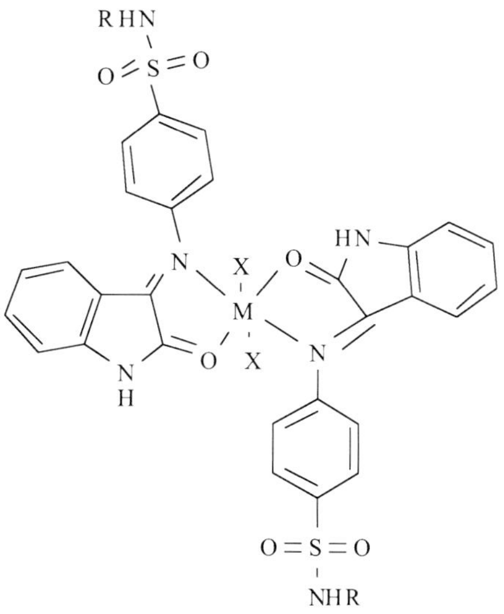

57a M = Co(II), X = Cl, R = L_1, L_2, L_3, L_4
57b M = Ni(II), X = Cl, R = L_1, L_2, L_3, L_4
57c M = Zn(II), X = Cl, R = L_1, L_2, L_3, L_4
57d M = Cu(II), R = L_1, L_2, L_3, L_4

56a M = Co(II), X = Cl
56b M = Ni(II), X = Cl
56c M = Zn(II), X = Cl
56d M = Cu(II)

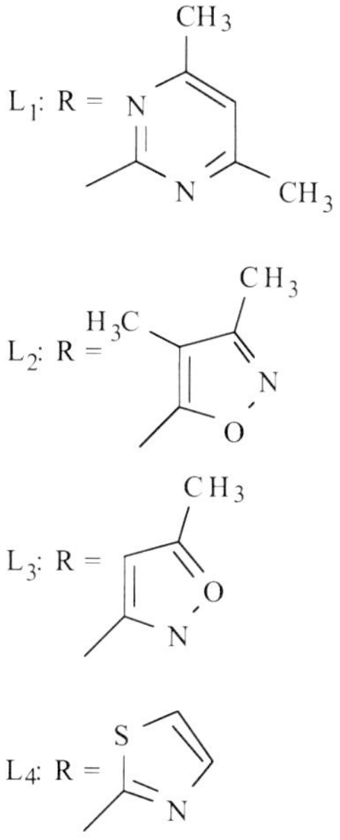

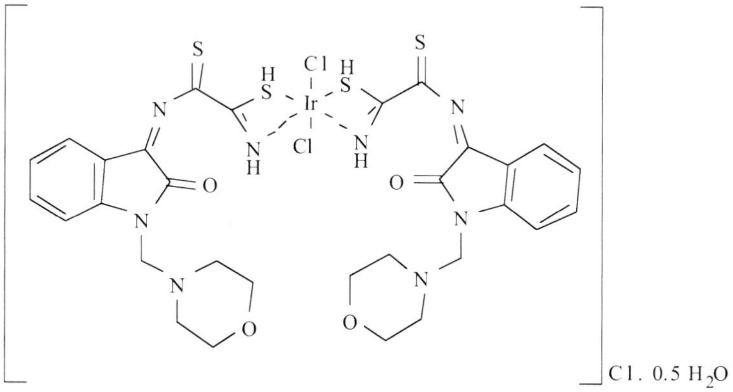

58

Fig. (19). Examples of isatin sulfonamide (**56** and **57**) metal complexes and an isatin-metal complex containing a Schiff base (**58**).

two Cu(II) complexes displayed potent cytotoxicity. The maximum activity observed was a LD_{50} value of 156 nM. The authors extended this work to include derivatised compounds of type **57** [139]. The four heterocyclic ligands were attached to each of the four metal complexes. Only the copper complexes (**57d**) displayed potent cytotoxicity against *Artemis salina* ($LD_{50} = 4.5 \times 10^{-4}$ - 6.4×10^{-4} μg/mL); the other metal complexes were deemed to be inactive.

Other new isatin-metal complexes include Schiff and Mannich base ligands coordinated to metal salts such as Co(II), Ni(II), Mn(II) and Ir(III) [140]. The complexes were evaluated against the Hep-2 larynx carcinoma cell line and the Ir(III) complex **58** (Fig. **19**) was found to be the most active complex, with cytotoxic activity increasing in a dose-dependent manner.

2.4.4. Isoindigo and Derivatives

Isoindigo (**59**, Fig. **20**) is the isomer of indirubin (**13**) containing two indolinone moieties. Glycosyl-isoindigo derivatives (**60**) have been prepared bearing benzyl or acetyl protecting groups on the sugar residue [141]. Protected analogues are speculated to enhance cellular penetration and therefore, display superior biological activity compared to the corresponding non-protected compounds. Acetylated glycosyl-isoindigo derivatives prepared by Sassatelli *et al.* displayed greater cytotoxicity against a panel of human solid tumour cell lines than the analogous benzylated compounds [141].

N-Methylisoindigo, more commonly known as meisoindigo (**61**), is approved for the treatment of CML [142] and induces apoptosis in the transformed human vein endothelial cell line, ECV304 [143]. Lee *et al.* have also investigated the potential of meisoindigo (**61**) against acute myeloid leukemia (AML) [144]. The compound is capable of inducing apoptosis in HL60 and other leukemic cells in a dose- and time-dependent manner. Further studies revealed **61** was also active in primary cells derived from eight AML patients and appears to exhibit moderate anti-AML activity in NOD/SCID mice.

Structural modifications to meisoindigo (**61**) have been prepared in an attempt to increase cytotoxicity. The *N*-substituent in **61** was replaced by arylalkyl substituents of varying chain lengths and alternative substituents being introduced to the phenyl ring of the phenethyl side chain [145]. *In vitro* results revealed the test compounds exhibited specificity for leukemic cells (HL60 and K562) rather than HCT-116 colon or HuH7 hepatoma cells. Additionally, the analogues displayed selectivity towards one leukemic cell line than the other after a 72 h exposure (K562: IC_{50} 1.4-8.5 μM; HL60: 3.8-16.6 μM). The introduction of a second *N*-methyl group to meisoindigo (**61**) significantly decreased cytotoxicity amongst all cell lines tested. It appears the presence of one lactam NH is imperative for activity as is an intact exocyclic double bond on the isoindigo core [145]. *N*-(Phenpropyl)-isoindigo (**62**) was determined to be the most cytotoxic compound of the series, with consistently greater potency than meisoindigo (**61**) amongst the four tumour cell lines.

Compounds integrating a 7'-azaisoindigo scaffold (**63**, Fig. **20**) have been recently synthesised [146, 147]. These compounds were discovered to exhibit micromolar IC_{50} values against the human buccal carcinoma cell line KB, and K562 and HL60 leukemic cell lines after 72 h, suggesting that the presence of an additional nitrogen atom to the isoindigo nucleus improves cytotoxicity. *N*-Alkylated analogues of 7'-azaisoindigo also display cytotoxic properties. Wang *et al.* reported that compounds possessing an isopropyl or butyl substituent at *N*1' (**64a-c**) were twice as cytotoxic (*i.e.* 8.3-9.1 μM) as meisoindigo (**61**) against DU-145 hormone-independent prostate carcinoma cells after a 24 h exposure [148]. The non-chlorinated analogue of **64a** has also exhibited micromolar activity against HeLa, A549, ECA-109 and HepG2 cell lines after a 48 h exposure [149].

2.4.5. Miscellaneous

Compounds incorporating a spirocycle at C3 on the isatin nucleus (also known as spiro-oxindoles) possess biological activities and the scaffold is common within the *Gelsemium* alkaloids such as 14-acetoxygelsenicine (**65**, Fig. **21**), which has an EC_{50} value of 0.25 μM against the A431 human epidermoid carcinoma after a 48 h exposure [150]. Spiro-oxindoles integrating silyl functionalities have been synthesised recently [151]. Two of these compounds, one including a tricyclic isatin core (**66**) and the other a *N*-benzylisatin analogue (**67**), were evaluated against A549 and HepG2 cell lines. Both compounds displayed comparable cytotoxicity towards the A549 cells after 24 h (EC_{50} = 42.8 μM and 42.6 μM respectively). However, when assessed against the HepG2 cell line, **67** exhibited twice the activity of the compound **66** (EC_{50} = 16.8 μM and 32.5 μM, respectively).

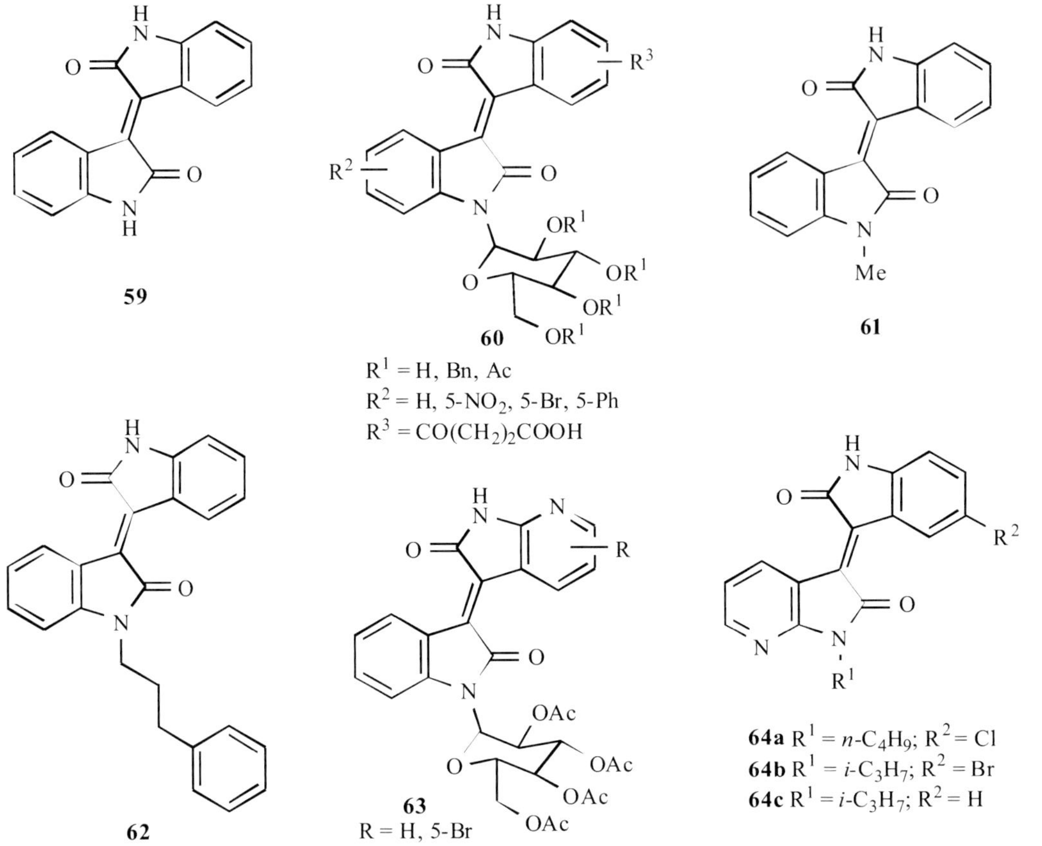

Fig. (20). Cytotoxic isoindigo and 7'-azaisoindigo derivatives.

Kaminskyy *et al.* have screened a variety of oxindoles incorporating a spiro-thiazolidinone moiety against 60 cancer cell lines from the NCI [152]. Derivatives **68a** and **68b** were identified as the most potent and displayed LC_{50} values < 4 μM against a range of cancer cell types in the panel.

Another class of oxindoles which have been evaluated for their anti-proliferative activity are the 3,3-diaryloxindoles which include oxyphenisatin (**69**, Fig. **21**). Uddin *et al.* demonstrated that the compound and its derivatives were potent antiproliferatives, particularly against the MDA-MB-468 cell line [153] (IC_{50} value of oxyphenisatin (**69**) is 112 nM). The two hydroxyl groups on **69** are essential for activity and cytotoxicity can be increased (to less than 10 nM) by replacing small and lipophilic substituents in the 6- and/or 7-position of the isatin moiety. The lead analogue was the 6,7-difluorooxyphenisatin which displayed an IC_{50} of 3 nM against MDA-MB-468 cells [153].

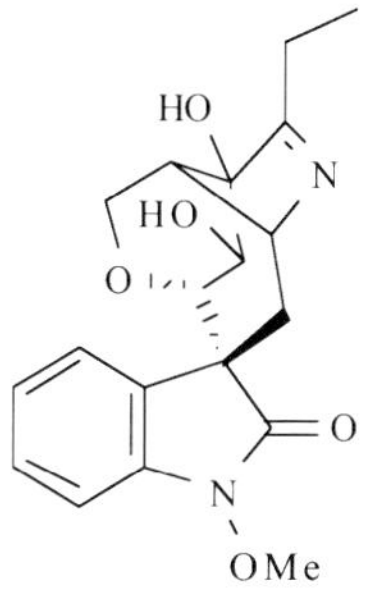

65

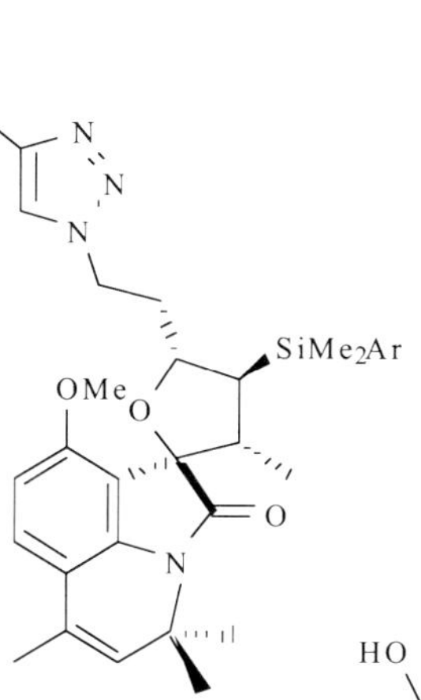

66

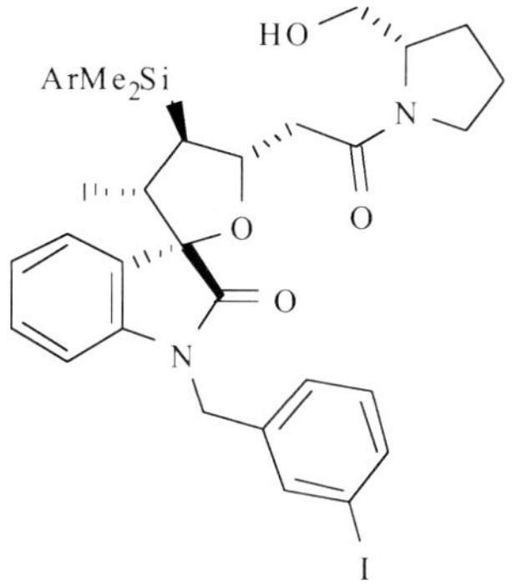

67

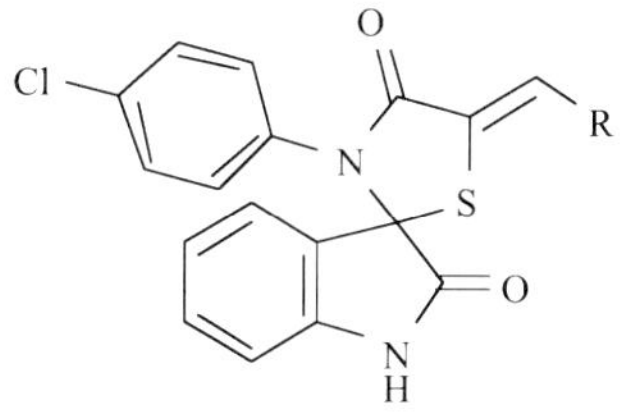

68a R = Ph
68b R = 4-*i*-Pr-Ph

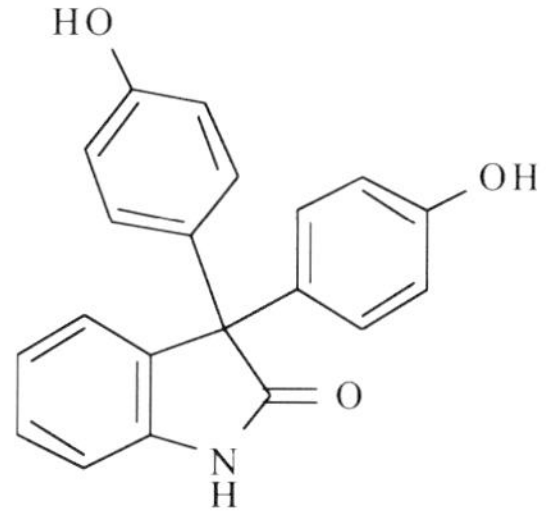

69

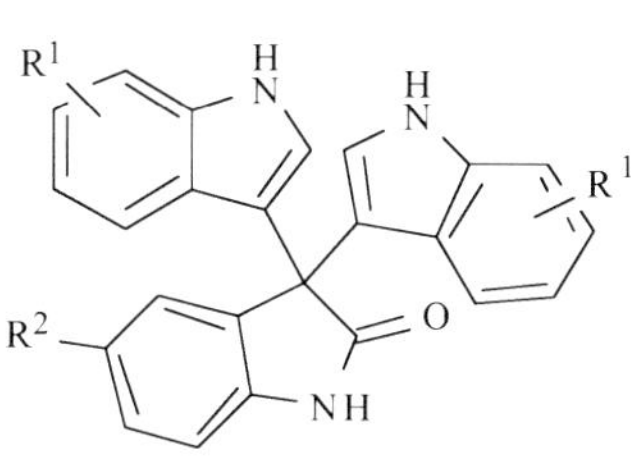

70a R^1 = 5-OCH$_3$, R^2 = H
70b R^1 = 6-OCH$_3$, R^2 = H
70c R^1 = 5-Br, R^2 = H
70d R^1 = 5-OCH$_3$, R^2 = F

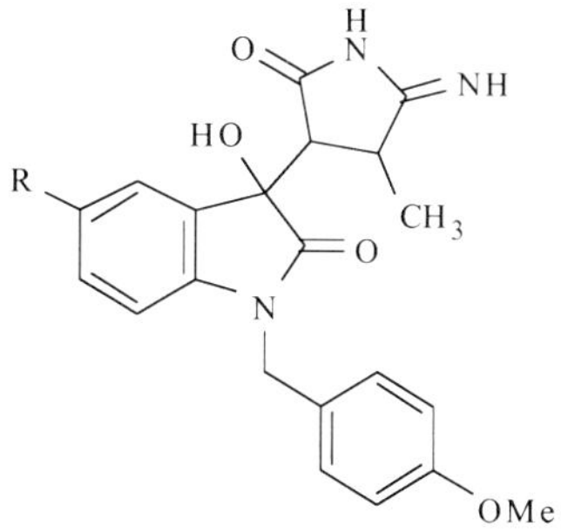

71a R = H
71b R = Cl

Fig. (21). Examples of biologically active spiro-oxindoles and 3,3-disubstituted oxindoles.

An extension of the 3,3-diaryloxindoles are the 3,3-diindolyloxindoles. This class of compounds (*e.g.* **70a-d**, Fig. **21**) were examined for cytotoxicity against five human cancer cell lines by Kamal *et al.* [154]. The 3,3-diindolyloxindoles were most susceptible towards DU-145 prostate cancer cells, with **70a-d** exhibiting IC_{50} values of < 5 μM after a 48 h exposure. Generally, introduction of methoxy groups onto the indole ring systems led to increased potency towards all cell lines, while a fluoro substituent at the 5-position on the oxindole core resulted in decreased potency, particularly against HepG2 liver cancer cells. Analogues containing nitro substituents on the indole ring systems displayed IC_{50} values of ~ 8 μM against DU-145 cells but were inactive against MCF-7 breast cancer cells. More recently, Subba Reddy *et al.* condensed isatin and 5-chloroisatin with 2- and/or 5-substituted indoles to prepare a new series of 3,3-diindolyloxindoles which exhibited sub-micromolar cytotoxicity against A549 lung cancer and SK-N-SH neuroblastoma cells, but were completely inactive against the MRC5 normal human lung cell line [155].

A series of *N*-alkylisatins containing a hydroxy substituent and a functionalised imidazole at the C3 position on isatin were evaluated for their cytotoxicity against 57 NCI cell lines [156]. Compounds **71a** and **71b** (Fig. **21**) exhibited growth inhibitory properties against 89% and 93% of all cancer cell lines in the panel respectively, with GI_{50} values in the range of 2-60 μM for **71a** and 0.19-30 μM for **71b**. Both compounds were capable of inhibiting the growth of the five leukemic cell lines in the panel with GI_{50} values in the range of 2-5 μM.

2.5. Isatin-Based Conjugates

The synthetic versatility of isatin has led to its further use in drug conjugate strategies whereby isatin or its analogues are chemically coupled to other bioactive and/or target specific molecules to improve drug efficacy and versatility of action. Two key approaches have been taken and are discussed further in sections 2.5.1 and 2.5.2.

2.5.1. Dual Action/Hybrid Agents

The hybridisation of two or more bioactive drug fragments with complementary functions or different mechanisms of action into a single molecule is a novel approach that often results in synergistic activity and enhanced drug efficacy. Solomon *et al.* was the first to report this dual action/hybrid pharmacophore strategy using isatin (**1**) by linking benzothiazole to isatin through its C3 carbonyl by Schiff formation [157] to yield compounds of type **72** (Fig. **22**). It was postulated that the combined anticancer activities of the isatin Mannich base derivatives and benzothiazole would yield highly potent targeted dual drugs for the treatment of breast cancer. Among the 30 isatin-benzothiazole derivatives screened, 4-chloro-1-dimethylaminomethyl-3-(6-methyl-benzothiazol-2-ylimino)-1,3-dihydroindol-2-one emerged as the most active against a panel of human breast cancer cell lines, with GI_{50} values in the range of 10.92 - 28.09 μM. Addition of the benzothiazole moiety increased activity by up to a factor of 12 over that of the unsubstituted isatin Mannich base.

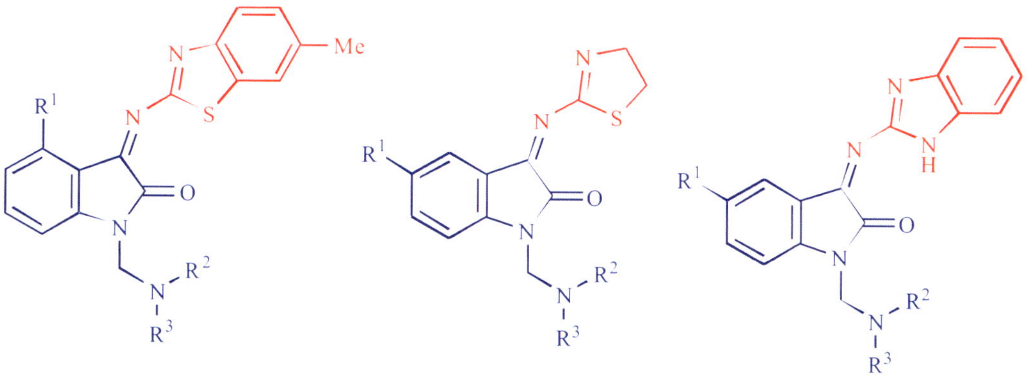

72
R^1 = H, Cl, Br
R^2R^3 = methyl, ethyl, phenyl, piperidinyl, morpholinyl

73
R^1 = H, Br
R^2R^3 = phenyl, piperazinyl, piperidinyl, morpholinyl

74
R^1 = H, Br
R^2R^3 = phenyl, piperazinyl, piperidinyl, morpholinyl

Fig. (22). Examples of isatin-benzothiazole (**72**), isatin-thiazoline (**73**) and isatin-benzimidazole (**74**) hybridised dual action derivatives.

Taher *et al.* further contributed to this work in the search for new anti-breast cancer agents through the synthesis of novel isatin-thiazoline and isatin-benzimedazole derivatives (compounds of type **73** and **74**, Fig. **22**) *via* condensation of isatin Mannich bases with either 2-aminothiazoline or 2-aminobenzimidazole, respectively [158]. Benzimidazole-based compounds have been reported to demonstrate cytotoxic activity against hormone-dependant breast cancer cells such as MCF-7 [159], while thiazoline derivatives possess both cytotoxic and cytostatic activity against a broad spectrum of cancer cell lines [160]. Of the 16 hybrid compounds prepared, 11 were screened for cytotoxic activity against a human breast adenocarcinoma cell line and all were found to be active in the nanomolar range. The most lethal compound, 3-(1*H*-benzimidazol-2-ylimino)-1-{[*N*,*N*-diphenyl-amino-1-yl]-methyl}indol-2(3*H*)-one, derived from the benzimidazole series **74**, showed potent activity with an IC_{50} of 22.59 nM against MCF-7 breast cancer cells [158].

Diazoles, such as pyrazoles and pyrazolines are small molecules that have also been found to exhibit remarkable anticancer activities and have been identified as inhibitors of CDKs [161], VEGF [162] and P-gp [163]. These observations led Lesyk and colleagues to synthesise new isatin-pyrazoline hybrids (**75a-d**, Fig. **23**) with the aim of discovering new active and selective compounds that elicit synergistic anticancer activity [164]. The further conjugation of isatin-pyrazoline hybrids with 4-thiazolidinones to from isatin-based hybrids with three distinct bioactive drug components (**76a-d**) builds on the work of Taher *et al.*, above. The synthesised hybrids were tested for anticancer activity in the NCI's 60 cell line screen and found the isatin-pyrazoline derivative 5-bromo-1-{2-[5-(4-chlorophenyl)-3-(4-methoxyphenyl)-4,5-dihydropyrazol-1-yl]-2-oxothyl}-1*H*-indole-2,3-dione (**75d**) to demonstrate the highest activity, particularly towards a leukemia subpanel with GI_{50} values in the range of 0.69 - 3.35 μM. SAR studies revealed that hybridisation of isatin with the pyrazoline ring system (**75a-d**) leads to enhanced anticancer activity and introduction of a bromine atom at the 5-position of the isatin fragment further enhances potency. However, condensation of the active isatin-pyrazoline hybrids with 4-thiazolidinones (**76a-d**) results in complete loss of activity [164].

Spiro thiazolidinone-isatin derivatives (**77a-f**, Fig. **23**) have also been explored and were found to exhibit modest activity *in vitro* (GI_{50} values in the range of 4.13 - 6.55 μM) against the NCI's full panel of 60 human cancer cell lines [165]. Despite the rationale behind this hybrid pharmacophore approach, all of the compounds described above were found to display novel modes of action and did not retain the mechanism of the individual fragments alone, as determined by the NCI's COMPARE Analysis Program [166, 167].

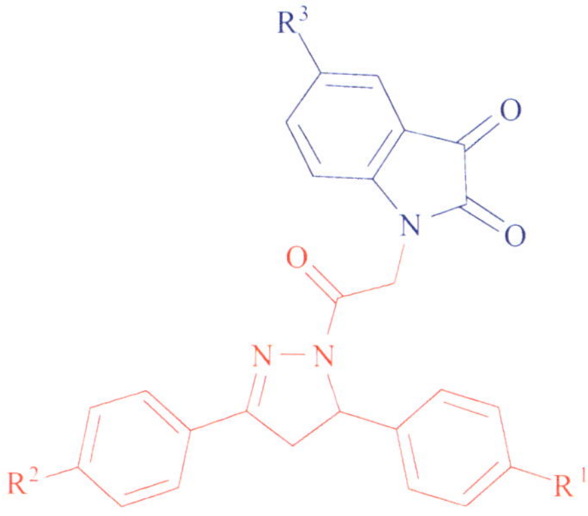

75

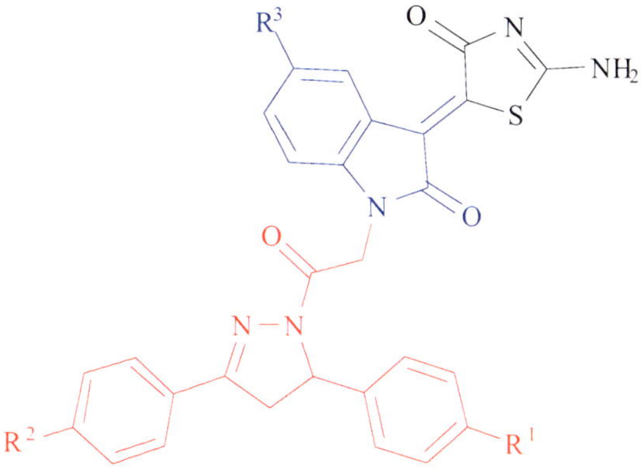

76

75/76a R^1 = OMe, R^2 = R^3 = H
75/76b R^1 = Cl, R^2 = R^3 = H
75/76c R^1 = Cl, R^2 = OMe, R^3 = H
75/76d R^1 = Cl, R^2 = OMe, R^3 = Br

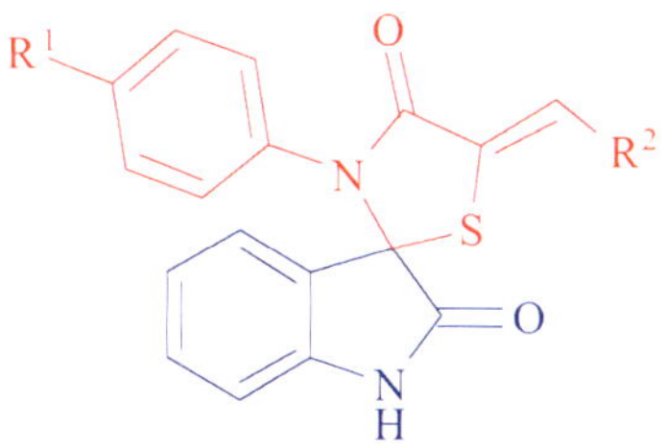

77

77a R^1 = Cl, R^2 = Ph
77b R^1 = Cl, R^2 = 4-*i*-Pr-Ph
77c R^1 = OH, R^2 = 4-(Me_2N)-Ph
77d R^1 = OH, R^2 = Ph-CH=CH-
77e R^1 = OH, R^2 = 3-MeO-4-$HOOCCH_2$-Ph
77f R^1 = OH, R^2 = 4-Br-Ph

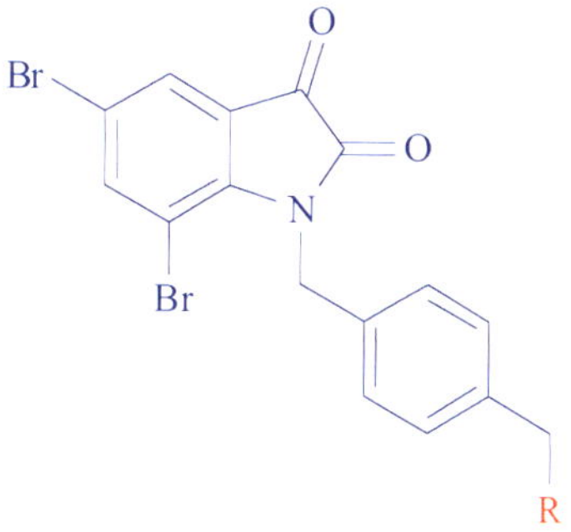

78 R = SCN
79 R = NCS

Fig. (23). Examples of pyrazoline-isatin hybridised dual action derivatives (**75** and **76**), spiro-thiazolidinone-isatin hybridised derivatives (**77**) and cytotoxic 5,7-dibromo-*N*-alkylisatins containing cyano-based substituents (**78** and **79**).

Conversely, hybridisation of thiocyanate, isothiocyanate or selenocyanate moieties (potent inhibitors of the PI3K/Akt pathway) to 5,7-dibromoisatin (**3h**) afforded 12 novel 5,7-dibromo-*N*-alkylisatin derivatives that concomitantly inhibit tubulin polymerisation and phosphorylation of Akt [168]. *In vitro* biological evaluation and SAR studies against a panel of human cancer cell lines found three of the isatin-selenocyanate analogues (containing a selenocyanate group in the alkyl chain) to be most active against the MCF-7 breast cancer cell line (IC_{50} 1.45 - 1.65 μM), while the isatin-thiocyanate and isatin-isothiocyanate derivatives (containing a thiocyanate or isothiocyanate group in the alkyl chain) were most active against the HT-29 colon (IC_{50} 1.09 - 3.24 μM), A549 lung (IC_{50} 2.13 - 5.53 μM) and UACC903 melanoma (IC_{50} 2.06 - 4.37 μM) cell lines. The two most active compounds, 5,7-dibromo-*N*-(*p*-thiocyanomethylbenzyl)isatin (**78**) and 5,7-dibromo-*N*-(*p*-isothiocyanatomethylbenzyl)isatin (**79**, Fig. **23**) emerged as promising dual inhibitors of microtubule assembly and Akt and are being further evaluated *in vivo* as antitumour agents for the treatment of colon cancer.

2.5.2. Selectively Deliverable Conjugates

Chemical conjugation of a potent cytotoxin to a tumour targeting moiety such as a protein, peptide or aptamer to increase the therapeutic index of the drug is another relatively new strategy used to confer high tumour selectivity and reduced toxicity to cytotoxic drugs. Vine *et al.* was the first to publish this approach using isatin whereby two potent *N*-alkylisatin-based microtubule destabilisers were coupled to the delivery agents, plasminogen activator inhibitor type-2 (PAI-2) or transferrin (Tf) [169, 170], to achieve site-specific drug delivery. Tf is an iron ferrying glycoprotein that has commonly been exploited to deliver potent chemotherapeutics to the intracellular space of cancer cells *via* the Tf receptor (TfR/CD71) [171], while PAI-2 is an irreversible, specific inhibitor of the proven metastatic marker urokinase plasminogen activator (uPA) [172]. Both ligands, upon interaction with appropriate cell surface receptors, are specifically endocytosed by the low density lipoprotein receptor family [171, 173] and can thus selectively deliver attached toxins to the intracellular space of targeted cells [174]. Exposure of the conjugate to high concentrations of lytic enzymes or the acidic conditions of the endosome or lysosome results in the selective release the cytotoxin and localised cell death (Fig. **24**).

In one report, 5,7-dibromo-*N*-(*p*-hydroxymethylbenzyl)isatin (**80**) was functionalised for attachment to Tf and PAI-2 *via* an esterase-labile succinate

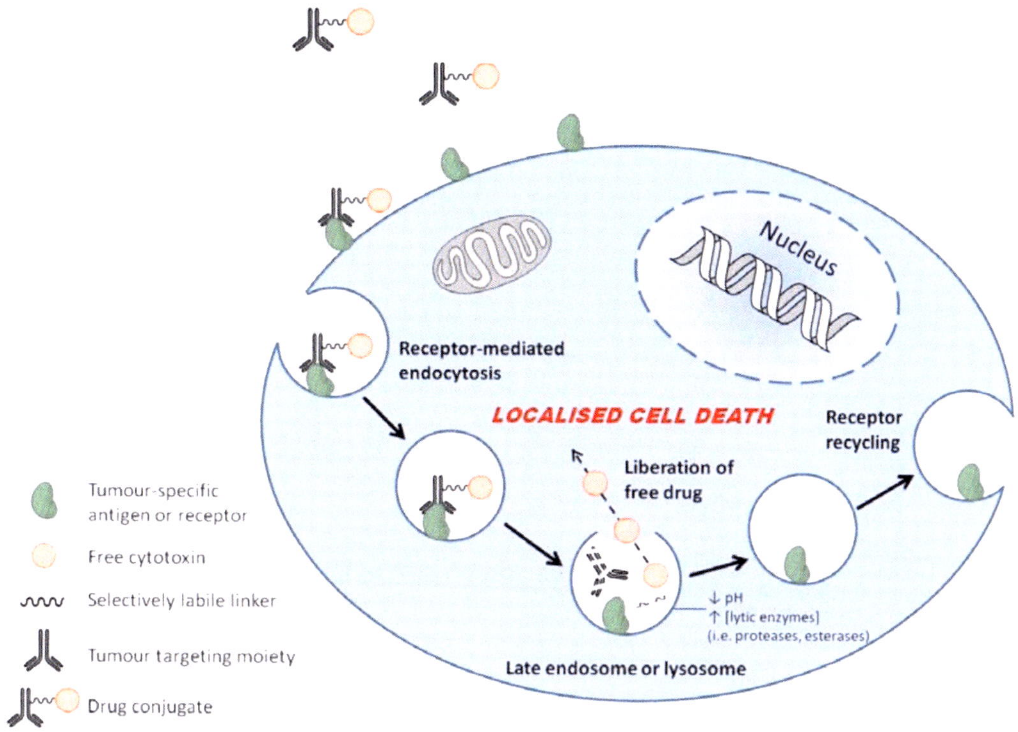

Fig. (24). Schematic representation of selectively deliverable drug conjugates. The drug conjugate is internalised by receptor-mediated endocytosis and then cleaved in the acidic environments of the late endosomes or lysosomes to release the free cytotoxin into the cytosol and cause cell death.

linker to form Tf- and PAI-2-*N*-alkylisatin conjugates (Tf-*N*-AIE and PAI-2-*N*-AIE, respectively) (**83**, Fig. **25**) [170]. Conjugation of the *N*-hydroxysuccinimide-derived active ester (**82**) to the targeting ligands Tf and PAI-2 was achieved by forming stable amide bonds between the ε-amino group of available surface lysine residues on the protein and the carboxylic acid group of the succinate linker on the functionalised *N*-alkylisatin (**81**). Tf-*N*-AIE was up to 24 times more active than the free drug (**80**) (IC_{50} 0.38 μM *vs* IC_{50} 9.01 μM) against the high TfR expressing MCF-7 breast cancer cell line and showed clear cytotoxicity patterns based on TfR levels. On the other hand, PAI-2-*N*-AIE showed equivalent activity compared to the parent drug (IC_{50} 1.02 μM *vs* IC_{50} 1.38 μM) against the high uPA/uPAR expressing MDA-MB-231 breast cancer cell line and strong selectivity patterns for uPA levels. Both Tf- and PAI-2-*N*-AIE conjugates exhibited impressive tumour growth delay in a metastatic, orthotopic human breast tumour xenograft mouse model and were efficacious at 1/20th and 1/10th of the dose of the free drug respectively, with no observable signs of toxicity [170].

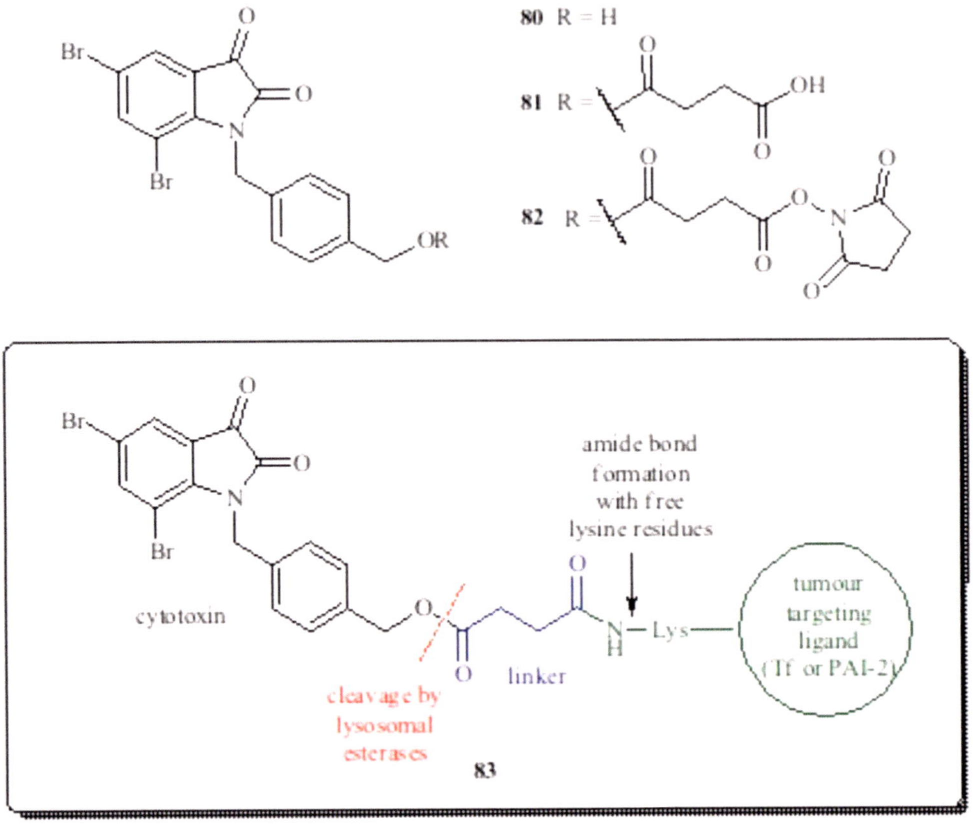

Fig. (25). The structures of Tf- and PAI-2-*N*-alkylisatin conjugates (**83**) and their precursor molecules (**80-82**).

In another report, 5,7-dibromo-*N*-(*p*-methoxybenzyl)isatin (**7k**) was conjugated to Tf *via* an acid-labile imine-functionalised (*para*-phenylpropionic acid) linker to form a novel *N*-alkylisatin-imine-Tf (NAI-imine-Tf) conjugate (**84**, Fig. **26**) [169]. The bifunctional linker was selected on the basis of hydrolytic studies led by Matesic *et al.* on a series of isatin-based imino acid derivatives [132]. The derivatives were functionalised at the C3 carbonyl group of 5,7-dibromo-*N*-(*p*-methoxybenzyl)isatin (**7f**) and were stable at physiological pH but readily cleaved at pH 4.5. Observed rates of hydrolysis for the embedded imine-acid moiety were in the order *para*-

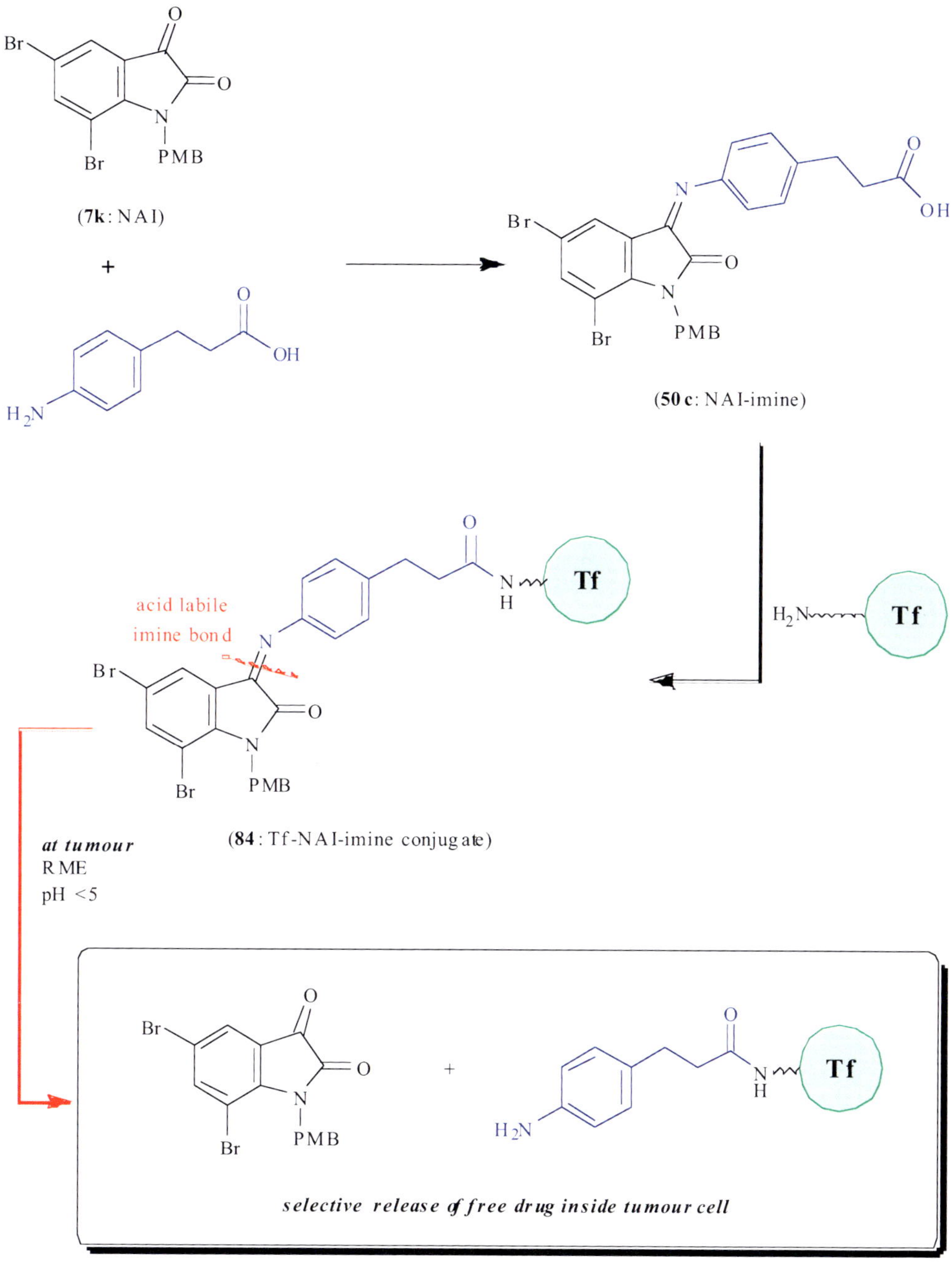

Fig. (26). *N*-Alkylisatin **7k** bound to the lysine residues of transferrin (Tf) *via* an acid-labile, imine linker (**84**). Upon receptor mediated endocytosis of the conjugate (**84**) at the target tumour, the free cytotoxin (**7k**) is selectively released inside the tumour cell along with modified protein.

phenylpropionic acid > phenylacetic acid (*para* > *meta*) > benzoic acid (*meta* > *para*). The half-life of the *para*-phenylpropionic acid derivative under acidic conditions was 17 min. The NAI-imine-Tf conjugate (**84**) was equipotent to the free drug (**7k**) against MCF-7 breast cancer cells (IC_{50} 2.00 μM *vs* IC_{50} 1.67 μM) and demonstrated clear receptor-dependent cytotoxicity [169].

2.6. Isatins in Combination Therapy

Combination chemotherapy is now the standard of care for the adjuvant (post-surgery) treatment of most solid and haematological cancers. The rationale behind this approach is two-fold: i) to minimise the dosage of each individual drug and therefore reduce non-specific toxicity and ii) through limited drug exposure, reduce the emergence of multi-drug resistance (MDR). Recently, the effect of combined administration of isatin (**1**) and the omega-3 fatty acid eicosapentaenoic acid (EPA), on a human breast cancer cell line was described [175]. In this study, EPA was found to significantly increase the cytotoxicity of isatin towards MDA-MB-231 cells *in vitro via* modulation of lipid peroxidation. Omega-3 fatty acids have previously been shown to increase the efficacy of various cancer chemotherapy drugs such as doxorubicin [176, 177], tamoxifen [178], and mitomycin C [179], as well as radiation therapy [180].

More recently, Vine *et al.* has demonstrated additivity and synergy with combinations of *N*-alkylisatin-based microtubule destabilisers and the commercial anticancer agents vinblastine, paclitaxel, 5-FU and colchicine. When combined at a molar ratio of 1:1 and concomitantly administered to either a MDR human uterine sarcoma cell line (MES-SA/Dx5) or a human histiocytic lymphoma cell line (U937), combinations were found to exhibit a significant increase in cytotoxicity over and above that of the individual drugs alone (Table **1**).

3. CONCLUSIONS

Isatin is the core nucleus of an array of cytotoxic and antineoplastic compounds. A SAR summary for the isatin derivatives discussed in this review is shown in Fig. (**27**). Derivatisation at X to form the mono- di- and tri-aryl ring substituted isatin series (see section 2.1) are generally found to induce cancer cell death *via* apoptosis in the mid-low micromolar range and necrosis in the high micromolar range. This is proposed to be linked to a reduction in ERK activity. Small electron-withdrawing groups at positions 5, 6 and/or 7 enhance, but are not essential for anti-tubulin or anti-kinase activity when found as part of a larger substituted compound (*i.e.* substitution at X with concomitant substitution at W, Y and Z). This is most likely due to increased cell permeability and hydrophobicity.

Table 1. Cytotoxicity (IC_{50}) of Single-Agent *vs* Combination Treatments in the Human U937 and MES-SA/Dx5 Cancer Cell Lines

Individual Drugs and Drug Combinations	*IC_{50} (μM)**	
	MES-SA/Dx5†	*U937*§
5,7-dibromo-N-(p-methoxybenzyl)isatin (**7k**)	*4.8*	-
5,7-dibromo-N-(p-trifluoromethylbenzyl)isatin (**7e**)	-	*1.24*
Vinblastine	*5.5*	*5*
Colchicine	*>10*	-
Paclitaxel	-	*>5*
5-fluorouracil (5-FU)	-	*>5*
(**7k**) + Vinblastine	*1.9*	-
(**7k**) + Colchicine	*2.9*	-
(**7e**) + Vinblastine	-	*0.42*
(**7e**) + Paclitaxel	-	*1.02*
(**7e**) + 5-FU	-	*0.98*

*IC_{50} values were calculated from sigmoidal dose response curves (variable slope), generated using GraphPad Prism V.5 software. Briefly, cells were incubated for 24 h in the presence of increasing concentrations of single agent or combinations (1:1) of drug and cell viability determined using the CellTiter 96 Aqueous One Cell Proliferation (MTS) Assay. Values are the means of triplicate determinations.
† MES-SA/Dx5 = MDR human uterine sarcoma.
§ U937 = human monocyte-like histiocytic lymphoma.
(-) = Not tested.

N-Alkylation at Y however, with no further substitution at W or Z, often results in cytotoxic compounds with sub-micromolar activity; inducing morphological change, G2/M cell cycle arrest and ultimately cell death *via* apoptosis (see section 2.2). The compounds discussed in this review appear to be tubulin specific and do not inhibit serine/threonine or tyrosine kinases [31]. A 1-3 carbon chain linker extending to an aromatic ring is optimal for potent microtubule disruption and small electron-withdrawing substituents on the ring in the *para* or *meta* position are favoured over the ortho position. Most importantly, and together with its specificity, this series of novel molecules are >10 times more active than the conventional cancer chemotherapeutics; 5-FU, vinblastine and paclitaxel on human monocytic lymphoma cells. In addition to the possibility that these compounds may bind to a novel site on tubulin, it suggests that the development of anticancer agents based on the *N*-alkylisatin scaffold may be beneficial in combination with clinically used anticancer agents for the treatment of MDR tumours in the future. Further development and preclinical assessment of this particular series of isatins is therefore warranted.

Substitution at W has by far resulted in the generation of the most structurally and biochemically diverse isatin-based compounds to date (see section 2.4). Yet despite over 1500 cytotoxic C3 substituted compounds reported in the literature, only one has made it to market as an anticancer drug. This is primarily due to their non-specific toxicity, as these molecules often target the ATP binding site of multiple kinases, therefore affecting a magnitude of cellular targets. For example, substitution at W on the 3'- and 4'-positions of the pyrrole ring of some arylidene derivatives, are regarded as favourable for CDK2 inhibition, while substituents in the 5'-position are beneficial for VEGFR-2 and PDGFR-β inhibition. 3-Substituted indolinones possessing the *Z* configuration are potent FGFR inhibitors, while compounds adopting the *E* configuration inhibit EGFR.

Finally, dimerisation at Z often results in ATP-competitive inhibition of CDK1, CDK2 and GSK3, as well as reduction in the activation and expression of, c-Src kinase and NF-κB (the most renowned modulators being the indirubins, see section 2.3). Although the early indirubin derivatives were plagued by poor water solubility, the addition of basic diamine side chains and the incorporation of a quaternary centre into the 3'-position markedly improved their water solubility, while retaining potency towards CDK2. Such small modifications have led to large advances in the development of this class of molecules as potential new anticancer agents. In general, the C2-substituted class of isatins is active in the micro to nanomolar range and extend from kinase inhibitors to potent anticancer antibiotics.

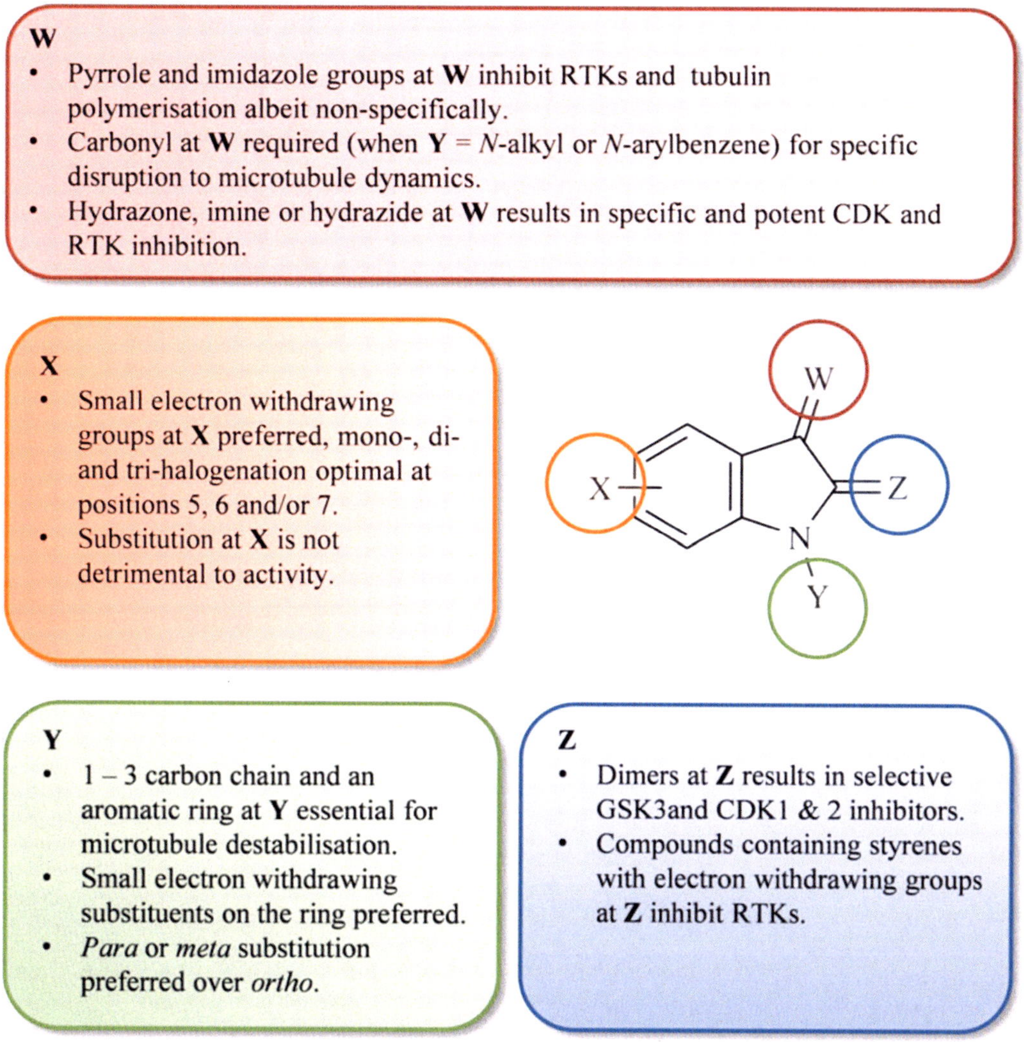

Fig. (27). A summary of the cytotoxic structure-activity relationship of isatin derivatives.

In summary, isatin has already proven to be an excellent scaffold for both the natural and synthetic construction of molecules with interesting biological activities. With the possibility of derivatising the N1, C2 and C3 positions, along with substitution on the aromatic ring, the synthetic permutations for isatin are almost endless. Despite the fact that isatins are well studied compounds, new derivatives are continually being discovered and known isatin-based compounds have been explored in combination therapy approaches, fused with other bioactive drug fragments and subsequently investigated as hybrid/dual action drugs and selectively targeted to cancer cells *via* conjugation to tumour targeting moieties. Isatin has proven to be a privileged scaffold in medicinal chemistry that warrants further exploration for the purpose of discovering new and exciting molecules with anticancer activity.

ABBREVIATIONS[1]

A549	=	Human non-small cell lung adenocarcinoma
AML	=	Acute mylogenous leukemia
CDK	=	Cyclin dependent kinase
CML	=	Chronic mylogenous leukemia
Colo-205	=	Human colon adenocarcinoma
DU-145	=	Hormone-independent prostate carcinoma
EAC	=	Ehrlich ascitic carcinoma
EC_{50}	=	Half maximal effective concentration
ECA-109	=	Human oesophageal carcinoma
EGF/R	=	Epidermal growth factor/receptor
EPA	=	Eicosapentaenoic acid
ERK	=	Extracellular signal-related protein kinase
GI_{50}	=	Concentration required to inhibit the growth a cellular population by 50%
GSK3	=	Glycogen synthase kinase 3
HCT-116	=	Human colon carcinoma
HeLa	=	Human cervical carcinoma
HepG2	=	Human liver hepatocellular carcinoma
HL60	=	Human promyleocytic leukemic cell line
HT-29	=	Human colon adenocarcinoma

[1]Only abbreviations that appear more than twice in the text are listed here.

IC_{50}	=	Concentration required for 50% inhibition of a biological or biochemical process *in vitro*
K562	=	Human myelogenous leukemia
KB-3-1	=	Human cervical carcinoma
LD_{50}	=	Median lethal dose
MCF-7	=	Human non-metastatic mammary gland adenocarcinoma
MDA-MB-231/468	=	Human metastatic/non-metastatic mammary gland adenocarcinoma
MDR	=	Multidrug resistance
NCI	=	National Cancer Institute
PAI-2	=	Plasminogen activator inhibitor type-2
PC-3	=	Human prostate adenocarcinoma
PDGF/R	=	Platelet-derived growth/receptor
P-gp	=	P-glycoprotein
RTK	=	Receptor tyrosine kinase
SAR	=	Structure activity relationship
SH-SY5Y	=	Human neuroblastoma
Tf/R	=	Transferrin/receptor
U937	=	Human monocyte-like histiocytic lymphoma
UCH-L1	=	Ubiquitin *C*-terminal hydrolase
uPA/R	=	Urokinase plasminogen activator/receptor
VEGF/R	=	Vascular endothelial growth factor/receptor

CONFLICT OF INTEREST

The authors declare that there is no conflict of interest.

ACKNOWLEDGEMENTS

We are grateful to the University of Wollongong for support through the Centre for Medical Bioscience, Centre for Medicinal Chemistry and a Vice Chancellor's

Postdoctoral Fellowship awarded to Dr. K. Vine. We also thank the Illawarra Cancer Carers Inc., Kiama, Minnamurra, and Gerringong Sunrise Rotary, the Robert East Memorial Fund, Prof. P. Clingan, and other private donors for funding assistance.

DISCLOSURE

This e-Book chapter is an updated version of the review article entitled "Cytotoxic and Anticancer Activities of Isatin and Its Derivatives: A Comprehensive Review from 2000-2008" published in *Anti-Cancer Agents in Medicinal Chemistry*, **2009**, *9*(4), 397-414.

REFERENCES

[1] Erdmann, O. L. Untersuchungen über den Indigo. *J. Prakt. Chem.* **1840**, *19*, 321-362.

[2] Laurent, A. Recherches sur l'indigo. *Ann. Chim. Phys.* **1840**, *3*, 393-434.

[3] Guo, Y.; Chen, F. *Zhongcaoyao* **1986**, *17*, 104.

[4] Bergman, J.; Lindström, J. O.; Tilstam, U. The structure and properties of some indolic constituents in *Couroupita guianensis* aubl. *Tetrahedron* **1985**, *41*, 2879-2881.

[5] Wei, L.; Wang, Q.; Liu, X. Application of thin-layer chromatography in quality control of Chinese medicinal preparations. II. Qualitative analysis of some Chinese medicinal preparations of Chansu. *Yaowu Fenxi Zazhi* **1982**, *2*, CA 98:95726b

[6] Kapadia, G. J.; Basak, S. P.; Shukla, Y. N.; Fales, H. M.; Sokoloski, E. A. Potential carcinogens.10. Melosatins, novel isatin alkaloids from *Melochia-tomentosa* roots. *Lloydia-the Journal of Natural Products* **1976**, *39*, 471.

[7] Kapadia, G. J.; Shukla, Y. N.; Basak, S. P.; Sokoloski, E. A.; Fales, H. M. Potential carcinogens.13. The melosatins - a novel class of alkaloids from *Melochia-tomentosa*. *Tetrahedron* **1980**, *36*, 2441-2447.

[8] Ansaasamoah, R.; Kapadia, G. J.; Lloyd, H. A.; Sokoloski, E. A. Picratidine, a new indole alkaloid from *Picralima nitida* seeds. *J. Nat. Prod.* **1990**, *53*, 975-977.

[9] Grafe, U.; Radics, L. Isolation and structure elucidation of 6-(3'-methyl-buten-2'-yl)isatin, an unusual metabolite from *Streptomyces-Albus*. *J. Antibiot.* **1986**, *39*, 162-163.

[10] Phelan, V. V.; Liu, W.-T.; Pogliano, K.; Dorrestein, P. C. Microbial metabolic exchange-the chemotype-to-phenotype link. *Nat. Chem. Biol.* **2012**, *8*, 26-35.

[11] Schunck, E. Notes on the purple of the ancients. 1. The chromogen of Purpura capillus. 2. Properties of the colouring matter formed by insolation from the chromogen of *Purpura capillus*. *J. Chem. Soc.* **1879**, *35*, 589-596.

[12] Letellier, A. Recherches sur la pourpre produite par le Purpura lapillus. *Arch. Zool. Exp. Gen., 2nde ser.* **1890**, *8*, 361-403.

[13] Baker, J. T.; Sutherland, M. D. Pigments of marine animals. VIII. Precursors of 6,6'-dibromoindigotin (tyrian purple) from the mollusc *Dicathais orbita* gmelin. *Tetrahedron Lett.* **1968**, *9*, 43-46.

[14] Benkendorff, K.; Bremner, J. B.; Davis, A. R. Indole derivatives from the egg masses of Muricid molluscs. *Molecules* **2001**, *6*, 70-78.

[15] Westley, C. B.; Vine, K. L.; Benkendorff, K. In: *Indirubin, the Red of Indigo*; L. Meijer; N. Guyard; L. A. Skaltsounis; G. Eisenbrand, (Eds.), Life in Progress Editions, Roscoff, France, **2006**; pp. 31-44.

[16] Hamaue, N.; Yamazaki, N.; Minami, M.; Endo, T.; Hirafuji, M.; Monma, Y.; Togashi, H.; Saito, H.; Parvez, S. H. Effect of isatin, an endogenous MAO inhibitor, on acetylcholine and dopamine levels in the rat striatum. *Biog. Amines* **1999**, *15*, 367-377.

[17] Gillam, E. M. J.; Notley, L. M.; Cai, H. L.; De Voss, J. J.; Guengerich, F. P. Oxidation of indole by cytochrome P450 enzymes. *Biochemistry* **2000**, *39*, 13817-13824.

[18] Pandeya, S. N.; Smitha, S.; Jyoti, M.; Sridhar, S. K. Biological activities of isatin and its derivatives. *Acta. Pharm.* **2005**, *55*, 27-46.

[19] Medvedev, A.; Igosheva, N.; Crumeyrolle-Arias, M.; Glover, V. Isatin: role in stress and anxiety. *Stress* **2005**, *8*, 175 -183.

[20] Medvedev, A.; Buneeva, O.; Glover, V. Biological targets for isatin and its analogues: implications for therapy. *Biol. Targets Ther.* **2007**, *1*, 151-162.

[21] Silva, J. F. M. d.; Garden, S. J.; Pinto, A. C. The chemistry of isatins: a review from 1975 to 1999. *J. Braz. Chem. Soc.* **2001**, *12*, 273-324.

[22] Sumpter, W. C. The chemistry of isatin. *Chem. Rev.* **1944**, *34*, 393-434.

[23] Popp, F. D.; Katritzky, A. R.; Boulton, A. J. *The Chemistry of Isatin*, in, Advances in Heterocyclic Chemistry, Academic Press, **1975**, pp. 1-58.

[24] Mesropyan, E. G.; Avetisyan, A. A. New isatin derivatives. *Russ. J. Org. Chem.* **2009**, *45*, 1583-1593.

[25] Ivashchenko, A. V.; Dziomko, V. M. Reactions of isatin and its derivatives with aromatic and heterocyclic ortho-diamines. *Uspekhi Khimii* **1977**, *46*, 228-238.

[26] Shvekhgeimer, M. G. A. Synthesis of heterocyclic compounds by the cyclization of isatin and its derivatives (review). *Chem. Heterocycl. Compd. (Engl. Transl.)* **1996**, *32*, 249.

[27] Joshi, K. C.; Joshi, R. Isatin: a versatile molecule for the synthesis of novel spiroheterocycles. *J. Indian Chem. Soc.* **1999**, *76*, 643-649.

[28] Chen, G.; Hao, X. Recent studies on the bioactivities of isatin. *Tianran Chanwu Yanjiu Yu Kaifa* **2010**, *22*, 356-360.

[29] Abele, E.; Abele, R.; Dzenitis, O.; Lukevics, E. Indole and isatin oximes: synthesis, reactions, and biological activity. *Chem. Heterocycl. Compd.* **2003**, *39*, 3-35.

[30] Karpenko, A.; Shibinskaya, M.; Zholobak, N.; Olevinskaya, Z.; Lyakhov, S.; Litvinova, L.; Spivak, M.; Andronati, S. Synthesis, DNA-binding, and interferon-inducing properties of isatin and benzoisatin hydrazones. *Pharm. Chem. J.* **2006**, *40*, 595-602.

[31] Vine, K. L.; Matesic, L.; Locke, J. M.; Ranson, M.; Skropeta, D. Cytotoxic and anticancer activities of isatin and its derivatives: a comprehensive review from 2000-2008. *Anti-Cancer Agents Med. Chem.* **2009**, *9*, 397-414.

[32] Pal, M.; Sharma, N. K.; Priyanka; Jha, K. K. Synthetic and biological multiplicity of isatin. *J. Adv. Sci. Res.* **2011**, *2*, 35-44.

[33] Bhrigu, B.; Pathak, D.; Siddiqui, N.; Alam, M. S.; Ahsan, W. Search for biological active Isatins: a short review. *Int. J. Pharm. Sci. Drug Res.* **2010**, *2*, 229-235.

[34] Tarek, A.-F.; Bin-Jubair, F. A. S. Anti-tubercular activity of isatin derivatives. *Int. J. Res. Pharm. Sci.* **2010**, *1*, 113-126.

[35] Harris, P. A. *Oxindole Inhibitors of Cyclin-Dependent Kinases as Anti-Tumor Agents*, Taylor and Francis Group, Boca Raton FL, USA, **2007**.

[36] Cerchiaro, G.; Ferreira, A. M. d. C. Oxindoles and copper complexes with oxindole-derivatives as potential pharmacological agents. *J. Braz. Chem. Soc.* **2006**, *17*, 1473-1485.

[37] Motzer, R. J.; Michaelson, M. D.; Redman, B. G.; Hudes, G. R.; Wilding, G.; Figlin, R. A.; Ginsberg, M. S.; Kim, S. T.; Baum, C. M.; DePrimo, S. E.; Li, J. Z.; Bello, C. L.; Theuer, C. P.; George, D. J.; Rini, B. I. Activity of SU11248, a multitargeted inhibitor of vascular endothelial growth factor receptor and platelet-derived growth factor receptor, in patients with metastatic renal cell carcinoma. *J. Clin. Oncol.* **2006**, *24*, 16-24.

[38] Prenen, H.; Cools, J.; Mentens, N.; Folens, C.; Sciot, R.; Schoffski, P.; Van Oosterom, A.; Marynen, P.; Debiec-Rychter, M. Efficacy of the kinase inhibitor SU11248 against gastrointestinal stromal tumor mutants refractory to imatinib mesylate. *Clin. Cancer. Res.* **2006**, *12*, 2622-2627.

[39] Vine, K. L.; Locke, J. M.; Ranson, M.; Benkendorff, K.; Pyne, S. G.; Bremner, J. B. *In vitro* cytotoxicity evaluation of some substituted isatin derivatives. *Bioorg. Med. Chem.* **2007**, *15*, 931-938.

[40] Hossain, M. M.; Islam, N.; Khan, R.; Islam, R. Cytotoxicity study of dimethylisatin and its heterocyclic derivatives. *Bangladesh J. Pharmacol.* **2007**, *2*, 66-70.

[41] Cane, A.; Tournaire, M. C.; Barritault, D.; Crumeyrolle-Arias, M. The endogenous oxindoles 5-hydroxyoxindole and isatin are antiproliferative and proapoptotic. *Biochem. Biophys. Res. Commun.* **2000**, *276*, 379-384.

[42] Igosheva, N.; Lorz, C.; O'Conner, E.; Glover, V.; Mehmet, H. Isatin, an endogenous monoamine oxidase inhibitor, triggers a dose- and time-dependent switch from apoptosis to necrosis in human neuroblastoma cells. *Neurochem. Int.* **2005**, *47*, 216-224.

[43] Nguyen, J. T.; Wells, J. A. Direct activation of the apoptosis machinery as a mechanism to target cancer cells. *Proc. Natl. Acad. Sci. U. S. A.* **2003**, *100*, 7533-7538.

[44] Liu, Y.; Lashuel, H. A.; Choi, S.; Xing, X.; Case, A.; Ni, J.; Yeh, L. A.; Cuny, G. D.; Stein, R. L.; Lansbury, P. T., Jr. Discovery of inhibitors that elucidate the role of UCH-L1 activity in the H1299 lung cancer cell line. *Chem. Biol.* **2003**, *10*, 837-846.

[45] Bacher, G.; Nickel, B.; Emig, P.; Vanhoefer, U.; Seeber, S.; Shandra, A.; Klenner, T.; Beckers, T. D-24851, a novel synthetic microtubule inhibitor, exerts curative antitumoral activity *in vivo*, shows efficacy toward multidrug-resistant tumor cells, and lacks neurotoxicity. *Cancer Res.* **2001**, *61*, 392-399.

[46] Sasaki, H.; Yukiue, H.; Moriyama, S.; Kobayashi, Y.; Nakashima, Y.; Kaji, M.; Fukai, I.; Kiriyama, M.; Yamakawa, Y.; Fujii, Y. Expression of the protein gene product 9.5, PGP9.5, is correlated with T-status in non-small cell lung cancer. *Jpn. J. Clin. Oncol.* **2001**, *31*, 532-535.

[47] Bittencourt Rosas, S. L.; Caballero, O. L.; Dong, S. M.; da Costa Carvalho Mda, G.; Sidransky, D.; Jen, J. Methylation status in the promoter region of the human PGP9.5 gene in cancer and normal tissues. *Cancer Lett.* **2001**, *170*, 73-79.

[48] Yamazaki, T.; Hibi, K.; Takase, T.; Tezel, E.; Nakayama, H.; Kasai, Y.; Ito, K.; Akiyama, S.; Nagasaka, T.; Nakao, A. PGP9.5 as a marker for invasive colorectal cancer. *Clin. Cancer Res.* **2002**, *8*, 192-195.

[49] Vine, K. L.; Locke, J. M.; Ranson, M.; Pyne, S. G.; Bremner, J. B. An investigation into the cytotoxicity and mode of action of some novel *N*-alkyl-substituted isatins. *J. Med. Chem.* **2007**, *50*, 5109-5117.

[50] Matesic, L.; Locke, J. M.; Bremner, J. B.; Pyne, S. G.; Skropeta, D.; Ranson, M.; Vine, K. L. N-phenethyl and N-naphthylmethyl isatins and analogues as *in vitro* cytotoxic agents. *Bioorg. Med. Chem.* **2008**, *16*, 3118-3124.

[51] Modi, N. R.; Shah, R. J.; Patel, M. J.; Suthar, M.; Chauhan, B. F.; Patel, L. J. Design, synthesis, and QSAR study of novel 2-(2,3-dioxo-2,3-dihydro-1H-indol-1-yl)-N-phenylacetamide derivatives as cytotoxic agents. *Med.l Chem. Res.* **2011**, *20*, 615-625.

[52] Singh, P.; Kaur, S.; Kumar, V.; Bedi, P. M.; Mahajan, M. P.; Sehar, I.; Pal, H. C.; Saxena, A. K. Synthesis and *in vitro* cytotoxic evaluation of N-alkylbromo and N-alkylphthalimido-isatins. *Bioorg. Med. Chem. Lett.* **2011**, *21*, 3017-3020.

[53] Solomon, V. R.; Hu, C. K.; Lee, H. Hybrid pharmacophore design and synthesis of isatin-benzothiazole analogs for their anti-breast cancer activity. *Bioorg. Med.l Chem.* **2009**, *17*, 7585-7592.

[54] Sabet, R.; Mohammadpour, M.; Sadeghi, A.; Fassihi, A. QSAR study of isatin analogues as *in vitro* anti-cancer agents. *Eur. J. Med. Chem.* **2010**, *45*, 1113-1118.

[55] Brancale, A.; Silvestri, R. Indole, a core nucleus for potent inhibitors of tubulin polymerization. *Med. Res. Rev.* **2007**, *27*, 209-238.

[56] Li, P. K.; Xiao, Z.; Hu, Z.; Pandit, B.; Sun, Y.; Sackett, D. L.; Werbovetz, K.; Lewis, A.; Johnsamuel, J. Conformationally restricted analogs of Combretastatin A-4 derived from SU5416. *Bioorg. Med. Chem. Lett.* **2005**, *15*, 5382-5835.

[57] Chen, Z.; Merta, P. J.; Lin, N. H.; Tahir, S. K.; Kovar, P.; Sham, H. L.; Zhang, H. A-432411, a novel indolinone compound that disrupts spindle pole formation and inhibits human cancer cell growth. *Mol. Cancer Ther.* **2005**, *4*, 562-568.

[58] Romagnoli, R.; Baraldi, P. G.; Cruz-Lopez, O.; Preti, D.; Bermejo, J.; Estevez, F. alpha-Bromoacrylamido N-Substituted Isatin Derivatives as Potent Inducers of Apoptosis in Human Myeloid Leukemia Cells. *ChemMedChem* **2009**, *4*, 1668-1676.

[59] Longcroft-Wheaton, G. R.; Higgins, B.; Bhandari, P. Flexible spectral imaging color enhancement and indigo carmine in neoplasia diagnosis during colonoscopy: a large prospective UK series. *Eur. J. Gastroenterol. Hepatol.* **2011**, *23*, 903-911.

[60] Hashimoto, K.; Higaki, S.; Nishiahi, M.; Fujiwara, K.; Gondo, T.; Sakaida, I. Does chromoendoscopy improve the colonoscopic adenoma detection rate? *Hepato-gastroenterol.* **2010**, *57*, 1399-1404.

[61] Hurlstone, D. P.; Fujii, T.; Lobo, A. J. Early detection of colorectal cancer using high-magnification chromoscopic colonoscopy. *Br. J. Surg.* **2002**, *89*, 272-282.

[62] Hurlstone, D. P.; George, R.; Brown, S. Novel clinical *in vivo* roles for indigo carmine: high-magnification chromoscopic colonoscopy. *Biotech. Histochem.* **2007**, *82*, 57-71.

[63] Potterat, O.; Hamburger, M. *Progress in Drug Research, Natural Compounds as Drugs*, F. Petersen; R. Amstutz, (Eds.); Birkhaeuser, **2008**, pp. 62-64.

[64] Meijer, L.; Guyard, N.; Skaltsounis, A.-L.; Eisenbrand, G. (Eds.) *Indirubin, the Red Shade of Indigo*, Station Biologique de Roscoff, **2006**.

[65] Meijer, L.; Shearer, J.; Bettayeb, K.; Ferandin, Y. Diversity of the intracellular mechanisms underlying the anti-tumor properties of indirubins. *Int. Congr. Ser.* **2007**, *1304*, 60-74.

[66] Eisenbrand, G.; Hippe, F.; Jakobs, S.; Muehlbeyer, S. Molecular mechanisms of indirubin and its derivatives: novel anticancer molecules with their origin in traditional Chinese phytomedicine. *J. Cancer Res. Clin. Oncol.* **2004**, *130*, 627-635.

[67] Karapetyan, G.; Chakrabarty, K.; Hein, M.; Langer, P. Synthesis and bioactivity of carbohydrate derivatives of indigo, its isomers and heteroanalogues. *ChemMedChem* **2011**, *6*, 25-37.

[68] Ferandin, Y.; Bettayeb, K.; Kritsanida, M.; Lozach, O.; Polychronopoulos, P.; Magiatis, P.; Skaltsounis, A.-L.; Meijer, L. 3'-Substituted 7-halogenoindirubins, a new class of cell death inducing agents. *J. Med. Chem.* **2006**, *49*, 4638-4649.

[69] Choi, S.-J.; Lee, J.-E.; Jeong, S.-Y.; Im, I.; Lee, S.-D.; Lee, E.-J.; Lee, S. K.; Kwon, S.-M.; Ahn, S.-G.; Yoon, J.-H.; Han, S.-Y.; Kim, J.-I.; Kim, Y.-C. 5,5'-Substituted indirubin-3'-oxime derivatives as potent cyclin-dependent kinase inhibitors with anticancer activity. *J. Med. Chem.* **2010**, *53*, 3696-3706.

[70] Wang, Z. H.; Li, W. Y.; Li, F. L.; Zhang, L.; Hua, W. Y.; Cheng, J. C.; Yao, Q. Z. Synthesis and antitumor activity of 7-azaindirubin. *Chin. Chem. Lett.* **2009**, *20*, 542-544.

[71] Cheng, X.; Rasque, P.; Vatter, S.; Merz, K.-H.; Eisenbrand, G. Synthesis and cytotoxicity of novel indirubin-5-carboxamides. *Bioorg. Med. Chem.* **2010**, *18*, 4509-4515.

[72] Libnow, S.; Methling, K.; Hein, M.; Michalik, D.; Harms, M.; Wende, K.; Flemming, A.; Koeckerling, M.; Reinke, H.; Bednarski, P. J.; Lalk, M.; Langer, P. Synthesis of indirubin-N'-glycosides and their anti-proliferative activity against human cancer cell lines. *Bioorg. Med. Chem.* **2008**, *16*, 5570-5583.

[73] Meijer, L.; Shearer, J.; Bettayeb, K.; Ferandin, Y. Diversity of the intracellular mechanisms underlying the anti-tumor properties of indirubins. *Int. Congr. Ser.* **2007**, *1304*, 60-74.

[74] Hoessel, R.; Leclerc, S.; Endicott, J. A.; Nobel, M. E.; Lawrie, A.; Tunnah, P.; Leost, M.; Damiens, E.; Marie, D.; Marko, D.; Niederberger, E.; Tang, W.; Eisenbrand, G.; Meijer, L. Indirubin, the active constituent of a Chinese antileukaemia medicine, inhibits cyclin-dependent kinases. *Nat. Cell. Biol.* **1999**, *1*, 60-67.

[75] Jautelat, R.; Brumby, T.; Schafer, M.; Briem, H.; Eisenbrand, G.; Schwahn, S.; Kruger, M.; Lucking, U.; Prien, O.; Siemeister, G. From the insoluble dye indirubin towards highly active, soluble CDK2-inhibitors. *ChemBioChem* **2005**, *6*, 531-540.

[76] Marko, D.; Schatzle, S.; Friedel, A.; Genzlinger, A.; Zankl, H.; Meijer, L.; Eisenbrand, G. Inhibition of cyclin-dependent kinase 1 (CDK1) by indirubin derivatives in human tumour cells. *Br. J. Cancer* **2001**, *84*, 283-289.

[77] Leclerc, S.; Garnier, M.; Hoessel, R.; Marko, D.; Bibb, J. A.; Snyder, G. L.; Greengard, P.; Biernat, J.; Wu, Y. Z.; Mandelkow, E. M.; Eisenbrand, G.; Meijer, L. Indirubins inhibit glycogen synthase kinase-3 beta and CDK5/P25, two protein kinases involved in abnormal tau phosphorylation in Alzheimer's disease - A property common to most cycline-dependent kinase inhibitors? *J. Biol. Chem.* **2001**, *276*, 251-260.

[78] Eisenbrand, G.; Hippe, F.; Jakobs, S.; Muehlbeyer, S. Molecular mechanisms of indirubin and its derivatives: novel anticancer molecules with their origin in traditional Chinese phytomedicine. *J. Cancer Res. Clin. Oncol.* **2004**, *130*, 627-635.

[79] Sethi, G.; Ahn, K. S.; Sandur, S. K.; Lin, X.; Chaturvedi, M. M.; Aggarwal, B. B. Indirubin enhances tumor necrosis factor-induced apoptosis through modulation of nuclear factor-kappa B signaling pathway. *J. Biol. Chem.* **2006**, *281*, 23425-23435.

[80] Adachi, J.; Mori, Y.; Matsui, S.; Takigami, H.; Fujino, J.; Kitagawa, H.; Miller, C. A.; Kato, T.; Saeki, K.; Matsuda, T. Indirubin and indigo are potent aryl hydrocarbon receptor ligands present in human urine. *J. Biol. Chem.* **2001**, *276*, 31475-31478.

[81] Spink, B. C.; Hussain, M. M.; Katz, B. H.; Eisele, L.; Spink, D. C. Transient induction of cytochromes P450 1A1 and 1B1 in MCF-7 human breast cancer cells by indirubin. *Biochem. Pharmacol.* **2003**, *66*, 2313-2321.

[82] Polychronopoulos, P.; Magiatis, P.; Skaltsounis, A. L.; Myrianthopoulos, V.; Mikros, E.; Tarricone, A.; Musacchio, A.; Roe, S. M.; Pearl, L.; Leost, M.; Greengard, P.; Meijer, L. Structural basis for the synthesis of indirubins as potent and selective inhibitors of glycogen synthase kinase-3 and cyclin-dependent kinases. *J. Med. Chem.* **2004**, *47*, 935-946.

[83] Choi, S.-J.; Lee, J.-E.; Jeong, S.-Y.; Im, I.; Lee, S.-D.; Lee, E.-J.; Lee, S. K.; Kwon, S.-M.; Ahn, S.-G.; Yoon, J.-H.; Han, S.-Y.; Kim, J.-I.; Kim, Y.-C. 5,5'-Substituted indirubin-3'-oxime derivatives as potent cyclin-dependent kinase inhibitors with anticancer activity, in, American Chemical Society, 2010, pp. MEDI-342.

[84] Zhang, X.; Song, Y.; Wu, Y.; Dong, Y.; Lai, L.; Zhang, J.; Lu, B.; Dai, F.; He, L.; Liu, M.; Yi, Z. Indirubin inhibits tumor growth by antitumor angiogenesis *via* blocking VEGFR2-mediated JAK/STAT3 signaling in endothelial cell. *Int. J. Cancer* **2011**, *129*, 2502-2511.

[85] Han, S.-Y.; Ahn, J. H.; Shin, C. Y.; Choi, S.-U. Effects of indirubin derivatives on the FLT3 activity and growth of acute myeloid leukemia cell lines. *Drug Dev. Res.* **2010**, *71*, 221-227.

[86] Yoon, H.-E.; Kim, S.-A.; Choi, H.-S.; Ahn, M.-Y.; Yoon, J.-H.; Ahn, S.-G. Inhibition of Plk1 and Pin1 by 5'-nitro-indirubinoxime suppresses human lung cancer cells. *Cancer Lett. (N. Y., NY, U. S.)* **2012**, *316*, 97-104.

[87] Kim, S.-A.; Kwon, S.-M.; Kim, J.-A.; Kang, K. W.; Yoon, J.-H.; Ahn, S.-G. 5'-Nitro-indirubinoxime, an indirubin derivative, suppresses metastatic ability of human head and neck cancer cells through the inhibition of Integrin β1/FAK/Akt signaling. *Cancer Lett.* **2011**, *306*, 197-204.

[88] Yoon, J.-H.; Kim, S.-A.; Kim, J.-I.; Park, J.-H.; Ahn, S.-G.; Yoon, J.-H. Inhibition of invasion and migration of salivary gland adenocarcinoma cells by 5'-nitro-indirubinoxime (5'-NIO). *Head Neck* **2010**, *32*, 619-625.

[89] Yoon, J.-H.; Kim, S.-A.; Kwon, S.-M.; Park, J.-H.; Park, H.-S.; Kim, Y.-C.; Yoon, J.-H.; Ahn, S.-G. 5'-Nitro-indirubinoxime induces G1 cell cycle arrest and apoptosis in salivary gland adenocarcinoma cells through the inhibition of Notch-1 signaling. *Biochim. Biophys. Acta, Gen. Subj.* **2010**, *1800*, 352-358.

[90] Saito, H.; Tabata, K.; Hanada, S.; Kanda, Y.; Suzuki, T.; Miyairi, S. Synthesis of methoxy- and bromo-substituted indirubins and their activities on apoptosis induction in human neuroblastoma cells. *Bioorg. Med. Chem. Lett.* **2011**, *21*, 5370-5373.

[91] Moon, M. J.; Lee, S. K.; Lee, J.-W.; Song, W. K.; Kim, S. W.; Kim, J. I.; Cho, C.; Choi, S. J.; Kim, Y.-C. Synthesis and structure-activity relationships of novel indirubin derivatives as potent anti-proliferative agents with CDK2 inhibitory activities. *Bioorg. Med. Chem.* **2006**, *14*, 237-246.

[92] Chan, Y.-K.; Kwok, H.-H.; Chan, L.-S.; Leung, K. S.-Y.; Shi, J.; Mak, N.-K.; Wong, R. N.-S.; Yue, P. Y.-K. An indirubin derivative, E804, exhibits potent angiosuppressive activity. *Biochem. Pharmacol.* **2012**, *83*, 598-607.

[93] Nam, S.; Buettner, R.; Turkson, J.; Kim, D.; Cheng, J. Q.; Muehlbeyer, S.; Hippe, F.; Vatter, S.; Merz, K.-H.; Eisenbrand, G.; Jove, R. Indirubin derivatives inhibit Stat3 signaling and induce apoptosis in human cancer cells. *Proc. Natl. Acad. Sci. U. S. A.* **2005**, *102*, 5998-6003.

[94] Nam, S.; Scuto, A.; Yang, F.; Chen, W.; Park, S.; Yoo, H.-S.; Konig, H.; Bhatia, R.; Cheng, X.; Merz, K.-H.; Eisenbrand, G.; Jove, R. Indirubin derivatives induce apoptosis of chronic myelogenous leukemia cells involving inhibition of Stat5 signaling. *Mol Oncol* **2012**.

[95] Wang, T. C.; Wei, J. Z.; Guo, C. S.; Zhang, H. B.; Fan, H. X. Design, synthesis and anti-proliferative studies of a novel series of indirubin derivatives. *Chin. Chem. Lett.* **2010**, *21*, 1407-1410.

[96] Carletti, I.; Banaigs, B.; Amade, P. Matemone, a new bioactive bromine-containing oxindole alkaloid from the indian ocean sponge iotrochota purpurea. *J.f Nat. Prod.* **2000**, *63*, 981-983.

[97] Wang, F. Z.; Fang, Y. C.; Zhu, T. J.; Zhang, M.; Lin, A. Q.; Gu, Q. Q.; Zhu, W. M. Seven new prenylated indole diketopiperazine alkaloids from holothurian-derived fungus *Aspergillus fumigatus*. *Tetrahedron* **2008**, *64*, 7986-7991.

[98] Gerby, B.; Boumendjel, A.; Blanc, M.; Bringuier, P. P.; Champelovier, P.; Fortune, A.; Ronot, X.; Boutonnat, J. 2-Arylidenedihydroindole-3-ones: design, synthesis, and biological activity on bladder carcinoma cell lines. *Bioorg. Med. Chem. Lett.* **2007**, *17*, 208-213.

[99] Griffith, R.; Brown, M. N.; McCluskey, A.; Ashman, L. K. Small molecule inhibitors of protein kinases in cancer - how to overcome resistance. *Mini-Rev. Med. Chem.* **2006**, *6*, 1101-1110.

[100] Pandit, B.; Sun, Y.; Chen, P.; Sackett, D. L.; Hu, Z.; Rich, W.; Li, C.; Lewis, A.; Schaefer, K.; Li, P.-K. Structure-activity-relationship studies of conformationally restricted analogs of Combretastatin A-4 derived from SU5416. *Bioorg. Med. Chem.* **2006**, *14*, 6492-6501.

[101] Atkins, M.; Jones, C. A.; Kirkpatrick, P. Sunitinib maleate. *Nat. Rev. Drug Discov.* **2006**, *5*, 279-280.

[102] Izzedine, H.; Buhaescu, I.; Rixe, O.; Deray, G. Sunitinib malate. *Cancer Chemother. Pharmacol.* **2007**, *60*, 357-364.

[103] Gao, N.; Kramer, L.; Rahmani, M.; Dent, P.; Grant, S. The three-substituted indolinone cyclin-dependent kinase 2 inhibitor 3-[1-(3*H*-imidazol-4-yl)-meth-(*Z*)-ylidene]-5-methoxy-1,3-dihydro-indol-2-one (SU9516) kills human leukemia cells *via* down-regulation of Mcl-1 through a transcriptional mechanism. *Mol. Pharmacol.* **2006**, *70*, 645-655.

[104] Harris, P. A. In: Inhib*itors of Cyclin-dependent Kinases as Anti-tumor Agents*; P. J. Smith; E. W. Yue, (Eds.); Taylor and Francis Group, Boca Raton FL, USA, **2007**, pp. 265-281.

[105] Li, H.-H.; Zhang, X.-H.; Tan, J.-Z.; Chen, L.-L.; Liu, H.; Luo, X.-M.; Shen, X.; Lin, L.-P.; Chen, K.-X.; Ding, J.; Jiang, H.-L. Design, synthesis, antitumor evaluations and molecular modeling studies of novel 3,5-substituted indolin-2-one derivatives. *Acta Pharmacol. Sin.* **2007**, *28*, 140-152.

[106] Klenke, F. M.; Abdollahi, A.; Bertl, E.; Gebhard, M.-M.; Ewerbeck, V.; Huber, P. E.; Sckell, A. Tyrosine kinase inhibitor SU6668 represses chondrosarcoma growth *via* antiangiogenesis *in vivo*. *BMC Cancer* **2007**, *7*, 49.

[107] Patyna, S.; Laird, A. D.; Mendel, D. B.; O'Farrell, A.-M.; Liang, C.; Guan, H.; Vojkovsky, T.; Vasile, S.; Wang, X.; Chen, J.; Grazzini, M.; Yang, C. Y.; Haznedar, J. O.; Sukbuntherng, J.; Zhong, W.-Z.; Cherrington, J. M.; Hu-Lowe, D. SU14813: A novel multiple receptor tyrosine kinase inhibitor with potent antiangiogenic and antitumor activity. *Mol. Cancer Ther.* **2006**, *5*, 1774-1782.

[108] Jin, Y. Z.; Fu, D. X.; Ma, N.; Li, Z. C.; Liu, Q. H.; Xiao, L.; Zhang, R. H. Synthesis and biological evaluation of 3-substituted-indolin-2-one derivatives containing chloropyrrole moieties. *Molecules* **2011**, *16*, 9368-9385.

[109] Lv, K.; Wang, L.-L.; Liu, M.-L.; Zhou, X.-B.; Fan, S.-Y.; Liu, H.-Y.; Zheng, Z.-B.; Li, S. Synthesis and antitumor activity of 5-[1-(3-(dimethylamino)propyl)-5-halogenated-2-oxoindolin-(3Z)-ylidenemethyl]-2,4-dimethyl-1H-pyrrole-3-carboxamides. *Bioorg. Med. Chem. Lett.* **2011**, *21*, 3062-3065.

[110] Luo, Y.; Xiao, F.; Qian, S. J.; He, Q. J.; Lu, W.; Yang, B. Synthesis and evaluation of novel 5-sulfonyl-indolin-2-ones as potent cytotoxic agents. *MedChemComm* **2011**, *2*, 1054-1057.

[111] Chiang, C. C.; Lin, Y. H.; Lin, S. F.; Lai, C. L.; Liu, C. W.; Wei, W. Y.; Yang, S. C.; Wane, R. W.; Teng, L. W.; Chuang, S. H.; Chang, J. M.; Yuan, T. T.; Lee, Y. S.; Chen, P. N.; Chi, W. K.; Yang, J. Y.; Huang, H. J.; Liao, C. B.; Huang, J. J. Discovery of pyrrole-indoline-2-ones as Aurora kinase inhibitors with a different inhibition profile. *J. Med. Chem.* **2010**, *53*, 5929-5941.

[112] Cho, T. P.; Dong, S. Y.; Jun, F.; Hong, F. J.; Liang, Y. J.; Lu, X. A.; Hua, P. J.; Li, L. Y.; Lei, Z.; Bing, H.; Ying, Z.; Qiong, L. F.; Bei, F. B.; Guang, L. L.; Shen, G. A.; Hong, S. G.; Hong, S. W.; Tai, M. X. Novel potent orally active multitargeted receptor tyrosine kinase inhibitors: synthesis, structure-activity relationships, and antitumor activities of 2-indolinone derivatives. *J. Med. Chem.* **2010**, *53*, 8140-8149.

[113] Islam, I.; Bryant, J.; Chou, Y.-L.; Kochanny, M. J.; Lee, W.; Phillips, G. B.; Yu, H.; Adler, M.; Whitlow, M.; Ho, E.; Lentz, D.; Polokoff, M. A.; Subramanyam, B.; Wu, J. M.; Zhu, D.; Feldman, R. I.; Arnaiz, D. O. Indolinone based phosphoinositide-dependent kinase-1 (PDK1) inhibitors. Part 1: Design, synthesis and biological activity. *Bioorg. Med. Chem. Lett.* **2007**, *17*, 3814-3818.

[114] Islam, I.; Brown, G.; Bryant, J.; Hrvatin, P.; Kochanny, M. J.; Phillips, G. B.; Yuan, S.; Adler, M.; Whitlow, M.; Lentz, D.; Polokoff, M. A.; Wu, J.; Shen, J.; Walters, J.; Ho, E.; Subramanyam, B.; Zhu, D.; Feldman, R. I.; Arnaiz, D. O. Indolinone based phosphoinositide-dependent kinase-1 (PDK1) inhibitors. Part 2: Optimization of BX-517. *Bioorg. Med. Chem. Lett.* **2007**, *17*, 3819-3825.

[115] Zou, H. B.; Zhang, L.; Ouyang, J. F.; Giulianotti, M. A.; Yu, Y. P. Synthesis and biological evaluation of 2-indolinone derivatives as potential antitumor agents. *Eur. J. Med. Chem.* **2011**, *46*, 5970-5977.

[116] Xiong, X. S.; Zhang, Y. W.; Gao, X.; Dong, Z. Y.; Li, L.; Ji, C. C.; Fu, L. L.; Luo, X. M.; Liu, H.; Mei, C. L. B5, a novel pyrrole-substituted indolinone, exerts potent antitumor efficacy through G2/M cell cycle arrest. *Invest. New Drugs* **2010**, *28*, 26-34.

[117] Zhang, W.; Go, M. L. Functionalized 3-benzylidene-indolin-2-ones: Inducers of NAD(P)H-quinone oxidoreductase 1 (NQO1) with antiproliferative activity. *Bioorg. Med. Chem.* **2009**, *17*, 2077-2090.

[118] Chen, G.; Hao, X. J.; Sun, Q. Y.; Ding, J. Rapid synthesis and bioactivities of 3-(nitromethylene)indolin-2-one analogues. *Chem. Pap.* **2010**, *64*, 673-677.

[119] Kulimova, E.; Oelmann, E.; Bisping, G.; Kienast, J.; Mesters, R. M.; Schwable, J.; Hilberg, F.; Roth, G. J.; Munzert, G.; Stefanic, M.; Steffen, B.; Brandts, C.; Muller-Tidow, C.; Kolkmeyer, A.; Buchner, T.; Serve, H.; Berdel, W. E. Growth inhibition and induction of apoptosis in acute myeloid leukemia cells by new indolinone derivatives targeting fibroblast growth factor, platelet-derived growth factor, and vascular endothelial growth factor receptors. *Mol. Cancer Ther.* **2006**, *5*, 3105-3112.

[120] Santos, E.; Gomez, J.; Raez, L. Targeting angiogenesis from multiple pathways simultaneously: BIBF 1120, an investigational novel triple angiokinase inhibitor. *Invest. New Drugs* **2012**, *30,* 1261-1269.

[121] Rizzi, E.; Cassinelli, G.; Dallavalle, S.; Linzi, C.; Cincinelli, R.; Nannei, R.; Cuccuru, G.; Zunino, F. Synthesis and RET protein kinase inhibitory activity of 3-arylureidobenzylidene-indolin-2-ones. *Bioorg. Med. Chem. Lett.* **2007**, *17*, 3962-3968.

[122] Sassatelli, M.; Debiton, E.; Aboab, B.; Prudhomme, M.; Moreau, P. Synthesis and antiproliferative activities of indolin-2-one derivatives bearing amino acid moieties. *Eur. J. Med. Chem.* **2006**, *41*, 709-716.

[123] Lawrence, H. R.; Pireddu, R.; Chen, L.; Luo, Y.; Sung, S.-S.; Szymanski, A. M.; Yip, M. L. R.; Guida, W. C.; Sebti, S. M.; Wu, J.; Lawrence, N. J. Inhibitors of Src homology-2 domain containing protein tyrosine phosphatase-2 (Shp2) based on oxindole scaffolds. *J. Med. Chem.* **2008**, *51*, 4948-4956.

[124] Pervez, H.; Iqbal, M. S.; Tahir, M. Y.; Nasim, F.-U.-H.; Choudhary, M. I.; Khan, K. M. *In vitro* cytotoxic, antibacterial, antifungal and urease inhibitory acitivities of some *N*4-substituted isatin-3-thiosemicarbazones. *J. Enzym. Inhib. Med. Chem.* **2008**, *23*, 848-854.

[125] Pervez, H.; Chohan, Z. H.; Ramzan, M.; Nasim, F. U. H.; Khan, K. M. Synthesis and biological evaluation of some new N4-substituted isatin-3-thiosemicarbazones. *J. Enzym. Inhib. Med. Chem.* **2009**, *24*, 437-446.

[126] Pervez, H.; Ramzan, M.; Yaqub, M.; Khan, K. M. Synthesis, cytotoxic and phytotoxic effects of some new N4-aryl substituted isatin-3-thiosemicarbazones. *Lett. Drug Des. Discov.* **2011**, *8*, 452-458.

[127] Pervez, H.; Saira, N.; Iqbal, M. S.; Yaqub, M.; Khan, K. M. Synthesis and toxicity evaluation of some N4-aryl substituted 5-trifluoromethoxyisatin-3-thiosemicarbazones. *Molecules* **2011**, *16*, 6408-6421.

[128] Hall, M. D.; Salam, N. K.; Hellawell, J. L.; Fales, H. M.; Kensler, C. B.; Ludwig, J. A.; Szakacs, G.; Hibbs, D. E.; Gottesman, M. M. Synthesis, activity, and pharmacophore development for isatin-*beta*-thiosemicarbazones with selective activity toward multidrug-resistant cells. *J. Med. Chem.* **2009**, *52*, 3191-3204.

[129] Hall, M. D.; Brimacombe, K. R.; Varonka, M. S.; Pluchino, K. M.; Monda, J. K.; Li, J. Y.; Walsh, M. J.; Boxer, M. B.; Warren, T. H.; Fales, H. M.; Gottesman, M. M. Synthesis and structure-activity evaluation of isatin-*beta*-thiosemicarbazones with improved selective activity toward multidrug-resistant cells expressing P-glycoprotein. *J. Med. Chem.* **2011**, *54*, 5878-5889.

[130] Abadi, A. H.; Abou-Seri, S. M.; Abdel-Rahman, D. E.; Klein, C.; Lozach, O.; Meijer, L. Synthesis of 3-substituted-2-oxoindole analogues and their evaluation as kinase inhibitors, anticancer and antiangiogenic agents. *Eur. J. Med. Chem.* **2006**, *41*, 296-305.

[131] Gudipati, R.; Anreddy, R. N. R.; Manda, S. Synthesis, characterization and anticancer activity of certain 3-{4-(5-mercapto-1,3,4-oxadiazole-2-yl) phenylimino}indolin-2-one derivatives. *Saudi Pharm. J.* **2011**, *19*, 153-158.

[132] Matesic, L.; Locke, J. M.; Vine, K. L.; Ranson, M.; Bremner, J. B.; Skropeta, D. Synthesis and hydrolytic evaluation of acid-labile imine-linked cytotoxic isatin model systems. *Bioorg. Med. Chem.* **2011**, *19*, 1771-1778.

[133] Matesic, L. PhD Thesis. Development of isatin-based compounds for use in targeted anti-cancer therapy, University of Wollongong, 2011.

[134] Jarrahpour, A.; Khalili, D.; De Clercq, E.; Salmi, C.; Brunel, J. M. Synthesis, antibacterial, antifungal and antiviral activity evaluation of some new bis-Schiff bases of isatin and their derivatives. *Molecules* **2007**, *12*, 1720-1730.

[135] Filomeni, G.; Cerchiaro, G.; Da Costa Ferreira, A. M.; De Martino, A.; Pedersen, J. Z.; Rotilio, G.; Ciriolo, M. R. Pro-apoptotic activity of novel isatin-Schiff base copper(II) complexes depends on oxidative stress induction and organelle-selective damage. *J. Biol. Chem.* **2007**, *282*, 12010-12021.

[136] Sathisha, M. P.; Revankar, V. K.; Pai, K. S. R. Synthesis, structure, electrochemistry, and spectral characterization of bis-isatin thiocarbohydrazone metal complexes and their antitumor activity against Ehrlich ascites carcinoma in Swiss albino mice. *Metal-Based Drugs* **2008**, *2008: 362105*.

[137] Karki, S. S.; Thota, S.; Darj, S. Y.; Balzarini, J.; De Clercq, E. Synthesis, anticancer, and cytotoxic activities of some mononuclear Ru(II) compounds. *Bioorg. Med. Chem.* **2007**, *15*, 6632-6641.

[138] Chohan, Z. H.; Shaikh, A. U.; Naseer, M. M. Metal-based isatin-bearing sulfonamides: their synthesis, characterization and biological properties. *Appl. Organomet. Chem.* **2006**, *20*, 729-739.

[139] Chohan, Z. H.; Supuran, C. T.; Ben Hadda, T.; Nasim, F. U. H.; Khan, K. M. Metal based isatin-derived sulfonamides: Their synthesis, characterization, coordination behavior and biological activity. *J. Enzym. Inhib. Med. Chem.* **2009**, *24*, 859-870.

[140] Abdulghani, A. J.; Abbas, N. M. Synthesis characterization and biological activity study of new Schiff and Mannich bases and some metal complexes derived from isatin and dithiooxamide. *Bioinorg. Chem. Appl.* **2011**, DOI: 10.1155/2011/706262.

[141] Sassatelli, M.; Bouchikhi, F.; Messaoudi, S.; Anizon, F.; Debiton, E.; Barthomeuf, C.; Prudhomme, M.; Moreau, P. Synthesis and antiproliferative activities of diversely substituted glycosyl-isoindigo derivatives. *Eur. J. Med. Chem.* **2006**, *41*, 88-100.

[142] Wang, L. K.; Mencher, S. K. In: *Indirubin, the Red Shade of Indigo*; L. Meijer; N. Guyard; L. A. Skaltsounis; G. Eisenbrand, (Eds.); Life in Progress Editions, Roscoff, France, **2006**, pp. 247-258.

[143] Xiao, Z.; Wang, Y.; Lu, L.; Li, Z.; Peng, Z.; Han, Z.; Hao, Y. Anti-angiogenesis effects of meisoindigo on chronic myelogenous leukemia *in vitro*. *Leuk. Res.* **2006**, *30*, 54-59.

[144] Lee, C. C.; Lin, C. P.; Lee, Y. L.; Wang, G. C.; Cheng, Y. C.; Liu, H. E. Meisoindigo is a promising agent with *in vitro* and *in vivo* activity against human acute myeloid leukemia. *Leuk. Lymphoma* **2010**, *51*, 897-905.

[145] Wee, X. K.; Yeo, W. K.; Zhang, B.; Tan, V. B. C.; Lim, K. M.; Tay, T. E.; Go, M. L. Synthesis and evaluation of functionalized isoindigos as antiproliferative agents. *Bioorg. Med. Chem.* **2009**, *17*, 7562-7571.

[146] Bouchikhi, F.; Anizon, F.; Moreau, P. Synthesis and antiproliferative activities of isoindigo and azaisoindigo derivatives. *Eur. J. Med. Chem.* **2008**, *43*, 755-762.

[147] Bouchikhi, F.; Anizon, F.; Moreau, P. Synthesis, kinase inhibitory potencies and *in vitro* antiproliferative activity of isoindigo and 7'-azaisoindigo derivatives substituted by Sonogashira cross-coupling. *Eur. J. Med. Chem.* **2009**, *44*, 2705-2710.

[148] Wang, Z. H.; Wang, T.; Yao, S. N.; Chen, J. C.; Hua, W. Y.; Yao, Q. Z. Synthesis and biological evaluation of 7-azaisoindigo derivatives. *Arch. Pharm.* **2010**, *343*, 160-166.

[149] Xu, J. J.; Dai, X. M.; Liu, H. L.; Guo, W. J.; Gao, J.; Wang, C. H.; Li, W. B.; Yao, Q. Z. A novel 7-azaisoindigo derivative-induced cancer cell apoptosis and mitochondrial dysfunction mediated by oxidative stress. *J. Appl. Toxicol.* **2011**, *31*, 164-172.

[150] Kitajima, M.; Nakamura, T.; Kogure, N.; Ogawa, M.; Mitsuno, Y.; Ono, K.; Yano, S.; Aimi, N.; Takayama, H. Isolation of gelsidine-type indole alkaloids from *Gelsenium elegans* and evaluation of the cytotoxic activity of *Gelsemium* alkaloids for A431 epidermoid carcinoma cells. *J. Nat. Prod.* **2006**, *69*, 715-718.

[151] Franz, A. K.; Dreyfuss, P. D.; Schreiber, S. L. Synthesis and cellular profiling of diverse organosilicon small molecules. *J. Am. Chem. Soc.* **2007**, *129*, 1020-1021.

[152] Kaminskyy, D.; Khyluk, D.; Vasylenko, O.; Zaprutko, L.; Lesyk, R. A facile synthesis and anticancer activity evaluation of spiro[thiazolidinone-isatin] conjugates. *Sci. Pharm.* **2011**, *79*, 763-777.

[153] Uddin, M. K.; Reignier, S. G.; Coulter, T.; Montalbetti, C.; Granas, C.; Butcher, S.; Krog-Jensen, C.; Fielding, J. Syntheses and antiproliferative evaluation of oxyphenisatin derivatives. *Bioorg. Med. Chem. Lett.* **2007**, *17*, 2854-2857.

[154] Kamal, A.; Srikanth, Y. V. V.; Khan, M. N. A.; Shaik, T. B.; Ashraf, M. Synthesis of 3,3-diindolyl oxyindoles efficiently catalysed by $FeCl_3$ and their *in vitro* evaluation for anticancer activity. *Bioorg. Med. Chem. Lett.* **2010**, *20*, 5229-5231.

[155] Subba Reddy, B. V.; Rajeswari, N.; Sarangapani, M.; Prashanthi, Y.; Ganji, R. J.; Addlagatta, A. Iodine-catalyzed condensation of isatin with indoles: A facile synthesis of di(indolyl)indolin-2-ones and evaluation of their cytotoxicity. *Bioorg. Med. Chem. Lett.* **2012**, *22*, 2460-2463.

[156] Penthala, N. R.; Yerramreddy, T. R.; Madadi, N. R.; Crooks, P. A. Synthesis and *in vitro* evaluation of *N*-alkyl-3-hydroxy-3-(2-imino-3-methyl-5-oxoimidazolidin-4-yl)indolin-2-one analogs as potential anticancer agents. *Bioorg. Med. Chem. Lett.* **2010**, *20*, 4468-4471.

[157] Solomon, V. R.; Hu, C.; Lee, H. Hybrid pharmacophore design and synthesis of isatin-benzothiazole analogs for their anti-breast cancer activity. *Bioorg. Med. Chem.* **2009**, *17*, 7585-7592.

[158] Taher, A. T.; Khalil, N. A.; Ahmed, E. M. Synthesis of novel isatin-thiazoline and isatin-benzimidazole conjugates as anti-breast cancer agents. *Arch. Pharm. Res.* **2011**, *34*, 1615-1621.

[159] Ramla, M. M.; Omar, M. A.; El-Khamry, A. M.; El-Diwani, H. I. Synthesis and antitumor activity of 1-substituted-2-methyl-5-nitrobenzimidazoles. *Bioorg. Med. Chem.* **2006**, *14*, 7324-7332.

[160] Rostom, S. A. Synthesis and *in vitro* antitumor evaluation of some indeno[1,2-c]pyrazol(in)es substituted with sulfonamide, sulfonylurea(-thiourea) pharmacophores, and some derived thiazole ring systems. *Bioorg. Med. Chem.* **2006**, *14*, 6475-6485.

[161] Lin, R.; Chiu, G.; Yu, Y.; Connolly, P. J.; Li, S.; Lu, Y.; Adams, M.; Fuentes-Pesquera, A. R.; Emanuel, S. L.; Greenberger, L. M. Design, synthesis, and evaluation of 3,4-disubstituted pyrazole analogues as anti-tumor CDK inhibitors. *Bioorg. Med. Chem. Lett.* **2007**, *17*, 4557-4561.

[162] Abadi, A. H.; Eissa, A. A.; Hassan, G. S. Synthesis of novel 1,3,4-trisubstituted pyrazole derivatives and their evaluation as antitumor and antiangiogenic agents. *Chem. Pharm. Bull. (Tokyo)* **2003**, *51*, 838-844.

[163] Manna, F.; Chimenti, F.; Fioravanti, R.; Bolasco, A.; Secci, D.; Chimenti, P.; Ferlini, C.; Scambia, G. Synthesis of some pyrazole derivatives and preliminary investigation of their affinity binding to P-glycoprotein. *Bioorg. Med. Chem. Lett.* **2005**, *15*, 4632-4635.

[164] Havrylyuk, D.; Kovach, N.; Zimenkovsky, B.; Vasylenko, O.; Lesyk, R. Synthesis and anticancer activity of isatin-based pyrazolines and thiazolidines conjugates. *Arch. Pharm. (Weinheim)* **2011**, *344*, 514-522.

[165] Kaminskyy, D.; Khyluk, D.; Vasylenko, O.; Zaprutko, L.; Lesyk, R. A facile synthesis and anticancer activity evaluation of spiro[thiazolidinone-isatin] conjugates. *Sci. Pharm.* **2011**, *79*, 763-777.

[166] Paull, K. D.; Shoemaker, R. H.; Hodes, L.; Monks, A.; Scudiero, D. A.; Rubinstein, L.; Plowman, J.; Boyd, M. R. Display and analysis of patterns of differential activity of drugs against human tumor cell lines: development of mean graph and COMPARE algorithm. *J. Natl. Cancer Inst.* **1989**, *81*, 1088-1092.

[167] Weinstein, J. N.; Myers, T. G.; O'Connor, P. M.; Friend, S. H.; Fornace, A. J., Jr.; Kohn, K. W.; Fojo, T.; Bates, S. E.; Rubinstein, L. V.; Anderson, N. L.; Buolamwini, J. K.; van Osdol, W. W.; Monks, A. P.; Scudiero, D. A.; Sausville, E. A.; Zaharevitz, D. W.; Bunow, B.; Viswanadhan, V. N.; Johnson, G. S.; Wittes, R. E.; Paull, K. D. An information-intensive approach to the molecular pharmacology of cancer. *Science* **1997**, *275*, 343-349.

[168] Krishnegowda, G.; Prakasha Gowda, A. S.; Tagaram, H. R.; Carroll, K. F.; Irby, R. B.; Sharma, A. K.; Amin, S. Synthesis and biological evaluation of a novel class of isatin analogs as dual inhibitors of tubulin polymerization and Akt pathway. *Bioorg. Med. Chem.* **2011**, *19*, 6006-6014.

[169] Indira Chandran, V.; Matesic, L.; Locke, J. M.; Skropeta, D.; Ranson, M.; Vine, K. L. Anti-cancer activity of an acid-labile N-alkylisatin conjugate targeting the transferrin receptor. *Cancer Lett.* **2012**, *316*, 151-156.

[170] Vine, K. L.; Chandran, V. I.; Locke, J. M.; Matesic, L.; Lee, J.; Skropeta, D.; Bremner, J. B.; Ranson, M. Targeting urokinase and the transferrin receptor with novel, anti-mitotic N-alkylisatin cytotoxin conjugates causes selective cancer cell death and reduces tumor growth. *Curr. Cancer Drug Targets* **2012**, *12*, 64-73.

[171] Qian, Z. M.; Li, H.; Sun, H.; Ho, K. Targeted drug delivery *via* the transferrin receptor-mediated endocytosis pathway. *Pharmacol. Rev.* **2002**, *54*, 561-587.

[172] Harris, L.; Fritsche, H.; Mennel, R.; Norton, L.; Ravdin, P.; Taube, S.; Somerfield, M. R.; Hayes, D. F.; Bast, R. C., Jr. American Society of Clinical Oncology 2007 update of recommendations for the use of tumor markers in breast cancer. *J. Clin. Oncol.* **2007**, *25*, 5287-5312.

[173] Croucher, D. R.; Saunders, D. N.; Stillfried, G. E.; Ranson, M. A structural basis for differential cell signaling by PAI-1 and PAI-2 in breast cancer cells. *Biochem. J.* **2007**, *408*, 203-210.

[174] Vine, K. L.; Locke, J. M.; Bremner, J. B.; Pyne, S. G.; Ranson, M. Selective targeting of 2 '-deoxy-5-fluorouridine to urokinase positive malignant cells *in vitro*. *Bioorg. Med. Chem. Lett.* **2010**, *20*, 2908-2911.

[175] Qiu, F.; Shu, H. Effect of combined administration with EPA and ISA on human breast cancer cell MDA-MB-231. *Yixue Linchuang Yanjiu* **2011**, *28*, 1172-1174.

[176] Hardman, W. E.; Avula, C. P.; Fernandes, G.; Cameron, I. L. Three percent dietary fish oil concentrate increased efficacy of doxorubicin against MDA-MB 231 breast cancer xenografts. *Clin. Cancer. Res.* **2001**, *7*, 2041-2049.

[177] Hardman, W. E.; Moyer, M. P.; Cameron, I. L. Dietary fish oil sensitizes A549 lung xenografts to doxorubicin chemotherapy. *Cancer Lett.* **2000**, *151*, 145-151.

[178] DeGraffenried, L. A.; Friedrichs, W. E.; Fulcher, L.; Fernandes, G.; Silva, J. M.; Peralba, J. M.; Hidalgo, M. Eicosapentaenoic acid restores tamoxifen sensitivity in breast cancer cells with high Akt activity. *Ann. Oncol.* **2003**, *14*, 1051-1056.

[179] Shao, Y.; Pardini, L.; Pardini, R. S. Dietary menhaden oil enhances mitomycin C antitumor activity toward human mammary carcinoma MX-1. *Lipids* **1995**, *30*, 1035-1045.

[180] Colas, S.; Paon, L.; Denis, F.; Prat, M.; Louisot, P.; Hoinard, C.; Le Floch, O.; Ogilvie, G.; Bougnoux, P. Enhanced radiosensitivity of rat autochthonous mammary tumors by dietary docosahexaenoic acid. *Int. J.Cancer* **2004**, *109*, 449-454.

Send Reprints Orders on reprints@benthamscience.net

Advances in Anticancer Agents in Medicinal Chemistry, 2013, Vol. *2*, 313-343

CHAPTER 6

Tripentones: A Promising Series of Potent Anti-Cancer Agents

Christophe Rochais, Sylvain Rault and Patrick Dallemagne*

Université de Caen Basse-Normandie, CERMN EA 4258 – FR CNRS 3038 INC3M – SF 4206 ICORE, Bd Becquerel 14032 Caen cedex, France

Abstract: The 8*H*-thieno[2,3-*b*]pyrrolizinones, some of which exert very potent cytotoxic activity against tumor cell lines *in vitro*, are a promising novel series of anti-cancer agents. These compounds belong to the tripentone family and are based on 9*H*-pyrrolo[1,2-*a*]indol-9-one derivatives and their heterocyclic isosteres. This paper inventories the different synthetic strategies for tripentones and reviews their biological effects and therapeutic potential.

Keywords: Tripentone, pyrrolizinone, pyrroloindolone, thiophene, cancer, pyrrole , heterocycles, clauson-kaas, acylation, ring closure.

INTRODUCTION

8*H*-Thieno[2,3-*b*]pyrrolizinones (Fig. **1**) are a promising series of novel compounds in cancer therapeutics. Several research groups have reported the very interesting antineoplastic effect of these tripentacyclic derivatives, as demonstrated by their *in vitro* cytotoxicity against tumor cells in the nanomolar range (Fig. **1**).

These anti-cancer properties seem to be clearly linked with the thienopyrrolizinone structural system, resulting in these compounds being named "tripentones". This vernacular term has been widely adopted and extended to all derivatives, including 9*H*-pyrrolo[1,2-*a*]indol-9-one derivatives—the first tripentones to be described in the literature—and their heterocyclic isosteres (Fig. **2**).

Here we report the different synthetic routes toward tripentone family members as well as the compounds' biological properties and therapeutic potential.

***Address correspondence to Patrick Dallemagne:** Université de Caen Basse-Normandie, CERMN EA 4258 – FR CNRS 3038 INC3M – SF 4206 ICORE, Bd Becquerel 14032 Caen cedex, France; Tel: 33 2 31 56 68 13; Fax: 33 2 31 56 68 03; E-mail: patrick.dallemagne@unicaen.fr

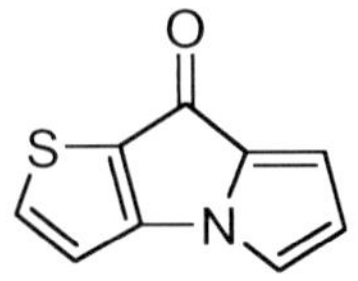

8*H*-thieno[2,3-*b*]pyrrolizin-8-ones

Fig. (1).

tripentones 9*H*-pyrrolo[1,2-*a*]indol-9-one

Fig. (2).

SYNTHESIS OF THE TRIPENTONE SYSTEM

The discovery of the important mitomycin anticancer agents in the 1950's [1] and elucidation of their pyrrolo[1,2-*a*]indole structure [2] spurred considerable interest in the 9*H*-pyrrolo[1,2-*a*]indol-9-one system and compelled many scientists to develop synthetic analogs of mitomycins called "mitosanes" (Fig. **3**).

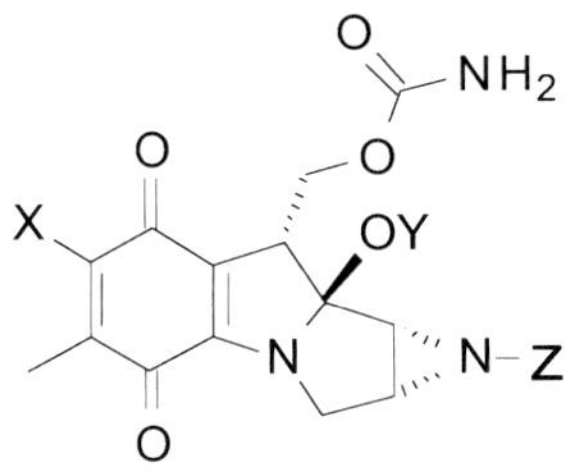

Mitomycin A : X = OCH_3, Y = CH_3, Z = H

Mitomycin B : X = OH, Y = CH_3, Z = CH_3

Mitomycin C : X = NH_2, Y = OCH_3, Z = H

Fig. (3).

Synthesis of 9*H*-pyrrolo[1,2-*a*]indol-9-one (**1**) was achieved according to four main pathways, starting either from various substituted phenylpyrroles (Routes A, B, C) or benzoylpyrroles (Route D) as depicted in Scheme **1**.

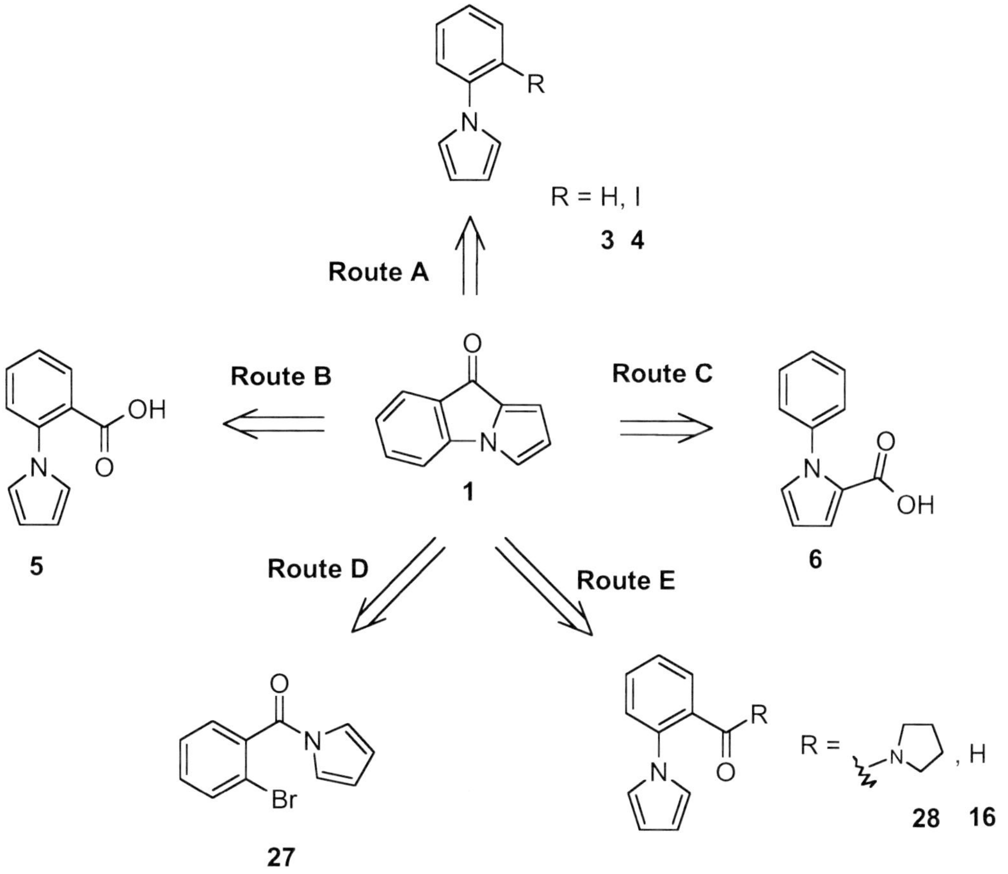

Scheme 1.

Route A: The first access to **1** was reported by Shirley *et al.* [3] in 1955 who incidentally synthesized it instead of the expected dicarboxylic acid (**2**). It was the only product of the bimetalation of 1-phenylpyrrole (**3**) by an excess of *n*-butyllithium, followed by a carbonylation reaction (Scheme **2**). This unforeseen method has been developed and improved more recently by the use of ethyl *N,N*-dimethylcarbamate in the place of CO_2 to produce **1** [4].

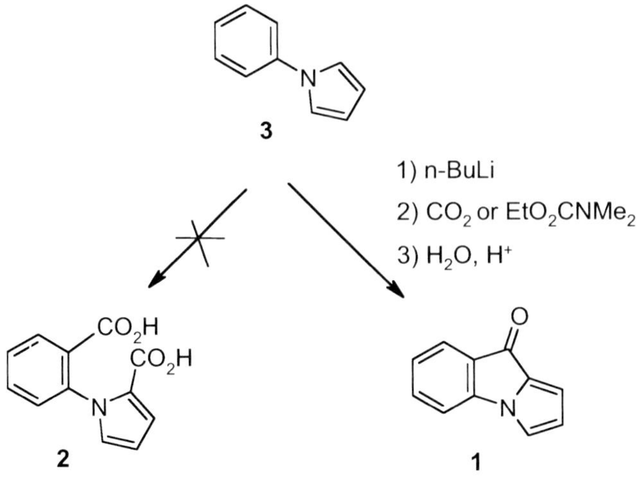

Scheme 2.

According to the same principle, a modern methodology developed for the synthesis of fluorenones has been applied to reach the pyrroloindolone system [5]. It proceeds through a palladium-catalyzed cyclocarbonylation of 1-(2-iodophenyl)pyrrole (**4**) leading to a quantitative yield of **1** (Scheme **3**).

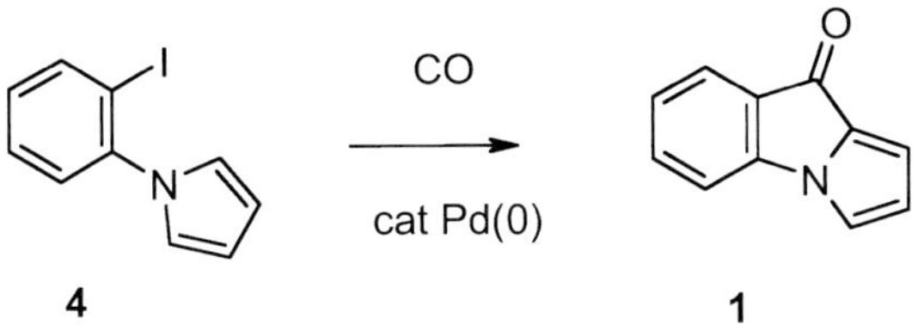

Scheme 3.

However, the most commonly used sequences to prepare **1** have involved isolating and subsequently cyclizing 2-(1*H*-pyrrol-1-yl)benzoic acids (**5**) (Route B) or 1-phenyl-1*H*-pyrrole-2-carboxylic acids (**6**) (Route C).

Route B: Intramolecular Friedel-Crafts acylation of **5** could be performed by the use of polyphosphoric acid, exploiting the electrophilicity of the alpha pyrrolic carbons to favor cyclization (Scheme **4**) [6]. Moreover, the originality of this pathway lies especially in the preparation of the starting material, **5**. Instead of the traditional reaction of anilines with mucic acid, 2-(1*H*-pyrrol-1-yl)benzoic acid

(**5**) was obtained for the first time according to the very useful method of Clauson-Kaas [7]. The latter involves reaction of methyl anthranilate (**7**) and 2,5-diethoxytetrahydrofuran in acetic acid to yield the new ester (**8**), which is then saponified into **5** in alkaline medium. Alternatively a novel procedure involves triphosgene as a novel reagent to cyclise **5** into **1** in good yield (80%) [8]. This method was further applied to some novel tripentones such as in naphthopyrrolizinone series.

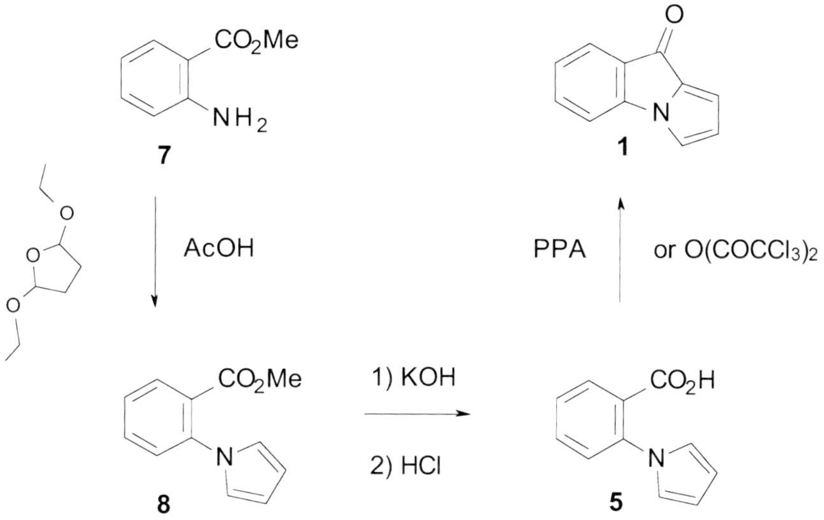

Scheme 4.

This approach was followed by using a Friedel-Crafts acylation to obtain substituted pyrrolo[1,2-*a*] indolones including an acylchloride (**9**), which was cyclized, this time by using $SnCl_4$ as a Lewis acid (Scheme **5**) [9].

Finally, it was recently shown that using boiling dioxane in the presence of 2 eq of 4-chloropyridine hydrochloride instead of acetic acid in Clauson-Kaas reaction not only improve the yield for the synthesis of **5** starting from anthranilic acid (**10**) but also perform the cyclisation of **5** into **1** according to a sequential one pot pyrrolation/cyclization sequence [10].

In a different approach, dimethyl derivatives of **1** were reached according to a multi-step sequence starting from methyl anthranilates (**7**) and first transforming them into sulfinyl-aminobenzoates (**11**) (Scheme **6**). The latter were then reacted with 2,3-dimethylbuta-1,3-diene to give the S-oxides of dimethylthiazinyl-benzoates (**12**) whose alkaline hydrolysis afforded dimethylpyrrolylbenzoic acids (**13**). Cyclization of **13** was achieved upon treatment with acetic anhydride and acetic acid [11-13].

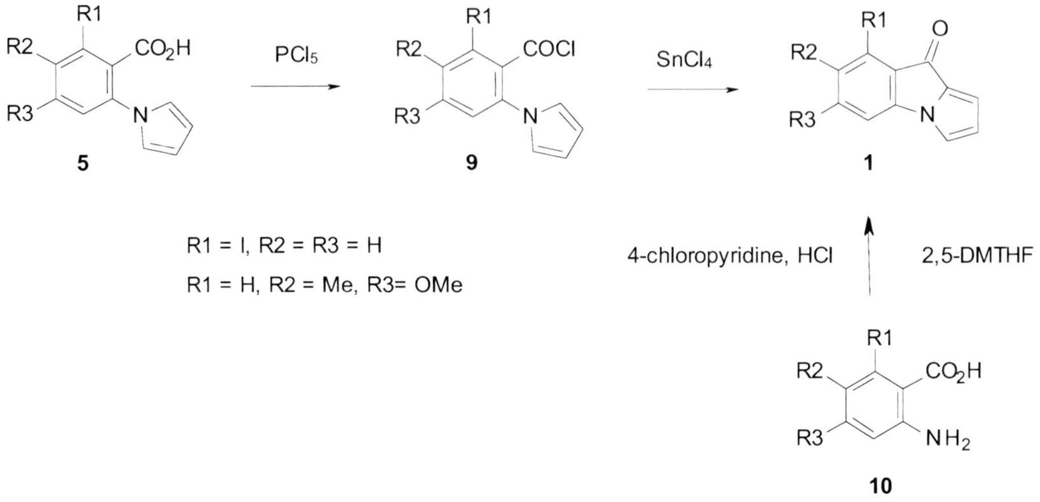

Scheme 5.

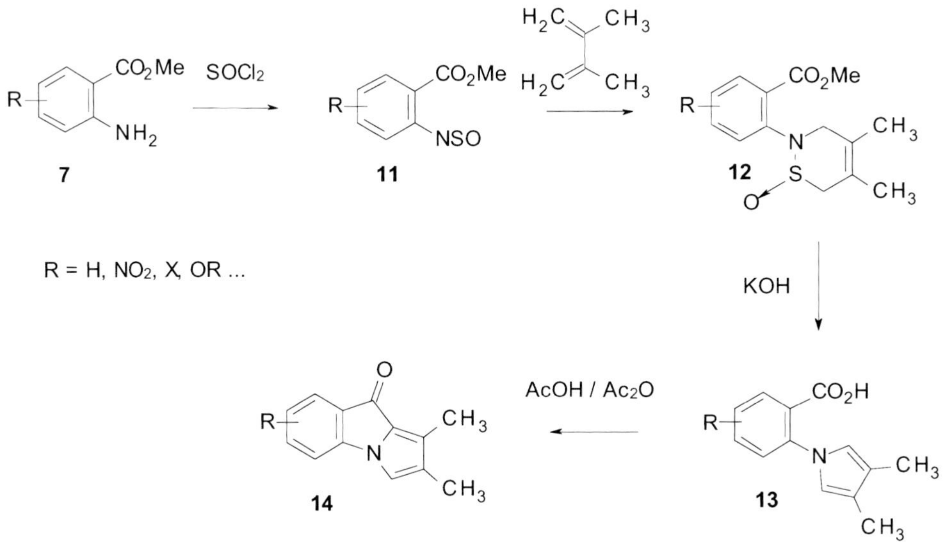

Scheme 6.

Route C: The side of the cyclization between the phenyl and pyrrole rings can be reversed, as demonstrated by Huisgen [14], who synthesized **1** (which he named "fluorazon") by a Friedel-Crafts acylation of a phenylpyrrole-2,3-dicarboxylic anhydride (**15**) and a subsequent decarboxylation of the resulting carboxylic acid intermediate (**16**) (Scheme **7**).

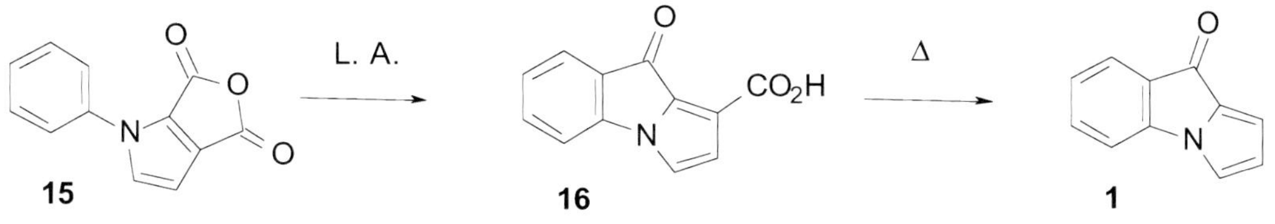

Scheme 7.

In a similar manner, 1-phenyl-1*H*-pyrrole-2-carboxylic acids (**6**), whose carboxylic acid groups were obtained by formylation of phenylpyrroles (**3**) and subsequent oxidation of the resulting phenypyrrolecarboxaldehydes (**17**), were cyclized into **1** according to a Friedel-Crafts procedure (Scheme **8**) [15].

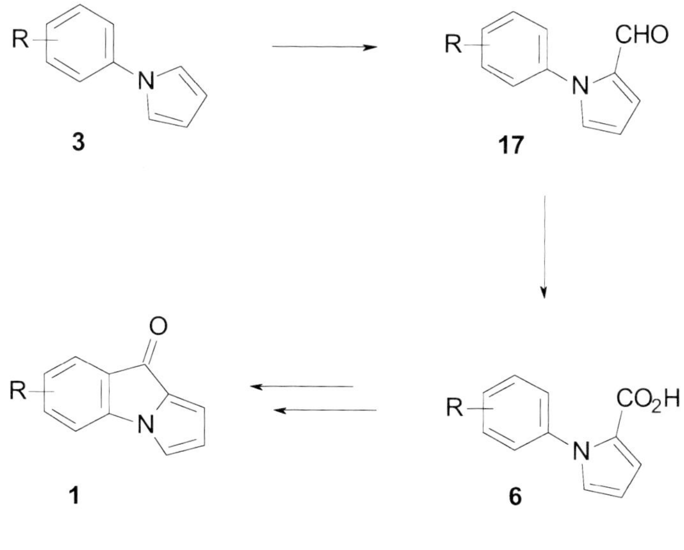

Scheme 8.

A similar process involved, first, reaction between 2,5-dimethoxyTHF-2-carboxylic acid and ortho-aminophenols (**18**) to form benzopyrroloxazinones (**19**).

These compounds were then rearranged under UV irradiation into 5-hydroxy-9*H*-pyrrolo[1,2-*a*]indol-9-ones (**20**) according to a meta-photo-Fries mechanism (Scheme **9**) [16,17].

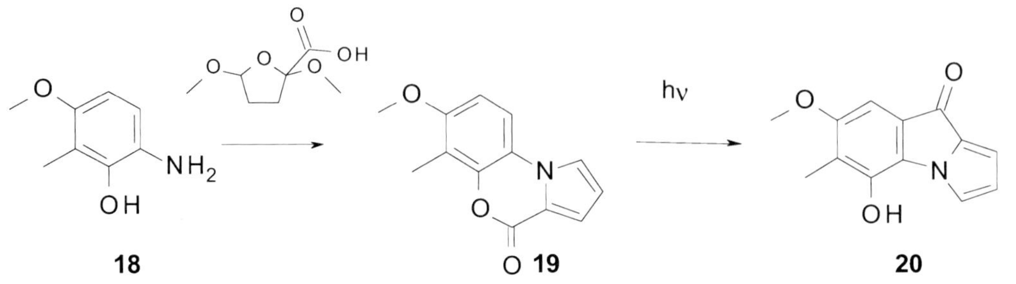

Scheme 9.

The same authors described another pathway to achieve the synthesis of 8-hydroxy-9*H*-pyrrolo[1,2-*a*]indol-9-ones (**21**) by reaction of the sodium salt of proline (**22**) with methylcyclohexanedione (**23**) (Scheme **10**) [18]. The resulting enamine (**24**) was cyclized in hot acetic anhydride into a tricyclic intermediate (**25**) before being subsequently aromatized on treatment with palladium charcoal.

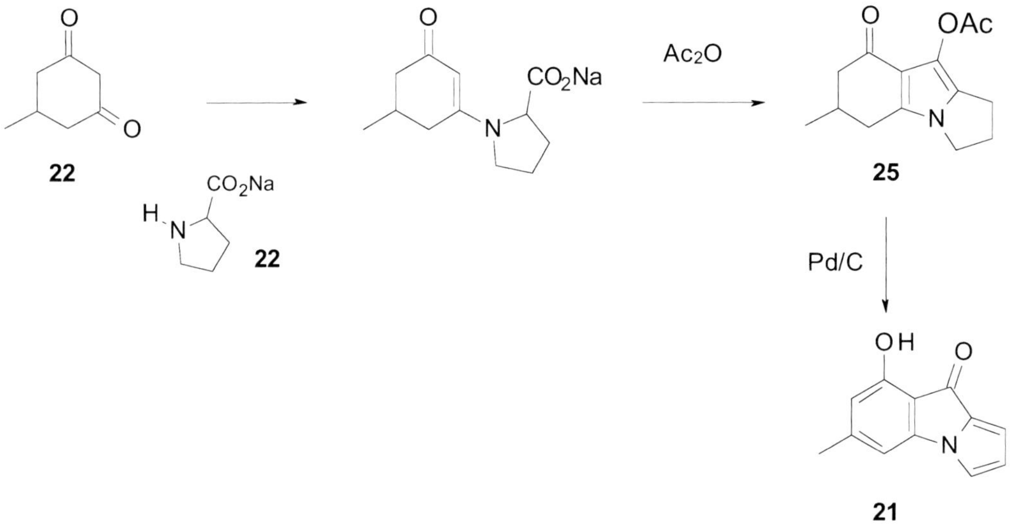

Scheme 10.

However, the Friedel-Crafts approach, mainly used according to routes B and C, has a disadvantage in this series, owing to the well-known sensitivity of the pyrrole ring toward the reagents used to activate the carboxylic acid group into an acylchloride, and notably toward $SOCl_2$. To circumvent this, two novel approaches were proposed.

Route D: This fourth pathway involves condensation of the acylchloride (**26**) with pyrrolylmagnesium iodide to afford the benzoylpyrrole (**27**). This is subsequently engaged in an intramolecular nucleophilic aromatic substitution to give a methoxymethyl derivative of **1** (Scheme **11**) [19].

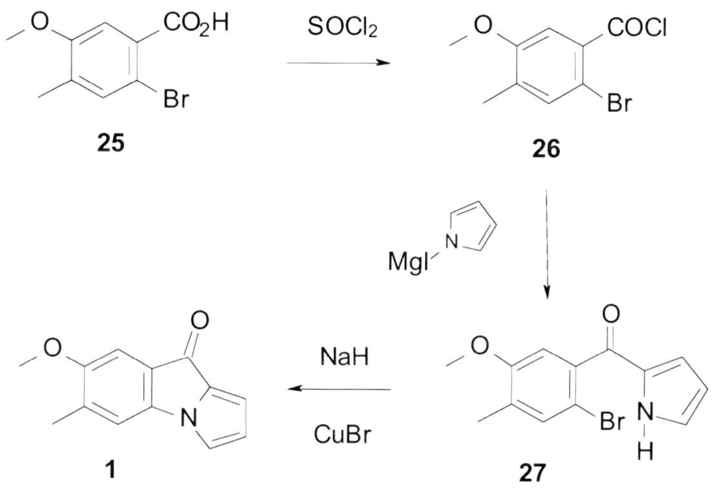

Scheme 11.

Route E: This method [20,21] employs a Vilsmeier-Haack acylation mechanism. For this process, a pyrrolidinecarboxamide (**28**), resulting from the corresponding ester (**8**), takes the place of DMF that is normally used in this reaction as a formylating reagent (Scheme **12**). The carboxamide is treated with phosphorus oxychloride to yield an iminium salt (**29**). The latter is very reactive and easily hydrolyzed in alkaline medium to obtain **1**. Various amines were studied, and the pyrrolidinecarboxamide appeared to be not only easy to synthesize, but also the most reactive in this cyclization process.

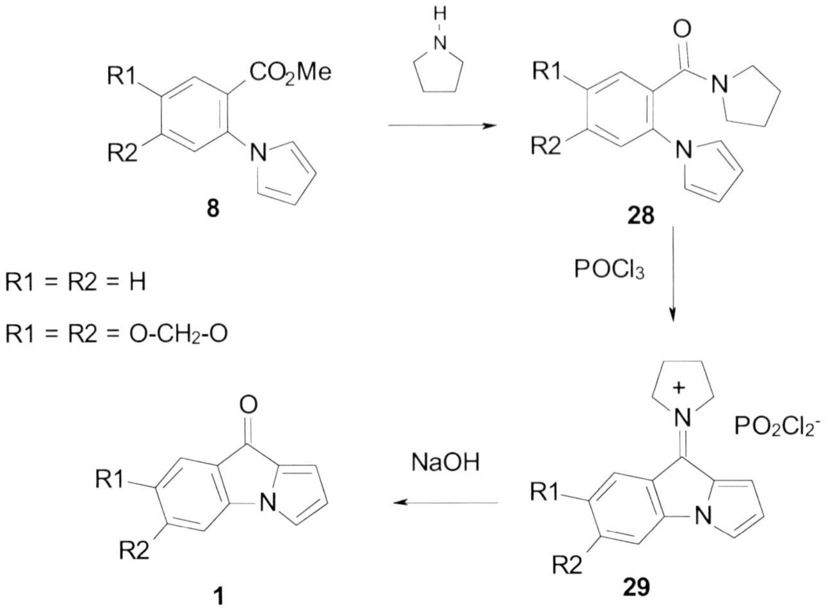

Scheme 12.

A more recent synthesis of 9*H*-pyrrolo[1,2-*a*]indol-9-ones (**1**), close to the latter method, proceeds through the acidic hydrolysis of 9-aryl-iminopyrroloindoles (**30**) resulting from the reaction between 2-(pyrrol-1-yl)benzaldehydes (**17**) and various arylamines (Scheme **13**) [22].

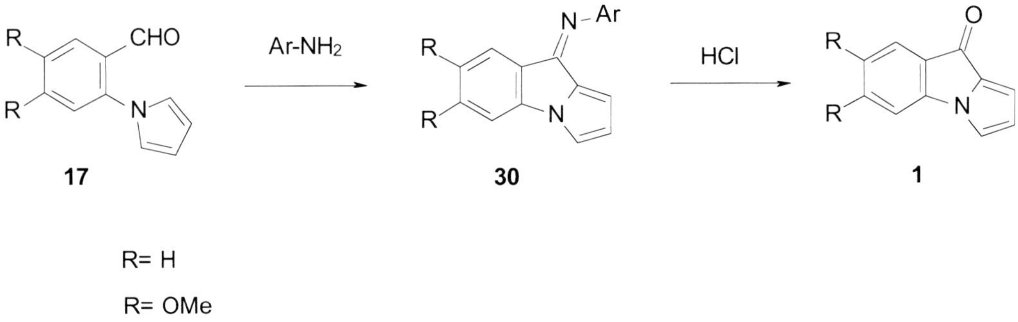

Scheme 13.

Finally, it was recently shown that it is possible to perform the one-pot cyclization of **1** starting from the alcohol (**31**) whose oxidation into **17**, using MnO_2 in refluxing toluene, is followed by a cyclization into the pyrroloindolol (**32**) which is itself oxidized into **1** (Scheme **14**) [23].

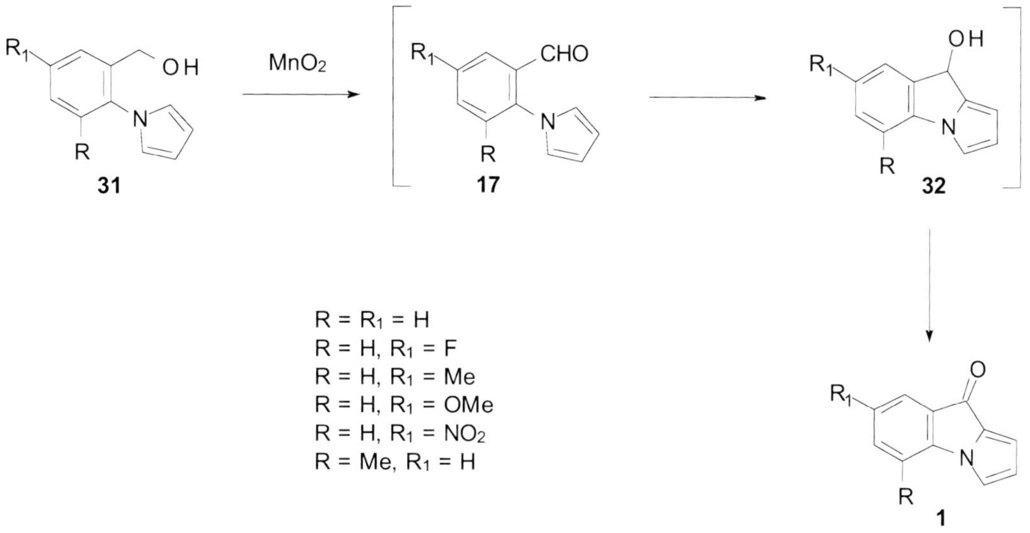

Scheme 14.

MISCELLANEOUS ROUTE

A recent miscellaneous annulation synthesis of **1** has been recently described in 54% yield by reacting arynes, generated *via* tetramethylammonium fluoride-induced elimination of *ortho*-silylphenyltriflate (**33**), with pyrrole-2-carboxylate (**34**) (Scheme **15**) [24].

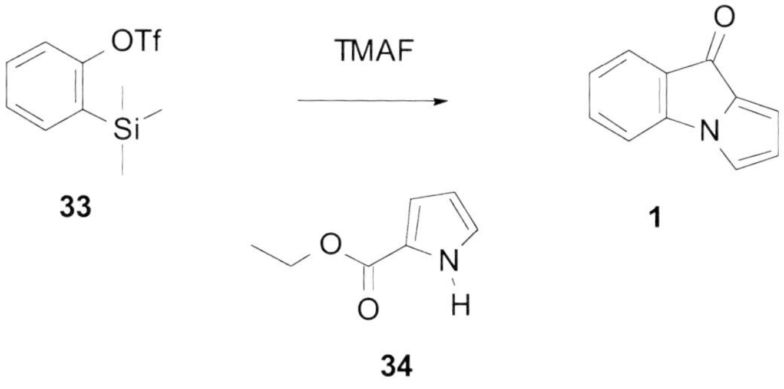

Scheme 15.

SYNTHESIS OF HETEROCYCLIC TRIPENTONES

The first synthesis of a heterocyclic isostere of the pyrrolo[1,2-*a*]indolone system was reported by Rault in 1983 in the thiophene series [25]. Some tetrahydrothienopyrrolizines had been previously reported but only as by-products of the cycloaddition reaction of thienylpyrrolidines with dimethyl acetylenedicarboxylate [26]. The pathway used in this synthesis follows the Vilsmeier-Haack approach. It starts by subjecting an aminothiophenecarboxylate (**35**) to a Clauson-Kaas reaction to produce a thienylpyrrolecarboxylate (**36**) (Scheme **16**). Cyclization of the latter generates the pyrrolidinecarboxamide (**37**), which is then treated with $POCl_3$ to yield the iminium salt (**38**) that is subsequently hydrolyzed into a thienopyrrolizinone. The first thiophenic tripentones, the two isomers *8*H-thieno[2,3-*b*]pyrrolizin-8-one (**39**) and *8*H-thieno[3,2-*b*]pyrrolizin-8-one (**40**), were obtained according to this sequence.

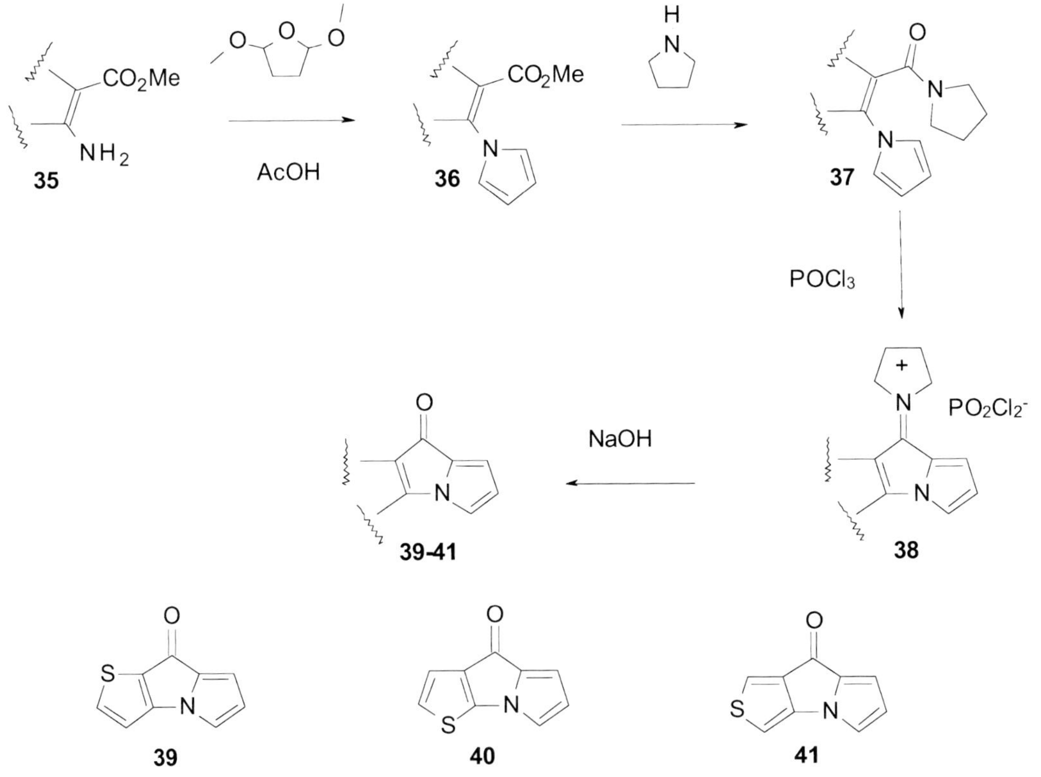

Scheme 16.

This useful methodology has also been successfully applied to the third and final *8*H-thieno[3,4-*b*]pyrrolizin-8-one series (**41**) [27] (Scheme 16) as well as to other heterocyclic tripentones, yielding pyrazino (**42**) [28], pyrazolo (**43**) [29], pyridothieno- (**44**), indolo (**45**) [30] or even more complex dimeric (**46**) [31] pyrrolizinones (Fig. **4**).

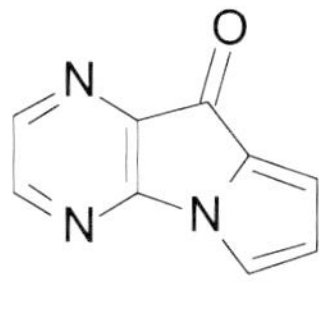

42

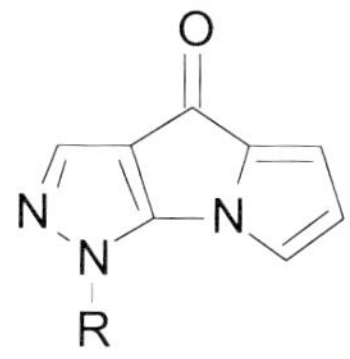

43

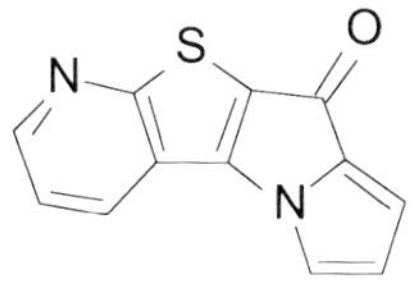

44

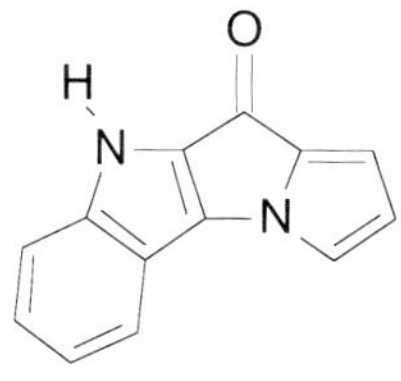

45

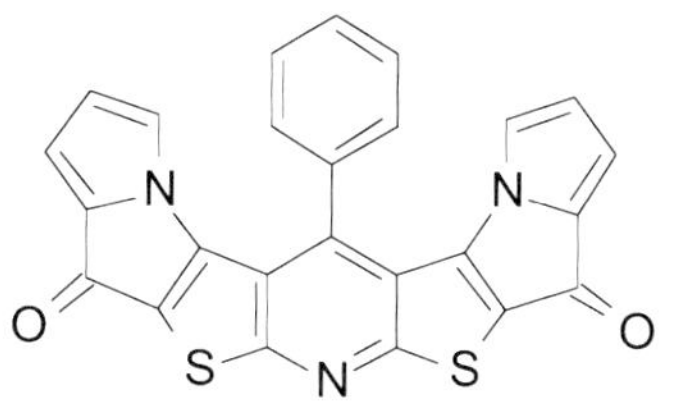

46

Fig. (4).

Pyridopyrrolizinones (**47**) seem not to be accessible through this pathway, because Ladurée [32] preferred Kametani's approach already used in the pyrroloindolone [16] and pyrazinopyrrolizinone [22] series (Scheme **17**).

Grande, however, recently reported the access to **47** using either the triphosgene or 2,5-diMeOTHF methods she previously described in pyrroloindolone series, starting from 2-pyrrolyl- (**48**) and 2-aminonicotinic (**49**) acids respectively (Scheme **17**) [8,10].

BIOLOGICAL PROPERTIES OF TRIPENTONES AND SAR

The first biological properties to be determined for the tripentone series concerned those of the dimethylpyrroloindolones such as compound **14** described above, which were identified as antidiabetic agents in 1974 [12,13]. Subsequently, a European patent claimed in 1984 that some spirosuccinimide derivatives (**50** and **51**) (Fig. **5**) had aldose reductase inhibitory activities able to prevent diabetic cataract [33].

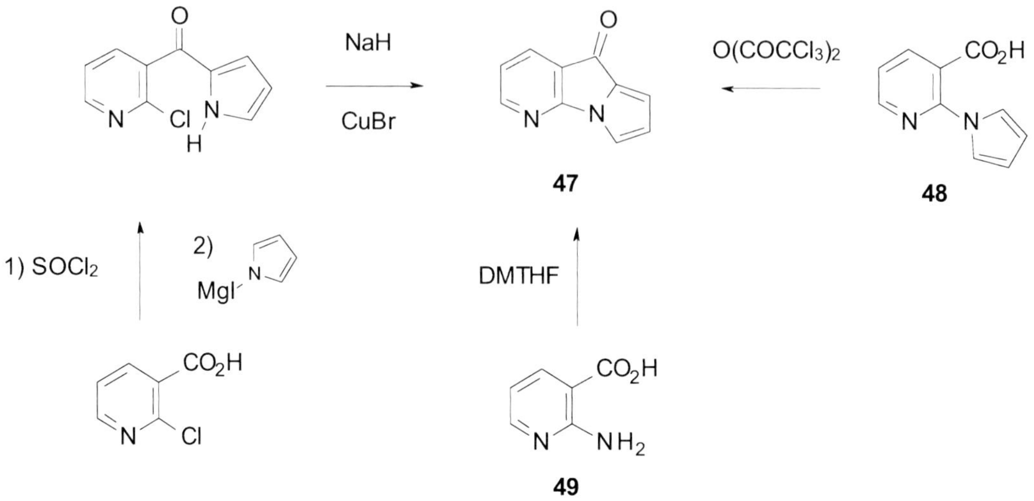

Scheme 17.

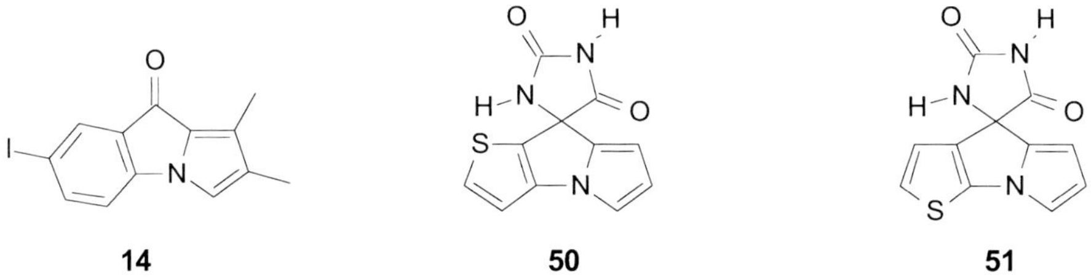

Fig. (5).

Also, some related pyrazolo[4,3-*b*]pyrrolizines (**52**) were described as being neuro-transmitter release enhancers useful in the treatment of cognitive disorders [34], and iminopyrroloindoles (**53**) (Fig. **6**) were reported as having non-amphetaminic stimulant activities on the central nervous system [35]. Oximino thiophene analogs of the latter, such as compound (**54**), were designed for their affinity for 5-HT_3 serotoninergic receptors. They were further used in defining the pharmacophore of this activity before being pharmacomodulated toward a more specific 5-HT transporter affinity [36-39].

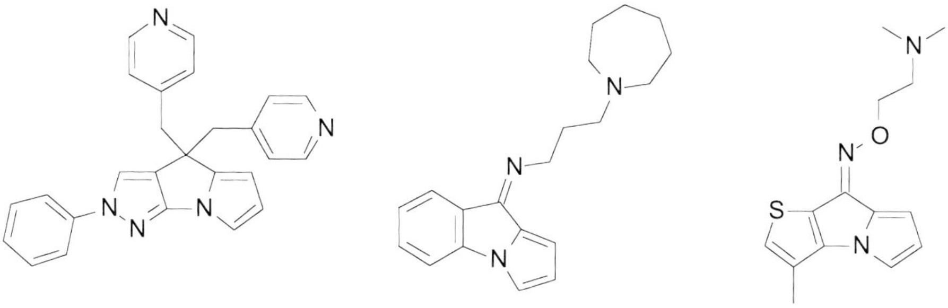

52 **53** **54**

Fig. (6).

However, it is in the anti-cancer field especially that compounds in the tripentone series have been studied as potential therapeutic agents. The cytotoxicity of the first training set of 3-aryl-*8*H-thieno[2,3-*b*]pyrrolizin-8-ones (**55**) was evaluated against the National Cancer Institute's 60 tumor-cell panel [40,41]. Their synthesis proceeded through convenient aminoesters (**56**) that are not commercially available, according to the original pathway as depicted in Scheme **18** [42-45].

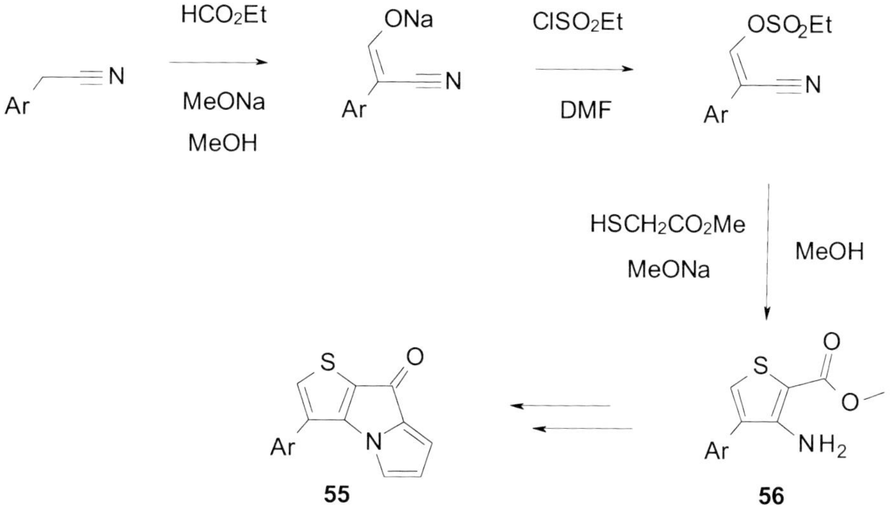

Scheme 18.

Among these tripentones, compound MR 16924 was selected because of its high anti-tumor activity, as evidenced by an IC_{50} in the submicromolar range (Table **1**).

Table 1. IC_{50} Values (μM) for MR 16924 Against a Selected Set of NCI Cell Lines

Compoud	MOLT4	EKVX	HCC2298	SF295	SKMEL2	OVCAR3	A498	DU145	HS578T
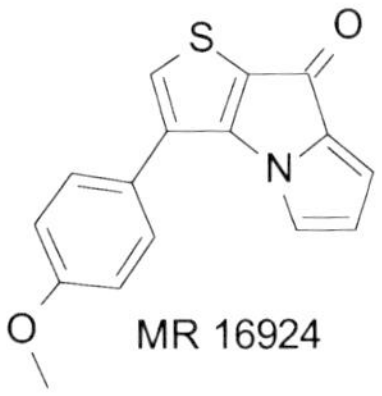 MR 16924	0.04	0.8	0.3	0.04	0.4	0.04	0.6	0.2	0.05

Subsequently, MR 16924 appeared as a hit and was pharmacomodulated with a view to transform it into a lead compound. To achieve this goal, three synthetic routes were elaborated to explore the influence of the thiophene ring (Route 1), the pyrrolizine core (Route 2), and the appendant phenyl ring (Route 3) on the activity of MR 16924 (Fig. **7**).

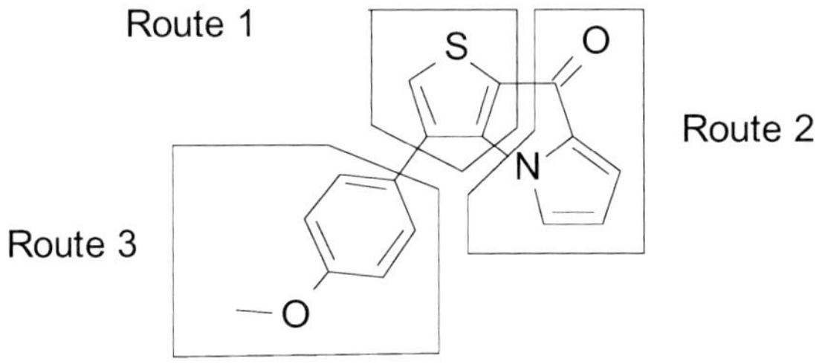

MR 16924

Fig. (7).

Route 1: Syntheses of pyrazolo (**57**, **58**) [46-48], pyrrolo (**59**) [49,50], furo (**60**) [41,51] and benzo (**61**) [41,52] analogs of MR 16964 were performed. The Vilsmeier-Haack methodology described above was used to achieve these syntheses. Again, appropriate arylaminoesters (**62-64**) appeared as crucial intermediates and were prepared from arylacetonitriles (**65**) as described for the preparation of the thiophene analogs (**55**) (Scheme **19**).

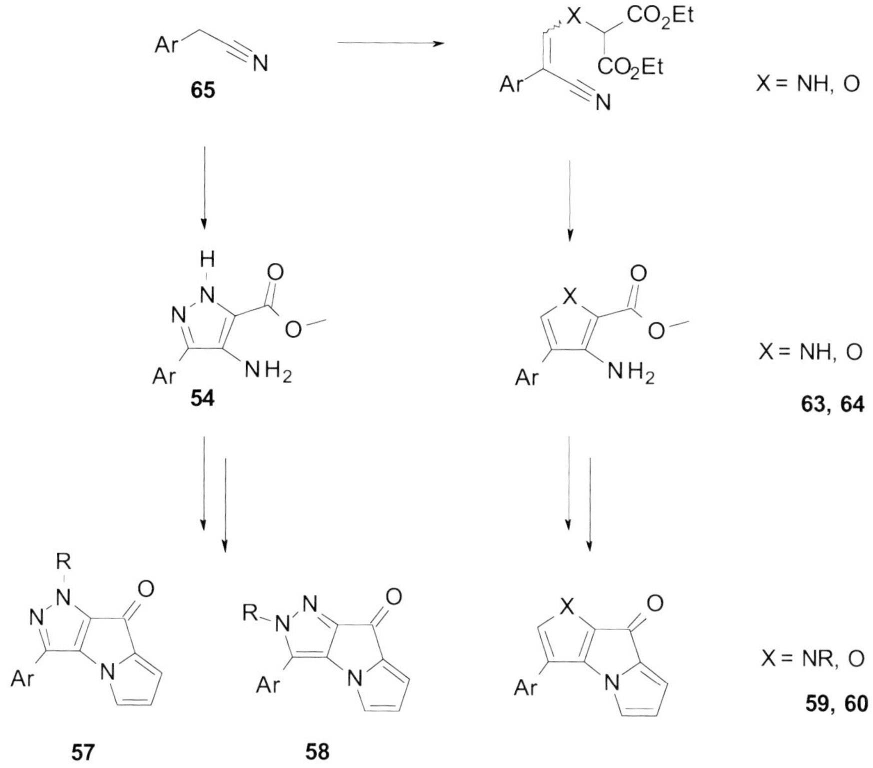

Scheme 19.

In the pyrroloindolone series, access to the 5-aryl derivatives (**61**) was achieved from 7-iodoisatin (**66**) as a precursor of the intermediate 3-iodoanthranilic acid (**67**) (Scheme **20**). The latter, after a Clauson-Kaas pyrrole ring formation, was cyclized under treatment with BBr_3 into a 5-iodotripentone (**68**) liable to engage in a Suzuki cross coupling with various arylboronic acids.

Although certain of these tripentones retained a cytotoxic effect against tumor cell lines (Leukemia L1210), albeit at a lower level, most were devoid of such activity, as illustrated for selected compounds in Table **2** [49]. The antiproliferative effect of MR 16924 thus appeared to be greatly linked to the thienopyrrolizinone core.

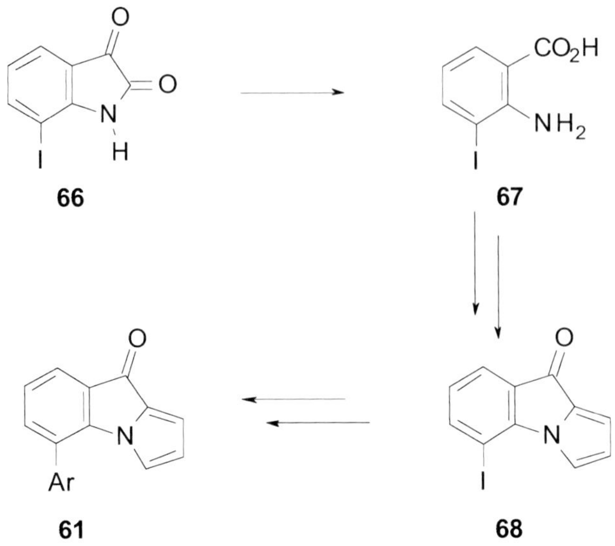

Scheme 20.

Route 2: Pharmacomodulation of the pyrrolizinone core of MR 16924 toward alcohols (**69**) and oximes (**70** and **71**) has been achieved by several teams (Fig. **8**) [41,53,54].

The compounds bearing both a substituted oximino group and a methylthio group on position 2 exhibited good activity against tumor cell lines such as Bel-7402, HT-1080, SGC-7901 and A549. Compound (**72**), especially, displayed promising antitumor activity, superior to that of cisplatin toward these tumor cells (Table **3**).

More drastic alteration to the pyrrolizinone core, consisting of deletion of the thiophene moiety (compound **73**) or enlargement of the pyrrolizine ring toward a pyrrolopyrazine one (compound **74**) (Fig. **9**) did not improve the antineoplastic activity (Table **4**) [41].

Route 3: The role of the 3-(*p*methoxyphenyl) ring on the activity of MR 16924 was also explored. The ring appears to be crucial, as evidenced by the total loss of cytotoxicity observed with the unsubstituted (**39**) and 3-methyl (**75**) tripentones against the L1210 cell line (Fig. **10**). The 2(-*p*methoxyphenyl) isomer (**76**) [55] exhibited a 50-fold lower antiproliferative effect than MR 16924 (IC_{50} = 9.4 µM *vs* 0.19 for MR 16924) [41].

Table 2. IC_{50} Values (μM) for Various Tripentones Against Leukemia L1210

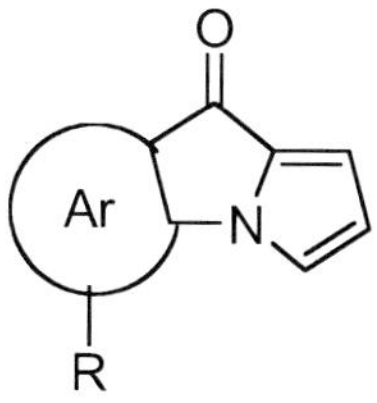

Ar	R	IC_{50} Against L1210 (μM)
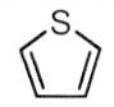	3-(*p*MeO-C_6H_4)	0.19
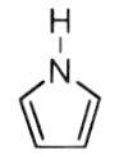	3-C_6H_5	36.9
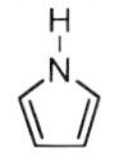	3-(*p*MeO-C_6H_4)	64.6
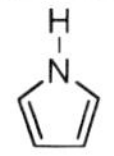	3-(*p*F-C_6H_4)	13.4
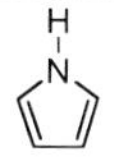	3-(*p*Me-C_6H_4)	10.9
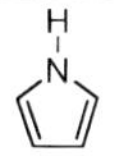	3-(*m,p*diOMe-C_6H_3)	11.8
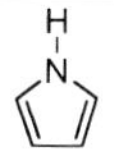	3-(thien-2-yl)	25.3
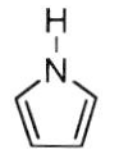	3-(thien-3-yl)	26.7
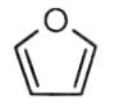	3-(*m,p*diOMe-C_6H_3)	24.2
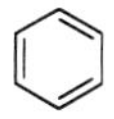	3-(*p*MeO-C_6H_4)	3.0
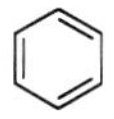	3-(*m,p*diOMe-C_6H_3)	72.2
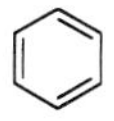	3-(thien-2-yl)	71.9
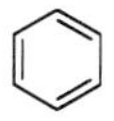	3-(fur-2-yl)	27.6

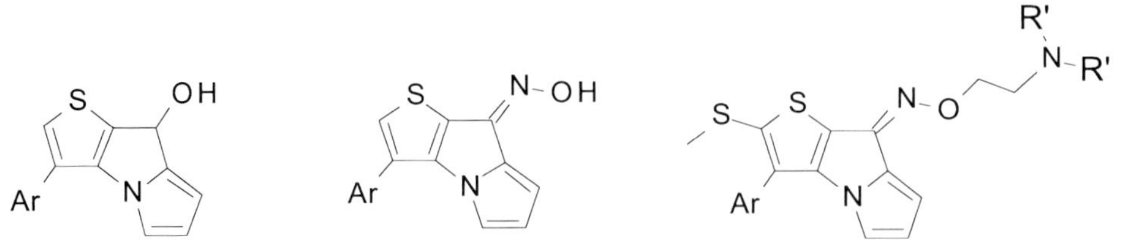

69 70 71

Fig. (8).

Table 3. IC_{50} Values (μM) for Compound 72 Against a Set of Cell Lines

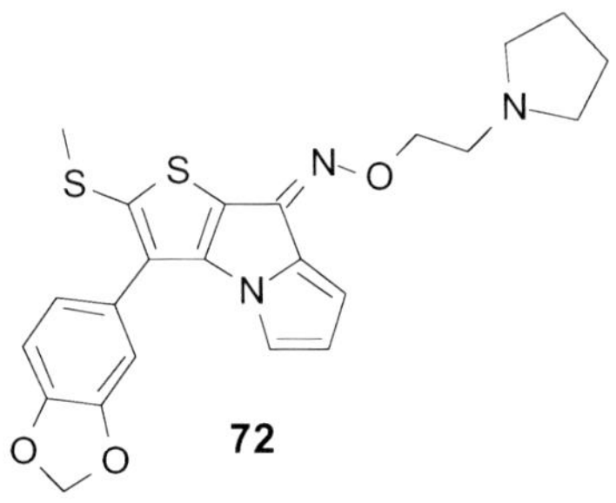

Compoud	Bel-7402	HT-1080	SGC-7901	A549
72	14.7	11.0	12.7	16.5
Cisplatin	25.2	16.7	13.3	23.3

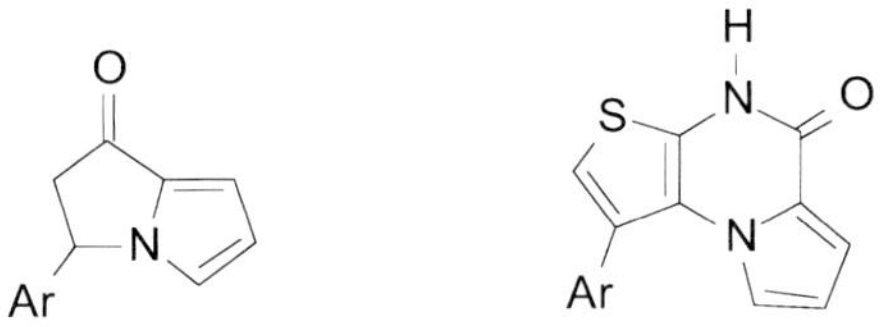

73 74

Fig. (9).

Considering the importance of both the nature and the position on the thienopyrrolizinone skeleton of the *p*-methoxyphenyl group, various alkoxy- and hydroxyphenyl derivatives were synthesized and evaluated against Leukemia L1210 (Table **4**) [56,41].

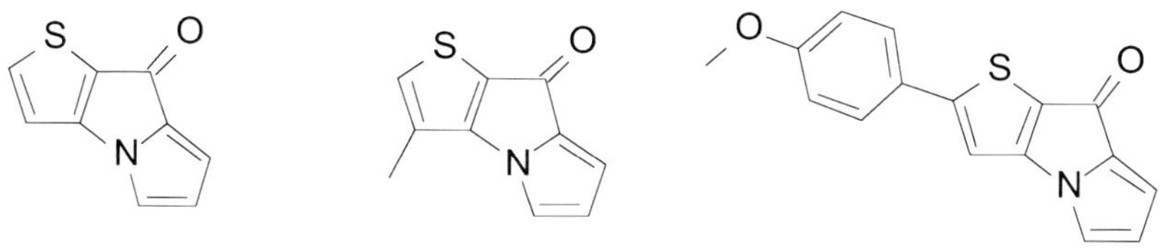

39 **75** **76**

Fig. (10).

Table 4. IC_{50} Values (μM) for Various Tripentones Against Leukemia L1210

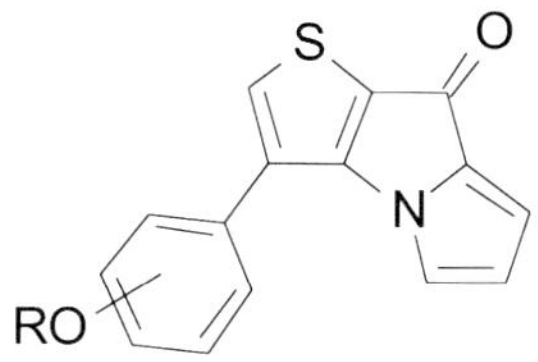

R	IC_{50} (μM)
*p*MeO-C_6H_4 **(MR 16924)**	0.19
*o*MeO-C_6H_4	18.9
*m*MeO-C_6H_4	5.2
*m,p*diMeO-C_6H_3	11.7
*o,m,p*triMeO-C_6H_2	36.4
m,pOCH_2O-C_6H_3	4.2
*m*BnO,*p*MeO-C_6H_3	5.4
*m*MeO,*p*BnO-C_6H_3	24.1
*m*HO,*p*MeO-C_6H_3 **(MR 22388)**	0.015
*m*MeO,*p*HO-C_6H_3	8
*o*HO-C_6H_4	3.7
*m*HO-C_6H_4	29
*p*HO-C_6H_4	30.1
*m,p*diHO-C_6H_3	0.28
*o,m,p*triHO-C_6H_2	12
*p*EtO-C_6H_4	0.43
pnC_3H_7O-C_6H_4	28.1
piC_3H_7O-C_6H_4	12.2
pnC_4H_9O-C_6H_4	29.6

These results, which identified three novel derivatives with sub-micromolar IC_{50} values, showed: (i) the para position of the phenyl ring is the best position for the methoxy group, (ii) the methoxy group is more favorable than larger alkoxy groups or hydroxyl groups, and (iii) an additional phenolic OH at the meta position of the phenyl ring greatly enhances the activity. Compound MR 22388 appeared to be the most cytotoxic in this series, with an IC_{50} of 15 nM. That is, MR 22388 is about 10-fold more potent than MR 16924 and 1000-fold more potent than its isomer (**77**) (Fig. **11**).

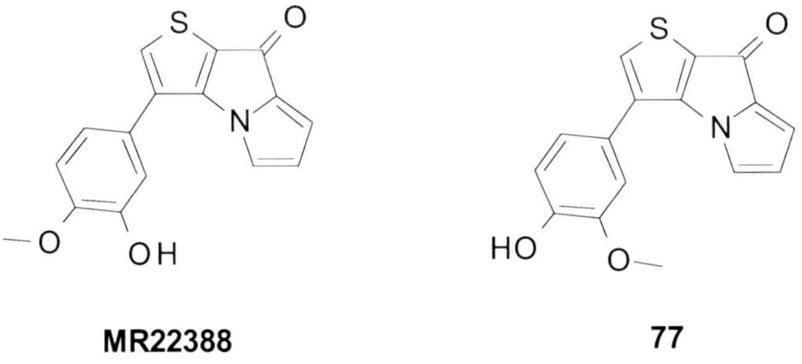

Fig. (11).

The cytotoxic activity of MR 22388 was confirmed against a set of selected tumor cell lines, including the resistant KBA1 cell line (Table **5**) [41]. Furthermore, it was established that the treated cells were arrested in the G2/M phase of the cell cycle with a significant percentage of cells having re-initiated a cycle of DNA synthesis (8N DNA content).

Table 5. IC_{50} Values (μM) for MR 22388 Against a Set of Tumor Cell Lines

B16	OVCAR3	A2780	DU145	A549	HT29	LS174T	KBA1	P388
0.023	0.031	0.040	0.043	0.045	0.71	0.89	0.015	0.021

This biological profile is consistent with an anti-tubulin effect and it was demonstrated that MR 22388 inhibits tubulin polymerization with the same range of magnitude as deoxypodophyllotoxin (IC_{50} = 2.9 *vs* 2.4 μM) (Fig. **12**).

This molecular target seems particularly sensitive to inhibitors bearing a *p*-methoxy-*m*-hydroxyphenyl ring such as combretastatin A-4 or certain synthetic compounds, including, for example, indolinone A-432411, anthracenone (**78**) and naphthothiophenone (**79**), which are known to mediate cytotoxic activities by binding with tubulin (Fig. **13**) [57-62].

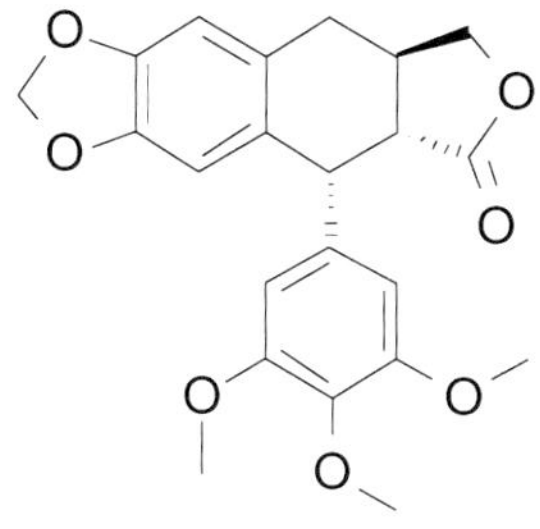

deoxypodophyllotoxin

Fig. (12).

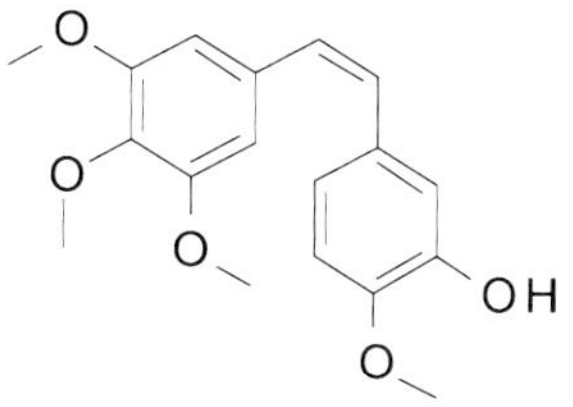

combretastatin A-4

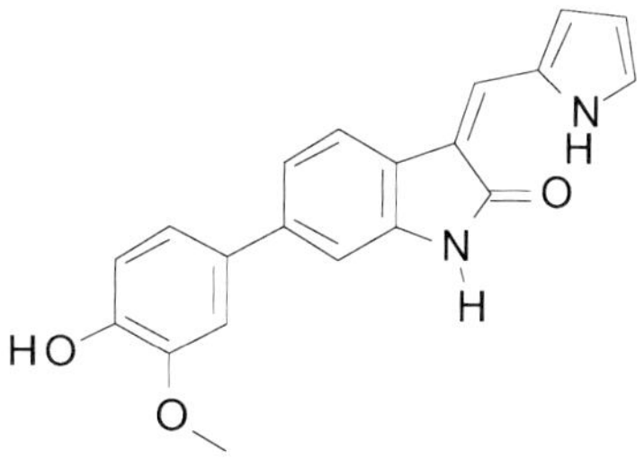

A-432411

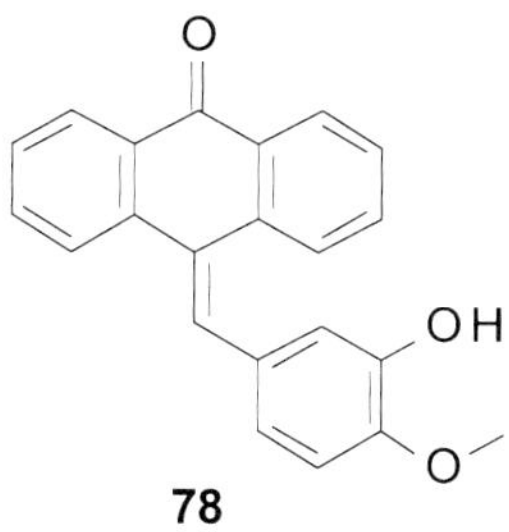

78

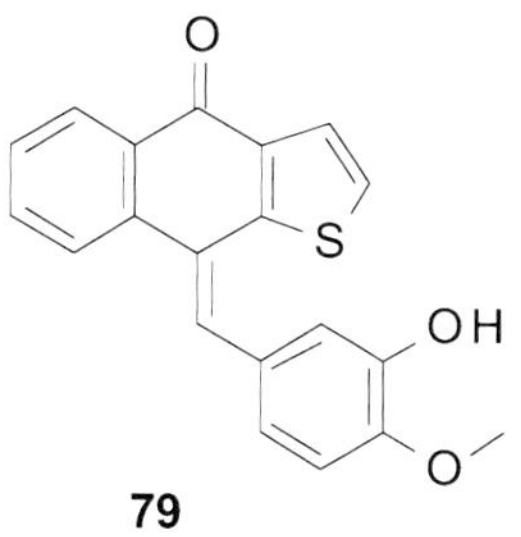

79

Fig. (13).

The crucial role played by the *p*-methoxy-*m*-hydroxyphenyl ring in the activity of MR 22388 was confirmed through the synthesis, by hydrogenative desulphurization of thienopyrrolizinones, of compound **80** which conserves a high cytotoxic effect against KB cells if it bears such a pending ring (Fig. **14**) [63]. This activity however was lost with compound **81**, which was synthesized as an analogue of combretastatin A4 [64].

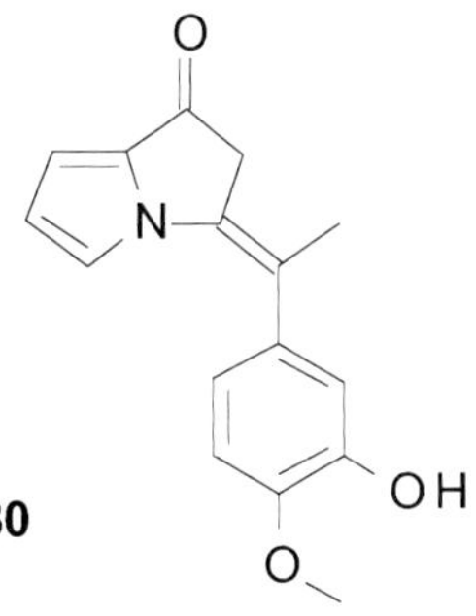

80

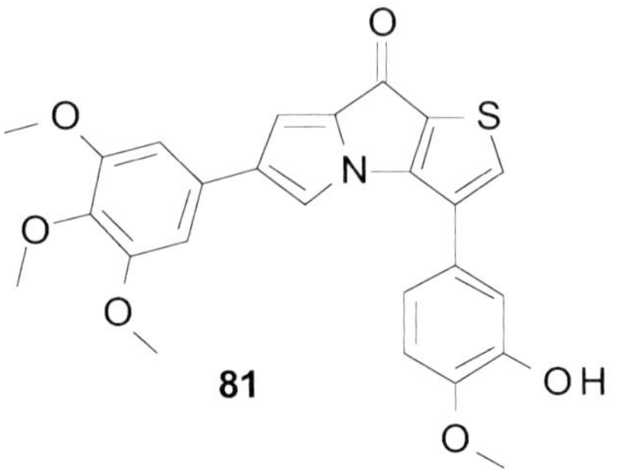

81

Fig. (14).

DEVELOPMENT OF MR 22388 AS A LEAD COMPOUND

The *in vivo* evaluation of MR 22388 in a P388 murine leukemia model appeared less conclusive than the results of the *in vitro* studies, probably due to the poor bioavailability of the tested drug as a consequence of its nearly total insolubility in water [41]. These results initiated a considerable effort to pharmacomodulate MR 22388 to improve its pharmacokinetic behavior. Two different methodologies were investigated to reach this goal.

The first entailed classical chemical pharmacomodulation of the series. A first attempt converted the OH phenolic group of MR 22388 into an ester, carbonate, phosphate or sulfamate group (Fig. **15**) [27]. However, the resulting compounds (**82**) seemed to be too rapidly hydrolyzed by cellular esterase(s), resulting in no significant gains in bioavailability. The derivatives showed *in vitro* cytotoxicity against L1210 cells, but this was probably due to presence of the parent compound.

The second effort aimed at improving the bioavailability of MR 22388 has lain in formulating the drug in lipidic nanoparticles by means of a phase inversion process [65]. Encapsulation of MR22388 in the colloidal carriers both significantly prolonged the drug's release profile and completely restored its potent antiproliferative activity on L1210 cells (Table **6**).

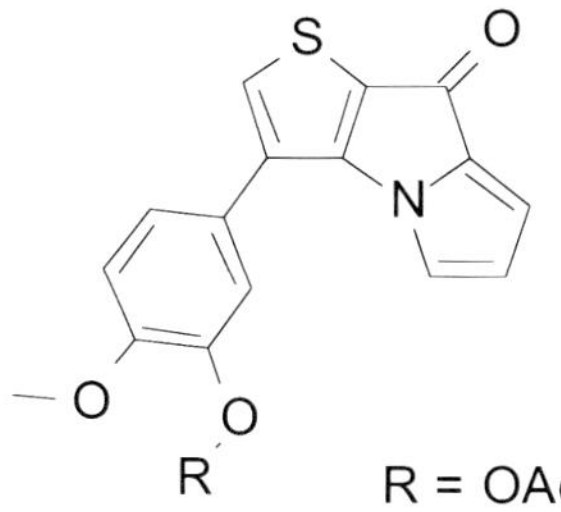

R = OAc, OCO_2Et, OCOtBu, $OP(O)OEt_2$, OSO_2NMe_2

82

Fig. (15).

Table 6. IC_{50} Values (μM) for Free MR 22388 and MR 22388 Loaded in Nanoparticles (NP) on L1210 Cells

Free MR 22388	Blank NP	MR 22388 NP
0.04	0.8	0.3

CONCLUSION

Tripentones are a novel, promising anti-cancer series whose possibilities for pharmacomodulation seem numerous. However, before any tripentone can emerge from an academic setting to become a potential commercial drug, it will be necessary to elucidate more fully the mechanism of tripentone action, which now appears to be more complex than solely the anti-tubulin activity that these compounds effectively exert. In particular, the poor correlation between the tubulin inhibitory effect and the cytotoxicity of MR 22388 suggests involvement of at least one other molecular target. Because diarylureapyrroloiosoindolones, such as compound (**83**) (Fig. **16**), have recently been designed as potent Cdk4/cyclin D inhibitors [66,67], some of the thiophene tripentones which show an antiproliferative effect were also evaluated against a set of kinases [27]. Among the tested compounds, MR 22388 exhibited the best inhibitory activity against Cdk1/cyclin B (IC_{50} = 5.5 μM) and GSK-3β (IC_{50} = 1.5 μM). Docking studies allowed both determination of the preferential orientation of MR 22388 inside the active site of GSK-3β and correlation of its affinity with those of some reference inhibitors [68].

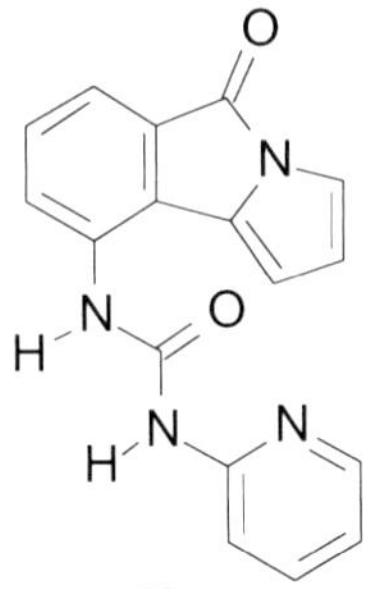

83

Fig. (16).

This kinase inhibitory effect of MR 22388, however, seems quite weak compared to its cytotoxic potency. Other molecular targets remain to be investigated in order to clearly identify the mechanism of the anti-cancer action of the tripentones. This goal remains an exciting challenge for motivated anti-cancer researchers.

CONFLICT OF INTEREST

The authors declare that there is no conflict of interest.

ACKNOWLEDGEMENTS

Declared none.

DISCLOSURE

This e-Book chapter is an updated version of the article entitled "Tripentones: A Promising Series of Potent Anti-Cancer Agents" published in 2009 in Anti-Cancer Agents in Medicinal Chemistry, 9(4), 369-380.

REFERENCES

[1] Hata, T.; Yoshimoto, S.; Sugawara, R.; Matsumae, A.; Kanamori, K.; Shima, T.; Hoshi, T. tomycin, a new antibiotic from Streptomyces. *J Antibiotics, (Tokyo), Ser. A.*, **1956**, *9(4)*, 141-6.

[2] Webb, J.S.; Cosulich, D.B.; Mowat, J.H.; Patrick, J.B.; Broschard, R.W.; Meyer, W.E.; lliams, R.P.; Wolf, C.F.; Fulmor, W.; Pidacks, D.; Lancaster, J.E. The Structures of tomycins A, B and C and Porfiromycin-Part I. *J. Am. Chem. Soc.*, **1962**, *84 (16)*, 3185-3187.

[3] Shirley, D.A.; Gross, B.H.; Roussel, P.A. Metalation of pyrrole, 1-methylpyrrole and 1-enylpyrrole with *n*-butyllithium. *J. Am. Chem. Soc.*, **1955**, *77 (20)*, 225-231.

[4] Kashulin, I.A.; Nifant'ev, I.E. Efficient method for the synthesis of hetareno-indanones based 3-arylhetarenes and their conversion into hetarenoindenes. *J. Org. Chem.*, **2004**, *69 (16)*, 76-5479.

[5] Campo, M.A.; Larock, R.C. Synthesis of fluoren-9-ones by the palladium-catalyzed clocarbonylation of *o*-halobiaryls. *J. Org. Chem.*, **2002**, *67 (16)*, 5616-5620.

[6] Josey, A.D.; Jenner, E.L. *N*-Functionnally substituted pyrroles. *J. Org. Chem.*, **1962**, *27 (7)*, 66-2470.

[7] Clauson-Kaas, N.; Tyle, Z. Preparation of *cis* and *trans* 2,5-dimethoxy-2-(acet-idomethyl)-2,5-dihydrofurans, of *cis* and *trans* 2,5-dimethoxy-2-(acetamidomethyl) rahydrofuran and of 1-phenyl-2-(acetamidomethyl)pyrrole. *Acta Chem. Scand.*, **1952**, *6*, 667-0.

[8] Aiello, F.; Garofalo, A.; Grande, F. Direct cyclization of *ortho*-(1*H*-pyrrol-1-yl)aryl and eroaryl carboxylic acids into fused pyrrolizinones. *Tetrahedron Lett.*, **2010**, *51*,6635-6636.

[9] Mazzola, V.J.; Bernardy, K.F.; Franck, R.W. 9*H*-pyrrolo[1,2-*a*]indoles. *J. Org. Chem.*, **1967**, *(2)*, 486–489.

[10] Aiello, F; Garofalo, A.; Grande, F. Convenient synthesis of fluorazone derivatives by one-pot rrolation/cyclization of anthranilic acids. *Tetrahedron Lett.*, **2011**, *52*, 5824-5826.

[11] Sugihara, H.; Matsumoto, N.; Kawamatsu, Y. Synthesis of pyrrolo[1,2-*a*]indole derivatives. *kagaku Zasshi*, **1974**, *94*, 181-188.

[12] Sugihara, H.; Matsumoto, N.; Hamuro, Y.; Kawamatsu, Y. Oral hypoglycaemic agents. 1-(2-rboxyphenyl)pyrroles. *Arzneimittel-Forsch.*, **1974**, *24*, 1560-1563.

[13] Kametani, T.; Takahashi, K. Synthesis of pyrrolo[1,2-*a*]indoles and related systems. *terocycles*, **1978**, *9(3)*, 293-351.

[14] Huisgen, R.; Laschtuvka, E. A new synthesis of derivatives of pyrrole. *Ber.*, **1960**, *93*, 65-81.

[15] Giuliano, R.; Porretta, G.C.; Scalzo, M.; Chimenti, F.; Artico, M.; Dolfini, E.; Morasca, L. tiblastic substances. I. Synthesis, cytotoxicity activity of 9*H*-pyrrolo[1,2-*a*]indole derivatives. *rmaco. Edizione Scientifica*, **1972**, *27*, 1091-1103.

[16] Siuta, G.J.; Franck, R.W.; Ozorio, A.A. Meta photo-Fries reaction. *J. Chem. Soc. Chem. mm.*, **1974**, *21*, 910.

[17] Crump, D.R.; Franck, R.W.; Gruska, R.; Ozorio, A.A.; Pagnotta, M.; Siuta, G.J.; White, J.G. proaches to the mitomycins. A meta photo-Fries reaction. *J. Org. Chem.*, **1977**, *42 (1)*, 105-8.

[18] Friary, R.J.; Gilligan, J.M.; Szajewski, R.P.; Falci, K.J.; Franck, R.W. Heterocyclic syntheses the intramolecular acylation of enamines derived from amino acids. *J. Org. Chem.*, **1973**, *33)*, 3487–3491.

[19] Kametani, T.; Ohsawa, T.; Takahashi, K.; Ihara, M.; Fukumoto, K. Photo-oxygenation of 9-o-7-methoxy-6-methyl-9*H*-pyrrolo[1,2-*a*]indole as a synthetic approach to the mitomycine. *terocycles*, **1976**, *4(10)*, 1637-1644.

[20] Rault, S.; Cugnon de Sevricourt, M.; Godard, A.; Robba, M. A Convenient synthesis of new inopyrroloindoles *via* an iminium salt. *Tetrahedron Lett.*, **1985**, *26 (19)*, 2305-2308.

[21] Bouyazza, L.; Lancelot, J.C.; Rault, S.; Robba, M.; Quermonne, M.A. A Convenient thesis of new aminomethylenedioxypyrroloindoles *via* an iminium salt, *J. Heterocycl. Chem.*, **91**, *28*, 373-377.

[22] Kobayashi, K.; Himei, Y.; Fukamachi, S.; Tanmatsu, M.; Morikawa, O.; Konishi, H. nthesis of 9-arylamino- and (*Z*)-9-arylimino-9*H*-pyrrolo[1,2-*a*]indoles by reaction of 2-rrol-1-yl)benzaldehydes with aryl amines. *Tetrahedron*, **2007**, *63 (20)*, 4356-4359.

[23] Aiello, F.; Garofalo, A.; Grande, F. Efficient synthesis of 9*H*-pyrrolo[1,2-*a*]indol-9-one rivatives based on active manganese dioxide promoted intramolecular cyclization. *rahedron*, **2010**, *66*, 274-277.

[24] Giacometti, R.D.; Ramtohul, Y.K. Synthesis of polycyclic indolone and pyrroloindolone erocycles *via* the annulation of indole- and pyrrole-2-carboxylate esters with arynes. *Synlett*, **09**, *12*, 2010-2016.

[25] Rault, S.; Lancelot, J.C.; Effi, Y.; Robba, M. Thiénopyrrolizines: New condensed eterocyclic systems. *Heterocycles*, **1983**, *20 (3)*, 477-480.

[26] Reinhoudt, D.N.; Trompenaars, W.P.; Geevers, J. Reactions of thiophenes with acetylenes in ar solvents; a novel annulation reaction. *Tetrahedron Lett.*, **1976**, *17 (51)*, 4777-4780.

[27] Rochais, C.; Lescot, E.; Lisowski, V.; Lepailleur, A.; Sopkova de Oliveira-Santos, J.; Bureau, Dallemagne, P.; Meijer, L.; Rault, S. Synthesis and biological evaluation of enopyrrolizines, a new family of CDK/GSK-3 inhibitors. *J. Enzyme Inhib. Med. Chem.*, **2004**, *(6)*,585-593.

[28] Ladurée, D.; El Kashef, H. ; Robba, M. Synthesis of 9*H*-pyrrolo[1,2-*a*]-1,4-diazaindol-9-one. *terocycles*, **1984**, *22 (2)*, 299-301.

[29] Massa, S.; Mai, A.; Artico, M. Heterocyclic system. XI. Synthesis of 1*H*,4*H*-pyrazolo[4,3-yrrolizine and 2*H*,4*H*-pyrazolo[4,3-*b*]pyrrolizine derivatives. *Heterocyclic Chem.*, **1990**, *27*, 05-1808.

[30] Diana, P.; Stagno, A.; Barraja, P.; Montalbano, A.; Carbone, A.; Parrino, B.; Cirrincione, G. nthesis of the new ring system pyrrolizino[2,3-*b*]indol-4(5*H*)-one. *Tetrahedron*, **2011**, *67*, 74-3379.

[31] Peinador, C.; Veiga, M.C.; Vilar, J.; Quintela, J.M. A synthesis of heterocyclic ring systems. rido[3',2':4,5]thieno[2,3-*b*]pyrrolizine and pyrido[6',5':4,5][3',2':4,5]di-thieno[2,3-*b'*:2,3-ipyrrolizine. *Heterocycles*, **1994**, *38 (6)*, 1299-1305.

[32] Ladurée, D.; Robba, M. Synthesis of 5*H*-pyrrolo[1,2-*a*]-1-azaindole and derivatives. *terocycles*, **1984**, *22 (2)*, 303-305.

[33] York, B.M. Spiro-tricyclicaromatic succinimide derivatives as inhibitors of aldose-reductase. *ropean Patent Appl. 84110855.8*, **1984**.

[34] Teleha, A.C.; Wilkerson, W.W. Novel polycyclic systems, and deriveratives thereof, as urotransmitter release enhancers useful in the treatment of cognitive disorders. *World Patent pl. 24131*, **1994**.

[35] Rault, S.; Lancelot, J.C.; Bouyazza, L.; Robba, M.; Quermonne, M.A.; Nammathao, B.; uchahi-Raoul, J.; Marcy, R. Synthèse et étude préliminaire de l'activité psychotrope lkylamino et iminopyrrolo[1,2-*a*] indoles. *Eur. J. Med. Chem.* **1991**, *26 (9)*, 939-946.

[36] Baglin, I.; Daveu, C.; Lancelot, J.C.; Bureau, R.; Dauphin, F.; Pfeiffer, B.; Renard, P.; lagrange, P.; S. Rault. First tricyclic oximino derivatives as 5-HT3 ligands. *Bioorg. Med. em. Lett.*, **2001**, *11 (4)*, 453-457.

[37] Bureau, R.; Daveu, C.; Baglin, I.; Sopkova-de Oliveira Santos, J.; Lancelot, J.C.; Rault, S. sociation of two 3D QSAR analyses. Application to the study of partial agonist serotonin-3 ands. *J. Chem. Inf. Comput. Sci.*, **2001**, *41 (3)*, 815-823.

[38] Bureau, R.; Daveu, C.; Lancelot, J.C.; Rault, S. Molecular design based on 3D-pharmacore. plication to 5-HT subtypes receptors. *J. Chem. Inf. Comput. Sci.*, **2002**, *42 (2)*, 429-436.

[39] Lepailleur, A.; Bureau, R.;Lemaître, S.; Dauphin, F.; Lancelot, J.C.; Contesse, V.; Lenglet, Delarue, C.; Vaudry, H.; Rault, S. Molecular design based on 3-D pharmacophore. plication to 5-HT7 receptors. *J. Chem. Inf. Comput. Sci.*, **2004**, *44 (3)*, 1148-1152.

[40] Lisowski, V.; Enguehard, C.; Lancelot, J.C.; Caignard, D.H.; Lambel, S.; Leonce, S.; Pierre, Atassi, G.; Renard, P.; Rault, S. Design, synthesis and antiproliferative activity of entones: A new series of antitubulin agents. *Bioorg. Med. Chem. Lett.*, **2001**, *11 (16)*, 2205-08.

[41] Lisowski, V.; Léonce, S.; Kraus-Berthier, L.; Sopkova-de-Oliveira Santos, J.; Pierré, A.; assi, G.; Caignard, D.H.; Renard, P.; Rault, P. Design, synthesis and evaluation of a novel enopyrrolizinone series as antitubulin agents. *J. Med. Chem.*, **2004**, *47 (6)*, 1448-1464.

[42] Fiesselman, H. Uber hydroxy- und aminothiophene (On hydroxy- and aminothiophene). *gew. Chem.*, **1959**, *11*, 377.

[43] Kirsch, G.; Cagniant, D.; Cagniant, P. Synthesis of 3-aminothiophenes from aryl and arylacetonitrile. *J. Heterocycl. Chem.*, **1982**, *19*, 443-445.

[44] Rault, S.; Lancelot, J.C.; Letois, B.; Robba, M.; Labat, Y. New derivatives of 3-mercapto-2-noic acid and process for their preparation. *French Patent Appl. 9203732*, **1992**.

[45] Lancelot, J.C.; Letois, B.; Rault, S.; Robba, M.; Rogosca, M. Thienopyrrolizines: new ndensed triheterocyclic systems. *J. Heterocycl. Chem.*, **1994**, *31*, 501-504.

[46] Tarzia, G.; Panzone, G.; De Paoli, A.; Schiatti, P.; Selva, D. Antiinflammatory properties of a ies of 4-amino-5-arylpyrazoles. *Farmaco. Edizione Scientifica*, **1984**, *39*, 618-636.

[47] Rochais, C.; Lisowski, V.; Dallemagne, P.; Rault, S. First synthesis of arylpyrrolo-and razolopyrrolizinones as useful agents with potential biological interest. *Tetrahedron Lett.*, **04**, *45 (33)*, 6353-6355.

[48] Rochais, C.; Sopkova-de Oliveira Santos, J.; Dallemagne, P.; Rault, S. Synthesis of novel razolopyrrolizinones as prospective anticancer agents. *Heterocycles*, **2006**, *68 (10)*, 2063-77.

[49] Rochais, C.; Lisowski, V.; Dallemagne, P.; Rault, S. First Synthesis of methyl 3-amino-4-t)aryl-1H-pyrrole-2-carboxylates as useful scaffolds in medicinal chemistry. *Tetrahedron*, **04**, *60 (9)*, 2267-2270.

[50] Rochais, C.; Lisowski, V.; Dallemagne, P.; Rault, S. Synthesis and biological evaluation of vel pyrrolopyrrolizinones as anticancer agents. *Bioorg. Med. Chem.*, **2006**, *14 (24)*, 8162-75.

[51] Lisowski, V.; Vu, D.N.; Feng, X.; Rault, S. Preparation of new ethyl 3-amino-4-arylfurane-2-boxylates. *Synthesis*, **2002**, *(6)*, 753-756.

[52] Lisowski, V.; Robba, M.; Rault, S. Efficient synthesis of new 3-(het) aryl-anthranilic acids a Susuki cross couping reaction of 7-iodoisatin with (het) arylboronic acids in water. *J. Org. em.*, **2000**, *65 (13)*, 4193-4194.

[53] Guo, S.; Zhao, Y.; Zhao, X.; Zhang, S.; Xie, L.; Kong, W., Gong, P. Synthesis and anti-tumor ivities of novel methylthio-, sulfinyl-, and sulfonyl-8*H*-thieno[2,3-*b*]pyrrolizin-8-oximino rivatives. *Arch. Pharm. Chem. Life. Sci.*, **2007**, *340 (8)*, 416-423.

[54] Guo, S.; Zhao, Y.; Li, R.; Xie, L.; Yang, Y.; Gong, P. Synthesis and biological evaluation of vel tricyclic oximino derivatives as antitumor agents. *Chem. Res. Chinese Universities*, **2008**, *(1)*, 47-53.

[55] Rault, S.; Robba, M.; Lancelot, J.C.; Prunier, H.; Renard, P.; Pfeiffer, B.; Guardiola-maître, B.; Rettori, M.C. Tricyclic oxime ether process for their preparation and armaceutical compositions containing them. *Eur. Pat. Appl. 0718299A1*, **1996**.

[56] Rault, S.; Enguehard, C.; Lancelot, J.C.; Robba, M.; Atassi, G.; Pierré, A.; Caignard, D.H.; nard, P. *Fr. Pat. Appl. 09552*, **1998**; *Eur. Patent 0982308*, **2000**; *Jpn. Kokai Tokkyo Koho 4572*, **2000**.

[57] Jordan, M.A. Mechanism of action of antitumor drugs that interact with microtubules and ulin. *Curr. Med. Chem. Anticancer Agents*, **2002**, *2 (1)*, 1-17.

[58] Li, Q.; Sham, H.L. Discovery and development of antimitotics agents that inhibit tubulin ymerisation for the treatment of cancer. *Expert Opin. Ther. Patents*, **2002**, *12 (11)*, 1663-02.

[59] Pettit, G.R.; Singh, S.B.; Hamel, E.; LIN, C.M.; Alberts, D.S.; Garcia-Kendall, D. Isolation d structure of the strong cell growth and tubulin inhibitor combretastatin A-4. *Experitientia*, **89**, *45(2)*, 209-211.

[60] Chen, Z.; Merta, P.J.; Lin, N.H.; Tahir, S.K.; Kovar, P.; Sham, H.L.; Zhang, H. A-432411, a vel indolinone compound that disrupts spindle pole formation and inhibits human cancer cell wth. *Mol. Cancer Ther.*, **2005**, *4(4)*, 562-568.

[61] Prinz, H.; Ishii, Y.; Hirano, T.; Stoiber, T.; Camacho-Gomez, J.A.; Schmidt, P.; Düssman, Burger, A.M.; Prehn, J.H.; Günther, E.G.; Umezawa, K. Novel benzylidene-9(10*H*)-hracenones as highly active antimicrotubule agents. Synthesis, antiproliferative activity, and ibition of tubulin polymerization. *J. Med. Chem.*, **2003**, *46(15)*, 3382-3394.

[62] Zuse, A.; Schmidt, P.; Baasner, S.; Böhm, K.J.; Müller, K.; Gerlach, M.; Günther, E.G.; ger, E.; Prinz, H. Sulfonate derivatives of naphtho[2,3-*b*]thiophen-4(9*H*)-one and 9(*10*H)-hracenone as highly active antimicrotubule agents. Synthesis, anti-proliferative activity, and ibition of tubulin polymerization. *J. Med. Chem.*, **2007**, *50 (24)*, 6059-6066.

[63] Perri, V.; Rochais, C.; Legay, R.; Cresteil, T.; Dallemagne, P.; Rault, S. Hydrogenative sulphurization of thienopyrrolizinones: an easy and selective access to (*Z*)-enethylidenepyrrolizinones with *in vitro* cytotoxic activity. *Eur. J. Med. Chem.*, **2010**, *45*, 46-1150.

[64] Perri, V.; Rochais, C.; Cresteil, T.; Dallemagne, P.; Rault, S. Synthesis, reactivity and logical evaluation of novel halogenated tripentones. *Bioorg. Med. Chem.*, **2009**, *17*, 7783–88.

[65] Malzert-Freon, A.; Vrignaud, S.; Saulnier, P.; Lisowski, V.; Benoît, J.P.; Rault, S. rmulation of substained release nanoparticles loaded with a tripentone, a new anticancer agent. *J. Pharm.*, **2006**, *320*, 157-164.

[66] Honma, T.; Hayashi, K.; Aoyama, T.; Hashimoto, N; Machida, T.; Fukasawa, K.; Iwama, T.; Ikeura, C.; Ikuta, M.; Suzuki-Takahashi, I.; Iwasawa, Y.; Hayama, T.; Nishimura, S.; Morishima, H. Structure-based generation of a new class of potent Cdk4 inhibitors: new *de novo* design strategy and library design. *J. Med. Chem*, **2001**, *44 (26)*, 4615-4627.

[67] Kawanishi, N.; Sugimoto, T.; Shibata, J., Nakamura, K.; Masutani, K.; Ikuta, M. Hirai, H. Structure-based drug design of a highly potent CDK1,2,4,6 inhibitor with novel macrcyclic quinoxalin-2-one structure. *Bioorg. Med. Chem. Lett.*, **2006**, *16 (19)*, 5122-5126.

[68] Lescot, E.; Bureau, R.; Sopkova-de Oliveira Santos, J.; Rochais, C.; Lisowski, V.; Lancelot, J.C.; Rault, S. ^{3}D-QSAR and docking studies of selectives GSK-3 inhibitors. Comparison with a thieno[2, 3-*b*]pyrrolizinones derivative, a new potential lead for GSK-3 Ligands. *J. Chem. Inf. Model.*, **2005**, *45 (3)*, 708-715.

CHAPTER 7

Selective Estrogen Receptor Modulators as Treatments and Preventives of Breast Cancer

Surojeet Sengupta[1], Jing Peng[2] and Virgil C. Jordan[*,1]

[1]Department of Oncology, Lombardi Cancer Center, Georgetown University Medical Center, Washington, DC 20057, USA; [2]Fox Chase Cancer Center, Philadelphia, PA 19111-2497, USA

Abstract: Estrogen is important in human health and diseases. Estrogen binds to estrogen receptors (ER), alpha and beta which subsequently function as transcription factors. Selective estrogen receptor modulators (SERMs) are synthetic molecules which bind to ER and can modulate its transcriptional capabilities in different ways in diverse estrogen target tissues. Tamoxifen, the first SERM, is extensively used for targeted therapy of ER positive breast cancers and is also approved as the first chemo-preventive agent for lowering breast cancer incidence in high risk women. The strategy for the therapeutic and preventive applications of tamoxifen was initially demonstrated in the laboratory which laid the foundation for its success in the clinic. Unfortunately, use of tamoxifen is associated with *de novo* and acquired resistance and some undesirable side effects. The molecular study of the resistance provides an opportunity to understand the mechanism of SERM action which may further help in designing new and improved SERMs. Clinical studies demonstrate that another SERM, raloxifene, used to treat post-menopausal osteoporosis, is also as efficient as tamoxifen in preventing breast cancers with fewer side effects. Overall, these findings provide opportunities for SERMs as a new class of drugs which not only can be used for therapeutic and preventive purposes of breast cancers but also for other disease states. The goal is to create new SERMs with a better therapeutic profile and fewer side effects.

Keywords: Breast cancer, osteoporosis, estrogen receptor, tamoxifen, raloxifene, SERMs, endocrine therapy, drug resistance.

1. INTRODUCTION

Breast cancer incidences and death rates have dropped significantly during recent years, which is associated strongly with improvement in early detection methods

***Address correspondence to Virgil C. Jordan:** Lombardi Comprehensive Cancer Center, Georgetown University Medical Center, 3970 Reservoir Rd NW, Washington, DC 20057, USA; Tel: 202.687.2897; Fax: 202.687.6402; E-mail: vcj2@georgetown.edu

Michelle Prudhomme (Ed)

and decrease of menopausal hormone replacement therapy (HRT) [1, 2]. HRT, in the form of estrogen alone or estrogen plus progesterone, had been widely used since the 1960s until recent years, to treat conditions associated with aging as well as unpleasant menopausal symptoms. HRT was also known to protect post-menopausal women from osteoporosis and also thought to protect women from heart disease and Alzheimer's disease. However, the Women's Health Initiative (WHI) study indicated that taking estrogen with or without progesterone for 5 or more years placed the women at higher risk of breast cancer, Alzheimer's disease, heart disease, blood clot and stroke, although HRT is effective to reduce the risks of osteoporosis and colon cancer [3, 4]. The Million Women Study (MWS) conducted in the UK also showed that women taking HRT were more likely to develop breast cancer [5], endometrial cancer [6] and ovarian cancer [7]. In the US, the use of estrogen-plus-progestin HRT has dropped almost 50% when the WHI announced their findings in 2002, and this was followed by a sharp 7% decrease of new breast cancers in 2003 [2]. Although the decrease of HRT uses is not the sole reason leading to less breast cancer incidences, much effort has been focused on finding more effective and safer compounds to replace HRT which not only relieve menopausal symptoms but also prevent and treat hormone-responsive cancers. One most promising approach is to use selective estrogen receptor modulators (SERMs).

SERMs are synthetic compounds that bind to estrogen receptors alpha and/or beta (ERα and/or ERβ) and exert estrogenic or antiestrogenic activities in a tissue/cell-specific manner. The first SERM that has been used successfully in the clinic to prevent and treat breast cancer is tamoxifen, a failed postcoital contraceptive that evolved into the "gold standard" for breast cancer treatment [8, 9]. Tamoxifen is estimated to have saved the lives of over 400,000 women with breast cancer [8]. The second generation SERM, raloxifene (formally called keoxifene), failed as a treatment for breast cancer but is effective against osteoporosis and prevents breast cancer at the same time. Raloxifene is as effective as tamoxifen to reduce invasive breast cancer risks without an increase in the risk of endometrial cancer observed with tamoxifen [10]. Indeed a recent study suggests that raloxifene might even be effective in preventing endometrial cancer [11]. These findings have acted as a catalyst for the search of new SERMs which are estrogen-like in bones and circulating lipids but antiestrogenic in women's reproductive organs and therefore are anti-cancer agents. However, there are problems associated with the current SERMs such as drug resistance and side effects. For example, both tamoxifen and raloxifene increase both hot flashes and blood clots [12].

Besides SERMs, other endocrine therapies target the ER indirectly to prevent and treat breast cancer. Aromatase inhibitors (AIs) that block the synthesis of estrogen from androgen in peripheral tissues have been extensively studied and show efficacy equivalent or superior to tamoxifen to treat postmenopausal breast cancer [13]. Since the mechanism for AIs to treat ER-positive breast cancer is to deplete estrogen in postmenopausal patients, they do not increase risks of endometrium cancer or blood clot and may be a better choice for postmenopausal breast cancer patients than tamoxifen. However, AIs are not effective in premenopausal women with actively functioning ovaries because AIs do not inhibit ovarian estrogen production. In addition, AIs lack the estrogenic protective function for cardiovascular diseases or osteoporosis. As a result, the side effects of AIs are mostly consistent with estrogen deprivation. AIs are associated with a greater incidence of bone loss and musculoskeletal symptoms, and probably higher risk of cardiovascular disease suggested by adjuvant trials comparing AIs and tamoxifen [14]. However, AIs are associated with a lower incidence of gynecological symptoms, thromboembolic diseases and hot flashes compared to tamoxifen in adjuvant setting [14]. Another strategy is to use selective estrogen receptor down-regulators (SERDs), such as fulvestrant, that cause degradation of ERs. Fulvestrant has been approved to treat advanced breast cancer after tamoxifen failure, and a recent phase III trial indicated that fulvestrant and AI exemestane were equally effective with a similar safety profile [15].

Resistance is a common problem associated with endocrine therapy therefore alternative treatment strategies without cross-resistance are necessary. Compared to the pure anti-estrogenic actions like AIs or fulvestrant, an ideal SERM with beneficial estrogenic effects has great potential for breast cancer prevention and treatment, especially in postmenopausal women as they often suffer from unpleasant symptoms resulting from lower estrogen. A perfect SERM would reduce the risk of breast cancer, ovarian cancer and uterine cancer, as well as strengthen the bone, prevent coronary heart disease, strokes and Alzheimer's disease, and relieve menopausal discomfort like hot flashes and vaginal atrophy [12].

The complicated outcome of SERMs action cannot just be explained by turning on or off the ERs and their downstream genes. Although much new knowledge is being developed, we are still evolving in our understanding of the detailed mechanism of SERMs and their interaction with the ERs. In the past decade, another group of protein factors, nuclear receptor coregulators, have been identified that are essential for modulating the functions of SERMs and ERs. In this article, we will review the evolving understanding of the molecular mechanisms of SERMs action in the context of other signal transduction pathways and nuclear receptor coregulators, as well as the problems associated with the application of SERMs as a treatment or preventative for breast cancer. Finally, the new SERMs with potential as new agents to treat or prevent breast cancer will be described.

2. MECHANISM OF ESTROGEN ACTION

2.1. Structure and Function of ER

The existence of estrogen binding protein was first predicted by Elwood Jensen and colleagues in early 1960's [16]. The first ER cDNA, now known as ERα, was later cloned in the mid-1980's [17, 18]. In 1996, an additional ER was cloned from rat prostate [19] and designated as ERβ. The action of estrogen in cells is therefore almost entirely mediated by these two related but distinct subtype of estrogen receptors, ERα and ERβ. Both receptors function as ligand activated transcription factors which can bind the cognate DNA sequences known as estrogen responsive elements (ERE), and activate transcription. The ER proteins can be structurally subdivided into six domains on the basis of the functions controlled by the region, as shown in Fig. (**1**). The A/B domain contains one of the two transcriptional activation functions (AFs), designated as AF1 which is involved in estrogen-independent activation of transcription. Another activation function domain, AF2, is located in the E domain which also harbors the ligand binding domain (LBD), and is involved in estrogen/ ligand dependent activation

[20, 21]. The ERβ has 97% homology in the DBD and 61% homology in the LBD with ERα suggesting differential ligand binding capability of ERs [21].

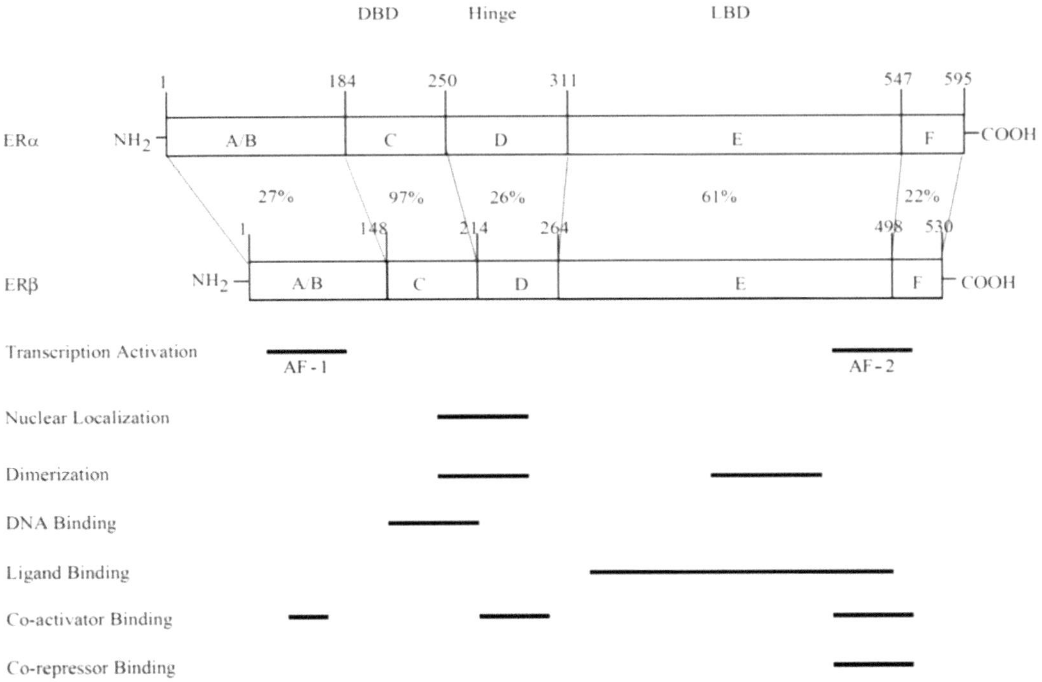

Fig. (1). Schematic comparison of human ER-α and ER-β structure. The structural domains are shown, and the percentage of amino acid identity shared by the two ERs is indicated for each domain. The horizontal bars highlight areas of different functions.

SERMs, the molecules which can bind to ERα and/or β and can either stimulate estrogen-like actions (agonist) or oppose estrogen actions (antagonist) in various estrogen target tissues and cells. This pharmacologic knowledge advanced studies to decipher the details of the molecular mechanism of estrogen action in different cell and tissue types.

The structural studies of a SERM complexed with the LBD of ERα and ERβ reveal that re-orientation of the AF2 helix (helix 12) after the binding of the SERM to the hydrophobic pocket of the LBD [22, 23]. The interaction of amino acid Asp351 of ERα with the alkylaminoethoxyphenyl side chain of tamoxifen or raloxifene is crucial to prevent the recruitment of coactivators to the SERM-receptor complex surface [22, 23]. Using different mutants of ERα for the amino acid Asp351, it was shown that shielding and neutralization of Asp351 by the side chain of raloxifene is critical in defining the antiestrogenicity of this SERM. Furthermore, it has been shown that changing the Asp351 from aspartate to glycine (D351G) abolishes the estrogen-agonist activity of the tamoxifen-ER complex, while retaining its antagonistic property. The AF2 region of the agonist-bound receptor is particularly important for the interactions of steroid receptor coactivators (SRCs 1-3) *via* the interacting amino acid motif LxxLL, known as nuclear receptor interacting domain (NRID). It is important to note that the affinity of ERs for these NRIDs of SRCs is highly dependent upon the ER subtype, α and β, and ligand bound to the ER [24-26]. Recruitment of these co-activator(s) is also responsible for facilitating the activation of estrogen responsive genes by modifying the chromatin structure and activating the transcriptional machinery. Additionally, SERMs may also show differential AF1 activity mediated by co-repressor binding. Using ERE-reporter constructs, it has been shown that the AF1 domain of ERα is actively involved in agonist-induced gene expression whereas the AF1 domain of ERβ is involved very weakly [27].

Estrogen can also modulate the expression of genes by another mechanism in which the receptor complex can interact with other transcription factors such as activating protein 1 (AP1) or stimulating protein 1 (Sp1) through a process known as a tethering mechanism. Intriguing differences are observed in the mechanism of action between ERα and ERβ through an AP1 site. In the presence of estrogen, ERα induces AP1 driven reporter activity but ERβ has no effect [28]. The raloxifene bound ERβ complex can induce transcriptional activity through the AP1 site but the activity through ERα bound to raloxifene is negligible.

ERs also act in a non-genomic manner initiated from the cell membrane. These actions are very fast (seconds to minutes) and occur without RNA or protein synthesis. They often mobilize second messenger molecules such as Ca^{2+} and cAMP, and are associated with protein kinase cascades such as PI3K/Akt and MAPK [29, 30]. Several explanations have been offered to explain these effects. There could be a subpopulation of nuclear ERs associate with the plasma membrane, either through posttranslational modification such as palmitoylation or mediated by scaffold proteins such as caveolin-1 and MNAR, since ERs do not have a transmembrane domain [29, 30]. Another membrane bound protein, G protein coupled receptor GPR30, was identified in recent years that mediates non-genomic actions of estrogen [31, 32]. The cellular localization of GPR30 is still controversial. Some evidence suggests it is at plasma membrane [33, 34] and other evidence suggests it is in the endoplasmic reticulum [32]. GPR30 binds to 17β-estradiol, tamoxifen and fulvestrant with high affinity [34] and is associated with breast cancer metastasis and transactivation of the epidermal growth factor receptor (EGFR) [35].

2.2. Co-Regulators

The co-regulators are protein molecules which can physically interact with the liganded or un-liganded ERs and modulate the transcription of the genes. The transcriptional activation or repression of the responsive genes is a combinatorial function of ligand-receptor interaction, recognition of cognate DNA sequence and recruitment of specific co-regulators onto the promoter of the gene. The assembly of the whole transcriptional complex is also dependent upon the affinity of the above mentioned individual components among themselves and their relative concentrations in the cell. Co-regulators play defining roles in the final tissue outcome in terms of transcriptional activation or repression mediated by estrogen or SERMs. The co-regulators can be broadly classified on the basis of their function, as co-activators which promote the activation of the transcriptional process, or co-repressors which are associated with repression of transcription of genes (Fig. **2**).

2.2.1. Co-Activators

Presently, around 200 co-activators are known, which are associated with 48 nuclear receptors [36]. The family of p160 proteins known as steroid receptor co-activators (SRCs) have been studied extensively. The relative abundance of SRC1 in uterine cells is responsible for the agonistic activity of tamoxifen, whereas in breast cancer cells, with low SRC1 levels, tamoxifen acts as an estrogen antagonist [37]. However, raloxifene, another related SERM, does not recruit SRC-1 even in the uterine cells [37], suggesting that the interaction with specific ligand which elicits a unique conformation of the receptor is critical for the

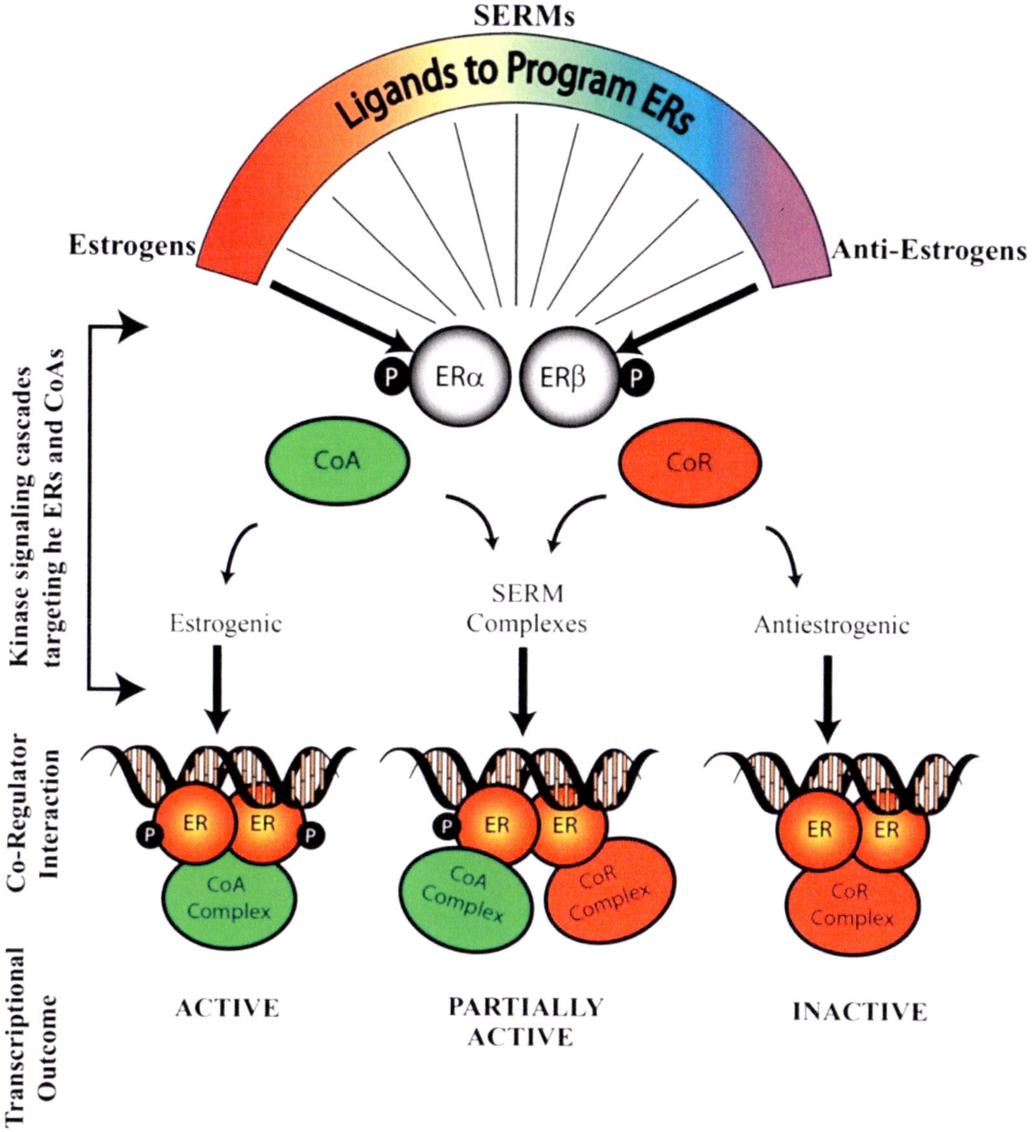

Fig. (2). Schematic representation of different liganded-ER complexes interacting with co-regulators and consequent transcriptional activities. ERs that bind to estrogenic ligands interact with co-activators (CoA) and activate transcription. Anti-estrogen liganded-ER complexes interact with co-repressors (CoR) and inactivate transcription of responsive genes. Selective estrogen receptor modulators (SERMs) bind to ERs and interact with either co-activator or co-repressor complexes eliciting partial transcriptional activity depending upon the cellular context.

interaction of co-regulators. These observations further provide an explanation for the earlier studies, where tamoxifen have been reported to induce growth of endometrial cancer cells but not of breast cancer cells in athymic mice [38] and also that estrogen agonistic properties of raloxifene is less in endometrial cancer cells [39]. These finding also translate very well to clinical experience [40, 41]. In addition, the SERMs can enhance the stability of the co-activators (SRC1 and SRC3) and thereby influence the transcriptional capability of other nuclear receptors [42]. Post-translational modifications of the co-activators, including but not limited to phosphorylation, methylation, ubiquitylation, sumoylation and acetylation, can also regulate the gene activation by influencing the ability of the co-activators to interact with ER and other components of the transcriptional complex [33, 35, 36]. The understanding of structure-function relationship of ligands at the ER has formed the basis of designing effective new SERMs with fewer side effects.

2.2.2. Co-Repressors

Co-repressors are functional counterparts of co-activators, which are associated with transcriptionally inactive promoters and help repress the expression of genes [43]. Fewer co-repressors have been reported compared to the co-activators. In the case of ER, the co-repressors are known to interact with the un-liganded and/or antagonist bound receptor. The two most extensively studied co-repressors in connection with ER are Nuclear receptor corepressor (NCoR) and silencing mediator of retinoic acid and thyroid hormone receptor (SMRT). The ER bound to raloxifene or 4-hydroxytamoxifen (a potent antagonist metabolite of tamoxifen) is known to recruit NCoR and SMRT to the promoters of estrogen responsive genes and repress transcription [37, 44, 45]. It has been shown that inhibition of NCoR or SMRT with monoclonal antibodies can enhance the agonistic property of 4-hydroxytamoxifen [46]. Moreover, using fibroblasts from NCoR null mice, 4-hydroxytamoxifen was shown to be a relatively potent ERα agonist [47]. The critical role of NCoR and SMRT in 4-hydroxytamoxifen-induced arrest of cell proliferation of ERα positive breast cancer cells is confirmed because 4-hydroxytamoxifen-stimulated cell cycle progression now occurs in NCoR-and-SMRT-deficient breast cancer cells [48]. However not all estrogen responsive genes are activated by 4-hydroxytamoxifen in NCoR and SMRT deficient cells, clearly indicating that additional molecules are important in SERM-induced repression of estrogen responsive genes. Indeed, there are several other corepressor proteins known for ER. Metastasis associated protein 1 (MTA1) is a corepressor found to mediate the ER transcriptional repression [49]. Another corepressor, known as repressor of estrogen action (REA) potentiates the inhibitory effects of anti-estrogens including 4-hydroxytamoxifen. Additionally, REA interacts with ER and competes with the co-activator SRC1 for binding to the estrogen bound ER [50, 51]. This again emphasizes the fact that the relative levels of co-regulators may be important in deciding the outcome of the SERM action. The proteasomal regulation of NCoR is another factor which may influence the SERM action. Degradation of NCoR occurs through the 26S proteasome, which is mediated by seven in absentia homologue 2 (Siah2) [52]. Interestingly, estrogen mediated upregulation of Siah2 in ER positive breast cancer cells has been implicated in the proteasomal degradation of NCoR, and subsequent de-repression of NCoR regulated genes [53].

In addition to acting as a "transcriptional adapter" between the receptors and the transcriptional machinery, the coregulator itself or its complex possess various enzymatic activities such as acetylation, phosphorylation, methylation or de-acetylation by which they are able to modify the local chromatin structure thereby making the local environment conducive for gene expression or repression. Intrinsic histone acetyl transferase activity was found to be associated with co-activator SRC1 which helps in the activation of transcriptional expression [54]. In contrast, the 4-hydroxytamoxifen bound ER complex which recruits the co-repressors NCoR and SMRT is associated with histone de-acetylases and other chromatin modifying enzymes [37, 55]. The deacetylase activity promotes transcriptional repression [37, 55]. Interestingly, another enzyme in the co-activator complex, CARM1 (coactivator associated arginine methyltransferase 1) has recently been implicated in modifying the coactivator itself and inducing the degradation of the complex [56]. This suggests the ability of the enzymes in the complex to modify other proteins in its own complex apart from a role in the modification of chromatin.

With this background of the molecular biology of SERM action, it is now appropriate to describe our evolving understanding about drug resistance. This is important not only because tumor drug resistance is the consequence of long term

SERM administration, but also because new knowledge will aid patients with the development of novel treatment strategies for SERM-resistant breast cancer.

3. DRUG RESISTANCE TO SERMs

There are three types of resistance to SERMs based on the mechanism: metabolic resistance, intrinsic resistance and acquired resistance [57].

3.1. Metabolic Resistance

Metabolic resistance to tamoxifen is mostly related to CYP2D6, an enzyme product that metabolizes tamoxifen into its active forms 4-hydroxytamoxifen and endoxifen [58]. This has been extensively reviewed recently and will only be briefly mentioned here [13, 59]. CYP2D6 is genetically polymorphic and 5-8% of Caucasian subjects are CYP2D6 "poor metabolizers" thus are less likely to benefit from tamoxifen treatment, although it has been shown that these women tolerate tamoxifen better and tend to remain on the drug for longer [59]. The genotype of CYP2D6 has been shown in some clinical trials to be directly related to the outcome of tamoxifen use, however, the results are not always consistent. Eight studies indicated that CYP2D6 "poor metabolizer" genotypes have worse outcome of breast cancer patients who received tamoxifen but two studies contradicted this conclusion [60]. In addition to the genotype of CYP2D6, it is important to consider that other drugs may interact with the enzyme system and block the metabolic activation of tamoxifen. Unfortunately, selective serotonin reuptake inhibitors (SSRIs) that are used to relieve the menopausal side effects of tamoxifen are also metabolized by CYP2D6 and block the metabolic activation of tamoxifen. The proper choice of SSRI may be important so as not to impair tamoxifen metabolism. The SSRI of choice is venlafaxine that has only a low affinity for the CYP2D6 enzyme [61]. Although these emerging data about CYP2D6 genotypes and the drug interaction between tamoxifen and SSRIs are important, it is perhaps too early to use CYP2D6 status to routinely choose between tamoxifen and aromatase inhibitors to treat postmenopausal women with breast cancer. At present, an international consortium is evaluating the overall CYP2D6 status of completed clinical trials with tamoxifen to assemble a large scale retrospective analysis of the worth of genotyping. The aim is to answer the question of whether "poor metabolizers" should avoid tamoxifen use.

3.2. Intrinsic Resistance

Approximately 30% ER-positive breast cancer patients do not respond to tamoxifen [62]. This type of resistance is referred to as "*de novo*" resistance or intrinsic resistance. Clinical studies showed that only 40% patients with ER-positive, progesterone receptor (PR)-negative breast cancers are responsive to anti-estrogen treatment (tamoxifen or endocrine ablation) compared to 80% responsive rate in ER-and-PR-positive patients [58, 59]. Historically, the status of PR has been regarded as an indicator of a functional ER pathway, since expression of PR is regulated by estrogen. On the other hand, recent evidence suggested that the absence of PR is associated with excessive growth factor signaling such as overexpression of HER2 [63, 64], which has been known to impair estrogen induction of PR and reduce the effectiveness of tamoxifen treatment for breast cancer [65]. However, the negative association between PR and HER2 seems more evident in older women (> 45 yrs) [66] and it remains controversial that PR-status could be used for clinical decision on choosing between tamoxifen or AIs [67].

Growth factor signaling, especially through epidermal growth factor (EGF) pathway, has been studied extensively in the past two decades and linked to SERM resistance. This has been recently reviewed [68] and will only be briefly summarized here. EGF binds to ErbB family of cell surface receptors that include four closely related receptor tyrosine kinases: EGFR (ErbB-1), HER2/c-neu (ErbB-2), HER3 (ErbB-3) and HER4 (ErbB-4). Overexpression of HER2 has been clinically linked to less response to endocrine therapies and worse prognosis [69-71], so has the overexpression of EGFR [72]. Different ErbB family members can form heterodimers and activate multiple signaling pathways including PI3K/Akt and MAPK. The major molecular mechanisms leading to SERM resistance can be summarized as follows: 1. Activation of downstream kinase cascade results in the phosphorylation of ER at key residues (Ser106/107, 118, 167, 305 and Thr 311) which activates transcription in a ligand-independent manner. Phosphorylation may change the binding of ER with ligands, DNA and coregulators, which may ultimately alter the activity of SERMs [73]. For example, phosphorylation of ER at Ser167 by Akt and Ser118 by the MAPK pathway both cause ligand-independent activation [74-76]. A recent study showed that phosphorylation of ER at Ser305 altered the orientation between the C-terminus of ER and SRC-1 that led to the recruitment of ER transcription coactivators and RNA polymerase II even in the presence of tamoxifen [77]. 2. Phosphorylation of ER co-regulators is equally important as the phosphorylation of ER itself, since phosphorylated co-activators have increased activity in the presence of SERMs [78-80]. Phosphorylation of co-repressors such as SMRT is associated with the co-repressor's nuclear export and impaired transcriptional suppressing function [81]. 3. Other than enhancing the transcriptional activity of the ER by phosphorylation, overexpression of EGFR or HER2 increases the non-genomic actions of ER, and SERMs may now act as estrogen agonists *via* the membrane effects of ER [82, 83]. In addition to the EGF signal pathway, the insulin-like growth factor (IGF) signal pathway is also involved in tamoxifen resistance [84]. It can activate PI3K/Akt pathway [71] and turn on genes that are otherwise activated by estrogen [85, 86].

Dysregulation of ER co-regulators is another major contributor to intrinsic SERM resistance. Overexpression of both AIB1 (SRC-3, ACTR, p/CIP, RAC3, TRAM-1) and HER2 have been shown to convert tamoxifen into an estrogen agonist in breast cancer cells [78]. Elevated AIB1 was found to associate with tamoxifen resistance, DNA-nondiploidy, high S-phase fraction and HER2 amplification in samples from clinical study [87]. Although a study indicated that high expression of AIB1 was not associated with relapse during tamoxifen treatment [88], AIB1 was shown to associate with tamoxifen resistance in breast cancers that overexpressed ErbB family proteins [88, 89]. AIB1 might be a predictor marker for tamoxifen ineffectiveness in ER-positive, HER2-positive and PR-negative breast cancer. On the other hand, low expression of ER co-repressor NcoR is associated with shorter relapse-free survival in breast cancer patients who only received tamoxifen after surgery [90]. Based on the emerging importance of co-regulators and tamoxifen resistance, one novel approach to overcome tamoxifen resistance is by the use of disulfide benzamide (DIBA) to disrupt the zinc finger in the ERα DNA binding domain. The approach facilitates ERα dissociation from coactivator AIB1 and concomitant association of corepressor NcoR without changing the phosphorylation of HER2, MAPK, Akt or AIB1 [91].

Another group of regulators associated with tamoxifen resistance are microRNAs (miRNA). These are naturally occurring single-stranded RNAs with the length of 21-23 nucleotides that do not code for proteins. They regulate gene expression mainly by inducing target mRNA degradation or inhibiting translation (protein synthesis). Dysregulation of miRNAs is associated with many cancers including breast cancer [92, 93]. Two recent studies show that miRNA-221/222 are upregulated in tamoxifen-resistant breast cancer cells and primary tumors, and they may contribute to tamoxifen resistance by down-regulating p27Kip1 or ERα [94, 95].

3.3. Acquired Resistance

Breast cancer patients who initially respond to tamoxifen later develop "acquired resistance" that is characterized by tamoxifen stimulated growth. This can be replicated in the laboratory with MCF-7 xenograft tumors implanted in ovariectomized athymic mice. Tamoxifen initially inhibits estrogen stimulated tumor growth but eventually some tumors start to grow during tamoxifen therapy [96]. These tumors now grow in response to either estrogen or tamoxifen and stop growing with no treatment or during treatment with fulvestrant [96]. The laboratory model is consistent with the clinic observation that aromatase inhibitor or fulvestrant are equally effective after the failure of tamoxifen treatment [97, 98]. It therefore appears that ER remains fully functional in the laboratory model of acquired tamoxifen resistance. In clinical studies, only 17-28% patients with acquired tamoxifen resistance have a loss of ER function [99, 100], and it is more likely that acquired resistance is associated with the stimulation of other growth/survival pathways [101]. For example, activated mammalian target of rapamycin (mTOR, downstream of PI3K/Akt and MAPK pathway) and c-Src (downstream of EGFR/HER2) were observed in breast cancer cells and mTOR and c-Src inhibitors can restore tamoxifen sensitivity in these cells, respectively [102, 103]. Several genes involved in cell proliferation and survival have altered expression level in breast cancer cells with acquired tamoxifen resistance. Examples of genes which down regulation is associated with acquired tamoxifen resistance include cyclin-dependent kinase inhibitors p21Cip [104] and p27Kip [105]. Examples of genes which upregulation is associated with tamoxifen acquired resistance include cyclin-dependent kinase 10 (CDK10) [106] and anti-apoptotic protein survivin [107].

Laboratory observation showed that acquired tamoxifen-resistant breast cancer cells/tumors respond differently to estrogen, and three phases of tamoxifen-resistance have been described, which seems to depend on the length of tamoxifen exposure [12]. Tumors with phase I resistance are stimulated by estrogen and tamoxifen but inhibited by AIs and fulvestrant; tumors with phase II resistance are stimulated by tamoxifen but are inhibited by estrogen due to apoptosis; tumors with phase III resistance (automatous growth) grow in a hormone-independent manner that is not responsive to either AIs or fulvestrant or SERMs, but estrogen still exerts apoptotic actions on those tumors [12]. The laboratory models suggest a new treatment strategy, in which limited duration, low-dose estrogen can be used to purge phase II- or phase III-resistant breast cancer cells so that the tumors will be responsive to antiestrogen therapy again. Phase II clinical study is ongoing to test this treatment plan [108].

Most studies on SERM-resistance are related to tamoxifen and little is known about raloxifene resistance. Based on a few studies on raloxifene resistance using cell culture and animal models, raloxifene-resistant tumors are likely to have similar properties as tamoxifen-resistant ones [109]. Raloxifene-resistant MCF7 cells generated by long-term exposure to raloxifene *in vitro* are also resistant to tamoxifen *in vitro* and *in vivo*. They exhibit phase II SERM-resistance as estradiol treatment causes tumor regression by inducing G2/M cell cycle arrest and apoptosis [110]. Another raloxifene-resistant breast tumor model generated by exposing MCF7 breast tumors to raloxifene *in vivo* exhibits phase I SERM-resistance whose growth is stimulated by tamoxifen, raloxifene and estrogen [109]. Interestingly, protein levels of EGFR and HER2 are also increased in this phase I raloxifene-resistant tumor model, which suggests raloxifene-resistant tumors share similar molecular mechanisms as tamoxifen-resistant ones [109].

Overall, the classifications of different forms of antihormonal drug resistance can be used as a basis to evaluate the pharmacology of new SERMs. The goal is to improve on tamoxifen, the pioneer that over the past 30 years found ubiquitous long term applications in the treatment and prevention of breast cancer.

4. NEW SERMs

The discovery of the first antibiotic penicillin initiated a search for further antibiotics to delay drug resistance and to target specific diseases. Similarly, the successful clinical application of tamoxifen in medicine has resulted in the investigation of numerous related molecules to develop the "ideal SERM". However, it has been challenging to find a SERM that is superior to tamoxifen, which retains or extends its benefit to treat and prevent breast cancer but with fewer side effects. Tamoxifen maintains bone density in animals [111] and humans [112] so SERMs are being developed to treat osteoporosis, but the potential to prevent breast cancer and uterine cancer will also increase their clinical value and commercial success. The core structures of SERMs are diverse, including triphenylethylene, benzothiophene, chromene (benzopyran), naphthalene, indole and steroid, but each of the newer SERM is really a mimic of tamoxifen, raloxifene or estradiol. The development of dozens of SERMs have been discontinued due to ineffectiveness for human disease or severe side effects, but several new SERMs are under active investigations with great potential in breast cancer treatment and/or prevention, alone or in combination with other type of drugs. In addition, since the identification of ERβ in 1996 [19], ER subtype selective SERMs have been developed which could potentially be used as breast cancer preventives. Thus this area of medicinal chemistry remains an important topic of interest as new ER regulated targets emerge. We will review the current status of several agents that are either approved or in the process of drug development (summarized in Table **1**).

4.1. Tamoxifen-Like SERMs

4.1.1. Toremifene (Fareston)

Toremifene (**2**) is a chlorinated tamoxifen analogue which has been approved in the US and several other countries for the treatment of metastatic breast cancer.

Table 1. Current Status of New SERMs

Drug Name	Category (Structure)	Effects	Preclinical Results	Clinical Status
Toremifene	Tamoxifen-like	Breast cancer treatment Heart protection Mastalgia treatment Prostate cancer prevention Relieve side effects of androgen deprivation therapy	Fewer genotoxic effects than tamoxifen [113], bone effects similar to tamoxifen [119]	FDA approved for metastatic breast cancer Phase II trial (65 women) better than tamoxifen regulating lipid metabolism [121, 122] Phase II trials (62 and 195 women) effective [126, 127] Phase II trial (514 men) decreases prostate cancer incidence [128] Phase III trial (1,389 men) improves lipid profiles [130] Phase III trial (1,392 men) increases bone mineral density [129]
Ospemifene	Tamoxifen-like	Vaginal atrophy treatment Osteoporosis treatment Breast cancer prevention	Estrogenic effects on vaginal epithelium that is not observed with tamoxifen or raloxifene [134-136] Inhibits tumor growth in animal models as effective as tamoxifen [140, 141]	Phase III trial (826 women) relieves vaginal dryness Phase II trial (118 women): Comparable to or slightly better than raloxifene [139] Phase III trial planned (detail not available) Not available
GW5638 (DPC974) & GW7604	Tamoxifen-like	Breast cancer treatment (2nd line therapy)	Works as a SERM and as a SERD [148], effective in tamoxifen-resistant tumors [144, 145]; functions as an ER agonist in bone and cardiovascular system but an antagonist in breast and endometrium [142]	Phase I trial (9 patients who failed first-line hormone therapy) low toxicity [ASCO meeting 2002, abstract 452]
Arzoxifene (LY353381)	Raloxifene-like	Breast cancer treatment Breast cancer prevention	Antiestrogenic in breast and endometrium, estrogenic in bone and lipids [150] Effective to prevent ER-positive and ER-negative mammary tumors especially in combination with LG100268 [140, 155]	Phase III trial (200 patients) inferior to tamoxifen [154] Phase I trials (50 and 76 women) low toxicity and favorable biomarker profile [156]

(Table 1) contd…..

Drug Name	Category (Structure)	Effects	Preclinical Results	Clinical Status
Lasofoxifene (CP-336156, Fablyn)	Raloxifene-like	Osteoporosis treatment and prevention Vaginal atrophy treatment Breast cancer treatment and prevention Heart disease prevention	Higher potency than tamoxifen and raloxifene [158]; higher oral bioavailability than raloxifene [160] Effects similar to tamoxifen to prevent and treat NMU-induced mammary tumor in rats [163]	Phase III trial (1,907 women) significantly increases bone mineral density compared to placebo, no endometrial effects, no association with thromboembolic disorder [159] Phase III trial to compare with raloxifene (CORAL trial, details not available) Phase III trial (445 patients) improves vaginal atrophy compared to placebo Phase III trial (PEARL trial with 8,556 women), reduces ER-positive breast cancer incidence compared to placebo; slightly decreases major coronary disease risk; reduces vertebral and non-vertebral fractures; increases risks of venous thromboembolic events but not stroke; no endometrial effects [SABCS 2008, abstract 11]
Pipendoxifene (ERA-923)	Raloxifene-like	Breast cancer treatment	Inhibits tamoxifen-sensitive and -resistant tumors in mice and rats no uterotrophic activities compared to raloxifene [167]	Phase II trial to treat tamoxifen-refractory breast cancer in postmenopausal women (details not available)
Bazedoxifene (TSE-424 WAY-140424)	Raloxifene-like	Osteoporosis treatment and prevention Breast cancer prevention	Increases bone density with little uterine or vasomotor effects Inhibits estrogen-stimulated breast cancer cells growth [169]	Phase III trial (7,492 women) reduces vertebral and non-vertebral fracture incidences, while raloxifene is not effective against non-vertebral fracture [171] Phase III trial (497 women) reduces endometrial thickness, unique property among known SERMs [170] Not available
Acolbifene (EM-652, SCH57068) & EM-800 (SCH57050)	Raloxifene-like	Breast cancer treatment (2nd line therapy) Breast cancer treatment (1st line therapy) Breast cancer prevention	Highest affinity for ER, inhibit growth of multiple breast cancer cells *in vitro* and *in vivo* [180]	Phase III trial, less effective than anastrozole to treat tamoxifen-resistance breast cancer, study halted [182] Phase III trial planned [182] Phase II trial (started in February, 2009) for premenopausal women

(Table 1) contd.....

Drug Name	Category (Structure)	Effects	Preclinical Results	Clinical Status
CHF4227	Raloxifene-like	Breast cancer and osteoporosis prevention	Prevents DMBA-induced mammary tumors and preserves bone mass in rats [184, 185];	Phase I trials (24 and 56 women) beneficial on bone markers and lipid metabolism; no effects on endometrium; not causing hot flashes
SP500263	Raloxifene-like	Breast cancer and osteoporosis treatment	Inhibits breast cancer cell growth *in vitro* and *in vivo* without stimulating uterine weight gain [188, 189], protects bone *in vitro* [190]	Not available
HMR3339	Steroidal	Osteoporosis and cardiovascular disease prevention	Better than raloxifene to protect cancellous bones [191]	Phase II trials (96 and 118 and 94 women) better than raloxifene at improving some beneficial cardiovascular markers [192-194]
PSK3471	Steroidal	Osteoporosis and breast cancer prevention and treatment	Prevents bone loss *in vivo*, inhibits growth of breast cancer cells *in vivo* [197]	Not available

Its structure is shown in Fig. (**3**). Toremifene is as effective as tamoxifen in the treatment of ER-positive breast cancer but with the potential of fewer genotoxic effects, since it does not produce DNA adducts in rat liver and human endometrium [113]. The mechanism for the reduced genotoxicity of toremifene can be explained as follows: Tamoxifen-DNA adducts are primarily formed *via* sulfonation of the α-hydroxylated tamoxifen metabolites, but the α-hydroxy metabolites of toremifene is poorly esterified or sulfonated, and even sulfonated α-hydroxy toremifene, α-sulfoxytoremifene, reacts poorly with DNA [114, 115]. However, there are some reports to show toremifene induces DNA damages and hepatocarcinogenesis in rats [116, 117].

The effects of toremifene and tamoxifen on bones are similar [118], as are the endometrial effects. However, a recent safety evaluation demonstrates that secondary endometrial cancer incidence is lower with toremifene than with tamoxifen and is similar to that with raloxifene [119]. Nevertheless, toremifene stimulates the growth of human endometrial cancer implanted in athymic mice in the same way as tamoxifen [120]. The positive effects of toremifene on lipid profiles are superior to tamoxifen's. Toremifene lowers the low-density lipoprotein (LDL) cholesterol to a level similar to that seen with tamoxifen, but unlike tamoxifen, toremifene slightly increases high-density lipoprotein (HDL) cholesterol and lowers triglycerides in the serum [121, 122].

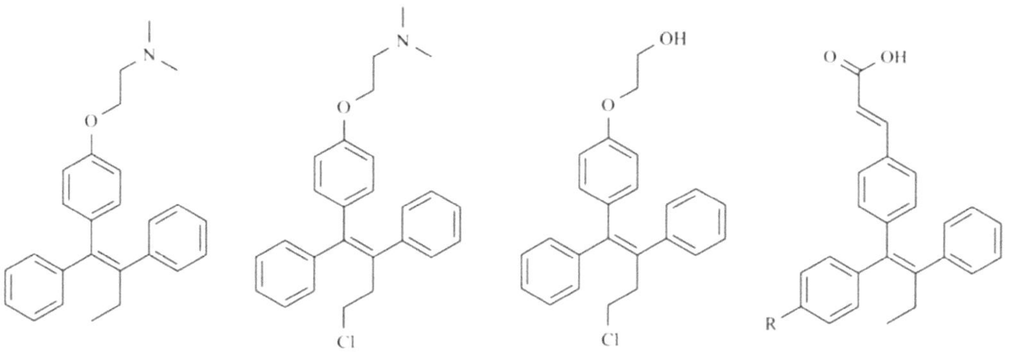

(**1**) Tamoxifen (**2**) Toremifene (**3**) Ospemifene (**4**) GW5638 R=H (**5**) GW7604 R=OH

Fig. (3). SERMs with a structure mimicking tamoxifen containing a triphenylethylene core.

Cross-resistance with tamoxifen is an important issue to consider when using toremifene for recurrent breast cancer because the majority of patients have received or failed adjuvant tamoxifen. Toremifene is completely cross-resistant with tamoxifen in human breast tumors implanted in athymic mice [123], as well as in breast cancer patients [124, 125]. Therefore, toremifene would not be effective as a second-line endocrine therapy after tamoxifen failure and may offer no therapeutic advantages over tamoxifen as an adjuvant therapy.

In recent years, toremifene has been developed to treat other estrogen-related diseases. Toremifene is effective to treat mastalgia in some small phase II trials [126, 127], and is also effective at decreasing prostate cancer incidences in a high-risk population [128]. In addition, a recent multicenter randomized phase III trial showed that toremifene increased bone density and improved lipid profile in men receiving androgen deprivation therapy for prostate cancer [129, 130].

4.1.2. Ospemifene (Deaminohydroxytoremifene, FC-1271a)

Ospemifene (**3**), or deaminohydroxytoremifene, is a metabolite of toremifene (Fig. **3**). Like toremifene, ospemifene is generally well tolerated and has a favorable safety profile. It does not induce DNA adducts in mice [131], rats [132] and monkey [133]. Ospemifene exerts a very weak estrogenic effect on endometrial histology, like raloxifene and decreases cholesterol [134]. However, unlike tamoxifen or raloxifene, ospemifene has significant estrogenic effects on vaginal epithelium [134-136] and is being developed for postmenopausal vaginal atrophy, a chronic condition experienced by about 40% postmenopausal women. Ospemifene is being evaluated in a phase III trial that has already recruited 826 women. Early results suggested that a 12-week course of ospemifene treatment significantly relieves symptoms of dryness in the vagina.

Ospemifene has showed promise in the prevention and treatment of osteoporosis. Cell culture studies indicated that ospemifene inhibits osteoclast formation and bone resorption and protects osteoblast-derived cells from apoptosis [137, 138]. In a recent phase II trial to compare effects of ospemifene and raloxifene on biochemical markers of bone turnover in postmenopausal women, ospemifene showed similar effects as raloxifene in regulating most of the bone markers examined, and at the 90-mg dose, ospemifene increased procollagen type I N propeptide (PINP) more than raloxifene [139]. Ospemifene is currently in phase III development for the treatment of postmenopausal osteoporosis.

Studies based on animal models suggest ospemifene might be effective in breast cancer prevention. Ospemifene prevented dimethylbenzanthracene (DMBA)-induced mammary tumors in female Sencar mice as effectively as tamoxifen, while raloxifene was not effective [140]. In a transplantable mouse model of ductal carcinoma *in situ* (DCIS), ospemifene had inhibitory effects equivalent to tamoxifen in terms of tumor growth and progression [141]. Nevertheless, the chemoprevention effects of ospemifene in breast cancer need to be further studied and substantiated by clinical trials.

4.1.3. GW5638 (DPC974) and GW7604

GW5638 (**4**) is a derivative of tamoxifen with an acrylate side chain in place of the dimethylaminoethoxy side chain in tamoxifen. GW7604 (**5**) is the 4-hydroxy version of GW5638, analogous to the major metabolite of tamoxifen, 4-hydroxytamoxifen. Their structures are shown in Fig. (**3**). GW5638 functions as a full ER agonist in bone and the cardiovascular system but as an antagonist in breast and endometrial system in rodent models [142].

Although the structures of tamoxifen and GW5638/GW7604 are similar, GW5638/GW7604 acts with a mechanism different from tamoxifen/4-hydroxy tamoxifen as suggested by the following evidence: 1). GW7604 acts as an antagonist in MDA-MB-231 cells transfected with wild-type ERα, but 4-hydroxytamoxifen acts as an agonist [143]; 2). Phage display experiments indicate that GW7604 bound ERα or ERβ is associated with different peptides from 4-hydroxytamoxifen, raloxifene or fulvestrant bound ERs [144]; 3). GW5638 inhibits the growth of tamoxifen-resistant breast tumor xenograft [144, 145]; 4). The crystal structure of the ERα LBD bound by GW5638 shows that GW5638 induces a distinct conformation of H12 in the ERα AF2 region, which increased exposure of hydrophobic residues and results in ERα destabilization in MCF7 cells [146].

GW5638 and GW7604 are also classified as selective estrogen receptor down-regulators (SERDs) because they induce ERα degradation, a property observed with the pure antiestrogen fulvestrant which was approved for the treatment of metastatic breast cancer [147]. However, a recent report [148] indicates that GW5638 induces ERα degradation through a different mechanism from fulvestrant and another SERD RU58,668, as the protein/protein interaction surface on ER required for fulvestrant-induced degradation is not necessary for GW5638-induced degradation. The fact that GW5638 has a unique mechanism to antagonize estrogen function and induces ER degradation in breast cancer cells makes it a possible second line therapy after tamoxifen failure and as an alternative to fulvestrant. Currently, GW5638 is under clinical development under the name DPC974 [148].

4.2. Raloxifene-Like SERMs

4.2.1. Arzoxifene (LY353381)

Arzoxifene (**7**) is a derivative of raloxifene with the ketone group replaced by an ether group and the hydroxy group is replaced by a methoxy group (Fig. **4**). These modifications have improved the pharmokinetic properties [149]. Arzoxifene has antiestrogenic effects on breast and endometrium but pro-estrogenic effects on bone and lipids [150]. Arzoxifene is cross-resistant in some but not all tamoxifen-stimulated breast tumor xenografts [151]. Phase II clinical trials indicate that arzoxifene is effective to treat tamoxifen-sensitive or tamoxifen-refractory patients with advanced or metastatic breast cancer [152] and patients with recurrent or advanced endometrial cancer [153] with minimal toxicity. However, a phase III trial showed arzoxifene was inferior to tamoxifen to treat patients with locally advanced and metastatic breast cancer [154]. The main role of arzoxifene may reside in its chemoprevention potential since it is more potent than raloxifene in pre-clinical studies [149].

The breast cancer chemoprevention property of arzoxifene has been studied with animal models and small short-term clinical trials. Arzoxifene effectively prevented nitrosomethylurea (NMU)-induced mammary tumor in rats [140] and induced apoptosis of breast cancer cells in rodent models especially when used in combination with rexinoid LG100268, a selective ligand for the retinoid X receptors (RXR) [155]. In two phase I clinical trials of women with newly diagnosed ductal carcinoma *in situ* or T1/T2 invasive cancer, arzoxifene did not demonstrate a significant reduction of tumor cell proliferation compared to placebo in 2-6 weeks treatment [156]. However, there were some favorable findings, such as a decrease of serum insulin like growth factor I (IGF-1) *vs* IGF binding protein 3 (IGFBP3) ratio and an increase of sex hormone binding globulin [156]. Another interesting aspect of the pharmacology of arzoxifene is that it might have chemopreventive properties for ER-negative breast cancer when used in combination with LG100268. A recent study showed that both SERMs arzoxifene and acolbifene alone prevent ER-negative mammary tumor in a mouse model and the effect is synergized with LG100268 [155]. Although the SERMs by themselves are not functional in the treatment of established tumors, together with LG100268 they inhibit proliferation and induce apoptosis in the ER-negative mammary tumors [155]. The mechanism how SERMs prevent tumorigenesis of ER-negative breast tissue is unknown, but the results suggest that arzoxifene has the potential for further clinical development as a chemoprevention drug of both ER-positive and negative breast cancer, especially in combination with rexinoids.

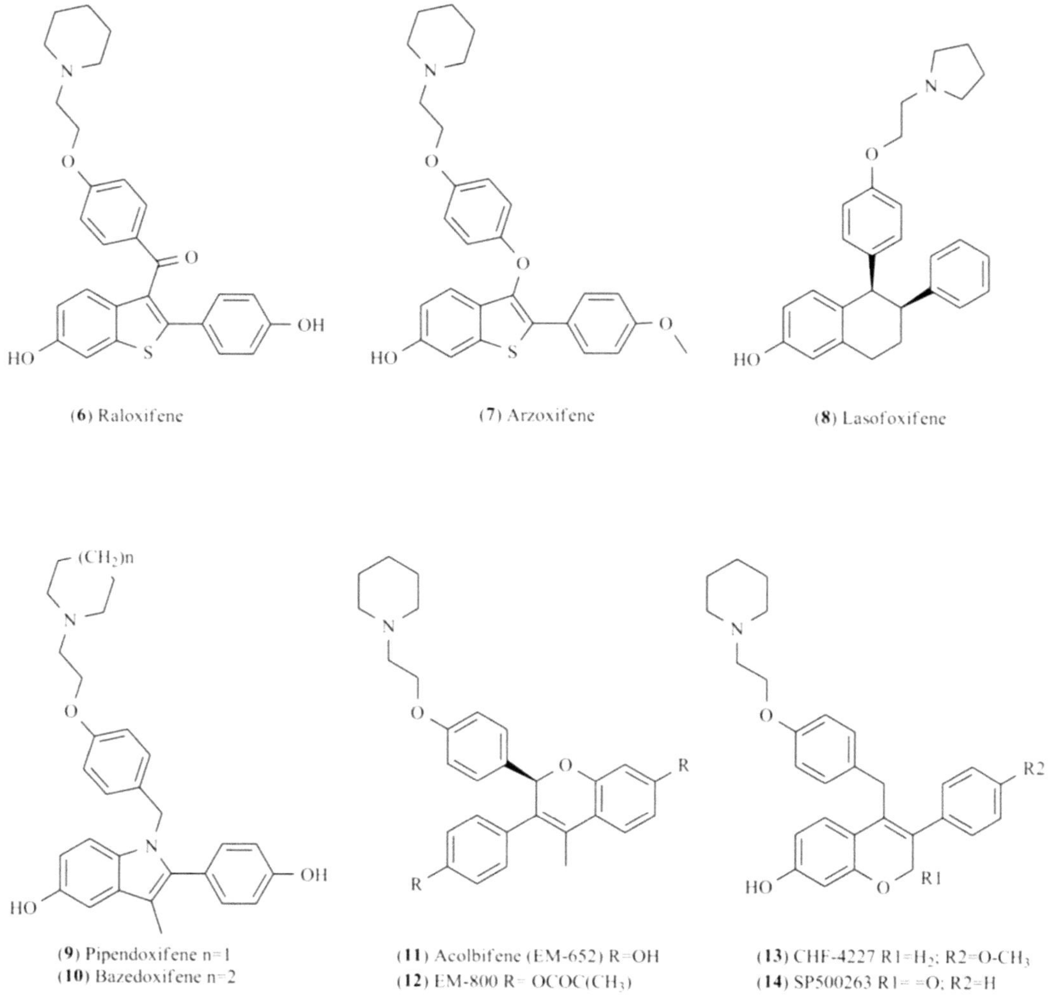

Fig. (4). SERMs with a structure mimicking raloxifene.

4.2.2. Lasofoxifene (CP-336156, Fablyn)

Lasofoxifene (**8**) has a naphthalene core structure, which is different from all the other SERMs discussed in this article (Fig. **4**). However, the crystal structure shows that lasofoxifene fits into the ERα LBD pocket in a similar manner as other ligands [157]. In addition, lasofoxifene-bound ERα LBD has similar conformational features as other SERM-bound ERα LBDs, such as tamoxifen or raloxifene, in which H12 in the "antagonist-bound" conformation and occludes the coactivator binding surface [157]. Lasofoxifene has a high affinity for ER with an IC_{50} of 1.5 nM, which is comparable to 17β-estradiol and higher than tamoxifen and raloxifene [158]. It preserves bone density and lowers serum cholesterol, and also has chemopreventive and chemotherapeutic effects in rat mammary tumor models without any uterine hypertrophic effects [159]. Lasofoxifene is currently undergoing an extensive clinical evaluation for the prevention and treatment of osteoporosis [159]. One advantage of lasofoxifene over raloxifene is its increased oral bioavailability due to the nonpolar naphthalene structure that makes it a poor substrate for intestinal wall glucuronidation [160]. In addition to its effects on bone, lasofoxifene significantly improves symptoms of vaginal atrophy [161] and a recently completed phase III trial indicated that lasofoxifene decreased vaginal pH and improved the vaginal-cell maturation index in osteoporotic postmenopausal women. These effects may be due to the increased vaginal ERβ and androgen receptor protein levels [162]. Lasofoxifene acts as a chemopreventive and treatment in the NMU-induced rat mammary tumor model. The results are similar to the comparator drug tamoxifen [163]. Phase III trials are currently ongoing to evaluate its ability to prevent breast cancer and cardiovascular diseases in postmenopausal women [164].

4.2.3. Pipendoxifene (ERA-923)

Pipendoxifene (**9**) has an indole core structure (Fig. **4**). It was designed by adding an alkylaminoethoxyphenyl side chain to zindoxifene (D-16726), a 2-phenylindol based SERM which failed as a treatment for breast cancer [165]. Pipendoxifene, also named ERA-923, mimics the structure of raloxifene and is devoid of uterotrophic activities in immature rats and ovariectomized mice compared to raloxifene [166]. It inhibits the growth of tamoxifen-sensitive and -resistant tumors in rats and mice [167] and is under phase II clinical development for the treatment of tamoxifen-resistant metastatic breast cancer. In a recent study, a combination of pipendoxifene and temsirolimus, which is a mammalian target of rapamycin (mTOR) inhibitor, synergistically inhibited growth of MCF-7 cells and xenograft models even at suboptimal doses, primarily by causing G1 cell cycle arrest [168]. This suggested that combination of a SERM and an mTOR inhibitor might be of clinic value as breast cancer treatments.

4.2.4. Bazedoxifene (TSE-424, WAY-140424)

Bazedoxifene (**10**) is another indole SERM, designed and synthesized at the same time as pipendoxifene with a slight structural difference, as shown in Fig. (**4**) [166]. This SERM is being actively developed to treat osteoporosis with the potential to prevent breast cancer. Bazedoxifene binds to ERα and ERβ with an affinity lower than raloxifene but is less selective for ERα [169]. It inhibits estrogen-mediated proliferation of breast cancer MCF7 cells and increases bone density with little uterine or vasomotor effects in rat models [169]. A Phase III trial with 497 healthy postmenopausal women showed that 6-month bazedoxifene treatment decreases endometrium thickness and uterine bleeding, suggesting antagonistic effects of bazedoxifene in endometrium [170]. Bazedoxifene is currently under review by the Food and Drug Administration (FDA) for the prevention and treatment of postmenopausal osteoporosis. The completed 3-year phase III trial which enrolled 7,492 postmenopausal women with moderate to severe osteoporosis showed bazedoxifene significantly reduced the incidences of vertebral and non-vertebral fracture compared to placebo, while raloxifene was not effective against non-vertebral fracture [171]. No safety concerns related to breast or endometrium were observed, however, a statistical insignificant increase of venous thromboembolic events was observed with groups treated with either bazedoxifene or raloxifene in the same study [172]. Based on studies using rodent models, combination of bazedoxifene and conjugated estrogens exerted positive vasomotor, lipid, and skeletal responses with minimal uterine stimulation [173]. This suggested that pairing SERMs and estrogen might be effective in the treatment of menopausal symptoms and prevention of osteoporosis. However, further studies are needed to examine the effectiveness of bazedoxifene in breast cancer prevention.

4.2.5. Acolbifene (EM-652, SCH57068) and EM-800 (SCH57050)

Acolbifene (EM-652) (**11**) and its orally active prodrug EM-800 (**12**) have a chromene core structure (Fig. **4**). They were initially misclassified as pure antiestrogens and their side chain was depicted by analogy with the pure antiestrogen fulvestrant [174]. However, the structure of acolbifene is actually similar to that of raloxifene, and unlike fulvestrant, the antiestrogenic side chain of acolbifene does not mask the mutant ER amino acid D351Y to produce an estrogenic action [175]. In addition, acolbifene and EM-800 act as antiestrogens in mammary and uterine tissues, but have estrogenic effects to prevent bone loss and have a favored function in the regulation of lipid metabolism by lowering plasma cholesterol and triglyceride in rodent models [176, 177]. Therefore, acolbifene and EM-800 should be classified as SERMs.

Acolbifene has the highest ER-binding affinity among all known compounds [178]. Preclinical studies indicated that acolbifene and EM-800 were more potent than tamoxifen, idoxifene, raloxifene, GW-5638, toremifene and droloxifene to inhibit the growth of breast cancer cell lines MCF-7, ZR-75-1, MCF-7 and T47D as well as ZR-75-1 xenograft in mice models [179, 180]. Interestingly, acolbifene caused disappearance of 65% ZR-75-1 xenograft in ovariectomized nude mice, while other SERMs tested (tamoxifen, toremifene, raloxifene, droloxifene, idoxifene and GW 5638) only decreased the tumor growth rate stimulated by estrone [180]. Acolbifene was evaluated as a second line therapy for tamoxifen-refractory breast cancers, since it was regarded as a pure anti-estrogen. In a small clinical trial involved 43 postmenopausal or ovariectomized women with breast cancer who had received tamoxifen for over a year but relapsed, the objective response to EM-800 was 12% with 1 complete response and 4 partial responses [181]. In a phase III trial to compare acolbifene with the aromatase inhibitor anastrozole in breast cancer patients who did not respond to tamoxifen, acolbifene did not show superior antitumor activity to anastrozole and the study was halted [182]. However, acolbifene and EM-800 may be more suitable as first line therapy and a phase III trial for untreated metastatic breast cancer patients is planned [182].

Recent studies indicate that acolbifene might be used in combination with other drugs. Acolbifene synergizes with rexinoid LG100268 in the prevention and treatment of mice with ER-negative mammary tumor [155]. It also synergizes with dehydroepiandrosterone (DHEA), which is a naturally produced prohormone for androgen and estrogen, in the prevention of dimethylbenzanthracene (DMBA)-induced mammary tumors in the rats [183]. A phase III trials of acolbifene plus DHEA for vaginal atrophy and uterine safety has been planned.

4.2.6. CHF4227

CHF4227 (**13**) is a SERM with a chromene (benzopyran) core structure, as shown in Fig. (**4**). Compared with raloxifene, CHF4227 binds to ERα and ERβ with higher affinity and inhibits the uterotropic action of 17alpha-ethynyl estradiol with more potency [184]. CHF4227 significantly prevents the development of DMBA-induced mammary tumors in rats [184]. It preserves bone mass without affecting uterine weight and decreases serum cholesterol and fat mass in ovariectomized rats [185]. A recent phase I study showed CHF4227 is well-tolerated, as 28 days of treatment has a positive effect on the serum lipid profile and bone markers without any negative effects on the endometrium or the fibrinolytic system. Additionally, CHF4227 does not cause vaginal bleeding or hot flashes [186]. These results suggest that CHF4227 is safe and worthy of further clinical development for osteoporosis and the chemoprevention of breast cancer.

4.2.7. SP500263

SP500263 (**14**) was discovered in a screen to identify ER agonist in bone cells [187]. It has a chromene core structure and binds to both ERα and ERβ with high affinity similar to raloxifene's (Fig. **4**) [187]. SP500263 inhibits the growth of breast cancer MCF7 cells and xenografts in nude mice, and does not stimulate uterine weight gain in immature rats or ovariectomized adult rats [188, 189]. SP500263 also blocks osteoclastogenesis in human bone cell model [190]. These preclinical results suggest that SP500263 has potential for the treatment of both breast cancer and osteoporosis. However, clinical value of this drug has yet to be determined.

4.3. Steroidal SERMs

4.3.1. HMR3339

All of the SERMs described to this point are non-steroidal. Recently, steroidal SERMs have been described (Fig. **5**). In rats, HMP3339 (**15**) not only increases bone mineral density but also restores the mechanical strength at multiple sites even after ovariectomy, and it affects both cortical and cancellous bones, while raloxifene was effective only at cancellous sites [191]. HMR3339 has entered clinical investigation for the prevention of osteoporosis and cardiovascular diseases. In a series of small phase II trials with healthy postmenopausal women, HMR3339 was found to reduce total cholesterol, LDL cholesterol, C-reactive protein (CRP, a pro-inflammatory cytokine and a cardiovascular disease risk factor), asymmetric dimethylarginine (AMDA, a nitric oxide synthase inhibitor) and homocysteine [192-194]. Elevation of AMDA or homocysteine is linked to a high incidence of cardiovascular disease but raloxifene treatment does not reduce the level of either AMDA or homocysteine [192]. HMR3339 reduces concentrations of procarboxypeptidase U (pro-CpU, an inhibitor of fibrinolysis), antithrombin and fibrinogen to a degree similar to raloxifene and shows beneficial effects on some markers of fibrinolysis [195, 196]. Therefore, HMR3339 has potential to prevent cardiovascular diseases and possibly also osteoporosis. However, whether or not there is potential as a cancer preventive has not been determined.

4.3.2. PSK3471

PSK3471 (**16**) is a newly developed SERM with a structure similar to HMR3339 (Fig. **5**). It was reported to prevent gonadectomy-induced bone loss in male and female mice, and antagonize estradiol-stimulated MCF-7 cell proliferation [197].

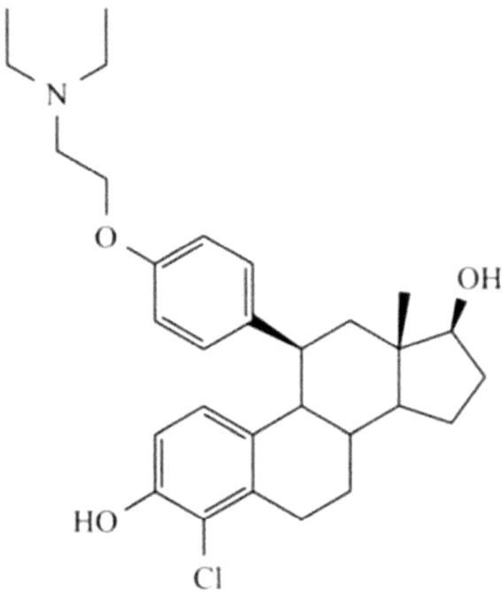

(**15**) HMR3339

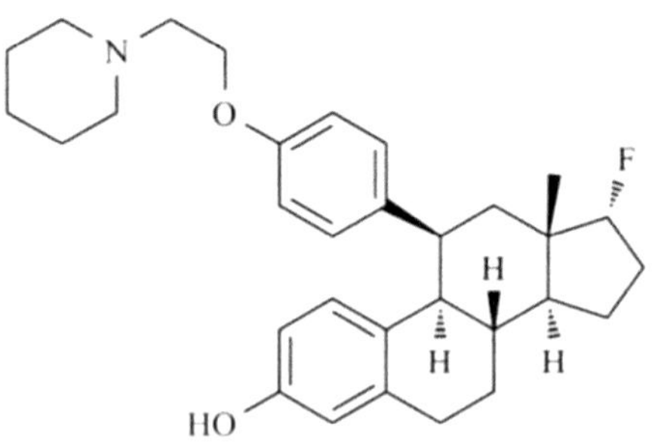

(**16**) PSK3471

Fig. (5). Steroidal SERMs.

4.4. ER Subtype Selective SERMs

ERα and ERβ have a different tissue distribution and have overlapping but distinct biological functions [198]. Unlike ERα, ERβ expression is not routinely examined in the clinic and its function in breast cancer remains unclear. ERβ expression is found in both normal and breast cancer specimens but does not correlate with ERα expression [199]. It seems that ERβ functions differently if it is expressed alone or co-expressed with ERα in breast cancers. In ERα-positive breast tumors, ERβ often antagonizes the pro-proliferation actions of ERα [200, 201] and its expression is associated with better response to endocrine therapy and a favorable clinical outcome in most cases [202]. Thus ERβ seems to function as a tumor suppressor. However in ERα-negative breast tumors, several studies indicated that the expression of ERβ correlates with proliferation markers such as Ki67 and cyclin A [202, 203], which suggested that ERβ might stimulate cancer growth. In the latter situation, ERβ could serve as an endocrine therapy target in those patients who would otherwise be regarded as ER-negative and have limited choice but chemotherapy. The presence of ERβ in ERα-negative breast cancers may partly explain why some “ER-negative” patients respond to SERMs. The reason that ERβ functions differently in the absence or presence of ERα might be due to the different activities between the ERα/β heterodimer and ERα or ERβ homodimers.

A new direction to consider is the estrogen related receptor (ERR) [204, 205]. There is emerging evidence that ERRα is critical for the growth of ER-negative breast-cancer MDA-MD-231 xenografts in mice [206], as ERRα appears to be involved in angiogenesis by inducing the expression of vascular endothelial growth factor (VEGF) [207, 208]. Novel therapeutic agents targeted to ERRα would be valuable to treat breast cancer.

Several ER-subtype selective SERMs have been reported, although it is difficult to design subtype selective ligands given the fact that only two amino acids are different in the ligand binding pocket between ERα and ERβ (despite that they have 61% amino acid identity in LBD). All the SERMs discussed previously were designed against ERα and have low subtype selection in terms of binding affinity. In contrast to the focus on ERα and breast cancer, most of ER subtype selective SERMs are developed for diseases other than breast cancer. In animal models,

ERβ-selective agonists ERB041 and diaryl-propionitrile (DPN) have been shown to have anti-inflammatory properties and antidepressant-like effects, respectively [209, 210]. An ERβ agonist, 8-vinylestra-1,3,5 (10)-triene-3,17β-diol, stimulates ovarian follicular development in hypophysectomized rats and gonadotropin-releasing hormone a tagonist-treated mice [211], thus this drug could be used to enhance fertility [198]. A few ERβ agonists are being developed for clinical applications in Alzheimer's disease and rheumatoid arthritis [212]. For breast cancer prevention and treatment, it is conceivable that ERβ agonist might have potential for ERα-and-β-positive tumors, especially in combination of an ERα selective antagonist, since the preclinical studies indicate a protective role of ERβ. However, this strategy poses a difficult pharmacologic issue of tissue pharmacodynamics. Nevertheless, a couple of ERβ modulators have been shown with positive effects to treat advanced postmenopausal breast cancer, which will be discussed below.

4.4.1. Discovery of New Properties of SERMs

The original discovery of SERMs provided both opportunities and challenges. The challenge is the control of hot flashes as this is a quality of life issue. No matter how good a medicine is at preventing a few spontaneous breast cancers in a large population, or controlling the increase in fractures noted with osteoporosis, if a woman does not accept the side effects of persistent hot flashes and stops taking the medicine- there is no advance. Numerous pharmaceutical companies are addressing the issue of hot flush control to create a more acceptable SERM.

Dainippon pharmaceuticals has employed spiro[indene-1,1'-indane]-5,5'-diol as a SERM core to design new SERM with all the traditional SERM effects on preserving bone, reducing circulating cholesterol with minimum effects on the breast and endometrium but preventing hot flashes. This is done assessing ovariectomized rat tail skin temperature [213]. They report a useful lead compound (Fig. **6**) that merits further investigation.

Eli Lilly has studied the structure activity relationships of oxachrysene derivative (Fig. **6**) to find a compound that binds to ERα and β, blocks the growth of MCF-7 breast cancer cells, Ishikawa endometrial cancer cells and is a powerful antagonist of estrogen-stimulated increases in rat uterine weight. In ovariectomized rats, bone density is maintained and there is a decrease in circulating cholesterol levels. Most importantly the compound was able to control temperature in a morphine dependent rat model [214].

Johnson and Johnson has a long standing program to address the issue of the control of hot flashes in novel SERMs. They originally reported that a chromene derived bisbenzopyran (Fig. **6**) had all the appropriate characteristics of a SERM plus alleviation of hot flashes (changes in the tail skin temperature during morphine withdrawal in the rat) and the alleviation of vaginal dryness [215]. Subsequently, the same group reported improved biology for a chromene derived selective ER modulator (Fig. **6**) [216] as an improved "back-up" to their original phase 2 development of the chromene based molecule.

Finally two additional innovations deserve mention. Eli Lilly has described a SERM targeted to premenopausal women for the treatment of leiomyomas [217]. Their compounds are naphthalene derivatives but their compound of interest LY2066948 (Fig. **7**) contains a methyl sulphone moiety that permits potent anti-uterotrophic activity but ensures the compound does not cross the blood brain barrier. They demonstrate that substitution of the methyl sulphone for fluorine (Fig. **7**) that passage of the blood brain barrier occurs resulting in 25 fold higher circulating estrogen. Thus LY2066948 could be a useful agent to stop the growth benign leiomyomas in premenopausal women.

Alzheimer's disease is a devastating neurodegenerative condition affecting 4.5 million people in the United States. Estrogen is known to stop the degeneration of neurons but current preparations have additional toxicological issue. Interestingly, there was a chance finding that the pure antiestrogen fulvestrant can mimic estrogen to stop neuronal degeneration [218] (Fig. **8**).

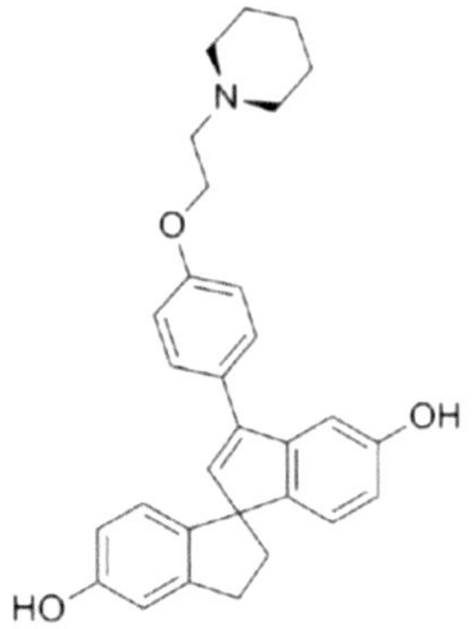

(**17**) Dainippon (+ enantiomer)

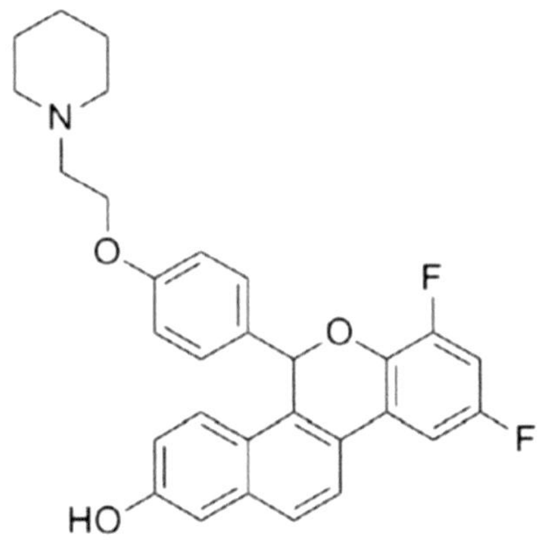

(**18**) Eli Lilly ((R)–(+) enantiomer)

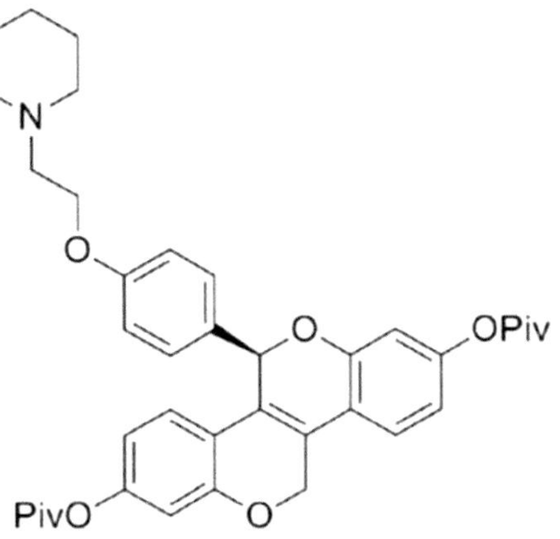

(**19**) Johnson and Johnson
(R enantiomer; original clinical candidate)

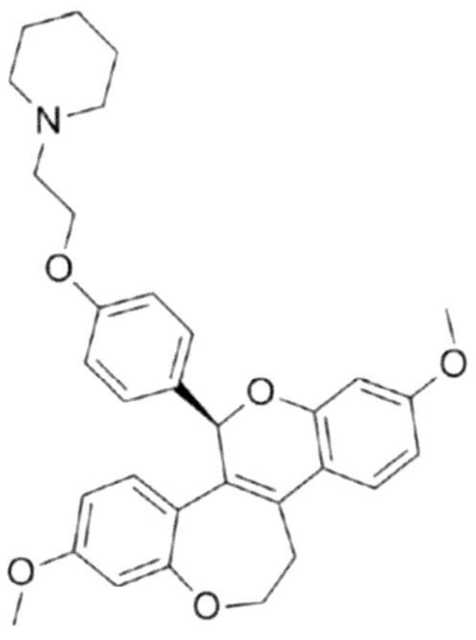

(**20**) Johnson and Johnson
(R enantiomer; back up)

Fig. (6). Ligands developed by various pharmaceutical companies for the treatment of 'hot flashes' in postmenopausal women.

Unfortunately, fulvestrant does not cross the blood brain barrier. A swap of the similar side chain of Vitamin E to the 7α position of fulvestrant demonstrates that it may be possible to create a "brain specific" estrogen [219] (Fig. **8**).

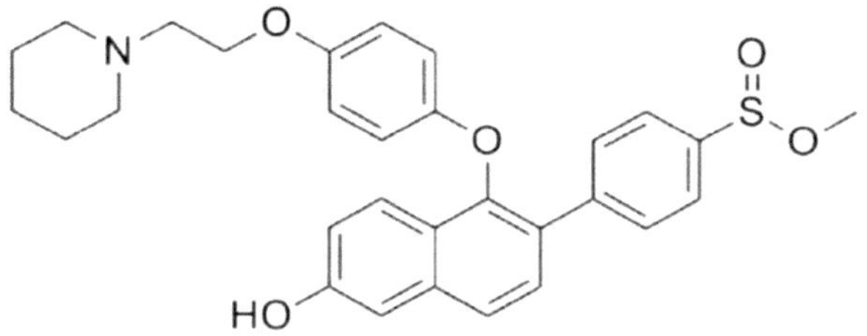

Eli Lilly (LY 2066948)

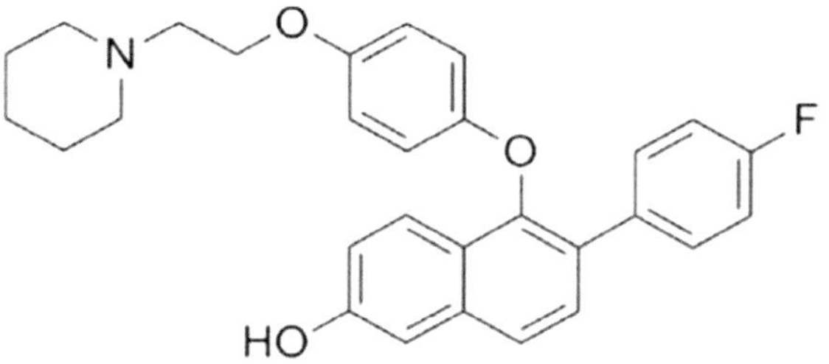

Eli Lilly (crosses blood brain barrier)

Fig (7). Chemical structure of SERM (LY 2066948) which could be used to treat leiyomyomas in premenopausal women. The molecule does not cross the blood brain barrier because of the methyl sulphone group. Exchange for fluorine allows passage of the blood brain barrier.

5. CONCLUDING REMARKS

Endocrine therapy targeting to ERα has been very successful in the treatment and prevention of breast cancer [220, 221]. It is very effective and less toxic compared to combinational cytotoxic chemotherapy that was the only option 30 years ago. In the ensuing period, multiple strategies have been developed to antagonize estrogen action. Most experience has accumulated with the competitive inhibitor of estrogen action tamoxifen, but targeting aromatase to deplete estrogen with AIs in postmenopausal patients or to induce ER degradation with SERDs have been valuable innovations in therapies. The goal for treatment is to create a "no-estrogen environment". However, SERMs that maintain the beneficial effects of estrogen but antagonize the harmful effects of estrogen have great potential in the prevention of multiple diseases in common. It is clear that many new SERMs are being developed that could provide better choices for patients in the future.

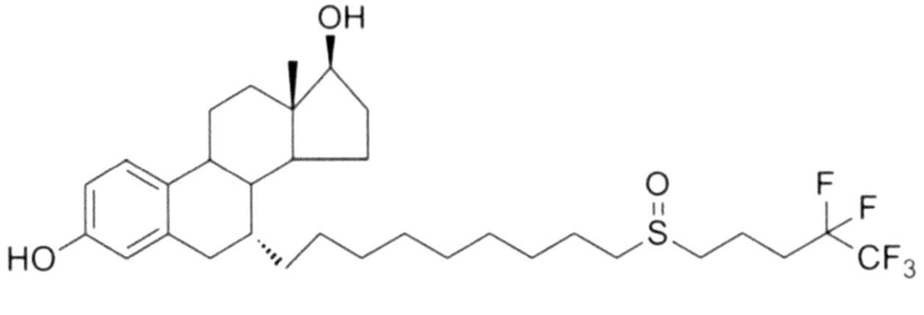

(**21**) Fulvestrant

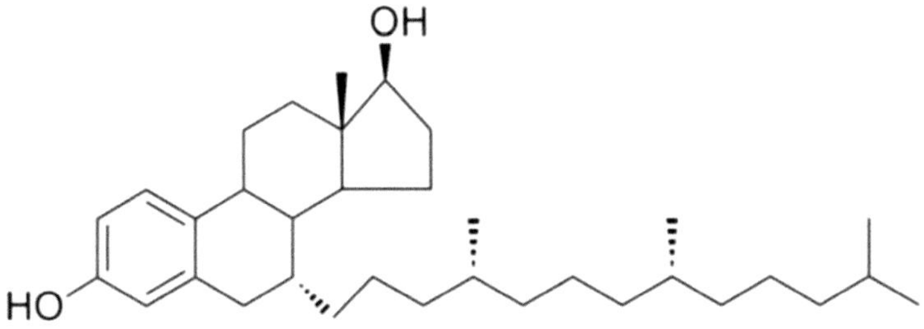

(**22**) Hybrid of 17β-estradiol and Vitamin E

Fig (8). Chemical structures of fulvestrant, and the hybrid molecule of 17β-estradiol and vitamin E which is capable of crossing the blood brain barrier and can function as a brain specific estrogen.

To overcome the unwanted side effects and problems with drug resistance, combination therapy might be another important direction in addition to the development of new SERMs. For example, combination of SERM acolbifene and DHEA could be protective against breast cancer and osteoporosis with beneficial effects to stimulate vaginal maturation and decrease skin dryness [182]. As traditional HRT is less acceptable to regulatory authorities because of the increased risk of breast cancer, a combination of HRT and a SERM may be a reasonable idea to relieve unpleasant menopausal effects while decrease breast cancer risks. With regards to avoiding drug resistance, combining a SERM and an inhibitor targeting significant survival signal transduction pathway is under active evaluation. By way of example, a combination of tamoxifen and inhibitors of the HER2 signal transduction pathway may prevent acquired tamoxifen resistance

[222]. Similarly, SERM pipendoxifene and mTOR inhibitor temsirolimus synergistically inhibits the proliferation of MCF7 breast cancer cells and xenograft at suboptimal concentrations [168]. Additionally, combinations of a SERM (arzoxifene or acolbifene) and a rexinoid LG100268 are effective to prevent and treat ER-negative mammary tumors in animal models [155]. The potential combination seems endless but the marriage of molecular biology and medicine holds great promise for advances in targeted therapeutics based on the SERM model.

In summary, it is clear that the original idea of targeting specific hormone receptor with selective medicine has proven its worth by advancing medicine with the SERMs tamoxifen and raloxifene. Now there are a whole range of new SERMs poised for clinical applications. But this is not the end of the story. Novel selective modulators of all members of the nuclear receptor superfamily are under investigation addressing the treatment or prevention of diseases never before considered possible [57, 221].

CONFLICT OF INTEREST

The authors declare that there is no conflict of interest.

ACKNOWLEDGEMENTS

Dr. Virgil C. Jordan is supported by the Department of Defense Breast Program under Award number W81XWH-06-1-0590 Center of Excellence; subcontract under the SU2C (AACR) Grant number SU2C-AACR-DT0409; the Susan G Komen For The Cure Foundation under Award number SAC100009; GHUCCTS CTSA (Grant # UL1RR031975) and the Lombardi Comprehensive Cancer Center Support Grant (CCSG) Core Grant NIH P30 CA051008. The content is solely the responsibility of the authors and does not necessarily represent the official views of the National Cancer Institute or the National Institutes of Health. Additionally, the views and opinions of the author(s) do not reflect those of the US Army or the Department of Defense."

DISCLOSURE

This e-Book chapter is an updated version of the review article entitled "Potential of Selective Estrogen Receptor Modulators as Treatments and Preventives of Breast Cancer" published in *Anti-Cancer Agents in Medicinal Chemistry*, **2009**, *9*(5), 481-499.

REFERENCES

[1] Berry DA.; Cronin KA.; Plevritis SK.; Fryback DG.; Clarke L.; Zelen M.; Mandelblatt JS.; Yakovlev AY.; Habbema JD.; Feuer EJ. Effect of screening and adjuvant therapy on mortality from breast cancer. *N Engl J Med*. **2005**, 353(17):1784-92.

[2] Ravdin PM.; Cronin KA.; Howlader N.; Berg CD.; Chlebowski RT.; Feuer EJ.; Edwards BK.; Berry DA. The Decrease in Breast-Cancer Incidence in 2003 in the United States. *N Engl J Med*. **2007**, 356(16):1670-4.

[3] Writing Group for the Women's Health Initiative I. Risks and Benefits of Estrogen Plus Progestin in Healthy Postmenopausal Women: Principal Results From the Women's Health Initiative Randomized Controlled Trial. *JAMA*. **2002**, 288(3):321-33.

[4] The Women's Health Initiative Steering C. Effects of Conjugated Equine Estrogen in Postmenopausal Women With Hysterectomy: The Women's Health Initiative Randomized Controlled Trial. *JAMA*. **2004**, 291(14):1701-12.

[5] Beral V. Breast cancer and hormone-replacement therapy in the Million Women Study. *Lancet*. **2003**, 362(9382):419-27.

[6] Beral V.; Bull D.; Reeves G. Endometrial cancer and hormone-replacement therapy in the Million Women Study. *Lancet*. **2005**, 365(9470):1543-51.

[7] Beral V.; Bull D.; Green J.; Reeves G. Ovarian cancer and hormone replacement therapy in the Million Women Study. *Lancet*. **2007**, 369(9574):1703-10.

[8] Jordan VC. Tamoxifen: a most unlikely pioneering medicine. *Nat Rev Drug Discov*. **2003**, 2(3):205-13.

[9] Veronesi U.; Boyle P.; Goldhirsch A.; Orecchia R.; Viale G. Breast cancer. *Lancet*. **2005**, 365(9472):1727-41.

[10] Cummings SR.; Eckert S.; Krueger KA.; Grady D.; Powles TJ.; Cauley JA.; Norton L.; Nickelsen T.; Bjarnason NH.; Morrow M.; Lippman ME.; Black D.; Glusman JE.; Costa A.; Jordan VC. The Effect of Raloxifene on Risk of Breast Cancer in Postmenopausal Women: Results From the MORE Randomized Trial. *JAMA*. **1999**, 281(23):2189-97.

[11] DeMichele A.; Troxel AB.; Berlin JA.; Weber AL.; Bunin GR.; Turzo E.; Schinnar R.; Burgh D.; Berlin M.; Rubin SC.; Rebbeck TR.; Strom BL. Impact of Raloxifene or Tamoxifen Use on Endometrial Cancer Risk: A Population-Based Case-Control Study. *J Clin Oncol*. **2008**, 26(25):4151-9.

[12] Jordan VC. Selective estrogen receptor modulation: concept and consequences in cancer. *Cancer Cell*. **2004**, 5(3):207-13.

[13] Jordan VC.; Brodie AM. Development and evolution of therapies targeted to the estrogen receptor for the treatment and prevention of breast cancer. *Steroids*. **2007**, 72(1):7-25.

[14] Perez EA. Safety profiles of tamoxifen and the aromatase inhibitors in adjuvant therapy of hormone-responsive early breast cancer. *Ann Oncol.* **2007**, 18(suppl_8):viii26-35.

[15] Chia S.; Gradishar W.; Mauriac L.; Bines J.; Amant F.; Federico M.; Fein L.; Romieu G.; Buzdar A.; Robertson JF.; Brufsky A.; Possinger K.; Rennie P.; Sapunar F.; Lowe E.; Piccart M. Double-blind, randomized placebo controlled trial of fulvestrant compared with exemestane after prior nonsteroidal aromatase inhibitor therapy in postmenopausal women with hormone receptor-positive, advanced breast cancer: results from EFECT. *J Clin Oncol.* **2008**, 26(10):1664-70.

[16] Jensen EV.; Jacobson HI. Basic guides to the mechanism of estrogen action. *Recent Prog Horm Res.* **1962**, 18:387-414.

[17] Green S.; Walter P.; Kumar V.; Krust A.; Bornert JM.; Argos P.; Chambon P. Human oestrogen receptor cDNA: sequence, expression and homology to v- erb-A. *Nature.* **1986**, 320(6058):134-9.

[18] Greene GL.; Gilna P.; Waterfield M.; Baker A.; Hort Y.; Shine J. Sequence and expression of human estrogen receptor complementary DNA. *Science.* **1986**, 231(4742):1150-4.

[19] Kuiper GG.; Enmark E.; Pelto-Huikko M.; Nilsson S.; Gustafsson JA. Cloning of a novel receptor expressed in rat prostate and ovary. *Proc Natl Acad Sci U S A.* **1996**, 93(12):5925-30.

[20] Tsai MJ.; O'Malley BW. Molecular mechanisms of action of steroid/thyroid receptor superfamily members. *Annu Rev Biochem.* **1994**, 63:451-86.

[21] MacGregor JI.; Jordan VC. Basic guide to the mechanisms of antiestrogen action. *Pharmacol Rev.* **1998**, 50(2):151-96.

[22] Brzozowski AM.; Pike AC.; Dauter Z.; Hubbard RE.; Bonn T.; Engstrom O.; Ohman L.; Greene GL.; Gustafsson JA.; Carlquist M. Molecular basis of agonism and antagonism in the oestrogen receptor. *Nature.* **1997**, 389(6652):753-8.

[23] Pike AC.; Brzozowski AM.; Hubbard RE.; Bonn T.; Thorsell AG.; Engstrom O.; Ljunggren J.; Gustafsson JA.; Carlquist M. Structure of the ligand-binding domain of oestrogen receptor beta in the presence of a partial agonist and a full antagonist. *Embo J.* **1999**, 18(17):4608-18.

[24] Bramlett KS.; Wu Y.; Burris TP. Ligands specify coactivator nuclear receptor (NR) box affinity for estrogen receptor subtypes. *Mol Endocrinol.* **2001**, 15(6):909-22.

[25] Wong CW.; Komm B.; Cheskis BJ. Structure-function evaluation of ER alpha and beta interplay with SRC family coactivators. ER selective ligands. *Biochemistry.* **2001**, 40(23):6756-65.

[26] Warnmark A.; Almlof T.; Leers J.; Gustafsson JA.; Treuter E. Differential recruitment of the mammalian mediator subunit TRAP220 by estrogen receptors ERalpha and ERbeta. *J Biol Chem.* **2001**, 276(26):23397-404.

[27] Hall JM.; McDonnell DP. The estrogen receptor beta-isoform (ERbeta) of the human estrogen receptor modulates ERalpha transcriptional activity and is a key regulator of the cellular response to estrogens and antiestrogens. *Endocrinology.* **1999**, 140(12):5566-78.

[28] Paech K.; Webb P.; Kuiper GG.; Nilsson S.; Gustafsson J.; Kushner PJ.; Scanlan TS. Differential ligand activation of estrogen receptors ERalpha and ERbeta at AP1 sites [see comments]. *Science.* **1997**, 277(5331):1508-10.

[29] Bjornstrom L.; Sjoberg M. Mechanisms of estrogen receptor signaling: convergence of genomic and nongenomic actions on target genes. *Mol Endocrinol.* **2005**, 19(4):833-42.

[30] Manavathi B.; Kumar R. Steering estrogen signals from the plasma membrane to the nucleus: two sides of the coin. *J Cell Physiol.* **2006**, 207(3):594-604.

[31] Filardo EJ.; Quinn JA.; Frackelton AR, Jr..; Bland KI. Estrogen action *via* the G protein-coupled receptor, GPR30: stimulation of adenylyl cyclase and cAMP-mediated attenuation of the epidermal growth factor receptor-to-MAPK signaling axis. *Mol Endocrinol.* **2002**, 16(1):70-84.

[32] Revankar CM.; Cimino DF.; Sklar LA.; Arterburn JB.; Prossnitz ER. A transmembrane intracellular estrogen receptor mediates rapid cell signaling. *Science.* **2005**, 307(5715):1625-30.

[33] Funakoshi T.; Yanai A.; Shinoda K.; Kawano MM.; Mizukami Y. G protein-coupled receptor 30 is an estrogen receptor in the plasma membrane. *Biochem Biophys Res Commun.* **2006**, 346(3):904-10.

[34] Thomas P.; Pang Y.; Filardo EJ.; Dong J. Identity of an estrogen membrane receptor coupled to a G protein in human breast cancer cells. *Endocrinology.* **2005**, 146(2):624-32.

[35] Filardo EJ.; Quinn JA.; Sabo E. Association of the membrane estrogen receptor, GPR30, with breast tumor metastasis and transactivation of the epidermal growth factor receptor. *Steroids.* **2008**, 73(9-10):870-3.

[36] Lonard DM.; O'Malley BW. The expanding cosmos of nuclear receptor coactivators. *Cell.* **2006**, 125(3):411-4.

[37] Shang Y.; Brown M. Molecular Determinants for the Tissue Specificity of SERMs. *Science.* **2002**, 295(5564):2465-8.

[38] Gottardis MM.; Robinson SP.; Satyaswaroop PG.; Jordan VC. Contrasting actions of tamoxifen on endometrial and breast tumor growth in the athymic mouse. *Cancer Res.* **1988**, 48(4):812-5.

[39] Gottardis MM.; Ricchio ME.; Satyaswaroop PG.; Jordan VC. Effect of steroidal and nonsteroidal antiestrogens on the growth of a tamoxifen-stimulated human endometrial carcinoma (EnCa101) in athymic mice. *Cancer Res.* **1990**, 50(11):3189-92.

[40] Vogel VG.; Costantino JP.; Wickerham DL.; Cronin WM.; Cecchini RS.; Atkins JN.; Bevers TB.; Fehrenbacher L.; Pajon ER, Jr..; Wade JL, 3rd.; Robidoux A.; Margolese RG.; James J.; Lippman SM.; Runowicz CD.; Ganz PA.; Reis SE.; McCaskill-Stevens W.; Ford LG.; Jordan VC.; Wolmark N. Effects of tamoxifen *vs* raloxifene on the risk of developing invasive breast cancer and other disease outcomes: the NSABP Study of Tamoxifen and Raloxifene (STAR) P-2 trial. *Jama.* **2006**, 295(23):2727-41.

[41] Vogel VG.; Costantino JP.; Wickerham DL.; Cronin WM.; Cecchini RS.; Atkins JN.; Bevers TB.; Fehrenbacher L.; Pajon ER.; Wade JL, 3rd.; Robidoux A.; Margolese RG.; James J.; Runowicz CD.; Ganz PA.; Reis SE.; McCaskill-Stevens W.; Ford LG.; Jordan VC.; Wolmark N. Update of the National Surgical Adjuvant Breast and Bowel Project Study of Tamoxifen and Raloxifene (STAR) P-2 Trial: Preventing breast cancer. *Cancer Prev Res (Phila).* **2010**, 3(6):696-706.

[42] Lonard DM.; Tsai SY.; O'Malley BW. Selective estrogen receptor modulators 4-hydroxytamoxifen and raloxifene impact the stability and function of SRC-1 and SRC-3 coactivator proteins. *Mol Cell Biol.* **2004**, 24(1):14-24.

[43] McKenna NJ.; Lanz RB.; O'Malley BW. Nuclear receptor coregulators: cellular and molecular biology. *Endocr Rev.* **1999**, 20(3):321-44.

[44] Shang Y.; Hu X.; DiRenzo J.; Lazar MA.; Brown M. Cofactor dynamics and sufficiency in estrogen receptor-regulated transcription. *Cell.* **2000**, 103(6):843-52.

[45] Smith CL.; Nawaz Z.; O'Malley BW. Coactivator and Corepressor regulation of the agonist/antagonist activity of the mixed antiestrogen, 4-hydroxytamoxifen. *Mol Endocrinol.* **1997**, 11:657-66.

[46] Lavinsky RM.; Jepsen K.; Heinzel T.; Torchia J.; Mullen TM.; Schiff R.; Del-Rio AL.; Ricote M.; Ngo S.; Gemsch J.; Hilsenbeck SG.; Osborne CK.; Glass CK.; Rosenfeld MG.; Rose DW. Diverse signaling pathways modulate nuclear receptor recruitment of N-CoR and SMRT complexes. *Proc Natl Acad Sci U S A.* **1998**, 95(6):2920-5.

[47] Jepsen K.; Hermanson O.; Onami TM.; Gleiberman AS.; Lunyak V.; McEvilly RJ.; Kurokawa R.; Kumar V.; Liu F.; Seto E.; Hedrick SM.; Mandel G.; Glass CK.; Rose DW.; Rosenfeld MG. Combinatorial roles of the nuclear receptor corepressor in transcription and development. *Cell.* **2000**, 102(6):753-63.

[48] Keeton EK.; Brown M. Cell cycle progression stimulated by tamoxifen-bound estrogen receptor-alpha and promoter-specific effects in breast cancer cells deficient in N-CoR and SMRT. *Mol Endocrinol.* **2005**, 19(6):1543-54.

[49] Mazumdar A.; Wang RA.; Mishra SK.; Adam L.; Bagheri-Yarmand R.; Mandal M.; Vadlamudi RK.; Kumar R. Transcriptional repression of oestrogen receptor by metastasis-associated protein 1 corepressor. *Nat Cell Biol.* **2001**, 3(1):30-7.

[50] Montano MM.; Ekena K.; Delage-Mourroux R.; Chang W.; Martini P.; Katzenellenbogen BS. An estrogen receptor-selective coregulator that potentiates the effectiveness of antiestrogens and represses the activity of estrogens. *Proc Natl Acad Sci U S A.* **1999**, 96(12):6947-52.

[51] Delage-Mourroux R.; Martini PG.; Choi I.; Kraichely DM.; Hoeksema J.; Katzenellenbogen BS. Analysis of estrogen receptor interaction with a repressor of estrogen receptor activity (REA) and the regulation of estrogen receptor transcriptional activity by REA. *J Biol Chem.* **2000**, 275(46):35848-56.

[52] Zhang J.; Guenther MG.; Carthew RW.; Lazar MA. Proteasomal regulation of nuclear receptor corepressor-mediated repression. *Genes Dev.* **1998**, 12(12):1775-80.

[53] Frasor J.; Danes JM.; Funk CC.; Katzenellenbogen BS. Estrogen down-regulation of the corepressor N-CoR: mechanism and implications for estrogen derepression of N-CoR-regulated genes. *Proc Natl Acad Sci U S A.* **2005**, 102(37):13153-7.

[54] Spencer TE.; Jenster G.; Burcin MM.; Allis CD.; Zhou J.; Mizzen CA.; McKenna NJ.; Onate SA.; Tsai SY.; Tsai MJ.; O'Malley BW. Steroid receptor coactivator-1 is a histone acetyltransferase. *Nature.* **1997**, 389(6647):194-8.

[55] Liu XF.; Bagchi MK. Recruitment of distinct chromatin-modifying complexes by tamoxifen-complexed estrogen receptor at natural target gene promoters *in vivo. J Biol Chem.* **2004**, 279(15):15050-8.

[56] Feng Q.; Yi P.; Wong J.; O'Malley BW. Signaling within a coactivator complex: methylation of SRC-3/AIB1 is a molecular switch for complex disassembly. *Mol Cell Biol.* **2006**, 26(21):7846-57.

[57] Jordan VC.; O'Malley BW. Selective Estrogen-Receptor Modulators and Antihormonal Resistance in Breast Cancer. *J Clin Oncol.* **2007**, 25(36):5815-24.

[58] Jin Y.; Desta Z.; Stearns V.; Ward B.; Ho H.; Lee KH.; Skaar T.; Storniolo AM.; Li L.; Araba A.; Blanchard R.; Nguyen A.; Ullmer L.; Hayden J.; Lemler S.; Weinshilboum RM.; Rae JM.; Hayes DF.; Flockhart DA. CYP2D6 genotype, antidepressant use, and tamoxifen metabolism during adjuvant breast cancer treatment. *J Natl Cancer Inst.* **2005**, 97(1):30-9.

[59] Weinshilboum R. Pharmacogenomics of endocrine therapy in breast cancer. *Adv Exp Med Biol.* **2008**, 630:220-31.

[60] Flockhart D. CYP2D6 genotyping and the pharmacogenetics of tamoxifen. *Clin Adv Hematol Oncol.* **2008**, 6(7):493-4.

[61] Borges S.; Desta Z.; Li L.; Skaar TC.; Ward BA.; Nguyen A.; Jin Y.; Storniolo AM.; Nikoloff DM.; Wu L.; Hillman G.; Hayes DF.; Stearns V.; Flockhart DA. Quantitative effect of CYP2D6 genotype and inhibitors on tamoxifen metabolism: implication for optimization of breast cancer treatment. *Clin Pharmacol Ther.* **2006**, 80(1):61-74.

[62] Harvell DM.; Richer JK.; Singh M.; Spoelstra N.; Finlayson C.; Borges VF.; Elias AD.; Horwitz KB. Estrogen regulated gene expression in response to neoadjuvant endocrine therapy of breast cancers: tamoxifen agonist effects dominate in the presence of an aromatase inhibitor. *Breast Cancer Res Treat.* **2008**.

[63] Arpino G.; Weiss H.; Lee AV.; Schiff R.; De Placido S.; Osborne CK.; Elledge RM. Estrogen receptor-positive, progesterone receptor-negative breast cancer: association with growth factor receptor expression and tamoxifen resistance. *J Natl Cancer Inst.* **2005**, 97(17):1254-61.

[64] Kim H-J.; Cui X.; Hilsenbeck SG.; Lee AV. Progesterone Receptor Loss Correlates with Human Epidermal Growth Factor Receptor 2 Overexpression in Estrogen Receptor-Positive Breast Cancer. *Clin Cancer Res.* **2006**, 12(3):1013s-8.

[65] Osborne CK.; Schiff R.; Arpino G.; Lee AS.; Hilsenbeck VG. Endocrine responsiveness: understanding how progesterone receptor can be used to select endocrine therapy. *Breast.* **2005**, 14(6):458-65.

[66] Huang HJ.; Neven P.; Drijkoningen M.; Paridaens R.; Wildiers H.; Van Limbergen E.; Berteloot P.; Amant F.; Christiaens MR.; Vergote I. Association between HER-2/neu and the progesterone receptor in oestrogen-dependent breast cancer is age-related. *Breast Cancer Res Treat.* **2005**, 91(1):81-7.

[67] Jordan VC.; Gelber RD. Problems With the Progesterone Receptor in Practice? *J Clin Oncol.* **2007**, 25(15):1957-9.

[68] Arpino G.; Wiechmann L.; Osborne CK.; Schiff R. Crosstalk between the estrogen receptor and the HER tyrosine kinase receptor family: molecular mechanism and clinical implications for endocrine therapy resistance. *Endocr Rev.* **2008**, 29(2):217-33.

[69] Slamon DJ.; Clark GM.; Wong SG.; Levin WJ.; Ullrich A.; McGuire WL. Human breast cancer: correlation of relapse and survival with amplification of the HER-2/neu oncogene. *Science.* **1987**, 235(4785):177-82.

[70] Konecny G.; Pauletti G.; Pegram M.; Untch M.; Dandekar S.; Aguilar Z.; Wilson C.; Rong HM.; Bauerfeind I.; Felber M.; Wang HJ.; Beryt M.; Seshadri R.; Hepp H.; Slamon DJ. Quantitative association between HER-2/neu and steroid hormone receptors in hormone receptor-positive primary breast cancer. *J Natl Cancer Inst.* **2003**, 95(2):142-53.

[71] De Laurentiis M.; Arpino G.; Massarelli E.; Ruggiero A.; Carlomagno C.; Ciardiello F.; Tortora G.; D'Agostino D.; Caputo F.; Cancello G.; Montagna E.; Malorni L.; Zinno L.; Lauria R.; Bianco AR.; De Placido S. A meta-analysis on the interaction between HER-2 expression and response to endocrine treatment in advanced breast cancer. *Clin Cancer Res.* **2005**, 11(13):4741-8.

[72] Tsutsui S.; Ohno S.; Murakami S.; Hachitanda Y.; Oda S. Prognostic value of epidermal growth factor receptor (EGFR) and its relationship to the estrogen receptor status in 1029 patients with breast cancer. *Breast Cancer Res Treat.* **2002**, 71(1):67-75.

[73] Likhite VS.; Stossi F.; Kim K.; Katzenellenbogen BS.; Katzenellenbogen JA. Kinase-Specific Phosphorylation of the Estrogen Receptor Changes Receptor Interactions with Ligand, Deoxyribonucleic Acid, and Coregulators Associated with Alterations in Estrogen and Tamoxifen Activity. *Mol Endocrinol.* **2006**, 20(12):3120-32.

[74] Bunone G.; Briand PA.; Miksicek RJ.; Picard D. Activation of the unliganded estrogen receptor by EGF involves the MAP kinase pathway and direct phosphorylation. *Embo J.* **1996**, 15(9):2174-83.

[75] Campbell RA.; Bhat-Nakshatri P.; Patel NM.; Constantinidou D.; Ali S.; Nakshatri H. Phosphatidylinositol 3-kinase/AKT-mediated activation of estrogen receptor alpha: a new model for anti-estrogen resistance. *J Biol Chem.* **2001**, 276(13):9817-24.

[76] Kato S.; Endoh H.; Masuhiro Y.; Kitamoto T.; Uchiyama S.; Sasaki H.; Masushige S.; Gotoh Y.; Nishida E.; Kawashima H.; *et al.* Activation of the estrogen receptor through phosphorylation by mitogen- activated protein kinase. *Science.* **1995**, 270(5241):1491-4.

[77] Zwart W.; Griekspoor A.; Berno V.; Lakeman K.; Jalink K.; Mancini M.; Neefjes J.; Michalides R. PKA-induced resistance to tamoxifen is associated with an altered orientation of ERalpha towards co-activator SRC-1. *Embo J.* **2007**, 26(15):3534-44.

[78] Font de Mora J.; Brown M. AIB1 is a conduit for kinase-mediated growth factor signaling to the estrogen receptor. *Mol Cell Biol.* **2000**, 20(14):5041-7.

[79] Lopez GN.; Turck CW.; Schaufele F.; Stallcup MR.; Kushner PJ. Growth factors signal to steroid receptors through mitogen-activated protein kinase regulation of p160 coactivator activity. *J Biol Chem.* **2001**, 276(25):22177-82.

[80] Wu RC.; Qin J.; Hashimoto Y.; Wong J.; Xu J.; Tsai SY.; Tsai MJ.; O'Malley BW. Regulation of SRC-3 (pCIP/ACTR/AIB-1/RAC-3/TRAM-1) Coactivator activity by I kappa B kinase. *Mol Cell Biol.* **2002**, 22(10):3549-61.

[81] Hong SH.; Privalsky ML. The SMRT corepressor is regulated by a MEK-1 kinase pathway: inhibition of corepressor function is associated with SMRT phosphorylation and nuclear export. *Mol Cell Biol.* **2000**, 20(17):6612-25.

[82] Schiff R.; Massarweh SA.; Shou J.; Bharwani L.; Mohsin SK.; Osborne CK. Cross-talk between estrogen receptor and growth factor pathways as a molecular target for overcoming endocrine resistance. *Clin Cancer Res.* **2004**, 10(1 Pt 2):331S-6S.

[83] Shou J.; Massarweh S.; Osborne CK.; Wakeling AE.; Ali S.; Weiss H.; Schiff R. Mechanisms of tamoxifen resistance: increased estrogen receptor-HER2/neu cross-talk in ER/HER2-positive breast cancer. *J Natl Cancer Inst.* **2004**, 96(12):926-35.

[84] Nicholson RI.; Hutcheson IR.; Knowlden JM.; Jones HE.; Harper ME.; Jordan N.; Hiscox SE.; Barrow D.; Gee JMW. Nonendocrine Pathways and Endocrine Resistance: Observations with Antiestrogens and Signal Transduction Inhibitors in Combination. *Clin Cancer Res.* **2004**, 10(1):346S-54.

[85] Creighton CJ.; Casa A.; Lazard Z.; Huang S.; Tsimelzon A.; Hilsenbeck SG.; Osborne CK.; Lee AV. Insulin-like growth factor-I activates gene transcription programs strongly associated with poor breast cancer prognosis. *J Clin Oncol.* **2008**, 26(25):4078-85.

[86] Lee AV.; Weng CN.; Jackson JG.; Yee D. Activation of estrogen receptor-mediated gene transcription by IGF-I in human breast cancer cells. *J Endocrinol.* **1997**, 152(1):39-47.

[87] Dihge L.; Bendahl PO.; Grabau D.; Isola J.; Lovgren K.; Ryden L.; Ferno M. Epidermal growth factor receptor (EGFR) and the estrogen receptor modulator amplified in breast cancer (AIB1) for predicting clinical outcome after adjuvant tamoxifen in breast cancer. *Breast Cancer Res Treat.* **2008**, 109(2):255-62.

[88] Kirkegaard T.; McGlynn LM.; Campbell FM.; Muller S.; Tovey SM.; Dunne B.; Nielsen KV.; Cooke TG.; Bartlett JM. Amplified in breast cancer 1 in human epidermal growth factor receptor - positive tumors of tamoxifen-treated breast cancer patients. *Clin Cancer Res*. **2007**, 13(5):1405-11.

[89] Osborne CK.; Bardou V.; Hopp TA.; Chamness GC.; Hilsenbeck SG.; Fuqua SA.; Wong J.; Allred DC.; Clark GM.; Schiff R. Role of the estrogen receptor coactivator AIB1 (SRC-3) and HER-2/neu in tamoxifen resistance in breast cancer. *J Natl Cancer Inst*. **2003**, 95(5):353-61.

[90] Girault I.; Lerebours F.; Amarir S.; Tozlu S.; Tubiana-Hulin M.; Lidereau R.; Bieche I. Expression Analysis of Estrogen Receptor {alpha} Coregulators in Breast Carcinoma: Evidence That NCOR1 Expression Is Predictive of the Response to Tamoxifen. *Clin Cancer Res*. **2003**, 9(4):1259-66.

[91] Wang LH.; Yang XY.; Zhang X.; An P.; Kim HJ.; Huang J.; Clarke R.; Osborne CK.; Inman JK.; Appella E.; Farrar WL. Disruption of estrogen receptor DNA-binding domain and related intramolecular communication restores tamoxifen sensitivity in resistant breast cancer. *Cancer Cell*. **2006**, 10(6):487-99.

[92] Iorio MV.; Ferracin M.; Liu CG.; Veronese A.; Spizzo R.; Sabbioni S.; Magri E.; Pedriali M.; Fabbri M.; Campiglio M.; Menard S.; Palazzo JP.; Rosenberg A.; Musiani P.; Volinia S.; Nenci I.; Calin GA.; Querzoli P.; Negrini M.; Croce CM. MicroRNA gene expression deregulation in human breast cancer. *Cancer Res*. **2005**, 65(16):7065-70.

[93] Lu J.; Getz G.; Miska EA.; Alvarez-Saavedra E.; Lamb J.; Peck D.; Sweet-Cordero A.; Ebert BL.; Mak RH.; Ferrando AA.; Downing JR.; Jacks T.; Horvitz HR.; Golub TR. MicroRNA expression profiles classify human cancers. *Nature*. **2005**, 435(7043):834-8.

[94] Miller TE.; Ghoshal K.; Ramaswamy B.; Roy S.; Datta J.; Shapiro CL.; Jacob S.; Majumder S. MicroRNA-221/222 confers tamoxifen resistance in breast cancer by targeting p27(Kip1). *J Biol Chem*. **2008**:M804612200.

[95] Zhao J-J.; Lin J.; Yang H.; Kong W.; He L.; Ma X.; Coppola D.; Cheng JQ. MicroRNA-221/222 negatively regulates ERalpha and associates with tamoxifen resistance in breast cancer. *J Biol Chem*. **2008**:M806041200.

[96] Gottardis MM.; Jordan VC. Development of tamoxifen-stimulated growth of MCF-7 tumors in athymic mice after long-term antiestrogen administration. *Cancer Res*. **1988**, 48(18):5183-7.

[97] Osborne CK.; Pippen J.; Jones SE.; Parker LM.; Ellis M.; Come S.; Gertler SZ.; May JT.; Burton G.; Dimery I.; Webster A.; Morris C.; Elledge R.; Buzdar A. Double-blind, randomized trial comparing the efficacy and tolerability of fulvestrant *versus* anastrozole in postmenopausal women with advanced breast cancer progressing on prior endocrine therapy: results of a North American trial. *J Clin Oncol*. **2002**, 20(16):3386-95.

[98] Howell A.; Robertson JF.; Quaresma Albano J.; Aschermannova A.; Mauriac L.; Kleeberg UR.; Vergote I.; Erikstein B.; Webster A.; Morris C. Fulvestrant, formerly ICI 182,780, is as effective as anastrozole in postmenopausal women with advanced breast cancer progressing after prior endocrine treatment. *J Clin Oncol*. **2002**, 20(16):3396-403.

[99] Johnston SR.; Saccani-Jotti G.; Smith IE.; Salter J.; Newby J.; Coppen M.; Ebbs SR.; Dowsett M. Changes in estrogen receptor, progesterone receptor, and pS2 expression in tamoxifen-resistant human breast cancer. *Cancer Res*. **1995**, 55(15):3331-8.

[100] Gutierrez MC.; Detre S.; Johnston S.; Mohsin SK.; Shou J.; Allred DC.; Schiff R.; Osborne CK.; Dowsett M. Molecular changes in tamoxifen-resistant breast cancer: relationship

between estrogen receptor, HER-2, and p38 mitogen-activated protein kinase. *J Clin Oncol.* **2005**, 23(11):2469-76.

[101] Normanno N.; Di Maio M.; De Maio E.; De Luca A.; de Matteis A.; Giordano A.; Perrone F. Mechanisms of endocrine resistance and novel therapeutic strategies in breast cancer. *Endocr Relat Cancer.* **2005**, 12(4):721-47.

[102] deGraffenried LA.; Friedrichs WE.; Russell DH.; Donzis EJ.; Middleton AK.; Silva JM.; Roth RA.; Hidalgo M. Inhibition of mTOR activity restores tamoxifen response in breast cancer cells with aberrant Akt Activity. *Clin Cancer Res.* **2004**, 10(23):8059-67.

[103] Chu I.; Sun J.; Arnaout A.; Kahn H.; Hanna W.; Narod S.; Sun P.; Tan CK.; Hengst L.; Slingerland J. p27 phosphorylation by Src regulates inhibition of cyclin E-Cdk2. *Cell.* **2007**, 128(2):281-94.

[104] Abukhdeir AM.; Vitolo MI.; Argani P.; De Marzo AM.; Karakas B.; Konishi H.; Gustin JP.; Lauring J.; Garay JP.; Pendleton C.; Konishi Y.; Blair BG.; Brenner K.; Garrett-Mayer E.; Carraway H.; Bachman KE.; Park BH. Tamoxifen-stimulated growth of breast cancer due to p21 loss. *Proceedings of the National Academy of Sciences.* **2008**:0710887105.

[105] Yuan Y.; Qin L.; Liu D.; Wu R-C.; Mussi P.; Zhou S.; Songyang Z.; Xu J. Genetic Screening Reveals an Essential Role of p27kip1 in Restriction of Breast Cancer Progression. *Cancer Res.* **2007**, 67(17):8032-42.

[106] Iorns E.; Turner NC.; Elliott R.; Syed N.; Garrone O.; Gasco M.; Tutt ANJ.; Crook T.; Lord CJ.; Ashworth A. Identification of CDK10 as an Important Determinant of Resistance to Endocrine Therapy for Breast Cancer. *Cancer Cell.* **2008**, 13(2):91-104.

[107] Moriai R.; Tsuji N.; Moriai M.; Kobayashi D.; Watanabe N. Survivin plays as a resistant factor against tamoxifen-induced apoptosis in human breast cancer cells. *Breast Cancer Res Treat.* **2008**.

[108] Jordan VC.; Lewis JS.; Osipo C.; Cheng D. The apoptotic action of estrogen following exhaustive antihormonal therapy: a new clinical treatment strategy. *Breast.* **2005**, 14(6):624-30.

[109] O'Regan RM.; Osipo C.; Ariazi E.; Lee ES.; Meeke K.; Morris C.; Bertucci A.; Sarker MA.; Grigg R.; Jordan VC. Development and therapeutic options for the treatment of raloxifene-stimulated breast cancer in athymic mice. *Clin Cancer Res.* **2006**, 12(7 Pt 1):2255-63.

[110] Liu H.; Lee ES.; Gajdos C.; Pearce ST.; Chen B.; Osipo C.; Loweth J.; McKian K.; De Los Reyes A.; Wing L.; Jordan VC. Apoptotic action of 17beta-estradiol in raloxifene-resistant MCF-7 cells *in vitro* and *in vivo*. *J Natl Cancer Inst.* **2003**, 95(21):1586-97.

[111] Jordan VC.; Phelps E.; Lindgren JU. Effects of anti-estrogens on bone in castrated and intact female rats. *Breast Cancer Res Treat.* **1987**, 10(1):31-5.

[112] Love RR.; Mazess RB.; Barden HS.; Epstein S.; Newcomb PA.; Jordan VC.; Carbone PP.; DeMets DL. Effects of tamoxifen on bone mineral density in postmenopausal women with breast cancer. *N Engl J Med.* **1992**, 326(13):852-6.

[113] Umemoto A.; Lin CX.; Ueyama Y.; Komaki K.; Santosh Laxmi YR.; Shibutani S. Absence of DNA adduct in the leukocytes from breast cancer patients treated with toremifene. *Chem Res Toxicol.* **2006**, 19(3):421-5.

[114] da Costa GG.; Pereira PC.; Churchwell MI.; Beland FA.; Marques MM. DNA adduct formation in the livers of female Sprague-Dawley rats treated with toremifene or alpha-hydroxytoremifene. *Chem Res Toxicol.* **2007**, 20(2):300-10.

[115] Shibutani S.; Ravindernath A.; Terashima I.; Suzuki N.; Laxmi YR.; Kanno Y.; Suzuki M.; Apak TI.; Sheng JJ.; Duffel MW. Mechanism of lower genotoxicity of toremifene compared with tamoxifen. *Cancer Res.* **2001**, 61(10):3925-31.

[116] Dragan VP.; Vaughan J.; Jordan VC.; Pitot HC. Comparison of the effects of tamoxifen and toremifene on liver and kidney tumor promotion in female rats. *Carcinogenesis.* **1995**, 16(11):2733-41.

[117] Sargent LM.; Dragan YP.; Sattler C.; Bahnub N.; Sattler G.; Martin P.; Cisneros A.; Mann J.; Thorgeirsson S.; Jordan VC.; Pitot HC. Induction of hepatic aneuploidy *in vivo* by tamoxifen, toremifene and idoxifene in female Sprague-Dawley rats. *Carcinogenesis.* **1996**, 17(5):1051-6.

[118] Erkkola R.; Mattila L.; Powles T.; Heikkinen J.; Toivola B.; Korhonen P.; Mustonen M. Bone mineral density and lipid changes during 5 years of follow-up in a study of prevention of breast cancer with toremifene in healthy, high-risk pre- and post-menopausal women. *Breast Cancer Res Treat.* **2005**, 93(3):277-87.

[119] Harvey HA.; Kimura M.; Hajba A. Toremifene: an evaluation of its safety profile. *Breast.* **2006**, 15(2):142-57.

[120] O'Regan RM.; Cisneros A.; England GM.; MacGregor JI.; Muenzner HD.; Assikis VJ.; Bilimoria MM.; Piette M.; Dragan YP.; Pitot HC.; Chatterton R.; Jordan VC. Effects of the antiestrogens tamoxifen, toremifene, and ICI 182,780 on endometrial cancer growth. *J Natl Cancer Inst.* **1998**, 90(20):1552-8.

[121] Kusama M.; Kaise H.; Nakayama S.; Ota D.; Misaka T.; Aoki T. Crossover trial for lipid abnormality in postmenopausal breast cancer patients during selective estrogen receptor modulators (SERMs) administrations. *Breast Cancer Res Treat.* **2004**, 88(1):9-16.

[122] Kusama M.; Miyauchi K.; Aoyama H.; Sano M.; Kimura M.; Mitsuyama S.; Komaki K.; Doihara H. Effects of toremifene (TOR) and tamoxifen (TAM) on serum lipids in postmenopausal patients with breast cancer. *Breast Cancer Res Treat.* **2004**, 88(1):1-8.

[123] Lee ES.; Schafer JM.; Yao K.; England G.; O'Regan RM.; De Los Reyes A.; Jordan VC. Cross-resistance of triphenylethylene-type antiestrogens but not ICI 182,780 in tamoxifen-stimulated breast tumors grown in athymic mice. *Clin Cancer Res.* **2000**, 6(12):4893-9.

[124] Stenbygaard LE.; Herrstedt J.; Thomsen JF.; Svendsen KR.; Engelholm SA.; Dombernowsky P. Toremifene and tamoxifen in advanced breast cancer--a double-blind cross-over trial. *Breast Cancer Res Treat.* **1993**, 25(1):57-63.

[125] Vogel CL.; Shemano I.; Schoenfelder J.; Gams RA.; Green MR. Multicenter phase II efficacy trial of toremifene in tamoxifen-refractory patients with advanced breast cancer. *J Clin Oncol.* **1993**, 11(2):345-50.

[126] Gong C.; Song E.; Jia W.; Qin L.; Guo J.; Jia H.; Hu X.; Su F. A double-blind randomized controlled trial of toremifen therapy for mastalgia. *Arch Surg.* **2006**, 141(1):43-7.

[127] Oksa S.; Luukkaala T.; Maenpaa J. Toremifene for premenstrual mastalgia: a randomised, placebo-controlled crossover study. *Bjog.* **2006**, 113(6):713-8.

[128] Price D.; Stein B.; Sieber P.; Tutrone R.; Bailen J.; Goluboff E.; Burzon D.; Bostwick D.; Steiner M. Toremifene for the prevention of prostate cancer in men with high grade prostatic intraepithelial neoplasia: results of a double-blind, placebo controlled, phase IIB clinical trial. *J Urol.* **2006**, 176(3):965-70; discussion 70-1.

[129] Smith MR.; Malkowicz SB.; Chu F.; Forrest J.; Price D.; Sieber P.; Barnette KG.; Rodriguez D.; Steiner MS. Toremifene increases bone mineral density in men receiving

androgen deprivation therapy for prostate cancer: interim analysis of a multicenter phase 3 clinical study. *J Urol.* **2008**, 179(1):152-5.

[130] Smith MR.; Malkowicz SB.; Chu F.; Forrest J.; Sieber P.; Barnette KG.; Rodriquez D.; Steiner MS. Toremifene improves lipid profiles in men receiving androgen-deprivation therapy for prostate cancer: interim analysis of a multicenter phase III study. *J Clin Oncol.* **2008**, 26(11):1824-9.

[131] Hellmann-Blumberg U.; Taras TL.; Wurz GT.; DeGregorio MW. Genotoxic effects of the novel mixed antiestrogen FC-1271a in comparison to tamoxifen and toremifene. *Breast Cancer Res Treat.* **2000**, 60(1):63-70.

[132] Qu Q.; Zheng H.; Dahllund J.; Laine A.; Cockcroft N.; Peng Z.; Koskinen M.; Hemminki K.; Kangas L.; Vaananen K.; Harkonen P. Selective estrogenic effects of a novel triphenylethylene compound, FC1271a, on bone, cholesterol level, and reproductive tissues in intact and ovariectomized rats. *Endocrinology.* **2000**, 141(2):809-20.

[133] Wurz GT.; Hellmann-Blumberg U.; DeGregorio MW. Pharmacologic effects of ospemifene in rhesus macaques: a pilot study. *Basic Clin Pharmacol Toxicol.* **2008**, 102(6):552-8.

[134] Komi J.; Lankinen KS.; Harkonen P.; DeGregorio MW.; Voipio S.; Kivinen S.; Tuimala R.; Vihtamaki T.; Vihko K.; Ylikorkala O.; Erkkola R. Effects of ospemifene and raloxifene on hormonal status, lipids, genital tract, and tolerability in postmenopausal women. *Menopause.* **2005**, 12(2):202-9.

[135] Rutanen EM.; Heikkinen J.; Halonen K.; Komi J.; Lammintausta R.; Ylikorkala O. Effects of ospemifene, a novel SERM, on hormones, genital tract, climacteric symptoms, and quality of life in postmenopausal women: a double-blind, randomized trial. *Menopause.* **2003**, 10(5):433-9.

[136] Voipio SK.; Komi J.; Kangas L.; Halonen K.; DeGregorio MW.; Erkkola RU. Effects of ospemifene (FC-1271a) on uterine endometrium, vaginal maturation index, and hormonal status in healthy postmenopausal women. *Maturitas.* **2002**, 43(3):207-14.

[137] Kallio A.; Guo T.; Lamminen E.; Seppanen J.; Kangas L.; Vaananen HK.; Harkonen P. Estrogen and the selective estrogen receptor modulator (SERM) protection against cell death in estrogen receptor alpha and beta expressing U2OS cells. *Mol Cell Endocrinol.* **2008**.

[138] Michael H.; Harkonen PL.; Kangas L.; Vaananen HK.; Hentunen TA. Differential effects of selective oestrogen receptor modulators (SERMs) tamoxifen, ospemifene and raloxifene on human osteoclasts *in vitro*. *Br J Pharmacol.* **2007**, 151(3):384-95.

[139] Komi J.; Lankinen KS.; DeGregorio M.; Heikkinen J.; Saarikoski S.; Tuppurainen M.; Halonen K.; Lammintausta R.; Vaananen K.; Ylikorkala O.; Erkkola R. Effects of ospemifene and raloxifene on biochemical markers of bone turnover in postmenopausal women. *J Bone Miner Metab.* **2006**, 24(4):314-8.

[140] Wurz GT.; Read KC.; Marchisano-Karpman C.; Gregg JP.; Beckett LA.; Yu Q.; Degregorio MW. Ospemifene inhibits the growth of dimethylbenzanthracene-induced mammary tumors in Sencar mice. *J Steroid Biochem Mol Biol.* **2005**, 97(3):230-40.

[141] Namba R.; Young LJ.; Maglione JE.; McGoldrick ET.; Liu S.; Wurz GT.; DeGregorio MW.; Borowsky AD.; MacLeod CL.; Cardiff RD.; Gregg JP. Selective estrogen receptor modulators inhibit growth and progression of premalignant lesions in a mouse model of ductal carcinoma *in situ*. *Breast Cancer Res.* **2005**, 7(6):R881-9.

[142] Willson TM.; Norris JD.; Wagner BL.; Asplin I.; Baer P.; Brown HR.; Jones SA.; Henke B.; Sauls H.; Wolfe S.; Morris DC.; McDonnell DP. Dissection of the molecular mechanism of action of GW5638, a novel estrogen receptor ligand, provides insights into the role of estrogen receptor in bone. *Endocrinology*. **1997**, 138(9):3901-11.

[143] Bentrem D.; Dardes R.; Liu H.; MacGregor-Schafer J.; Zapf J.; Jordan V. Molecular mechanism of action at estrogen receptor alpha of a new clinically relevant antiestrogen (GW7604) related to tamoxifen. *Endocrinology*. **2001**, 142(2):838-46.

[144] Connor CE.; Norris JD.; Broadwater G.; Willson TM.; Gottardis MM.; Dewhirst MW.; McDonnell DP. Circumventing tamoxifen resistance in breast cancers using antiestrogens that induce unique conformational changes in the estrogen receptor. *Cancer Res*. **2001**, 61(7):2917-22.

[145] Dardes RC.; O'Regan RM.; Gajdos C.; Robinson SP.; Bentrem D.; De Los Reyes A.; Jordan VC. Effects of a new clinically relevant antiestrogen (GW5638) related to tamoxifen on breast and endometrial cancer growth *in vivo*. *Clin Cancer Res*. **2002**, 8(6):1995-2001.

[146] Wu YL.; Yang X.; Ren Z.; McDonnell DP.; Norris JD.; Willson TM.; Greene GL. Structural basis for an unexpected mode of SERM-mediated ER antagonism. *Mol Cell*. **2005**, 18(4):413-24.

[147] Fan M.; Rickert EL.; Chen L.; Aftab SA.; Nephew KP.; Weatherman RV. Characterization of molecular and structural determinants of selective estrogen receptor downregulators. *Breast Cancer Res Treat*. **2007**, 103(1):37-44.

[148] Wittmann BM.; Sherk A.; McDonnell DP. Definition of functionally important mechanistic differences among selective estrogen receptor down-regulators. *Cancer Res*. **2007**, 67(19):9549-60.

[149] Sporn MB. Arzoxifene: a promising new selective estrogen receptor modulator for clinical chemoprevention of breast cancer. *Clin Cancer Res*. **2004**, 10(16):5313-5.

[150] Munster PN. Arzoxifene: the development and clinical outcome of an ideal SERM. *Expert Opin Investig Drugs*. **2006**, 15(3):317-26.

[151] Schafer JM.; Lee ES.; Dardes RC.; Bentrem D.; O'Regan RM.; De Los Reyes A.; Jordan VC. Analysis of cross-resistance of the selective estrogen receptor modulators arzoxifene (LY353381) and LY117018 in tamoxifen-stimulated breast cancer xenografts. *Clin Cancer Res*. **2001**, 7(8):2505-12.

[152] Buzdar A.; O'Shaughnessy JA.; Booser DJ.; Pippen JE, Jr..; Jones SE.; Munster PN.; Peterson P.; Melemed AS.; Winer E.; Hudis C. Phase II, randomized, double-blind study of two dose levels of arzoxifene in patients with locally advanced or metastatic breast cancer. *J Clin Oncol*. **2003**, 21(6):1007-14.

[153] McMeekin DS.; Gordon A.; Fowler J.; Melemed A.; Buller R.; Burke T.; Bloss J.; Sabbatini P. A phase II trial of arzoxifene, a selective estrogen response modulator, in patients with recurrent or advanced endometrial cancer. *Gynecol Oncol*. **2003**, 90(1):64-9.

[154] Deshmane V.; Krishnamurthy S.; Melemed AS.; Peterson P.; Buzdar AU. Phase III Double-Blind Trial of Arzoxifene Compared With Tamoxifen for Locally Advanced or Metastatic Breast Cancer. *J Clin Oncol*. **2007**, 25(31):4967-73.

[155] Liby K.; Rendi M.; Suh N.; Royce DB.; Risingsong R.; Williams CR.; Lamph W.; Labrie F.; Krajewski S.; Xu X.; Kim H.; Brown P.; Sporn MB. The combination of the rexinoid, LG100268, and a selective estrogen receptor modulator, either arzoxifene or acolbifene, synergizes in the prevention and treatment of mammary tumors in an estrogen receptor-negative model of breast cancer. *Clin Cancer Res*. **2006**, 12(19):5902-9.

[156] Fabian CJ.; Kimler BF.; Anderson J.; Tawfik OW.; Mayo MS.; Burak WE, Jr..; O'Shaughnessy JA.; Albain KS.; Hyams DM.; Budd GT.; Ganz PA.; Sauter ER.; Beenken SW.; Grizzle WE.; Fruehauf JP.; Arneson DW.; Bacus JW.; Lagios MD.; Johnson KA.; Browne D. Breast cancer chemoprevention phase I evaluation of biomarker modulation by arzoxifene, a third generation selective estrogen receptor modulator. *Clin Cancer Res.* **2004**, 10(16):5403-17.

[157] Vajdos FF.; Hoth LR.; Geoghegan KF.; Simons SP.; LeMotte PK.; Danley DE.; Ammirati MJ.; Pandit J. The 2.0 A crystal structure of the ERalpha ligand-binding domain complexed with lasofoxifene. *Protein Sci.* **2007**, 16(5):897-905.

[158] Ke HZ.; Paralkar VM.; Grasser WA.; Crawford DT.; Qi H.; Simmons HA.; Pirie CM.; Chidsey-Frink KL.; Owen TA.; Smock SL.; Chen HK.; Jee WS.; Cameron KO.; Rosati RL.; Brown TA.; Dasilva-Jardine P.; Thompson DD. Effects of CP-336,156, a new, nonsteroidal estrogen agonist/antagonist, on bone, serum cholesterol, uterus and body composition in rat models. *Endocrinology.* **1998**, 139(4):2068-76.

[159] Gennari L. Lasofoxifene: a new type of selective estrogen receptor modulator for the treatment of osteoporosis. *Drugs Today (Barc).* **2006**, 42(6):355-67.

[160] Rosati RL.; Da Silva Jardine P.; Cameron KO.; Thompson DD.; Ke HZ.; Toler SM.; Brown TA.; Pan LC.; Ebbinghaus CF.; Reinhold AR.; Elliott NC.; Newhouse BN.; Tjoa CM.; Sweetnam PM.; Cole MJ.; Arriola MW.; Gauthier JW.; Crawford DT.; Nickerson DF.; Pirie CM.; Qi H.; Simmons HA.; Tkalcevic GT. Discovery and preclinical pharmacology of a novel, potent, nonsteroidal estrogen receptor agonist/antagonist, CP-336156, a diaryltetrahydronaphthalene. *J Med Chem.* **1998**, 41(16):2928-31.

[161] Gass M.; Kagan R.; Simon J.; Spino C.; Barcomb L. Objective Measures of Vaginal Atrophy Are Improved With Lasofoxifene, A Next-Generation Selective Estrogen Receptor Modulator. *Obstetrics & Gynecology.* **2005**, 105(4):71S.

[162] Wang XN.; Simmons HA.; Salatto CT.; Cosgrove PG.; Thompson DD. Lasofoxifene enhances vaginal mucus formation without causing hypertrophy and increases estrogen receptor beta and androgen receptor in rats. *Menopause.* **2006**, 13(4):609-20.

[163] Cohen LA.; Pittman B.; Wang CX.; Aliaga C.; Yu L.; Moyer JD. LAS, a novel selective estrogen receptor modulator with chemopreventive and therapeutic activity in the N-nitroso-N-methylurea-induced rat mammary tumor model. *Cancer Res.* **2001**, 61(24):8683-8.

[164] Vogelvang TE.; van der Mooren MJ.; Mijatovic V.; Kenemans P. Emerging selective estrogen receptor modulators: special focus on effects on coronary heart disease in postmenopausal women. *Drugs.* **2006**, 66(2):191-221.

[165] Stein RC.; Dowsett M.; Cunningham DC.; Davenport J.; Ford HT.; Gazet JC.; von Angerer E.; Coombes RC. Phase I/II study of the anti-oestrogen zindoxifene (D16726) in the treatment of advanced breast cancer. A Cancer Research Campaign Phase I/II Clinical Trials Committee study. *Br J Cancer.* **1990**, 61(3):451-3.

[166] Miller CP.; Collini MD.; Tran BD.; Harris HA.; Kharode YP.; Marzolf JT.; Moran RA.; Henderson RA.; Bender RH.; Unwalla RJ.; Greenberger LM.; Yardley JP.; Abou-Gharbia MA.; Lyttle CR.; Komm BS. Design, synthesis, and preclinical characterization of novel, highly selective indole estrogens. *J Med Chem.* **2001**, 44(11):1654-7.

[167] Greenberger LM.; Annable T.; Collins KI.; Komm BS.; Lyttle CR.; Miller CP.; Satyaswaroop PG.; Zhang Y.; Frost P. A new antiestrogen, 2-(4-hydroxy-phenyl)-3-methyl-1-[4-(2-piperidin-1-yl-ethoxy)-benzyl]-1H-in dol-5-ol hydrochloride (ERA-923),

inhibits the growth of tamoxifen-sensitive and -resistant tumors and is devoid of uterotropic effects in mice and rats. *Clin Cancer Res.* **2001**, 7(10):3166-77.

[168] Sadler TM.; Gavriil M.; Annable T.; Frost P.; Greenberger LM.; Zhang Y. Combination therapy for treating breast cancer using antiestrogen, ERA-923, and the mammalian target of rapamycin inhibitor, temsirolimus. *Endocr Relat Cancer.* **2006**, 13(3):863-73.

[169] Komm BS.; Kharode YP.; Bodine PV.; Harris HA.; Miller CP.; Lyttle CR. Bazedoxifene acetate: a selective estrogen receptor modulator with improved selectivity. *Endocrinology.* **2005**, 146(9):3999-4008.

[170] Ronkin S.; Northington R.; Baracat E.; Nunes MG.; Archer DF.; Constantine G.; Pickar JH. Endometrial effects of bazedoxifene acetate, a novel selective estrogen receptor modulator, in postmenopausal women. *Obstet Gynecol.* **2005**, 105(6):1397-404.

[171] Silverman SL.; Christiansen C.; Genant HK.; Vukicevic S.; Zanchetta JR.; de Villiers TJ.; Constantine GD.; Chines AA. Efficacy of Bazedoxifene in Reducing New Vertebral Fracture Risk in Postmenopausal Women With Osteoporosis: Results From a 3-Year, Randomized, Placebo- and Active-Controlled Clinical Trial*. *J Bone Miner Res.* **2008**.

[172] Bazedoxifene: Bazedoxifene Acetate, TSE 424, TSE-424, WAY 140424. *Drugs R D.* **2008**, 9(3):191-6.

[173] Kharode Y.; Bodine PVN.; Miller CP.; Lyttle CR.; Komm BS. The Pairing of a Selective Estrogen Receptor Modulator, Bazedoxifene, With Conjugated Estrogens as a New Paradigm for the Treatment of Menopausal Symptoms and Osteoporosis Prevention. *Endocrinology.* **2008**:en.2008-0817.

[174] Tremblay A.; Tremblay GB.; Labrie C.; Labrie F.; Giguere V. EM-800, a novel antiestrogen, acts as a pure antagonist of the transcriptional functions of estrogen receptors alpha and beta. *Endocrinology.* **1998**, 139(1):111-8.

[175] Schafer JI.; Liu H.; Tonetti DA.; Jordan VC. The interaction of raloxifene and the active metabolite of the antiestrogen EM-800 (SC 5705) with the human estrogen receptor. *Cancer Res.* **1999**, 59(17):4308-13.

[176] Martel C.; Picard S.; Richard V.; Belanger A.; Labrie C.; Labrie F. Prevention of bone loss by EM-800 and raloxifene in the ovariectomized rat. *J Steroid Biochem Mol Biol.* **2000**, 74(1-2):45-56.

[177] Lemieux C.; Gelinas Y.; Lalonde J.; Labrie F.; Richard D.; Deshaies Y. Hypocholesterolemic action of the selective estrogen receptor modulator acolbifene in intact and ovariectomized rats with diet-induced hypercholesterolemia. *Metabolism.* **2006**, 55(5):605-13.

[178] Martel C.; Provencher L.; Li X.; St Pierre A.; Leblanc G.; Gauthier S.; Merand Y.; Labrie F. Binding characteristics of novel nonsteroidal antiestrogens to the rat uterine estrogen receptors. *J Steroid Biochem Mol Biol.* **1998**, 64(3-4):199-205.

[179] Simard J.; Labrie C.; Belanger A.; Gauthier S.; Singh SM.; Merand Y.; Labrie F. Characterization of the effects of the novel non-steroidal antiestrogen EM-800 on basal and estrogen-induced proliferation of T-47D, ZR-75-1 and MCF-7 human breast cancer cells *in vitro*. *Int J Cancer.* **1997**, 73(1):104-12.

[180] Gutman M.; Couillard S.; Roy J.; Labrie F.; Candas B.; Labrie C. Comparison of the effects of EM-652 (SCH57068), tamoxifen, toremifene, droloxifene, idoxifene, GW-5638 and raloxifene on the growth of human ZR-75-1 breast tumors in nude mice. *Int J Cancer.* **2002**, 99(2):273-8.

[181] Labrie F.; Champagne P.; Labrie C.; Roy J.; Laverdiere J.; Provencher L.; Potvin M.; Drolet Y.; Pollak M.; Panasci L.; L'Esperance B.; Dufresne J.; Latreille J.; Robert J.; Samson B.; Jolivet J.; Yelle L.; Cusan L.; Diamond P.; Candas B. Activity and Safety of the Antiestrogen EM-800, the Orally Active Precursor of Acolbifene, in Tamoxifen-Resistant Breast Cancer. *J Clin Oncol.* **2004**, 22(5):864-71.

[182] Labrie F. Future perspectives of selective estrogen receptor modulators used alone and in combination with DHEA. *Endocr Relat Cancer.* **2006**, 13(2):335-55.

[183] Luo S.; Sourla A.; Labrie C.; Belanger A.; Labrie F. Combined effects of dehydroepiandrosterone and EM-800 on bone mass, serum lipids, and the development of dimethylbenz(A)anthracene-induced mammary carcinoma in the rat. *Endocrinology.* **1997**, 138(10):4435-44.

[184] Galbiati E.; Caruso PL.; Amari G.; Armani E.; Ghirardi S.; Delcanale M.; Civelli M. Pharmacological actions of a novel, potent, tissue-selective benzopyran estrogen. *J Pharmacol Exp Ther.* **2002**, 303(1):196-203.

[185] Armamento-Villareal R.; Sheikh S.; Nawaz A.; Napoli N.; Mueller C.; Halstead LR.; Brodt MD.; Silva MJ.; Galbiati E.; Caruso PL.; Civelli M.; Civitelli R. A new selective estrogen receptor modulator, CHF 4227.01, preserves bone mass and microarchitecture in ovariectomized rats. *J Bone Miner Res.* **2005**, 20(12):2178-88.

[186] Civelli M.; Preti AP.; Cenacchi V.; Rondelli I.; Guastalla D.; Tarral A.; Dostert P.; Guillevic Y.; Homery MC. Single and multiple ascending dose studies of a novel tissue-selective oestrogen receptor modulator, CHF 4227, in healthy postmenopausal women. *Br J Clin Pharmacol.* **2007**, 64(3):304-16.

[187] Brady H.; Doubleday M.; Gayo-Fung LM.; Hickman M.; Khammungkhune S.; Kois A.; Lipps S.; Pierce S.; Richard N.; Shevlin G.; Sutherland MK.; Anderson DW.; Bhagwat SS.; Stein B. Differential response of estrogen receptors alpha and beta to SP500263, a novel potent selective estrogen receptor modulator. *Mol Pharmacol.* **2002**, 61(3):562-8.

[188] Brady H.; Desai S.; Gayo-Fung LM.; Khammungkhune S.; McKie JA.; O'Leary E.; Pascasio L.; Sutherland MK.; Anderson DW.; Bhagwat SS.; Stein B. Effects of SP500263, a novel, potent antiestrogen, on breast cancer cells and in xenograft models. *Cancer Res.* **2002**, 62(5):1439-42.

[189] Sutherland MK.; Brady H.; Gayo-Fung LM.; Leisten J.; Lipps SG.; McKie JA.; O'Leary E.; Patnaik N.; Anderson DW.; Bhagwat SS.; Stein B. Effects of SP500263, a novel selective estrogen receptor modulator, on bone, uterus, and serum cholesterol in the ovariectomized rat. *Calcif Tissue Int.* **2003**, 72(6):710-6.

[190] Kung Sutherland MS.; Lipps SG.; Patnaik N.; Gayo-Fung LM.; Khammungkune S.; Xie W.; Brady HA.; Barbosa MS.; Anderson DW.; Stein B. SP500263, a novel SERM, blocks osteoclastogenesis in a human bone cell model: role of IL-6 and GM-CSF. *Cytokine.* **2003**, 23(1-2):1-14.

[191] Ammann P.; Bourrin S.; Brunner F.; Meyer JM.; Clement-Lacroix P.; Baron R.; Gaillard M.; Rizzoli R. A new selective estrogen receptor modulator HMR-3339 fully corrects bone alterations induced by ovariectomy in adult rats. *Bone.* **2004**, 35(1):153-61.

[192] Vogelvang TE.; Mijatovic V.; Kenemans P.; Teerlink T.; van der Mooren MJ. HMR 3339, a novel selective estrogen receptor modulator, reduces total cholesterol, low-density lipoprotein cholesterol, and homocysteine in healthy postmenopausal women. *Fertil Steril.* **2004**, 82(6):1540-9.

[193] Vogelvang TE.; Mijatovic V.; Kenemans P.; Schalkwijk CG.; van der Mooren MJ. Effect of HMR 3339, a novel selective estrogen receptor modulator, on C-reactive protein levels in healthy postmenopausal women. *Am J Cardiol.* **2004**, 94(9):1205-8.

[194] Verhoeven MO.; Teerlink T.; Kenemans P.; Vogelvang TE.; van der Mooren MJ. Effects on asymmetric dimethylarginine of HMR 3339, a novel selective estrogen receptor modulator: a 12-week, randomized, placebo-controlled, double-blind, dose-ranging study in healthy postmenopausal women. *Menopause.* **2007**, 14(2):235-42.

[195] Vogelvang TE.; Leurs JR.; Mijatovic V.; Willemse J.; van der Mooren MJ. HMR 3339, a novel selective estrogen receptor modulator, reduces concentrations of procarboxypeptidase U, an inhibitor of fibrinolysis. A randomized, placebo-controlled study in postmenopausal women. *J Thromb Haemost.* **2005**, 3(5):1090-2.

[196] Vogelvang TE.; Mijatovic V.; Kenemans P.; Emeis JJ.; Heijst JA.; van der Mooren MJ. The effects of 12 weeks of HMR 3339, a novel selective estrogen receptor modulator, on markers of coagulation and fibrinolysis: a randomized, placebo-controlled, double-blind, dose-ranging study in healthy postmenopausal women. *Am J Obstet Gynecol.* **2005**, 193(4):1384-94.

[197] Windahl SH.; Galien R.; Chiusaroli R.; Clement-Lacroix P.; Morvan F.; Lepescheux L.; Nique F.; Horne WC.; Resche-Rigon M.; Baron R. Bone protection by estrens occurs through non-tissue-selective activation of the androgen receptor. *J Clin Invest.* **2006**, 116(9):2500-9.

[198] Zhao C.; Dahlman-Wright K.; Gustafsson JA. Estrogen receptor beta: an overview and update. *Nucl Recept Signal.* **2008**, 6:e003.

[199] Skliris GP.; Leygue E.; Watson PH.; Murphy LC. Estrogen receptor alpha negative breast cancer patients: estrogen receptor beta as a therapeutic target. *J Steroid Biochem Mol Biol.* **2008**, 109(1-2):1-10.

[200] Chang EC.; Frasor J.; Komm B.; Katzenellenbogen BS. Impact of estrogen receptor beta on gene networks regulated by estrogen receptor alpha in breast cancer cells. *Endocrinology.* **2006**, 147(10):4831-42.

[201] Lin CY.; Strom A.; Li Kong S.; Kietz S.; Thomsen JS.; Tee JB.; Vega VB.; Miller LD.; Smeds J.; Bergh J.; Gustafsson JA.; Liu ET. Inhibitory effects of estrogen receptor beta on specific hormone-responsive gene expression and association with disease outcome in primary breast cancer. *Breast Cancer Res.* **2007**, 9(2):R25.

[202] Murphy LC.; Watson PH. Is oestrogen receptor-beta a predictor of endocrine therapy responsiveness in human breast cancer? *Endocr Relat Cancer.* **2006**, 13(2):327-34.

[203] Rosa FE.; Caldeira JR.; Felipes J.; Bertonha FB.; Quevedo FC.; Domingues MA.; Moraes Neto FA.; Rogatto SR. Evaluation of estrogen receptor alpha and beta and progesterone receptor expression and correlation with clinicopathologic factors and proliferative marker Ki-67 in breast cancers. *Hum Pathol.* **2008**, 39(5):720-30.

[204] Ariazi EA.; Jordan VC. Estrogen-related receptors as emerging targets in cancer and metabolic disorders. *Curr Top Med Chem.* **2006**, 6(3):203-15.

[205] Stein RA.; McDonnell DP. Estrogen-related receptor {alpha} as a therapeutic target in cancer. *Endocr Relat Cancer.* **2006**, 13(Supplement_1):S25-32.

[206] Stein RA.; Chang C-y.; Kazmin DA.; Way J.; Schroeder T.; Wergin M.; Dewhirst MW.; McDonnell DP. Estrogen-Related Receptor {alpha} Is Critical for the Growth of Estrogen Receptor-Negative Breast Cancer. *Cancer Res.* **2008**, 68(21):8805-12.

[207] Arany Z.; Foo SY.; Ma Y.; Ruas JL.; Bommi-Reddy A.; Girnun G.; Cooper M.; Laznik D.; Chinsomboon J.; Rangwala SM.; Baek KH.; Rosenzweig A.; Spiegelman BM. HIF-independent regulation of VEGF and angiogenesis by the transcriptional coactivator PGC-1alpha. *Nature*. **2008**, 451(7181):1008-12.

[208] Ao A.; Wang H.; Kamarajugadda S.; Lu J. Involvement of estrogen-related receptors in transcriptional response to hypoxia and growth of solid tumors. *Proc Natl Acad Sci U S A*. **2008**, 105(22):7821-6.

[209] Leventhal L.; Brandt MR.; Cummons TA.; Piesla MJ.; Rogers KE.; Harris HA. An estrogen receptor-beta agonist is active in models of inflammatory and chemical-induced pain. *Eur J Pharmacol*. **2006**, 553(1-3):146-8.

[210] Meyers MJ.; Sun J.; Carlson KE.; Marriner GA.; Katzenellenbogen BS.; Katzenellenbogen JA. Estrogen receptor-beta potency-selective ligands: structure-activity relationship studies of diarylpropionitriles and their acetylene and polar analogues. *J Med Chem*. **2001**, 44(24):4230-51.

[211] Hegele-Hartung C.; Siebel P.; Peters O.; Kosemund D.; Muller G.; Hillisch A.; Walter A.; Kraetzschmar J.; Fritzemeier KH. Impact of isotype-selective estrogen receptor agonists on ovarian function. *Proc Natl Acad Sci U S A*. **2004**, 101(14):5129-34.

[212] Barker S. Non-steroidal anti-estrogens in the treatment of breast cancer. *Curr Opin Investig Drugs*. **2006**, 7(12):1085-91.

[213] Watanabe N.; Ikeno A.; Minato H.; Nakagawa H.; Kohayakawa C.; Tsuji J. Discovery and preclinical characterization of (+)-3-[4-(1- piperidinoethoxy)phenyl]spiro[indene- 1,1'-indane]-5,5'-diol hydrochloride: a promising nonsteroidal estrogen receptor agonist for hot flush. *J Med Chem*. **2003**, 46(19):3961-4.

[214] Wallace OB.; Lauwers KS.; Dodge JA.; May SA.; Calvin JR.; Hinklin R.; Bryant HU.; Shetler PK.; Adrian MD.; Geiser AG.; Sato M.; Burris TP. A selective estrogen receptor modulator for the treatment of hot flushes. *J Med Chem*. **2006**, 49(3):843-6.

[215] Jain N.; Kanojia RM.; Xu J.; Jian-Zhong G.; Pacia E.; Lai MT.; Du F.; Musto A.; Allan G.; Hahn D.; Lundeen S.; Sui Z. Novel chromene-derived selective estrogen receptor modulators useful for alleviating hot flushes and vaginal dryness. *J Med Chem*. **2006**, 49(11):3056-9.

[216] Jain N.; Xu J.; Kanojia RM.; Du F.; Jian-Zhong G.; Pacia E.; Lai MT.; Musto A.; Allan G.; Reuman M.; Li X.; Hahn D.; Cousineau M.; Peng S.; Ritchie D.; Russell R.; Lundeen S.; Sui Z. Identification and structure-activity relationships of chromene-derived selective estrogen receptor modulators for treatment of postmenopausal symptoms. *J Med Chem*. **2009**, 52(23):7544-69.

[217] Hummel CW.; Geiser AG.; Bryant HU.; Cohen IR.; Dally RD.; Fong KC.; Frank SA.; Hinklin R.; Jones SA.; Lewis G.; McCann DJ.; Rudmann DG.; Shepherd TA.; Tian H.; Wallace OB.; Wang M.; Wang Y.; Dodge JA. A selective estrogen receptor modulator designed for the treatment of uterine leiomyoma with unique tissue specificity for uterus and ovaries in rats. *J Med Chem*. **2005**, 48(22):6772-5.

[218] Zhao L.; O'Neill K.; Brinton RD. Estrogenic agonist activity of ICI 182,780 (Faslodex) in hippocampal neurons: implications for basic science understanding of estrogen signaling and development of estrogen modulators with a dual therapeutic profile. *J Pharmacol Exp Ther*. **2006**, 319(3):1124-32.

[219] Zhao L.; Jin C.; Mao Z.; Gopinathan MB.; Rehder K.; Brinton RD. Design, synthesis, and estrogenic activity of a novel estrogen receptor modulator--a hybrid structure of 17beta-estradiol and vitamin E in hippocampal neurons. *J Med Chem.* **2007**, 50(18):4471-81.

[220] Jensen EV.; Jordan VC. The estrogen receptor: a model for molecular medicine. *Clin Cancer Res.* **2003**, 9(6):1980-9.

[221] Jordan VC. Tamoxifen: catalyst for the change to targeted therapy. *Eur J Cancer.* **2008**, 44(1):30-8.

[222] Massarweh S.; Osborne CK.; Creighton CJ.; Qin L.; Tsimelzon A.; Huang S.; Weiss H.; Rimawi M.; Schiff R. Tamoxifen Resistance in Breast Tumors Is Driven by Growth Factor Receptor Signaling with Repression of Classic Estrogen Receptor Genomic Function. *Cancer Res.* **2008**, 68(3):826-33.

Send Reprints Orders on reprints@benthamscience.net

Advances in Anticancer Agents in Medicinal Chemistry, **2013, Vol.** *2*, **397-409** **397**

CHAPTER 8

Targeting Leukemia Stem Cells with Novel Therapeutic Agents

Yaoyu Chen[1,3], Cong Peng[1,4], Dongguang Li[2] and Shaoguang Li[*,1]

[1]Division of Hematology/Oncology, Department of Medicine, University of Massachusetts Medical School, 364 Plantation Street, Worcester, MA 01605, USA

[2]School of Computer and Security Science, Edith Cowan University, 2 Bradford Street, Mount Lawley, WA 6050, Australia

[3]Current address: Novartis Institutes for BioMedical Research, Oncology, Cambridge, MA 02139, USA

[4]Current address: Department of Hematology/Oncology, Children's Hospital Boston, Harvard Medical School, Boston, MA 02115, USA

Abstract: Chronic myeloid leukemia (CML) is induced by the BCR-ABL oncogene, a product of Philadelphia (Ph) chromosome. The BCR-ABL kinase inhibitor imatinib is a standard treatment for Ph+ leukemia, and has been shown to induce a complete hematologic and cytogenetic response in most chronic phrase CML patients. However, imatinib does not cure CML, and one of the reasons is that imatinib does not kill leukemia stem cells (LSCs) in CML both *in vitro* and *in vivo*. Recently, several new targets or drugs have been reported to inhibit LSCs in cultured human CD34+ CML cells or in mouse model of BCR-ABL induced CML, including an Alox5 pathway inhibitor, Hsp90 inhibitors, omacetaxine, hedgehog inhibitor and BMS-214662. Specific targeting of LSCs but not normal stem cell is a correct strategy for developing new anticancer therapies in the future.

Keywords: Chronic myeloid leukemia (CML), BCR-ABL oncogene, Philadelphia (Ph) chromosome, BCR-ABL kinase inhibitor, leukemia stem cells (LSCs), Hsp90 inhibitors, omacetaxine, hedgehog inhibitor, BMS-214662, Alox5 inhibitor.

INTRODUCTION

Chronic myeloid leukemia (CML) is a myeloproliferative disease characterized by massive expansion of granulocytic cells, leading to high white blood cell (WBC)

***Address correspondence to Shaoguang Li:** University of Massachusetts Medical School, Department of Medicine, 364 Plantation Street, Worcester, MA 01605, USA; Tel: 508-856-1691, Fax: 508-856-7969; E-mail: shaoguang.li@umassmed.edu counts and marked splenomegaly. A chromosomal translocation between chromosome 9 and 22 [t(9;22)(q34;q11)], resulting in the formation of Philadelphia chromosome and at the molecular level, a chimeric gene known as BCR-ABL responsible for CML initiation by causing a clonal expansion of BCR-ABL-expressing hematopoietic stem cells. CML often initiates in a chronic phase, and without intervention, eventually progresses to a terminal blastic phase [1]. In general, based on their molecular weights, there are three types of human BCR-ABL chimeric genes: P190, P210 and P230; each form of the BCR-ABL oncogene is mainly associated with a distinct type of human leukemia. For example, P190 is always present in B-cell acute lymphoblastic leukemia (B-ALL) [2]; P210 is mainly involved in CML and some acute lymphoid and myeloid leukemias in blast crisis [2]; P230 is associated with a very mild form of CML [3]. BCR-ABL activates many signaling pathways, including Ras, MAPK, STAT, JNK/SAPK, PI-3 kinase, NF-kB and c-Myc, through which BCR-ABL promotes survival and proliferation and reduces apoptosis of leukemia cells [4]. BCR-ABL is a non-receptor tyrosine kinase, and it is obvious that a straightforward strategy for treating CML is to use drugs that shut down BCR-ABL kinase activity.

The BCR-ABL kinase inhibitor imatinib mesylate (Gleevec) is a standard of care for Ph^+ leukemia, and has been shown to induce a complete hematologic and cytogenetic response in most chronic phrase CML patients [5]. Although it is very effective in treating chronic phase CML patients, imatinib will unlikely provide a cure to these patients for two obvious reasons. One reason is that BCR-ABL develops imatinib-resistant mutations in its kinase domains. Recently, other BCR-ABL kinase inhibitors have been developed to overcome imatinib resistance, including dasatinib and nilotinib. However, these drugs are still ineffective to BCR-ABL-T315I mutant that is present in about 15-20% of imatinib-resistant patients [6]. Another reason is that leukemia stem cells in CML are insensitive to imatinib treatment [6,7].

LEUKEMIA STEM CELLS

Stem cells have two unique functions: self-renewal that produces themselves and differentiation that gives rise to mature functional cells in variable tissues in the body [8]. Leukemia stem cells (LSCs) are defined as a small cell population required for the initiation and maintenance of leukemia [8-12]. In CML patients, born marrow $CD34^+Lin^-$ cells, in which normal hematopoietic stem cells (HSCs) reside, are thought to contain CML stem cells and be responsible for disease initiation, progression and resistance to imatinib [6,7]. Similarly, in mice with BCR-ABL induced CML, LSCs are phenotypically similar to normal hematopoietic stem cells (HSC) and BCR-ABL-expressing HSCs ($GFP^+Lin^-c\text{-}Kit^+Sca\text{-}1^+$) are able to induce CML in secondary recipient mice [13]. It has been shown that human $CD34^+$ CML stem cells cannot be effectively killed by BCR-ABL kinase inhibitor imatinib treatment both *in vitro* [7] and *in vivo* [6]. Specifically, in a cell culture assay, $CD34^+$ CML stem cells, especially the undivided $CD34^+$ cell population, are not sensitive to inhibition by imatinib [7]. Furthermore, BCR-ABL transcripts are still detectable in $CD34^+$ bone marrow cells from CML patients after a long-term treatment with imatinib [6], suggesting that these LSCs cannot be eradicated through inhibiting BCR-ABL kinase activity. Similarly, imatinib does not eradicate LSCs in CML mice, because total numbers and percentages of LSCs in bone marrow of imatinib treated mice continued to increase during the treatment [14]. It is important to point out that the insensitivity of LSCs to imatinib is not associated with the development of imatinib-resistant mutations on BCR-ABL [15]. Together, these results indicate that some unknown pathways contribute to the maintenance of survival and self-renewal of LSCs, and identification of novel genes that play critical role in regulating the function of LSCs will help to develop new therapeutic strategies through targeting LSCs.

NOVEL THERAPEUTIC DRUGS AGAINST LSCs

The best way to identify stem cell targets in CML is to fully understand CML-initiating genetic changes. BCR-ABL is believed to be the main genetic alteration that represents a major difference between normal HSCs and BCR-ABL-expressing LSCs, although the molecular differences between HSCs and LSCs are still unclear. We speculate that a series of aberrantly expressed genes regulated by BCR-ABL exist and collectively turn a normal HSC into a LSC, although both of them express similar phenotypic markers on cell surface. To reach a goal of curing CML, therapeutic strategies aiming to target LSCs must be developed. Towards this goal, two general strategies have been tested. One strategy is to inhibit genes that play roles in functional regulation of both normal HSCs and LSCs. The examples include Hedgehog, Wnt/β-catenin, Bim-1[15-18]. Another strategy is to inhibit genes that play crucial roles in functional regulation of LSCs but not normal HSCs. Following these two strategies, several LSC target genes and drugs have been reported (Fig. **1**). In Table **1**, some representative anti-LSC agents and underlying mechanisms.

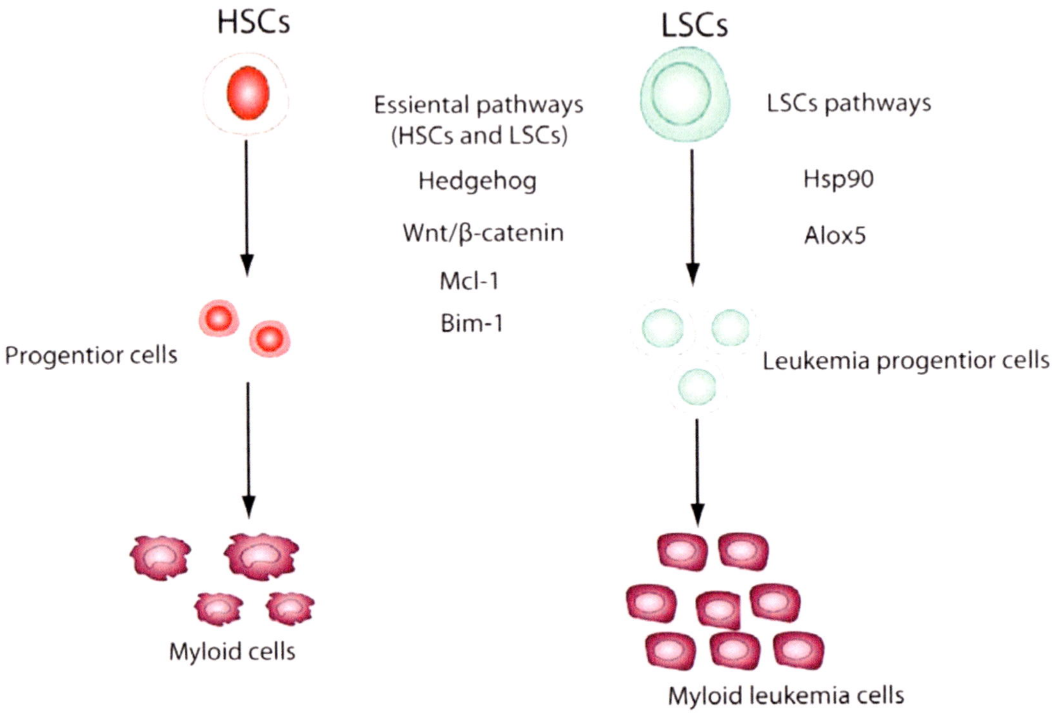

Fig. (1). Strategies to cure CML.

Alox5 Inhibitor

The Alox5 gene has been shown to regulate numerous physiological and pathological progresses, including inflammation and cancer [19-21]. Alox5 is differentially expressed in $CD34^+$ human CML cells and an *in vitro* study shows that an Alox5 inhibitor suppresses proliferation and induces apoptosis of K562 cells (a human CML cell line) [22-24], although an off-target effect of the Alox5 inhibitor needs to be ruled out. These data suggest a possibility that Alox5 is involved in CML development. However, it has never been thought that Alox5 may regulate the function of LSCs in CML until a recent discovery of the essential role of Alox5 in survival and self-renewal of LSCs. In this recent study, Alox5 is identified as a key gene that regulates the function of LSCs in CML mice, as BCR-ABL cannot induce CML in mice in the absence of the Alox5 gene. This striking discovery provides a unique opportunity to develop a novel anti-stem cell therapy for CML [25].

Table 1. Some Representative Anti LSC-Agents and Underlying Mechanism

Target Gene	Drug Name	Mechanism
Alox5	Zileuton	An inhibitor of 5-lipoxygenase, and thus inhibiting leukotrienes formation
Hsp90	IPI-504	A selective Hsp90 chaperone inhibitor
MCl-1	Omacetaxine	Inhibit BCR-ABL, Mcl- and Hsp90
PKCβ	BMS-214662	A farneysyltransferase inhibitor and activate PKC β
Hedgehog	Cyclopamine	Locks Smo in its inactive conformation

The function of Alox5 in leukemia stem cells was further linked to a cell surface receptor macrophage scavenger receptor (*Msr1*), which suppressing self-renew and proliferation of LSCs and being up-regulated by loss of *Alox5*. *Msr1* is a member of scavenger receptor family and is mostly expressed in hematopoietic cells [26]. *Msr1* is important for mediating host-cell interactions, macrophage adhesion and phagocytosis of apoptotic cells [27]. In CML mouse model, *Msr1* is down-regulated by *BCR-ABL* and this down-regulation is partially restored by *Alox5* deletion, and that *Msr1* deletion causes acceleration of CML development [28]. *Msr1* deletion markedly increases LSC function through its effects on cell cycle progression and apoptosis. In human CML cell lines, over-expression of Msr1also suppresses the proliferation of leukemia cells. In addition, *Msr1* affects CML development by regulating the PI3K-AKT pathway and β-Catenin [28].

Zileuton, a drug that has been currently used to treat human asthma, specifically inhibits the enzymatic activity of arachidonate 5-lipoxygenase (5-LO), the product of the Alox5 gene [29]. To test its therapeutic effect on CML, BCR-ABL transduced bone marrow cells were transplanted into recipient mice to induce

CML, and then the CML mice were treated with a placebo, Zileuton or imatinib alone, or two agents in combination. All placebo-treated mice developed and died of CML within 4 weeks after the induction of CML by BCR-ABL, and Zileuton alone was even more effective than imatinib in prolonging survival of CML mice. About 7 weeks after the treatment with Zileuton, $GFP^{+}Gr\text{-}1^{+}$leukemia cells in peripheral blood of the mice gradually declined and dropped from over 50% to less than 2%, indicating that myeloid leukemia is eventually eliminated. Treatment of CML mice with both Zileuton and imatinib had a better therapeutic effect than with either Zileuton or Imatinib alone in prolonging survival of the mice. At the early stage of CML development, Zileuton treatment only caused a less marked reduction of white blood cell counts than did imatinib treatment. This therapeutic effect of Zileuton on CML is caused by inhibiting LSCs. LT (long-term)-LSCs were found to accumulate in bone marrow of the treated mice; however, ST (short-term)-LSCs and MPP (multiple potent progenitor) cells were gradually depleted, suggesting that inhibition of 5-LO by Zileuton causes the blockade of differentiation of LT-LSCs. The inhibitory effect of Zileuton are consistent with those from above-described genetic studies using $Alox5^{-/-}$ mice, demonstrating that targeting of the Alox5 pathway is potentially curative for CML, and this idea needs to tested in human CML patients.

Hsp90 Inhibitors

Hsp90 is a ubiquitously expressed chaperone protein which accounts for about 1-2% of total cellular protein in mammalian cells [30]. It is a chaperone of several oncoproteins such as Her2 [31], v-Src [32], BCR-ABL [33], and plays a role in regulating survival, proliferation apoptosis of cancer cells. Hsp90 is constitutively expressed at a level that is 2-10 folds higher in tumor cells than in their normal stem cell counterparts, suggesting that Hsp90 is a potential therapeutic target in cancers. The benzoquinone ansamycin geldanamycin (GA) is the first inhibitor of Hsp90 [32] and it destructs the v-Src-Hsp90 herterprotein complex to inhibit the v-Src mediated transformation *in vitro*. BCR-ABL has also been shown to be a major client protein of Hsp90 in a study using human K562 CML cells [33]. In this study, after the cells were briefly exposed to GA, BCR-ABL was dissociated with Hsp90 and P23. 17-allylamino-17-demethoxygeldanamycin (17-AAG) is a less toxic analogue of GA, and it induces cytosolic accumulation of cytochrome c and cleavage of caspase-9 and caspase-3, triggering apoptosis of HL-60/ BCR-ABL and K562 cells [34]. 17-AAG down-regulates intracellular BCR-ABL and c-Raf proteins, and reduces activity of Akt kinase in K562 cells [34]. Although GA or 17-AAG shows their inhibitory effect on cultured leukemia cells, their poor solubility and complex organic formulations make it likely that it is necessary to develop better Hsp90 inhibitors. Thus, a new analogue of 17-AAG, IPI-504, has been produced [35]. IPI-504 is a hydrochloride salt, and can be purified and stored at low temperatures under N2 atmosphere as a solid, resulting in a high aqueous solubility (250 mg/ml), and stability in acidic aqueous buffers (pH 3, >10 h) [35]. These characteristics indicate that IPI-504 is a more applicable drug for therapy.

It has been shown that IPI-504 efficiently induces dissociation of BCR-ABL and Hsp90 in BCR-ABL-expressing 32D cells as quickly as 30 min after the treatment. Because the stability of BCR-ABL is shown *in vitro* to be more dependent on Hsp90 when it carries imatinib-resistant mutations [36], the dependence of mutant BCR-ABL on Hsp90 has been tested further *in vivo*. In mice with CML induced by wild type BCR-ABL or the BCR-ABL-T315I mutant, treatment with IPI-504 alone significantly prolonged the survival of mice with wild-type BCR-ABL-induced CML, but more markedly prolonged the survival of mice with BCR-ABL-T315I-induced CML [37]. The markedly prolonged survival of the IPI-504-treated mice with BCR-ABL-T315I-induced CML correlates with the more significant *in vivo* degradation of the mutant BCR-ABL than that of wild type BCR-ABL. In CML mice, HSCs harboring BCR-ABL (GFP^+) function as LSCs [13]. Using this mouse CML stem cell model, bone marrow cells from mice with T315I-induced CML were isolated from the mice, and cultured under the conditions that support survival and growth of HSCs. During the culture, the bone marrow cells were treated with IPI-504. Six days after the treatment, FACS analysis shows that compared with the untreated group, imatinib treatment did not lower the percentage and the number of LSCs, whereas IPI-504 treatment had a dramatic inhibitory effect on the stem cells [37]. To assess the effect of IPI-504 on LSCs *in vivo*, CML mice were treated with IPI-504, and the number of LSCs in bone marrow was analyzed 6 days after the treatment. Consistent with the *in vitro* data, IPI-504 treatment had a dramatic inhibitory effect on LSCs in CML mice. These studies demonstrate that inhibition of Hsp90 can effectively inhibit the survival and proliferation of LSCs.

Because knocking down Hsp90a and Hsp90b are embryonic lethal, it is still not possible to genetically prove the importance of Hsp90a and Hsp90b in LSCs. However, it is a very important approach to take to investigate the role of Hsp90 in regulating the function of LSCs.

Omacetaxine

Omacetaxine (formerly homoharringtonine) is a cephalotaxine ester derived from the evergreen tree, Cephalotaxus harringtonia, native to China. Omacetaxine has shown clinical activity alone and in combination with imatinib in CML patients resistant to imatinib or other tyrosine kinase inhibitors; although it is not clear whether this drug could be effective in inhibiting LSCs for a while [38-40]. Recently, omacetaxine has been shown to have the ability to kill LSCs effectively *in vitro* and *in vivo* [41]. After treating LSCs from CML mice with omacetaxine for 6 days, LSCs ($GFP^+Lin^-cKit^+Sca\text{-}1^+$) were inhibited by omacetaxine in a dose-dependent manner. The effect of omacetaxine on LSCs on CML mice was also examined. Mice with BCR-ABL-induced CML were treated with omacetaxine for 4 days from day 10 after BMT, and Omacetaxine treatment resulted in a great reduction of the numbers of both LSCs and total leukemia cells. Because of its mechanism that is different from tyrosine kinase inhibitors, Omacetaxien also showed an inhibitory effect on LSCs harboring BCR-ABL-T315I. This inhibitory on BCR-ABL-T315I induced CML was more effective than on wild-type BCR-ABL induced CML, which is supported by an earlier *in vitro* study [42]. The underlying mechanism for the inhibitory effect of Omacetaxine on LSCs is still unknown, although several potential pathways are thought to be involved. The clues come from this study using Omacetaxine. First, the expression of BCR-ABL is reduced by omacetaxine, likely through affecting Hsp90 that stabilizes BCR-ABL proteins. Second, an important short-lived *anti*-apoptotic BCL-2 family protein MCL-1 is found to be down-regulated after treatment with omacetaxine. It is reasonable to think that omacetaxine could act by directly or indirectly inhibiting the BCR-ABL, MCL-1 and HSP90 in CML cells. In addition, the clinical efficacy of omacetaxine in CML could be due, at least in part, to its inhibitory activity on LSCs [15, 41].

Hedgehog Inhibitor

Hedgehog (Hh) signaling is involved in regulation of normal development and oncogenesis of many tissue types, and has been shown to play a role in preserving and increasing the short-term repopulating capacity of human HSCs [43]. Recently, Hh signaling has been demonstrated as a required functional pathway for CML stem cells, as a loss of this pathway impairs leukemia progression [16, 44]. In these studies, $Smo^{-/-}$ mice (lacking the receptor for Hh) were used to induce CML. Wild-type bone marrow cells transduced with BCR–ABL caused CML in 94% of recipients within 3 months, whereas BCR-ABL transduced $Smo^{-/-}$ cells caused CML in only 47% of recipients. The frequency of LSCs ($Lin^-c\text{-}Kit^+Sca\text{-}1^+$) was significantly reduced in the absence of the Hh receptor. These results suggest that CML stem cells depend on the Hh pathway for survival and self-renewal, raising a possibility that these stem cells may be targeted by pharmacological blockade of Hh signaling [44]. Because cyclopamine inhibits Hh signaling by stabilizing Smo in its inactive form, BCR-ABL induced CML mice were further treated with cyclopamine [44, 45]. The control animals died of CML within 4 weeks; however, 60% of the cyclopamine-treated mice were still alive after 7 weeks. In addition, cyclopamine-treated mice had up to a 14-fold reduction in the CML stem cell population. Targeting of CML stem cells by cyclopamine appeared to be most effective when it was used at early stages after CML induction in mice. Furthermore, cyclopamine was tested on imatinib-resistant CML in mice. BCR-ABL-T315I induced leukemia cells were unresponsive to imatinib, but their growth was reduced by 2.5-fold after treatment with cyclopamine. Cyclopamine was also effective in treating mice with BCR-ABL-T315I induced CML. These results indicate that the Hh pathway is required for the functional regulation of CML stem cells, and cyclopamine may be an effective drug for treating human CML, although its effect on normal HSCs needs to be examined.

BMS-214662

BMS-214662 is a cytotoxic farnesyltransferase inhibitor and is reported to kill nonproliferating tumor cells [46]. In this study, BMS-214662, alone or in combination with imatinib or dasatinib, induces apoptosis of both proliferating and quiescent primitive $CD34^+CD38^-$ CML stem cells. In contrast, normal $CD34^+$ HSCs were much less sensitive to BMS-214662 inhibition, suggesting a selectivity of this compound for CML stem cells. The selective inhibitory effect of BMS214662 on CML stem cells was unique to BMS-214662, as BMS-225975, a structurally similar farnesyltransferase inhibitor, did not inhibit CML stem cells, suggesting that the effect of BMS-214662 on CML stem cells is mediated through a mechanism not associated with its farnesyltransferase activity. It is likely that there are several apoptotic pathways involved, such as Bax conformational changes, loss of mitochondrial membrane potential, generation of reactive oxygen species, release of Cytochrome c, and Caspase-9/3 activation. These changes were coupled with up-regulation of protein kinase Cβ (PKCβ), down-regulation of E2F1 and phosphorylation of Cyclin A-associated Cyclin-dependent kinase 2. Co-treatment of CML $CD34^+$ and $CD34^+CD38^-$ cells with PKC modulators, bryostatin-1 or hispidin, markedly decreased these early biochemical events and the subsequent apoptosis. These data indicate that BMS-214662 may provide a molecular framework for development of novel therapeutic strategies [47, 48].

CONCLUSIONS

These ideas discussed in this review emphasize several points. First, specific inhibition of LSCs in CML is a feasible and reasonable approach to developing a cure for CML in the future. Second, several target gene required by LSCs have been identified and shown to be good targets for inhibiting LSCs, and among them, Alox5 is particularly important because it is much more specifically required for LSCs comparing to other genes discussed in this review. Third, several promising drugs are available for inhibiting CML stem cells in future clinical trials, inhibitors of Alox5, Hedgehog and Hsp90 inhibitor have better specificity on LSCs. The mechanisms by which these target genes regulate the function of LSCs need to be further studied.

CONFLICT OF INTEREST

The authors declare that there is no conflict of interest.

ACKNOWLEDGEMENTS

Declared none.

DISCLOSURE

This e-Book chapter is an updated version of the article entitled "Novel Therapeutic Agents Against Cancer Stem Cells of Chronic Myeloid Leukemia" published in 2010 in *Anti-Cancer Agents in Medicinal Chemistry,* 10 (2), 111-115.

REFERENCES

[1] Bartram, C.R.; de Klein, A.; Hagemeijer, A.; van Agthoven, T.; Geurts van Kessel, A.; Bootsma, D.; Grosveld, G.; Ferguson-Smith, M.A.; Davies, T.; Stone, M.; *et al., Nature,* 1983, *306,* (5940), 277-280.
[2] Deininger, M.W.; Goldman, J.M.; Melo, J.V., *Blood,* 2000, *96,* (10), 3343-3356.
[3] Pane, F.; Frigeri, F.; Sindona, M.; Luciano, L.; Ferrara, F.; Cimino, R.; Meloni, G.; Saglio, G.; Salvatore, F.; Rotoli, B., *Blood,* 1996, *88,* (7), 2410-2414.
[4] Sattler, M.; Griffin, J.D., *Seminars in hematology,* 2003, *40,* (2 Suppl 2), 4-10.
[5] Druker, B.J.; Talpaz, M.; Resta, D.J.; Peng, B.; Buchdunger, E.; Ford, J.M.; Lydon, N.B.; Kantarjian, H.; Capdeville, R.; Ohno-Jones, S.; Sawyers, C.L., *The New England journal of medicine,* 2001, *344,* (14), 1031-1037.
[6] Bhatia, R.; Holtz, M.; Niu, N.; Gray, R.; Snyder, D.S.; Sawyers, C.L.; Arber, D.A.; Slovak, M.L.; Forman, S.J., *Blood,* 2003, *101,* (12), 4701-4707.
[7] Graham, S.M.; Jorgensen, H.G.; Allan, E.; Pearson, C.; Alcorn, M.J.; Richmond, L.; Holyoake, T.L., *Blood,* 2002, *99,* (1), 319-325.
[8] Reya, T.; Morrison, S.J.; Clarke, M.F.; Weissman, I.L., *Nature,* 2001, *414,* (6859), 105-111.
[9] Jordan, C.T.; Guzman, M.L.; Noble, M., *The New England journal of medicine,* 2006, *355,* (12), 1253-1261.
[10] Pardal, R.; Clarke, M.F.; Morrison, S.J., *Nature reviews,* 2003, *3,* (12), 895-902.
[11] Rossi, D.J.; Jamieson, C.H.; Weissman, I.L., *Cell,* 2008, *132,* (4), 681-696.
[12] Wang, J.C.; Dick, J.E., *Trends in cell biology,* 2005, *15,* (9), 494-501.
[13] Hu, Y.; Swerdlow, S.; Duffy, T.M.; Weinmann, R.; Lee, F.Y.; Li, S., *Proceedings of the National Academy of Sciences of the United States of America,* 2006, *103,* (45), 16870-16875.
[14] Hu, Y.; Chen, Y.; Douglas, L.; Li, S., *Leukemia,* 2009, *23,* (1), 109-116.
[15] Chen, Y.; Peng, C.; Sullivan, C.; Li, D.; Li, S., *Leukemia,* 2010, *24,* (9), 1545-1554.
[16] Dierks, C.; Beigi, R.; Guo, G.R.; Zirlik, K.; Stegert, M.R.; Manley, P.; Trussell, C.; Schmitt-Graeff, A.; Landwerlin, K.; Veelken, H.; Warmuth, M., *Cancer cell,* 2008, *14,* (3), 238-249.
[17] Zhao, C.; Blum, J.; Chen, A.; Kwon, H.Y.; Jung, S.H.; Cook, J.M.; Lagoo, A.; Reya, T., *Cancer cell,* 2007, *12,* (6), 528-541.
[18] Lessard, J.; Sauvageau, G., *Nature,* 2003, *423,* (6937), 255-260.

[19] Catalano, A.; Rodilossi, S.; Caprari, P.; Coppola, V.; Procopio, A., *The EMBO journal,* 2005, *24*, (1), 170-179.
[20] Chen, X.S.; Sheller, J.R.; Johnson, E.N.; Funk, C.D., *Nature,* 1994, *372*, (6502), 179-182.
[21] Radmark, O.; Werz, O.; Steinhilber, D.; Samuelsson, B., *Trends in biochemical sciences,* 2007, *32*, (7), 332-341.
[22] Graham, S.M.; Vass, J.K.; Holyoake, T.L.; Graham, G.J., *Stem cells (Dayton, Ohio),* 2007, *25*, (12), 3111-3120.
[23] Radich, J.P.; Dai, H.; Mao, M.; Oehler, V.; Schelter, J.; Druker, B.; Sawyers, C.; Shah, N.; Stock, W.; Willman, C.L.; Friend, S.; Linsley, P.S., *Proceedings of the National Academy of Sciences of the United States of America,* 2006, *103*, (8), 2794-2799.
[24] Anderson, K.M.; Seed, T.; Plate, J.M.; Jajeh, A.; Meng, J.; Harris, J.E., *Leukemia research,* 1995, *19*, (11), 789-801.
[25] Chen, Y.; Hu, Y.; Zhang, H.; Peng, C.; Li, S., *Nature genetics,* 2009, *41*, (7), 783-792.
[26] Rohrer, L.; Freeman, M.; Kodama, T.; Penman, M.; Krieger, M., *Nature,* 1990, *343*, (6258), 570-572.
[27] Platt, N.; Gordon, S., *The Journal of clinical investigation,* 2001, *108*, (5), 649-654.
[28] Chen, Y.; Sullivan, C.; Peng, C.; Shan, Y.; Hu, Y.; Li, D.; Li, S., *Blood,* 2011, *118*, (2), 390-400.
[29] Knapp, H.R., *The New England journal of medicine,* 1990, *323*, (25), 1745-1748.
[30] Scheibel, T.; Buchner, J., *Biochemical pharmacology,* 1998, *56*, (6), 675-682.
[31] Solit, D.B.; Zheng, F.F.; Drobnjak, M.; Munster, P.N.; Higgins, B.; Verbel, D.; Heller, G.; Tong, W.; Cordon-Cardo, C.; Agus, D.B.; Scher, H.I.; Rosen, N., *Clin Cancer Res,* 2002, *8*, (5), 986-993.
[32] Whitesell, L.; Mimnaugh, E.G.; De Costa, B.; Myers, C.E.; Neckers, L.M., *Proceedings of the National Academy of Sciences of the United States of America,* 1994, *91*, (18), 8324-8328.
[33] An, W.G.; Schulte, T.W.; Neckers, L.M., *Cell Growth Differ,* 2000, *11*, (7), 355-360.
[34] Nimmanapalli, R.; O'Bryan, E.; Bhalla, K., *Cancer research,* 2001, *61*, (5), 1799-1804.
[35] Ge, J.; Normant, E.; Porter, J.R.; Ali, J.A.; Dembski, M.S.; Gao, Y.; Georges, A.T.; Grenier, L.; Pak, R.H.; Patterson, J.; Sydor, J.R.; Tibbitts, T.T.; Tong, J.K.; Adams, J.; Palombella, V.J., *Journal of medicinal chemistry,* 2006, *49*, (15), 4606-4615.
[36] Gorre, M.E.; Ellwood-Yen, K.; Chiosis, G.; Rosen, N.; Sawyers, C.L., *Blood,* 2002, *100*, (8), 3041-3044.
[37] Peng, C.; Brain, J.; Hu, Y.; Goodrich, A.; Kong, L.; Grayzel, D.; Pak, R.; Read, M.; Li, S., *Blood,* 2007, *110*, (2), 678-685.
[38] Kantarjian, H.M.; Talpaz, M.; Santini, V.; Murgo, A.; Cheson, B.; O'Brien, S.M., *Cancer,* 2001, *92*, (6), 1591-1605.
[39] Luo, C.Y.; Tang, J.Y.; Wang, Y.P., *Hematology,* 2004, *9*, (4), 259-270.
[40] Quintas-Cardama, A.; Kantarjian, H.; Garcia-Manero, G.; O'Brien, S.; Faderl, S.; Estrov, Z.; Giles, F.; Murgo, A.; Ladie, N.; Verstovsek, S.; Cortes, J., *Cancer,* 2007, *109*, (2), 248-255.
[41] Chen, Y.; Hu, Y.; Michaels, S.; Segal, D.; Brown, D.; Li, S., *Leukemia,* 2009, *23*, (8), 1446-1454.
[42] Legros, L.; Hayette, S.; Nicolini, F.E.; Raynaud, S.; Chabane, K.; Magaud, J.P.; Cassuto, J.P.; Michallet, M., *Leukemia,* 2007, *21*, (10), 2204-2206.
[43] Taipale, J.; Beachy, P.A., *Nature,* 2001, *411*, (6835), 349-354.

[44] Zhao, C.; Chen, A.; Jamieson, C.H.; Fereshteh, M.; Abrahamsson, A.; Blum, J.; Kwon, H.Y.; Kim, J.; Chute, J.P.; Rizzieri, D.; Munchhof, M.; VanArsdale, T.; Beachy, P.A.; Reya, T., *Nature,* 2009, *458*, (7239), 776-779.

[45] Chen, J.K.; Taipale, J.; Cooper, M.K.; Beachy, P.A., *Genes & development,* 2002, *16*, (21), 2743-2748.

[46] Manne, V.; Lee, F.Y.; Bol, D.K.; Gullo-Brown, J.; Fairchild, C.R.; Lombardo, L.J.; Smykla, R.A.; Vite, G.D.; Wen, M.L.; Yu, C.; Wong, T.W.; Hunt, J.T., *Cancer research,* 2004, *64*, (11), 3974-3980.

[47] Pellicano, F.; Copland, M.; Jorgensen, H.G.; Mountford, J.; Leber, B.; Holyoake, T.L., *Blood,* 2009.

[48] Copland, M.; Pellicano, F.; Richmond, L.; Allan, E.K.; Hamilton, A.; Lee, F.Y.; Weinmann, R.; Holyoake, T.L., *Blood,* **2008**, *111*, (5), 2843-2853.

410 *Advances in Anticancer Agents in Medicinal Chemistry*, 2013, Vol. 2, 410-443

CHAPTER 9

Targeting Migrating Cells in Glioblastoma

Ranjith Babu, Chunhui Di, Austin K. Mattox, Steve Harward and Cory Adamson*

Preston Robert Tisch Brain Tumor Center, Departments of Surgery (Neurosurgery) and Neurobiology, Duke University; Neurosurgery Section, Durham VA Medical Center, NC 27710, USA

Abstract: Glioblastoma multiforme (GBM) is the most common and aggressive primary brain tumor in humans. Despite aggressive surgical resection using state-of-the-art neuroimaging and radiochemotherapy, the prognosis of GBM remains poor, with an estimated median survival of 12-14 months. At presentation, tumor cells have already have migrated into normal brain tissue beyond the main tumor mass. This accounts for the inability of surgery to cure this tumor. It is therefore imperative to better understand how inhibit GBM cell migration. In this review, we describe various potential targets that may be exploited to inhibit the migration GBM cells.

Keywords: Glioblastoma, migration, signaling, stem cell.

INTRODUCTION

Malignant gliomas have an annual incidence of approximately 5 cases per 100,000 people, with glioblastoma (GBM) accounting for 60-70% of these cases [1]. The majority of malignant gliomas consist of high grade astrocytomas, namely WHO grade III anaplastic astrocytomas and grade IV GBMs. GBMs are the most common and aggressive primary brain tumor in humans, with a median survival of 12-14 months. Due to their robust cellular invasion and universal recurrence, there are currently no effective treatments for the management of these aggressive tumors.

Cell migration is a highly regulated and complex process which is essential to the development and maintenance of normal and abnormal tissue. For example, tissue formation during embryonic development, immune responses, tumor maintenance,

***Address correspondence to Cory Adamson:** Neurosurgery Section, Durham VA Medical Center, DUMC Box 2624, Durham, NC 27710, USA; Tel: 919-698-3152; E-mail: cory.adamson@duke.edu and wound healing all require the coordinated movement of cells to specific locations *via* a variety of internal and external regulating factors. Errors during migration may have serious and diverse consequences including vascular disease, mental retardation, and tumor progression to noncontiguous sites. A primary feature of malignant gliomas is their ability to infiltrate the brain beyond the primary tumor mass. Understanding the factors and mechanisms involved in cell migration, some of which likely overlaps with normal biology, is therefore necessary to identify therapeutic targets that can decrease tumor progression and improve patient survival. This review focuses on intracellular and cell surface proteins and their associated signaling pathways to elucidate their involvement in GBM cell migration and potential as therapeutic targets.

The inability of surgeons to entirely resect GBM tumors is due to their aggressive and diffusely invasive nature. At the cellular level, tumors cell migration has characteristic hallmarks, with this morphological pattern of invasion known as the secondary structures of Scherer [2]. Migrating gliomas cells are most easily appreciated at pial margins (subpial invasion), around neurons (perineural satellitosis) and blood vessels (perivascular satellitosis), and trailing along white matter tracts (intrafacicular spread). An example of this intrafacicular spread is seen when frontal lobe GBMs spread into the contralateral frontal lobe *via* the anterior corpus callosum, forming the classic "butterfly GBM". At the cellular level, glioma cell migration is regulated by a complex cascade of events (Fig. **1**) including cell interactions with adjacent cells and extra-cellular matrix (ECM) factors, and other biochemical processes which support cell movement. The process of initiating cell motility initially requires the up- and down-regulation of cell adhesion molecules. For example, neural cell adhesion molecules and E-cadherin are down-regulated [3], while N-cadherin and CD44 are up-regulated [4]. ECM factors also participate in these steps with a multitude of key ECM-related proteins (tenascin, integrins, fibronectin, collagen, and vitronectin) being localized to the perivascular spaces where glioma cell invasion typically occurs. Transmembrane heterodimeric proteins such as integrins are important for cell migration and invasion by regulating cell–ECM interactions and mediating signaling pathways which control cytoskeletal organization. The ionotropic transmembrane protein AMPAR (a-Amino-3-hydroxy-5-methylisoxazole-4-

propionic acid receptor) is highly expressed and has been found at the invading edges of GBM tumors, suggesting an important role in promoting tumor invasion. Additional studies have shown AMPAR to promote glioma cell invasion *via* b1 integrin–dependent adhesion to the ECM [5]. An important question is why and how GBM cells favor the secondary structures of Scherer, possibly depending on glioma cell-specific changes and ECM factors. Matrix-metalloproteinases (MMPs) are zinc-dependent endopeptidases which degrade various types of ECM proteins and are also thought to play an important role in glioma cell migration. They are involved in the cleavage of cell surface receptors, chemokine/cytokine regulation, and the release of apoptotic ligands such as the FAS ligand, functions which all assist in the creation of avenues for invading glioma cells [6]. Once the many barriers to migration are removed, glioma cells must be able to enter the spaces created by the rearrangement of cytoskeletal networks by forming filopodia and lamellipodia, a process thought to be regulated by the Rho family of GTPases. For example, RECK has been shown to act as a transformation suppressor gene which can effect ECM barriers to movement. It can inhibit glioma cell migration and invasion by decreasing MMP-2 and MMP-9. However, microRNA21 (miR21) is upregulated in gliomas and targets RECK, contributing to the decreased RECK expression in gliomas compared to normal brain tissue [7]. Another molecule, TWIST1 has also been shown to be upregulated in GBM, with *in vitro* and *in vivo* studies showing that TWIST1 can promote cell migration and invasion *via* actin cytoskeletal reorganization and by increasing movement toward fibronectin substrates [8].

These complex processes clearly involve a variety of cellular activities acting in synchrony. However, a few signaling factors are known to be important in glioma cell migration, including the Transforming Growth Factor β (TGF-β), Epidermal Growth Factor Receptor (EGFR) and other GFs, Immunoglobulins (Ig), Integrins, cytokines, G Protein-Coupled Receptors (GPCRs), GBM stem cell factors, and other poorly understood factors such Adherens Junctional Associated Protein (AJAP1). These alterations most likely depend on various cells in the brain as while glioma cells secrete factors that act in an autocrine fashion such as EGF, other cells also play an important role by secreting factors that function in a paracrine role (*e.g.* VEGF from altered endothelium and cytokines from migroglia). Tumor microglia and endothelia are typically not altered quantitatively, rather being modified qualitatively. For example, the immune system in and around GBM tumors is dysfunctional and significantly altered as killer T cells exhibit little anti-tumoral activity.

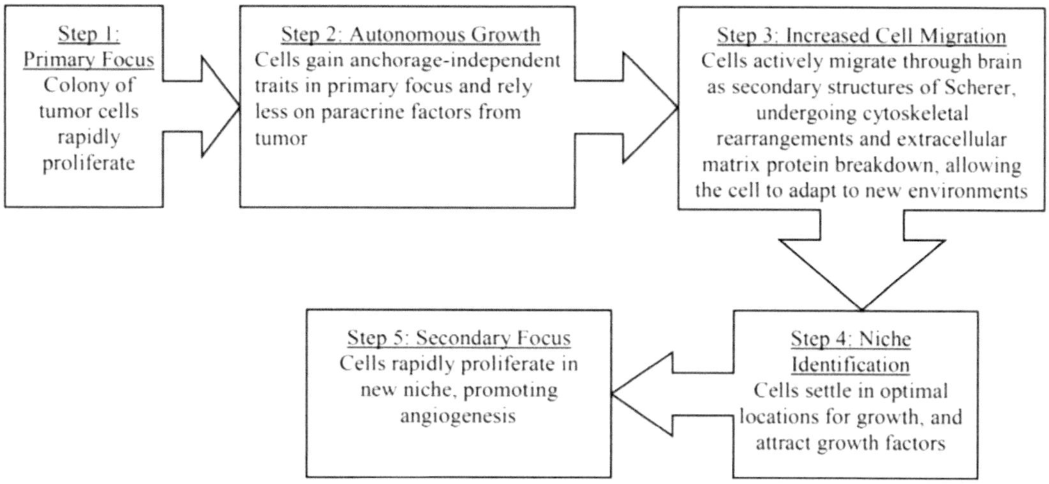

Fig. (1). Proposed steps in GBM migration. Step 1 (Primary Focus): colony of tumor cells rapidly proliferate; Step 2 (Autonomous Growth): cells gain anchorage-independent traits due to growing hypoxia and hypovascularity in primary focus and rely less on paracrine factors from tumor colony; Step 3 (Increased Cell Migration): cells actively migrate through brain as secondary structures of Scherer, undergoing cytoskeletal rearrangements and extracellular matrix protein breakdown, allowing the cell to adapt to new environments; Step 4 (Niche Identification): cells settle in optimal locations for growth, and attract growth factors; Step 5 (Secondary Focus): cells rapidly proliferate in new niche, promoting angiogenesis. Blue circle = GBM cell; ovoid circle = GBM cell having undergone cytoskeletal changes amongst ECM alterations, facilitating increased migration; red bars = new blood vessels.

EGFR AND RELATED GROWTH FACTOR PATHWAYS

EGFR signaling pathways are the best characterized in all of gliomagenesis and are important in cell migration (Fig. **2**) [9]. EGFRs are receptor tyrosine kinases (RTKs) that function as high-affinity cell surface receptors for a variety of cytokines, polypeptide GFs, and hormones. RTKs have been shown to be important factors in normal cellular processes and in the development and progression of various cancers [10]. Other RTKs include Eph receptor, hepatocyte growth factor/scatter factor (HGF/SF) receptor (aka Met), and fibroblast growth factor receptor (FGFRs). Other non-RTK pathways include signal transducers and activators of transcription (STATs), platelet-derived growth factor (PDGF), receptor protein tyrosine phosphatase ζ (RPTP ζ) and glial cell line-derived neurotrophic factor (GDNF). Approximately one hundred unique tyrosine kinase genes have been identified in the human genome, with 58 encoding functional RTKs [11]. While a few RTKs exist in multimeric complexes, most function as single subunit receptors. Each monomer contains a hydrophobic transmembrane-spanning domain containing approximately 30 amino acids, an intracellular C-terminal region, and an extracellular N-terminal region. The extracellular N-terminal region contains various conserved elements including fibronectin type III repeats, EGF-like or Ig-like domains, and cysteine-rich regions which are characteristic for each subfamily of RTKs. These domains contain a ligand-binding site which binds extracellular ligands [10]. The intracellular C-terminal region has the highest level of conservation and contains the catalytic domains which are responsible for the kinase activity of these receptors, catalyzing tyrosine and RTK substrate phosphorylation and receptor autophosphorylation [10]. Receptor binding of adaptor or ligand proteins results in the autophosphorylation of intracellular tyrosine residues or activates GTPase pathways, and the stimulation of membrane-bound Ras. Ras is a diversion point in signaling cascades and activates PI3K and Raf pathways, which both promote cell migration [12]. Recently, it has been shown that the catalytic PI3K isoform p110δ is expressed at high levels in gliomas and is a key regulator in cell migration [13].

The specific ErbB protein family or EGFR family consists of four structurally related RTKs: EGFR (HERI, ErbBI), ErbB2 (HER2), ErbB3 (HER3), and ErbB4 (HER4). TGF-α, EGF, HB-EGF, betacellulin, amphiregulin, epiregulin and epigen can all bind to EGFR (ErbBI). Currently, no ligand has been identified that binds to ErbB2. ErbB3 has been shown to interact with neuregulin 1 [14], neuregulin2 [14b], PA2G4 [15], and RGS4 [16]. STAT5A [17], while DLG4 [18], neuregulin-1β1(NRG1β1), and YAP1 are known ligands for ErbB4. Ligand binding to ErbB4 leads to the phosphorylation of AKT [19] EGFRvIII is a mutant variant of EGFR and is missing exons 2-7. It is the most common and best characterized mutation in GBM [20]. It has been shown to confer an invasive advantage *via* the myristoylated alanine-rich protein kinase C substrate (MARCKS) [21]. Amplification of the EGFR gene is known to occur in up to

70% of primary GBMs, with 70 to 90% of these tumors having overexpressed protein [22].

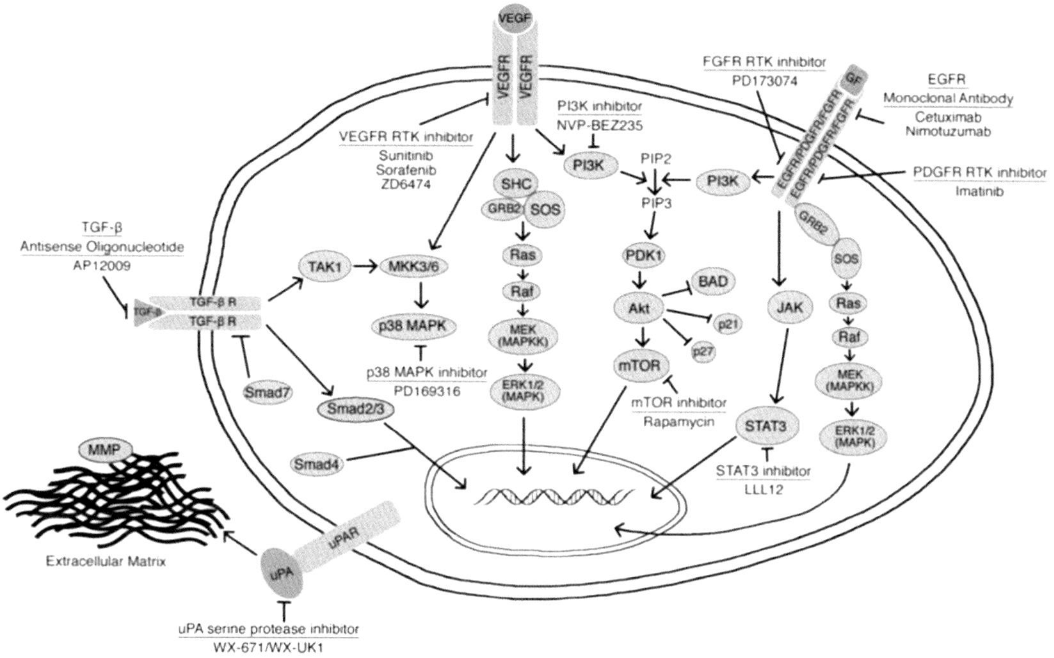

Fig. (2). Major molecular pathways implicated in GBM migration. Cytoskeletal rearrangements, ECM breakdown, and alterations in the signaling cascade of various paracrine and autocrine factors are thought to contribute to GBM migration. Notable implicated proteins include EGFR, PDGF, integrins, and MMPs and many of these proteins are chemotherapeutically targetable.

Up to 70% of GBM tumors have been shown to have alterations in RTK/PI3K signaling [23]. Ras activates PI3K by interacting with its Ras binding domain [24]. Binding of the p85 regulatory subunit to phosphotyrosine in a YXXM consensus motif can also activate PI3K. PI3K is negatively regulated by phosphatase and tensin homolog (PTEN) which converts PIP3 back to PIP2 [25]. PI3K is activated by the CD95 ligand which recruits the Src family member Yes and the p85 subunit of PI3K, signaling invasion *via* the glycogen synthase kinase 3-β pathway and subsequent expression of MMPs [26]. AKT is a downstream effector of PI3K activation and regulates the activity of a variety of molecules including transcription factors, kinases, and other regulatory molecules [27]. AKT activation has also been implicated in the transformation of anaplastic astrocytomas (WHO grade III) to GBM, potentially reflecting increased migratory activities [28]. Another molecule important in various processes such as cell survival, migration, angiogenesis, invasion, and cell growth is sphingosine-1-phosphate (Sph1P), a potent sphingolipid mediator [29]. Sphingosine kinase 1 (SphK1), one of the two isoenzymes that produce Sph1P, is overexpressed in GBM tumors and has been shown to be a poor prognostic factor in patients. Inhibitors of SphK1 are able to inhibit glioma cell migration and invasion by reducing AKT phosphorylation, suggesting that isozyme-specific inhibitors of SphK1 may function as effective therapeutic agents.

Activation of invasion-promoting pathways *via* PI3K and MAPK occurs byt the alteration of EGFR signaling. However, other factors may also play a similar role. Urokinase plasminogen activator (uPA) can activate a variety of proteases which result in ECM degradation and attenuate cell-matrix and cell-cell interactions *via* the c-Src/MEK/MAPK pathway, thereby acting as a regulator of glioma cell invasion [30]. PI3K and MEK inhibitors can block EGF/EGFR-mediated colony formation and cell invasion *via* MMP-9, suggesting that MMP-9 is involved in PI3K/AKT and EGFR/Ras/MEK pathway-mediated anchorage-independent growth and cell invasion [31]. MARCKS has also been shown to play a role in glioma cell invasion and adhesion [21]. As the reduction of MARCKS expression in glioma cells results in a decrease in adhesion to fibronectin and collagen, but not to laminin, cell adhesion mechanisms may depend on the environment of the ECM. While cell adhesion in ECM areas rich with laminin is mediated *via* MARCKS-independent pathways, adhesion in areas abundant with fibronectin and collagen is mediated *via* MARCKS-dependent pathways. Additionally, MARCKS-mediated cell attachment and spreading is independent of EGFRvIII signaling. This is consistent with studies showing that a reduction of MARCKS results in the inhibition of cell spreading. EGFRvIII is able to regulate MARCKS phosphorylation and expression *via* PKC-a, while EGFRvIII and MARCKS can regulate PKC, thereby modulating cell invasion [21]. Another molecule, CRMP1, has decreased expression in EGFRvIII positive GBM cells. While the overexpression of EGFRvIII in wild-type EGFR-expressing glioma cells results in the reduced expression of CRMP1 and promotes cell invasion, rescue of CRMP1 expression has been shown to inhibit the invasion of the EGFRvIII-expressing glioma cells by regulating the balance between Rho and Rac [32]. Recent studies have shown EGFRvIII to stimulate Rac1 signaling by inducing Src family kinase-dependent phosphorylation of Dock180, a guanine nucleotide exchange factor for Rac1. Inhibition of Src family kinases has been shown to reduce Rac1 activity and cell migration [33]. EGFRvIII also promotes invasion *via* MMP13 in glioma cells [34].

The PDGF family is comprised of PDGF-A, -B, -C and -D, which can form homo- or heterodimers. PDGF-BB has been shown to be involved in GBM cell migration, with PDGFR being overexpressed in 24% of astrocytomas [35]. Upon binding of PDGF to its receptor, PDGFR is activated, resulting in the phosphorylation of the eight tyrosine residues of its intracellular domain. The binding sites and ligands of PDGRF are well defined. While Src binds to tyrosine residues Y-579 and Y-581, GRB2 and phospholipase C-γ (PLCγ) bind to residues Y-716 and Y-1021, respectively. Also, p120-GAP (GTPase activating protein), a negative regulator of Ras, binds at residue Y-771, with the SH2-domain containing phosphatase-2 (SH-PTP2 or SHP2, previously known as Syp, PTP1D or PTP2C) binds at residue Y-1009. Finally, PI3K and Shc (*src* homologous collagen-like protein) can both bind at residues Y-740 and Y-751 [36]. The use of sunitinib to inhibit PDGFR expression has been shown to reduce glioma cell migration and invasion *via* blockade of Src and focal adhesion kinase (FAK) [37]. PDGFR overexpression in glial progenitor cells has a potent oncogenic effect, resulting in tumors with robust proliferative and invasive properties [38].

The fibroblast growth factor receptors (FGFRs) consist of an intracellular domain with tyrosine kinase activity, a transmembrane helix domain, and an extracellular ligand domain composed of three Ig-like domains. A key factor in FGFR signaling is the FGFR-associated substrate 2a (FRS2a), which after phosphorylation, activates adaptor molecules such as Shp2 and Grb2. This relays signals to the PI3K/AKT or Ras/mitogen-activated protein kinase (MAPK) pathways, regulating glioma cell migration [39].

Ephrin (Eph) receptors are the largest sub-family of RTKs, with studies suggesting their strong involvement in various aspects of tumorigenesis, including invasion [40]. While not found in the normal brain, EphA2 is found in up to 90% of GBM tumors. It is phosphorylated and regulated by ephA1 in glioma cells, with invasion being negatively affected by EphA2 expression [41]. EphrinB3 is expressed in glioma cells, with ephrin B3 phosphorylation, signaling and expression *via* Rac1 being important for glioma cell invasion [42]. Stable expression of EphB2 in glioma cells also results in marked invasive growth in *ex vivo* rat brain slice models [43]. Studies have shown EphB2 to regulate glioma cell growth, invasion and adhesion *via* R-Ras signaling. The overexpression of EphA4 in glioma cells results in FGF2-mediated proliferation and migration, with enhanced FGF 2-triggered AKT and MAPK phosphorylation. Activation of AKT results in AKT-dependent EphA2 phosphorylation of residue S897 [44]. The result, P-EphA2$_{S897}$, is required for lamellipodia formation and thus cell migration. Also, active forms of Cdc42 and Rac1 are up-regulated in cells overexpressing EphA4. Additionally, FGFR-mediated downstream signaling is potentiated after EphA4 forms a heteroreceptor complex with FGFR1. EphA4 therefore enhances cell proliferation and migration by accelerating FGFR signaling pathways, playing an important role in malignant phenotype of GBM [39]. High expression of fibroblast growth factor 5 (FGF5) and its high-affinity receptor (FGFR1 IIIc) is found in GBM cells and tumors. While the expression of FGF5 can affect cell growth, it has a stronger effect on cell migration [45]. Interestingly, while EphA2 overexpression results in increased invasion, activation of EphA2 kinase by ephrin-A1 results in tumor suppression [46]. This may occur by the down-regulation of these receptors following exposure to ephrin-A1, resulting in reduced migration and proliferation [47]. As GBM cells have low levels of ephrin-A1, this may explain the overexpression of EphA2. Recent studies have shown EphA2 to act as a tumor suppressor following activation by ephrin-A1, but a tumor promoter when phosphorylated by Akt *via* ligand-independent signaling [44]. Ephrin-A1 is thought to inhibition migration by disrupting EphA2-AKT complexes, preventing the formation of P-EphA2$_{S897}$. Also Hsp90 has been shown to increase glioma cell motility by interacting with EphA2 [48]. This is thought to occur by the maintenance of AKT activation and thus formation of P-EphA2$_{S897}$.

Met, the receptor for the hepatocyte growth factor/scatter factor (HGF/SF) ligand, is a potent inducer of gliomas cell invasion [49]. HGF/SF is able to regulate GBM cell invasion and proliferation *via* the Myc and MAPK pathways. The induction of uPA by HGF/SF is also known to play an important role in cell invasion [50]

Also the restoration of PTEN has been shown to block HGF-induced changes of signal transduction proteins such as JNK, mTOR, AKT, and GSK-3, in addition to cell cycle regulatory proteins E2F-1, cyclin E, and p27, inhibiting these HGF-induced factors that are involved in the invasion and migration glioma cells [51]. CXCR4 also plays an important role in glioma cell migration, as its expression is induced in hypoxic conditions *via* HGF. This induction by HGF occurs through NF-κB, resulting in glioma cell migration [52].

Signal transducers and activators of transcription (STATs) are downstream transcription factors (TFs) of RTKs, interacting in Jak-independent and -dependent pathways [53]. STATs that are phosphorylated form homo- or heterodimers *via* their SH2 domains, then translocating to the nucleus. The expression of a constitutive active form of STAT3 in PTEN deficient glioma cells has been shown to inhibit cell invasiveness, proliferation, and spreading on myelin [54]. STAT3 is mostly expressed in GBM primary tumors and stem cells. This expression is regulated by a variety of proteins. GRIM-19, a novel gene essential for normal development interacts with STAT3 and inhibits its transcriptional activity [55]. The expression of a variety of STAT3-dependent genes are also regulated by GRIM-19. Inhibition of STAT3 has been shown to decrease the proliferation of glioma stem cells and prevent neurosphere formation. LLL12, a STAT3 inhibitor, is able to inactivate STAT3 function to reduce tumor migration and proliferation, suggesting the importance of this factor in stem cells and glioma migration [56]. STAT3 may function as a promoter for invasion by increasing expression of YKL-40 (chitinase 3-like 1/human cartilage glycoprotein 39/breast regression protein 39), a secreted glycoprotein [57]. This protein has been shown to induce VEGF expression in GBM, and regulate migration and invasion in glioma cells.

Glial cell line-derived neurotrophic factor (GDNF) is a member of the growing GDNF family of ligands (GFL). GDNF interacts with GDNF family receptor alpha 1 and 2 (GFRA). GDNF and GFRA2 both stimulate cell migration through p38 MAPK, ERK-1/2 and JNK signaling pathways [58].

Receptor protein tyrosine phosphatase ζ (RPTP ζ) is also able to promote glioma cell invasion. The only soluble ligand that can bind RPTP ζ is pleiotrophin (PTN).

PTN inactivates the phosphatase activity of RPTP ζ, resulting in an increase in the phosphorylation of Fyn, beta-adducin, and beta-catenin, proteins that disrupt the stability of the cellular cytoskeleton and increase cell motility. The expression of PTN and RPTP ζ has been shown to be higher in GBM tumors compared to normal brain [38].

TRANSFORMING GROWTH FACTOR β (TGF-β) RECEPTORS

TGF-β is involved is a variety of aspects of gliomagenesis – immune response, differentiation, and cell growth. However, its most important role may be in cell migration (Fig. **2**) [59]. TGF-β has three surface receptors Tb-RI, -RII, -RIII, which all activate intracellular Smads [60]. The receptor-regulated Smads (R-Smads), the inhibitory Smads (I-Smads) and the co-mediator Smads (Co-Smads) are three classes of Smads. Tb-R1 only directly phosphorylates R-Smads. Co-Smads and R-Smads form a complex and translocate to the nucleus to regulate downstream genes, such as VEGF and PAI-1 which both regulate glioma cell invasion and migration [61].

TGF-β also induces glioma cell invasiveness and migration [62] by stimulating the Sp1 family of transcription factors and increasing integrin expression. Additionally, TGF-β can induce both MMP-2 and MMP-9 to induce glioma cell migration. Endo180, a collagen internalization receptor, is overexpressed in GBM and can be directly enhanced by TGF-β1, promoting glioma cell invasion [63]. CX3CL1, a chemokine, is found in primary cell cultures and glioma cell lines, and can regulate cell invasion and migration *via* TGF-β1 signaling [64]. Recent studies have also suggested that TGF-β1 induces glioma cell migration by stimulating TNF-α converting enzyme (TACE/ADAM17) [65]. This enzyme, in addition to releasing the soluble form of TNF-α, cleaves collagen IV and releases a variety of integrins from the cell surface, increasing cell motility [66]. Also ADAM17 is an upsteam component of many EGFR proligands, resulting in the activation of MEK/ERK and PI3K/AKT pathways [67].

INTEGRINS

Integrins are heterodimers of two glycosylated subunits α and β that interact with proteins in the ECM (Fig. **2**) [68]. The use of antibodies to blocking the α and β subunits have been shown to inhibit glioma cell migration *via* a variety of ECM components [69]. Each integrin subunit has a short cytoplasmic domain and crosses the membrane once. Some integrins also bind to the RGD (Arg-Gly-Asp) motif in collagen, laminin, vitronectin and fibronectin. Others bind to the Ig-superfamily of co-receptors and participate in cell–cell adhesion. Integrin can activate FAK and result in its autophosphorylation at the Y397 site. This creates a binding site for the recruitment of SH2-containing proteins such as PLCg, p85, Fyn and Src [70]. The activation of FAK turns on various downstream pathways, such as the PI3K/AKT and Ras/Erk pathways. Pyk2, a FAK homology protein, can also activate many proteins such as FAK [71]. The inhibition and overexpression of FAK in glioma cell lines decreases and increases cell migration and invasion, respectively [72]. Gene expression studies have shown ECM-related molecules and their receptors to play an important role in the glioma cell invasion process, including cell migration and adhesion to the surrounding microenvironment [73]. A recent study elucidated the role of integrins involving multiple levels of ECM-based signaling in gliomas cell invasion [74]. The level of MMP12 has been seen to increase with glioma grade, with a reduction in MMP12 expression mitigating glioma cell invasion *via* its interaction with tenascin-C [75]. Various pro-invasive ECM factors are upregulated in the glioma microenvironment as the ECM of malignant gliomas can promote NSC migration [76].

Both cysteine-rich angiogenic inducer 61 (Cyr61) and angiopoietin 2 (Ang2) can bind to integrins. Ang2 activates JNK, ERK 1/2, CAS, and FAK and enhances MMP-2 expression and secretion [77]. The overexpression of Cyr61 results in the upregulation of integrin-linked kinase (ILK), anb3, and integrin expression [78]. Galectin-1 regulates vimentin, PKCe, and integrin-β1 localization. The loss of galectin-1 expression results in the loss of integrin-β1 on the cell membrane at points of focal adhesion complexes coincident with increased integrin-b1 intracellular levels. Also, galectin-1 can bind integrin-b1, modulating FAK activation and adhesion while inhibiting cell growth through the Ras/MEK/ERK pathway [79].

Secreted protein acidic and rich in cysteine (SPARC) is found in both low and high grade astrocytomas, including GBM. Though it may supress glioma growth, it promotes invasion and migration by mediating RTKs, integrin, and their downstream effectors [80]. Additional studies have shown PTEN reconstitution to decrease migration *via* the suppression of ERK, RAF, SHC, AKT and FAK activation in SPARC-expressing glioma cells. The expression of PTEN is able to inhibit invasion of control gliomas and SPARC-expressing cells. While PTEN expression has been seen to extend survival in control and SPARC-expressing tumors, the longest survival occurs in tumors which express PTEN and SPARC.

IMMUNOGLOBULIN FAMILY

Immunoglobulins (Igs) are gamma globulin proteins used by the immune system to identify and neutralize foreign entities. CD44 is an Ig which interacts with hyaluronic acid (HA) and is released into the surroundings by MMPs, stimulating cell motility [81]. CD44 can also bind to ErbB2 and EGFR in glioma cells (Fig. **2**). It promotes ADAM10 cleavage and cell migration *via* the modulation of MMP-9 on the cell surface and Rac-mediated cytoskeletal rearrangement [82,83]. CD155, another Ig protein, is involved in cell motility and functions as a cell adhesion molecule, binding poliovirus to host cells [84]. High levels of CD155 is seen in glioma cell lines and primary tumors, with inactivation inhibiting glioma cell migration [85]. Additionally, the expression of CD155 decreases focal adhesion density, cell spreading, substrate adhesion, and the number of actin stress fibers in a substrate-dependent manner [86]. It enhances the adhesion-induced activation of p130c and paxillin in cells adhering to vitronectin, and increases Src/FAK signaling in a substrate-dependent manner [87]. A cell surface immunoglobulin superfamily 3 (IGSF3), EWI-2, has decreased expression in glioma cell lines compared to normal brain tissue. The overexpression of EWI-2 results in the inhibition of tumor growth. EWI-2 is thought to function by reorganizing CD81 and CD9 protein complexes. This is accompanied by the reorganization of other CD81 and CD9 partner proteins (*e.g.*, signaling molecules, adhesion receptors, proteases), leading to decreased glioma cell growth, motility, and invasion.

G PROTEIN-COUPLED RECEPTORS (GPCRs)

G protein-coupled receptors (GPCRs) are seven-transmembrane domain receptors (G protein-linked receptors, serpentine receptor, heptahelical receptors, and 7TM receptors) (Fig. **2**). There are two primary signal transduction pathways involving the G protein-coupled receptors: the PI and cAMP signal pathways. Stromal cell derived factor 1 (CXCL12/SDF-1) and its receptor, CXCR4, are involved in glioma cell migration and proliferation *via* the Akt and ERK1/2 pathways [88]. Through similar pathways, CXCL12 increases chemotaxis, proliferation, upregulation of proMMP-2 and invasion [89]. CXCL12 promotes invasion through MT2-MMP, but not *via* MMP-2 or MMP-9 [90]. However, CXCL12 – mediated migration has been shown to require activation of intermediate conductance Ca^{2+}-activated K channels as blockade of these channels completely eliminated CXCL12 induced migration [91]. Both sphingosine-1-phosphate (S1P) and lipophosphatidic acid (LPA) can regulate GPCRs. Cleavage of lipophosphatidylcholine (LPC) and sphingosylphosphorylcholine (SPC) produces ATX, stimulating the invasion of glioma cells [92]. S1P promotes glioma cell migration *via* S1P1 and S1P3 receptors [29a, 29d, 93]. S1P2 is able to mediate glioma cell migration *via* G12/13-proteins/Rho signaling pathways [29b]. (G-protein coupled receptor 56) GPCR56 (TM7XN1) is an adhesion GPCR better characterized as HE6 (human epididymis-specific protein 6). The up-regulation of GPR56 occurs in GBM tumors [94], co-localizing with a-actinin, and playing a role in cell migration and adhesion. The activation of TCF and PAI-1 reporters by GPR56 is implicated in β-catenin and vitronectin/integrin GPR56 signaling [95]. Once activated, S1P and SphK can affect glioma cell invasion *via* a variety of mechanisms. S1P promotes glioma cell invasion through S1P2/CCN1 signaling, and regulates glioma cell motility *via* S1P1 and S1P3. SphK1 maintains basal levels of glioma invasiveness and stimulates uPA and uPAR enhanced cell migration [29c].

SIGNALING MOLECULES

Tumor necrosis factor-alpha (TNF-alpha) and TNF receptors are members of the TNF ligand and receptor families (Fig. **2**). MMP-2 and MMP-9 are produced in glioma cells by stimulation of IL1 and TNF through nuclear factor kappa-light-chain-enhancer of activated B cells (NFkB) or PKCζ [96]. CD95 (Fas, Apo-1), a member of subfamily of TNF receptors named death receptors, is known to be a regulator of apoptosis [97,98]. Additional studies however have shown CD95-induced signaling pathways to promote glioma cell invasion [99]. The interaction of CD95L with CD95 on glioma cells results in the recruitment of the p85 subunit of PI3K and the Src family member Yes to CD95. This promotes invasion *via* the GSK3b pathway due to the expression of MMPs. Fn14, another member of TNF receptor family, and its endogenous (TNF-like weak inducer of apoptosis, TWEAK) ligand both regulate cell migration [100]. PTEN inactivation results in increased translation of TRAIL and FLIPS resistance through the mTOR pathway. The FLIPS protein has been seen to have a longer half-life in PTEN mutant glioma cells compared to PTEN-deficient cells, correlating with decreased FLIPS polyubiquitination. The inhibition of AIP4 levels by RNAi in PTEN wild-type cells decreases FLIPS decrease, enhances TRAIL resistance, and extends FLIPS half-life. Also, the activation of Akt that was seen to increase TRAIL resistance did not alter AIP4 levels. It instead increased FLIPS steady-state levels, increased AIP4 ubiquitination, and suppressed FLIPS ubiquitination. This confirms that FLIPS ubiquitination, TRAIL sensitivity, and FLIP S stability are controlled by PTEN-Akt-AIP4 pathway [101].

Granulocyte macrophage colony-stimulating factor (GM-CSF) and granulocyte-colony stimulating factor (G-CSF) are secreted glycoproteins that can stimulate glioma cell migration *via* GM-CSF receptors. G-CSF has been shown to be widely expressed in gliomas of various grades and is implicated progression and recurrence of these tumors [102]. The reduction of cytokine expression with small RNA interference has been seen to inhibit cell migration. Similar evidence of GM-CSF has been found in mouse glioma cell migration [103]. Recent studies have shown G-CSF to affect cell migration by regulating the activation of STAT3 and expression of its downstream effectors [102]. Interlukin-10 (IL-10), a suppressor of immune responses, is overexpressed in GBM and can enhance glioma cell invasion [104] Two natural forms (PTN15 and 18) of pleiotrophin (PTN) can bind cell surface receptors: the anaplastic lymphoma kinase (ALK) and the protein tyrosine phosphatase receptor ζ (PTPRZ1). These receptors are frequently overexpressed in GBM [105]. PTN15 induces the phosphorylation of MAPK and Akt in ALK-expressing glioma cells in a dose-dependent manner, enhancing migration in PTPRZ1 expressing glioma cells. The two forms of PTN can mediate migration through PTPRZ1 and mitogenic activity through ALK. PTN and its receptor-associated pathways are potential therapeutic targets for the invasive and proliferative characteristics of GBM [106]. An IL-6 family cytokine, Oncostatin M (OSM), has been tested in GBM. TNF-a protein expression can be detected in the supernatants from microglia treated with OSM, with p65 phosphorylation being detected as early as 15 min following treatment. Also, IL-27 can inhibit OSM-mediated p65 activation and recruitment to the iNOS and TNF-α promoters [107].

Bradykinin (BK) is a member of the kinin family of signaling molecules and is upregulated in gliomas [108]. BK can bind to two bradykinin receptors (BR), both of which trigger a variety of processes including activating PKC and mobilizing calcium. BK activation of B2R has been shown to cause oscillations in intracellular Ca^{2+}, enhancing cell motility [109]. Additionally BK has been shown to function as a chemoattactant, guiding infiltrating glioma cells toward blood vessels. As pharmalogical inhibition of B2R reduces the number of cells along blood vessels, BK and its associated receptors may provide targets for inhibiting glioma cell migration.

Another family of secreted molecules involved in cell migration and invasion is the Wnt proteins. These proteins regulate cell growth and motility by acting *via* B-catenin-dependent and –independent pathways [110]. Recent studies have shown that some Wnt proteins such as Wnt-5a are overexpressed in malignant gliomas, with expression correlating with clinical grade and MMP-2 levels [111]. As knockdowns of Wnt-5a resulted in decreased expression of MMP-2 and thus decreased migration and invasion, these molecules may also serve as therapeutic targets.

GBM STEM CELLS

Glioma stem cells (GSCs) comprise a small percentage of the tumor cell population. These cells are able to undergo asymmetric cell division into self-renewing GSCs and daughter cells which can differentiate and acquire various phenotypes, then losing their multipotent ability [112]. Isolated GSCs express CD133 are varying levels and can form highly vascular and/or invasive tumors following intracranial implantation into immunodeficient mice [113]. Integrin α6 has recently been found to be co-expressed with conventional GSC markers and allows for the enrichment of GSCs [114]. Targeting integrin α6 is able to inhibit the tumor formation capacity, proliferation, and self-renewal ability of GSCs. Additional studies have shown integrin α6 to regulate downstream molecules such as c-myc and Akt, factors critical for the maintenance of GSCs. Hypoxia inducible factor 1 (HIF-1) is also a key factor for the maintenance of cancer stem cell (CSC) characteristics. It also promotes the self-renewal potential and survival of CSCs. HIF-1 also plays an important role in cell migration as inhibiting HIF-1 prevents tumor sphere formation and decreases the migration ability [115]. HIF-1α has recently been shown to be induced by IDH2 (isocitrate dehydrogenase) mutations, resulting in secretion of pro-MMP-2 and pro-MMP-9, increasing migration [116]. IGFBP2 is another gene related to GBM cell migration. It is overexpressed in GSCs and promotes GSC expansion and keeps a restricted self-renewal trait. Additionally, IGFBP2 promotes the activation of Akt and the expression of stem cell and cell cycle genes [117]. A20 (TNFAIP3), a regulator of the NFkB pathway and cell survival is also overexpressed in GSCs. It regulates apoptosis and promotes cell invasion through the TNF-α pathway [118].

OTHER MECHANISMS RESPONSIBLE FOR MIGRATION

Recently other factors have been identified to play a significant role in glioma cell invasion. Stomatin-like protein 2 (STOML2), a member of the stomatin family, has been shown to be significantly upregulated in glioma cell lines and tissues [119]. This overexpression results in increased levels of NFkB and MMP-9, increasing migration. Silencing of STOML2 has been shown to decrease invasion and migratory speed of glioma cells. RTVP-1, also known as gliomas pathogenesis-related protein (GLIPR1), is highly expressed in malignant gliomas and has been shown to also increase cell invasion, migration, and anchorage-independent growth of gliomas [120]. The expression of this protein has been shown to be regulated by PKC, and the transcription factor serum response factor (SRF). Connective tissue growth factor (CTGF) has also been shown to play a role in the highly invasive nature of glioma tumor stem cells [121]. CTGF binds to beta 1 integrin (ITGB1) and the tyrosine kinase receptor type A (TrkA), resulting in NFkB transcriptional activation. This leads to the binding of ZEB-1 to the E-cadherin promoter, resulting in E-cadherin suppression. As TrkA is only expressed in infiltrative glioma cells, with CTGF secretion by the surrounding reactive astrocytes, the activation of ITGB1 and TrkA plays a role in the invasiveness of malignant gliomas. Another factor thought to play a role in glioma cell migration is aquaporin-4 (AQP4), an integral membrane protein involved in maintaining water and ion homeostasis [122]. AQP4 has been shown to be overexpressed in malignant gliomas, with expression correlating with MMP-2 levels. Additionally AQP4 is able to modulate cell adhesion, with downregulation increasing the expression of beta-catenin and connexin 43, reducing cell motility. Other genes including CDH11, PCSK6, and SH3GL3 have also been idenfitied as invasion-associated genes [123].

Some factors have also been shown to be downregulated in gliomas. The Runt family of transcription factors consists of RUNX1-RUNX3, and has been shown to act as tumor suppressors in a variety of cancers [124]. Recently, decreased RUNX3 expression was found in gliomas, with re-expression decreasing MMP-2 production and enzymatic activity, resulting in decreased cell invasion and migration. Another molecule, p27, is a cell cycle inhibitor which has shown to be downregulated in gliomas [125]. Loss of p27 has been shown to enhance tumor progression and decrease survival in PDGF-expressing gliomas [126]. However, these studies did not show tumor invasion into the surrounding brain tissue. Further studies have shown that p27 deficient cells that originate from the subventricular zone are unable to invade parenchyma, suggesting that p27 downregulation results in migration defects in gliomas [127]. However, as the inhibition of Rho reverses the non-invasive nature of gliomas with p27 deficiency, it supports the notion that deregulation of Rho is caused by the absence of p27, modulating migration [128]. Additionally, the location of p27 has been shown to affect cell motility and survival, with the exclusion of p27 from the nucleus or its retention in the cytoplasm resulting in cell invasion. This is supported by studies showing cytoplasmic p27 to be an independent poor prognostic factor, while nuclear p27 resulted in greater survival in those with gliomas [129].

UNEXPLORED FACTORS IN MIGRATION

Using genome-wide screens, the loss of *AJAP1* expression in GBM was identified. The expression of this protein was seen to be lost in more than 85% of GBM patients. Studies of AJAP1 suggested it to have an important role in glioma cell migration as AJAP1 loss in glioma cell lines results in increased cell invasion and migration. In contrast, the restoration of AJAP1 expression inhibits both cell invasion and migration. Additionally, AJAP1 overexpression results in reduced tumor growth and increased survival in mouse glioma xenografts. *AJAP1* has also been thought to act as a tumor suppressor gene in other types of tumors. A study by White *et al.* found a loss in 25% of primary neuroblastomas at a region on 1p36.3 which contains approximately 30 genes including *AJAP1* [130]. Also Dong *et al.* discovered a smaller region deleted at 1p36.3 containing *AJAP1* and 8 other genes in 52 oligodendrogliomas [131]. *AJAP1* is thought to encode a transmembrane protein which does not belong to any known protein family. While it is known to interact with beta-catenin/E-cadherin complexes at adherens junctions in polarized epithelial cells, little is known regarding its function [132]. In polarized epithelial cells, adherens junctions are known to form adhesion belts around interacting cells. Cadherins form homodimers in the membrane where the extracellular domain of one dimer binds to the extracellular domain of a dimer in an adjacent cell. The intracellular domains bind anchor proteins such as vinvulin, actinin, and catenin that connect them to a contractile band of actin filaments running along the cytoplasmic surface. Currently how AJAP1 functions in the protein complex is unclear. A study by Bharti *et al.* showed that AJAP1 does not interact with these proteins in nonpolarized, invasive and highly migratory epithelial cells. This gene is widely and preferentially expressed in the developing adult cortex, cerebellum, spinal cord, and spleen [130, 133]. While E-cadherin is not commonly expressed in brain tumors (except in benign choroid plexus papillomas and meningiomas), beta-catenin and N-cadherin are found at cell-cell junctions in malignant gliomas [134,134b]. However, E-cadherin expression is frequently lost during the transformation of benign meningiomas to more invasive and malignant meningiomas [134a, 135]. Recently, Schreiner *et al.* demonstrated that AJAP1 can interact with CD147, a regulatory subunit of gamma-secretase and inducer of MMP activity in endometrial cells [133]. Currently, the interaction of AJAP1 with other signaling pathways and proteins in the normal brain is unknown as it may not function in the context of adherens junctions. As mentioned above, the loss of AJAP1 expression is found in neuroblastoma, oligodendroglioma and GBM tumors, with loss of gene expression not occurring in the normal brain surrounding oligodendrogliomas [136]. Interestingly, AJAP1 overexpression in tumor cells results in decreased cell motility. *AJAP1* may therefore be a novel invasion-related gene in glial cells where its function and molecular mechanism may differ from the mesenchymal and epithelial cells found outside the brain. AJAP1 may therefore be a potential therapeutic target for the treatment of GBM.

CONCLUSIONS: TREATMENT OUTLOOK AND PROMISING DEVELOPMENTS

Glioblastoma is a devastating disease which has a median survival of slightly more than a year. Despite surgical resection of all visible tumor, recurrence is universal due to the progression of cells that have migrated into the brain parenchyma and secondary structures of Scherer. The past decade, there has been a rapid growth in our understanding of the important molecular factors that support this invasive nature, along with molecular inhibitors which target these pathways (Fig. **3**). We now understand that gliomagenic signaling pathways do not exist in isolation but instead there are many opportunities for "cross-talk". For example, EGFR, an important member of RTKs, regulates various downstream pathways by either binding with ligands or *via* constitutive activation (*e.g.* EGFRvIII) to promote cell invasion and proliferation [137]. It is important to understand that the downstream signaling molecules including components of the PI3K and MAPK pathways are shared among not only RTKs, but also immunoglobulins, cytokine receptors, integrins, and GPCRs. Integrins can phosphorylate and at least partially activate GFRs including PDGFR, c-Met, and EGFR in the absence of growth ligands [138]. Also PI3K pathways regulate various gliomagenic phenotypes including invasion, proliferation, and uncontrolled cell growth. S1P functions to regulate cell surface signaling pathways through a group of five GPCRs to activate PI3K and Rac, initiating glioma migration and invasion [139].

The need to develop therapies which target glioma cell migration have become even more important due to changes in therapeutic options. While the current standard of care utilizing temozolomide for GBM was FDA approved in 2005, a therapeutic antibody for GBM that targets VEGF (bevacizumab) was approved by the FDA in 2009. Due to its success in treating other cancers and the neoangiogenic characteristics of GBM tumors, bevacizumab provided an exciting option for therapy-resistant GBM. However, several reports have suggested that bevacizumab-treated GBMs may recur with a more invasive phenotype that may preclude additional resections.

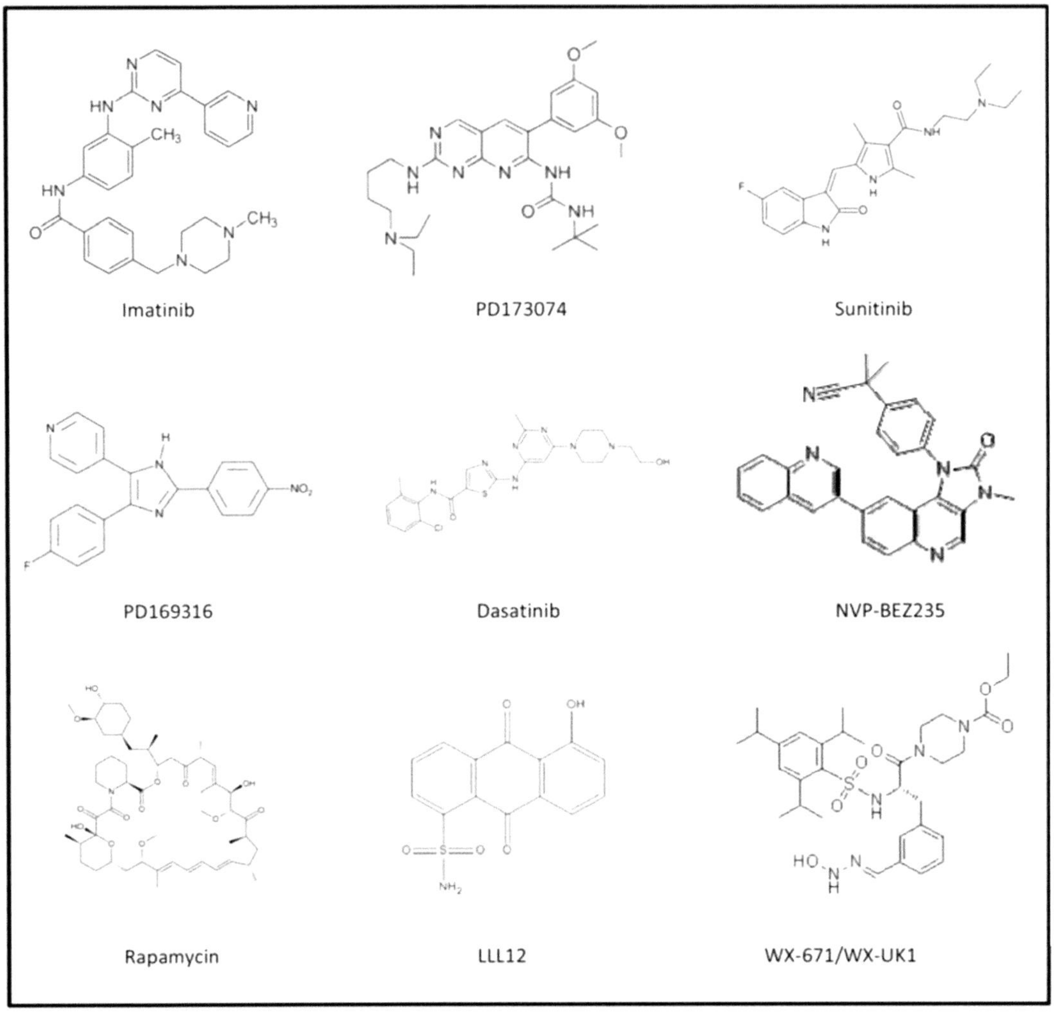

Fig. (3). Structures of inhibitors currently under study in GBM therapy. Chemical structures for most small molecular inhibitors under study in GBM therapeutics are known, which should lead to even more rapid exploitation of ways to use them. A few have yet to be published.

Table 1. There are multiple, well-established factors and pathways that promote invasion of GBM cells, with targeted therapies currently in clinical trials

Gene	Pathway	Role	Inhibitor
EGFR	EGFR Signaling Pathway	Binds cell surface receptors	Erlotinib, gefitinib, lapatinib, BIBW2992, nimotuzumab, cetuximab and AEE788
PDGF	PDGF Signaling Pathway	Binds PDGFR to regulate GBM cell migration	Dasatinib, imatinib, tandutinib and pazopanib
FGFR	FGFR Signaling Pathway	Regulates GBM cell migration through Ras/MAPK or PI3K/AKT pathways	AZD4547
Met	Met Signaling Pathway	Induces GBM cell invasion *via* MAPK and Myc pathways.	XL184
STATs	JAK-STAT Signaling Pathway	Activates Jak-dependent and Jak-independent pathways.	WP-1034 and LLL12
AKT	PI3K/AKT signaling Pathway	Activates PI3K/AKT signaling pathway to promote cell invasion.	Perifosine
PI3K	PI3K/AKT signaling Pathway	Activates PI3K/AKT signaling pathway to promote cell invasion.	BEZ235 and XL765
Ras	Ras/Raf signaling Pathway	Activates PI3K/AKT signaling pathway to promote cell invasion.	TLN-4601
Raf	Ras/Raf signaling Pathway	Activates MAPK/ERK signaling pathway.	Sorafenib
uPA	c-Src/ MEK/MAPK signaling pathway	Degrades ECM and attenuates cell-cell and cell-matrix interactions.	WX-671
MAPK	MAPK/ERK signaling Pathway	Promotes cell motility.	PD169316
TGF-β	TGF-β Signaling Pathway	Activates R-smad and Co-smad *via* regulation of MMPs and integrins.	AP12009
VEGF	VEGF Signaling Pathway	Binds VEGFR and activates PI3K and Ras/Raf pathways.	PTK787 and semaxanib
mTOR	mTOR signaling Pathway	Interacts with S6K to induce GBM cell migration.	Everolimus, sirolimus, temsirolimus, deforolimus and rapamycin
Src	c-Src/MEK/MAPK pathway	Degrades ECM and attenuates cell-cell and cell-matrix interactions.	Dasatinib

GBM cell migration and invasion is complex and is influenced by various signaling cascades. The current dogma among most neuro-oncology scientists is that future therapies will need to target multiple pathways, using either single agents at "cross-talk" junctions or with multiple agents at divergent pathways. However these drugs will need to be highly specific and result in minimal toxicity. Fortunately, a variety of therapies are currently in clinical trials and now target various factors involved in invasion, specifically at critical "crossroad" sites (Table **1**, Fig. **2**). These targeted therapies will hopefully be less toxic and more effective that current chemotherapies in mitigating glioma cell migration. As surgeons can typically resect the primary tumor focus, effective anti-invasive inhibitors may allow patients to be cured of this aggressive disease.

CONFLICT OF INTEREST

The authors declare that there is no conflict of interest.

ACKNOWLEDGEMENTS

Declared none.

DISCLOSURE

This chapter represents an updated version of this topic previously published in *Anti-Cancer Agents in Medicinal Chemistry*, **2010**, *10*, 543-555.

REFERENCES

[1] Wen, P. Y.; Kesari, S. Malignant gliomas in adults. *The New England journal of medicine* **2008**, *359* (5), 492-507.

[2] Scherer, H. J. *Brain* **1940**, *40*, 631-635.

[3] (a) Cavallaro, U.; Christofori, G. Cell adhesion and signalling by cadherins and Ig-CAMs in cancer. *Nature Reviews Cancer* **2004**, *4* (2), 118-132; (b) Sasaki, H.; Yoshida, K.; Ikeda, E.; Asou, H.; Inaba, M.; Otani, M.; Kawase, T. Expression of the neural cell adhesion molecule in astrocytic tumors. *Cancer* **1998**, *82* (10), 1921-1931.

[4] Ranuncolo, S. M.; Ladeda, V.; Specterman, S.; Varela, M.; Lastiri, J.; Morandi, A.; Matos, E.; Joffe, E. B. D. K.; Puricelli, L.; Pallotta, M. G. CD44 expression in human gliomas. *Journal of Surgical Oncology* **2002**, *79* (1), 30-36.

[5] Piao, Y.; Lu, L.; de Groot, J. AMPA receptors promote perivascular glioma invasion *via* β1 integrin–dependent adhesion to the extracellular matrix. *Neuro-Oncology* **2009**, *11* (3), 260-273.

[6] Van Lint, P.; Libert, C. Chemokine and cytokine processing by matrix metalloproteinases and its effect on leukocyte migration and inflammation. *J Leukoc Biol* **2007**, *82* (6), 1375-1381.

[7] Silveira Corrêa, T. C.; Massaro, R. R.; Brohem, C. A.; Taboga, S. R.; Lamers, M. L.; Santos, M. F.; Maria-Engler, S. S. RECK-mediated inhibition of glioma migration and invasion. *Journal of Cellular Biochemistry* **2010**, *110* (1), 52-61.

[8] Mikheeva, S.; Mikheev, A.; Petit, A.; Beyer, R.; Oxford, R.; Khorasani, L.; Maxwell, J.-P.; Glackin, C.; Wakimoto, H.; Gonzalez-Herrero, I.; Sanchez-Garcia, I.; Silber, J.; Horner, P.; Rostomily, R. TWIST1 promotes invasion through mesenchymal change in human glioblastoma. *Molecular Cancer* **2010**, *9* (1), 194.

[9] (a) Engebraaten, O.; Bjerkvig, R.; Pedersen, P.; Laerum, O. Effects of EGF, bFGF, NGF and PDGF(bb) on cell proliferative, migratory and invasive capacities of human brain-tumour biopsies *in vitro*. *Int J Cancer* **1993**, *53* (2), 209-214; (b) Pedersen, P.-H.; Ness, G.; Engebraaten, O.; Bjerkvig, R.; Lillehaug, J.; Laerum, O. Heterogeneous response to the growth factors [EGF, PDGF (bb), TGF-a, bFGF, IL-2] on glioma spheriod growth, migration and invasion. *Int J Cancer* **1994**, *56* (2), 255-261; (c) Koochekpour, S.; Merzak, A.; Pilkington, G. J. Growth factors and gangliosides stimulate laminin production by human glioma cells *in vitro*. *Neuroscience Letters* **1995**, *186* (1), 53-56.

[10] Zwick, E.; Bange, J.; Ullrich, A. Receptor tyrosine kinase signalling as a target for cancer intervention strategies. *Endocr Relat Cancer* **2001**, *8* (3), 161-173.

[11] Robinson, D. R.; Wu, Y.-M.; Lin, S.-F. The protein tyrosine kinase family of the human genome. *Oncogene* **2000**, *19* (49), 5548-5557.

[12] Schlessinger, J. Cell Signaling by Receptor Tyrosine Kinases. *Cell* **2000**, *103* (2), 211-225.

[13] Luk, S. K.; Piekorz, R. P.; Nurnberg, B.; Tony To, S. S. The catalytic phosphoinositol 3-kinase isoform p110delta is required for glioma cell migration and invasion. *Eur J Cancer* **2012**, *48* (1), 149-57.

[14] (a) Singer, E.; Landgraf, R.; Horan, T.; Slamon, D.; Eisenberg, D. Identification of a Heregulin Binding Site in HER3 Extracellular Domain. *Journal of Biological Chemistry* **2001**, *276* (47), 44266-44274; (b) Carraway III, K. L.; Weber, J. L.; Unger, M. J.; Ledesma, J.; Yu, N.; Gassmann, M.; Lai, C. Neuregulin-2, a new ligand of ErbB3/ErbB4-receptor tyrosine kinases. *Nature* **1997**, *387* (6632), 512-516.

[15] Yoo, J.-Y.; X W Wang; Rishi, A. K.; Lessor, T.; Xia, X.-M.; Gustafson, T. A.; Hamburger, A. W. Interaction of the PA2G4 (EBP1) protein with ErbB-3 and regulation of this binding by heregulin. *Br J Cancer* **2000**, *82* (3), 683-690.

[16] Thaminy, S.; Auerbach, D.; Arnoldo, A.; Stagljar, I. Identification of Novel ErbB3-Interacting Factors Using the Split-Ubiquitin Membrane Yeast Two-Hybrid System. *Genome Research* **2003**, *13* (7), 1744-1753.

[17] (a) Williams, C. C.; Allison, J. G.; Vidal, G. A.; Burow, M. E.; Beckman, B. S.; Marrero, L.; Jones, F. E. The ERBB4/HER4 receptor tyrosine kinase regulates gene expression by functioning as a STAT5A nuclear chaperone. *The Journal of Cell Biology* **2004**, *167* (3), 469-478; (b) Schulze, W. X.; Deng, L.; Mann, M. Phosphotyrosine interactome of the ErbB-receptor kinase family. *Mol Syst Biol* **2005**, *1*.

[18] (a) Garcia, R. A. G.; Vasudevan, K.; Buonanno, A. The neuregulin receptor ErbB-4 interacts with PDZ-containing proteins at neuronal synapses. *Proceedings of the National Academy of Sciences of the United States of America* **2000**, *97* (7), 3596-3601; (b) Huang, Y. Z.; Won, S.; Ali, D. W.; Wang, Q.; Tanowitz, M.; Du, Q. S.; Pelkey, K. A.; Yang, D. J.; Xiong, W. C.; Salter, M. W.; Mei, L. Regulation of Neuregulin Signaling by PSD-95 Interacting with ErbB4 at CNS Synapses. *Neuron* **2000**, *26* (2), 443-455.

[19] Gambarotta, G.; Garzotto, D.; Destro, E.; Mautino, B.; Giampietro, C.; Cutrupi, S.; Dati, C.; Cattaneo, E.; Fasolo, A.; Perroteau, I. ErbB4 Expression in Neural Progenitor Cells (ST14A) Is Necessary to Mediate Neuregulin-1β1-induced Migration. *Journal of Biological Chemistry* **2004**, *279* (47), 48808-48816.

[20] Davies, G. C.; Ryan, P. E.; Rahman, L.; Zajac-Kaye, M.; Lipkowitz, S. EGFRvIII undergoes activation-dependent downregulation mediated by the Cbl proteins. *Oncogene* **2006**, *25* (49), 6497-6509.

[21] Micallef, J.; Taccone, M.; Mukherjee, J.; Croul, S.; Busby, J.; Moran, M. F.; Guha, A. Epidermal Growth Factor Receptor Variant III-Induced Glioma Invasion Is Mediated through Myristoylated Alanine-Rich Protein Kinase C Substrate Overexpression. *Cancer Research* **2009**, *69* (19), 7548-7556.

[22] Huang, P. H.; Xu, A. M.; White, F. M. Oncogenic EGFR Signaling Networks in Glioma. *Science Signaling* **2009**, *2* (87), re6.

[23] Cancer Genome Atlas Research Network, Comprehensive genomic characterization defines human glioblastoma genes and core pathways. *Nature* **2008**, *455* (7216), 1061-8.

[24] Gough, N. R. From Ras to PI3K. *Science Signaling* **2006**, *2006* (362), tw397.

[25] Abounader, R. Interactions between PTEN and receptor tyrosine kinase pathways and their implications for glioma therapy. *Expert Review of Anticancer Therapy* **2009**, *9* (2), 235-245.

[26] Kleber, S.; Sancho-Martinez, I.; Wiestler, B.; Beisel, A.; Gieffers, C.; Hill, O.; Thiemann, M.; Mueller, W.; Sykora, J.; Kuhn, A.; Schreglmann, N.; Letellier, E.; Zuliani, C.; Klussmann, S.; Teodorczyk, M.; Gröne, H.-J.; Ganten, T. M.; Sültmann, H.; Tüttenberg, J.; von Deimling, A.; Regnier-Vigouroux, A.; Herold-Mende, C.; Martin-Villalba, A. Yes and PI3K Bind CD95 to Signal Invasion of Glioblastoma. *Cancer Cell* **2008**, *13* (3), 235-248.

[27] Sansal, I.; Sellers, W. R. The Biology and Clinical Relevance of the PTEN Tumor Suppressor Pathway. *Journal of Clinical Oncology* **2004**, *22* (14), 2954-2963.

[28] Sonoda, Y.; Ozawa, T.; Aldape, K. D.; Deen, D. F.; Berger, M. S.; Pieper, R. O. Akt Pathway Activation Converts Anaplastic Astrocytoma to Glioblastoma Multiforme in a Human Astrocyte Model of Glioma. *Cancer Research* **2001**, *61* (18), 6674-6678.

[29] (a) Van Brocklyn, J. R.; Young, N.; Roof, R. Sphingosine-1-phosphate stimulates motility and invasiveness of human glioblastoma multiforme cells. *Cancer Letters* **2003**, *199* (1), 53-60; (b) Malchinkhuu, E.; Sato, K.; Maehama, T.; Mogi, C.; Tomura, H.; Ishiuchi, S.; Yoshimoto, Y.; Kurose, H.; Okajima, F. S1P2 receptors mediate inhibition of glioma cell migration through Rho signaling pathways independent of PTEN. *Biochemical and Biophysical Research Communications* **2008**, *366* (4), 963-968; (c) Young, N.; Pearl, D. K.; Van Brocklyn, J. R. Sphingosine-1-Phosphate Regulates Glioblastoma Cell Invasiveness through the Urokinase Plasminogen Activator System and CCN1/Cyr61. *Molecular Cancer Research* **2009**, *7* (1), 23-32; (d) Young, N.; Van Brocklyn, J. R. Roles of sphingosine-1-phosphate (S1P) receptors in malignant behavior of glioma cells.

Differential effects of S1P2 on cell migration and invasiveness. *Experimental Cell Research* **2007**, *313* (8), 1615-1627.

[30] Amos, S.; Redpath, G. T.; diPierro, C. G.; Carpenter, J. E.; Hussaini, I. M. Epidermal Growth Factor Receptor-Mediated Regulation of Urokinase Plasminogen Activator Expression and Glioblastoma Invasion *via* C-SRC/MAPK/AP-1 Signaling Pathways. *Journal of Neuropathology & Experimental Neurology* **2010**, *69* (6), 582-592.

[31] Zhao, Y.; Xiao, A.; diPierro, C. G.; Carpenter, J. E.; Abdel-Fattah, R.; Redpath, G. T.; Lopes, M.-B. S.; Hussaini, I. M. An Extensive Invasive Intracranial Human Glioblastoma Xenograft Model: Role of High Level Matrix Metalloproteinase 9. *American Journal of Pathology* **2010**, *176* (6), 3032-3049.

[32] Mukherjee, J.; DeSouza, L. V.; Micallef, J.; Karim, Z.; Croul, S.; Siu, K. W. M.; Guha, A. Loss of Collapsin Response Mediator Protein1, as Detected by iTRAQ Analysis, Promotes Invasion of Human Gliomas Expressing Mutant EGFRvIII. *Cancer Research* **2009**, *69* (22), 8545-8554.

[33] Feng, H.; Hu, B.; Jarzynka, M. J.; Li, Y.; Keezer, S.; Johns, T. G.; Tang, C. K.; Hamilton, R. L.; Vuori, K.; Nishikawa, R.; Sarkaria, J. N.; Fenton, T.; Cheng, T.; Furnari, F. B.; Cavenee, W. K.; Cheng, S. Y. Phosphorylation of dedicator of cytokinesis 1 (Dock180) at tyrosine residue Y722 by Src family kinases mediates EGFRvIII-driven glioblastoma tumorigenesis. *Proc Natl Acad Sci U S A* **2012**, *109* (8), 3018-23.

[34] Gan, H. K.; Kaye, A. H.; Luwor, R. B. The EGFRvIII variant in glioblastoma multiforme. *Journal of Clinical Neuroscience* **2009**, *16* (6), 748-754.

[35] Hata, N.; Shinojima, N.; Gumin, J.; Yong, R.; Marini, F.; Andreeff, M.; Lang, F. F. Platelet-Derived Growth Factor BB Mediates the Tropism of Human Mesenchymal Stem Cells for Malignant Gliomas. *Neurosurgery* **2010**, *66* (1), 144-157.

[36] Feldkamp, M. M.; Lau, N.; Guha, A. Signal transduction pathways and their relevance in human astrocytomas. *Journal of Neuro-Oncology* **1997**, *35* (3), 223-248.

[37] de Boüard, S.; Herlin, P.; Christensen, J. G.; Lemoisson, E.; Gauduchon, P.; Raymond, E.; Guillamo, J.-S. Antiangiogenic and anti-invasive effects of sunitinib on experimental human glioblastoma. *Neuro-Oncology* **2007**, *9* (4), 412-423.

[38] Hoelzinger, D. B.; Demuth, T.; Berens, M. E. Autocrine Factors That Sustain Glioma Invasion and Paracrine Biology in the Brain Microenvironment. *Journal of the National Cancer Institute* **2007**, *99* (21), 1583-1593.

[39] Fukai, J.; Yokote, H.; Yamanaka, R.; Arao, T.; Nishio, K.; Itakura, T. EphA4 promotes cell proliferation and migration through a novel EphA4-FGFR1 signaling pathway in the human glioma U251 cell line. *Molecular Cancer Therapeutics* **2008**, *7* (9), 2768-2778.

[40] (a) Dodelet, V. C.; Pasquale, E. B. Eph receptors and ephrin ligands: embryogenesis to tumorigenesis. *Oncogene* **2000**, *19* (49), 5614-5619; (b) Wimmer-Kleikamp, S. H.; Lackmann, M. Eph-modulated Cell Morphology, Adhesion and Motility in Carcinogenesis. *IUBMB Life* **2005**, *57* (6), 421 - 431.

[41] Wykosky, J.; Debinski, W. The EphA2 Receptor and EphrinA1 Ligand in Solid Tumors: Function and Therapeutic Targeting. *Molecular Cancer Research* **2008**, *6* (12), 1795-1806.

[42] Nakada, M.; Drake, K. L.; Nakada, S.; Niska, J. A.; Berens, M. E. Ephrin-B3 ligand promotes glioma invasion through activation of Rac1. *Cancer Res* **2006**, *66* (17), 8492-500.

[43] Nakada, M.; Niska, J. A.; Miyamori, H.; McDonough, W. S.; Wu, J.; Sato, H.; Berens, M. E. The phosphorylation of EphB2 receptor regulates migration and invasion of human glioma cells. *Cancer Res* **2004**, *64* (9), 3179-85.

[44] Miao, H.; Li, D. Q.; Mukherjee, A.; Guo, H.; Petty, A.; Cutter, J.; Basilion, J. P.; Sedor, J.; Wu, J.; Danielpour, D.; Sloan, A. E.; Cohen, M. L.; Wang, B. EphA2 mediates ligand-dependent inhibition and ligand-independent promotion of cell migration and invasion *via* a reciprocal regulatory loop with Akt. *Cancer Cell* **2009**, *16* (1), 9-20.

[45] Allerstorfer, S.; Sonvilla, G.; Fischer, H.; Spiegl-Kreinecker, S.; Gauglhofer, C.; Setinek, U.; Czech, T.; Marosi, C.; Buchroithner, J.; Pichler, J.; Silye, R.; Mohr, T.; Holzmann, K.; Grasl-Kraupp, B.; Marian, B.; Grusch, M.; Fischer, J.; Micksche, M.; Berger, W. FGF5 as an oncogenic factor in human glioblastoma multiforme: autocrine and paracrine activities. *Oncogene* **2008**, *27* (30), 4180-4190.

[46] Wykosky, J.; Gibo, D. M.; Stanton, C.; Debinski, W. EphA2 as a novel molecular marker and target in glioblastoma multiforme. *Molecular cancer research : MCR* **2005**, *3* (10), 541-51.

[47] Liu, D. P.; Wang, Y.; Koeffler, H. P.; Xie, D. Ephrin-A1 is a negative regulator in glioma through down-regulation of EphA2 and FAK. *International journal of oncology* **2007**, *30* (4), 865-71.

[48] Gopal, U.; Bohonowych, J. E.; Lema-Tome, C.; Liu, A.; Garrett-Mayer, E.; Wang, B.; Isaacs, J. S. A novel extracellular Hsp90 mediated co-receptor function for LRP1 regulates EphA2 dependent glioblastoma cell invasion. *PloS one* **2011**, *6* (3), e17649.

[49] Koochekpour, S.; Jeffers, M.; Rulong, S.; Taylor, G.; Klineberg, E.; Hudson, E. A.; Resau, J. H.; Vande Woude, G. F. Met and hepatocyte growth factor/scatter factor expression in human gliomas. *Cancer Res* **1997**, *57* (23), 5391-8.

[50] Xie, Q.; Gao, C.-F.; Shinomiya, N.; Sausville, E.; Hay, R.; Gustafson, M.; Shen, Y.; Wenkert, D.; Woude, G. F. V. Geldanamycins exquisitely inhibit HGF//SF-mediated tumor cell invasion. *Oncogene* **2005**, *24* (23), 3697-3707.

[51] Li, Y.; Guessous, F.; DiPierro, C.; Zhang, Y.; Mudrick, T.; Fuller, L.; Johnson, E.; Marcinkiewicz, L.; Engelhardt, M.; Kefas, B.; Schiff, D.; Kim, J.; Abounader, R. Interactions between PTEN and the c-Met pathway in glioblastoma and implications for therapy. *Molecular Cancer Therapeutics* **2009**, *8* (2), 376-385.

[52] Esencay, M.; Newcomb, E.; Zagzag, D. HGF upregulates CXCR4 expression in gliomas *via* NF-κB: implications for glioma cell migration. *Journal of Neuro-Oncology* **2010**, *99* (1), 33-40.

[53] (a) Ihle, J. N.; Kerr, I. M. Jaks and Stats in signaling by the cytokine receptor superfamily. *Trends in Genetics* **1995**, *11* (2), 69-74; (b) Bromberg, J.; Chen, X. STAT proteins: signal tranducers and activators of transcription. *Methods Enzymol* **2001**, *333*, 138-151.

[54] de la Iglesia, N.; Konopka, G.; Lim, K.-L.; Nutt, C. L.; Bromberg, J. F.; Frank, D. A.; Mischel, P. S.; Louis, D. N.; Bonni, A. Deregulation of a STAT3-Interleukin 8 Signaling Pathway Promotes Human Glioblastoma Cell Proliferation and Invasiveness. *Journal of Neuroscience* **2008**, *28* (23), 5870-5878.

[55] Zhang, Y.; Hao, H.; Zhao, S.; Liu, Q.; Yuan, Q.; Ni, S.; Wang, F.; Liu, S.; Wang, L.; Hao, A. Downregulation of GRIM-19 promotes growth and migration of human glioma cells. *Cancer science* **2011**, *102* (11), 1991-9.

[56] Lin, L.; Hutzen, B.; Li, P.-K.; Ball, S.; Zuo, M.; DeAngelis, S.; Foust, E.; Sobo, M.; Friedman, L.; Bhasin, D.; Cen, L.; Li, C.; Lin, J. A Novel Small Molecule, LLL12, Inhibits STAT3 Phosphorylation and Activities and Exhibits Potent Growth-Suppressive Activity in Human Cancer Cells. *Neoplasia* **2010**, *12* (1), 39-50.

[57] Singh, S. K.; Bhardwaj, R.; Wilczynska, K. M.; Dumur, C. I.; Kordula, T. A complex of nuclear factor I-X3 and STAT3 regulates astrocyte and glioma migration through the secreted glycoprotein YKL-40. *The Journal of biological chemistry* **2011**, *286* (46), 39893-903.

[58] Song, H.; Moon, A. Glial cell-derived neurotrophic factor (GDNF) promotes low-grade Hs683 glioma cell migration through JNK, ERK-1/2 and p38 MAPK signaling pathways. *Neuroscience Research* **2006**, *56* (1), 29-38.

[59] Weller, M.; Fontana, A. The failure of current immunotherapy for malignant glioma. Tumor-derived TGF-beta, T-cell apoptosis, and the immune privilege of the brain. *Brain Research Reviews* **1995**, *21* (2), 128-151.

[60] Wrana, J.; Attisano, L.; Wieser, R.; Ventura, F.; Massagué, J. Mechanism of activation of the TGF-beta receptor. *Nature* **1994**, *370*, 341-347.

[61] Hjelmeland, M. D.; Hjelmeland, A. B.; Sathornsumetee, S.; Reese, E. D.; Herbstreith, M. H.; Laping, N. J.; Friedman, H. S.; Bigner, D. D.; Wang, X.-F.; Rich, J. N. SB-431542, a small molecule transforming growth factor-β-receptor antagonist, inhibits human glioma cell line proliferation and motility. *Molecular Cancer Therapeutics* **2004**, *3* (6), 737-745.

[62] (a) Merzak, A.; McCrea, S.; Koocheckpour, S.; Pilkington, G. J. Control of human glioma cell growth, migration and invasion *in vitro* by transforming growth factor beta 1. *Br J Cancer* **1994**, *70* (2), 199-203; (b) Nakano, A.; Tani, E.; Miyazaki, K.; Yamamoto, Y.; Furuyama, J.-i. Matrix metalloproteinases and tissue inhibitors of metalloproteinases in human gliomas. *Journal of Neurosurgery* **2009**, *83* (2), 298-307.

[63] Huijbers, I. J.; Iravani, M.; Popov, S.; Robertson, D.; Al-Sarraj, S.; Jones, C.; Isacke, C. M. A Role for Fibrillar Collagen Deposition and the Collagen Internalization Receptor Endo180 in Glioma Invasion. *PloS one* **2010**, *5* (3), e9808.

[64] Sciumè, G.; Soriani, A.; Piccoli, M.; Frati, L.; Santoni, A.; Bernardini, G. CX3CR1/CX3CL1 axis negatively controls glioma cell invasion and is modulated by transforming growth factor-beta1. *Neuro-Oncology* **2010**, *12* (7), 701-710.

[65] Lu, Y.; Jiang, F.; Zheng, X.; Katakowski, M.; Buller, B.; To, S. S.; Chopp, M. TGF-beta1 promotes motility and invasiveness of glioma cells through activation of ADAM17. *Oncology reports* **2011**, *25* (5), 1329-35.

[66] Wildeboer, D.; Naus, S.; Amy Sang, Q. X.; Bartsch, J. W.; Pagenstecher, A. Metalloproteinase disintegrins ADAM8 and ADAM19 are highly regulated in human primary brain tumors and their expression levels and activities are associated with invasiveness. *Journal of neuropathology and experimental neurology* **2006**, *65* (5), 516-27.

[67] Zheng, X.; Jiang, F.; Katakowski, M.; Zhang, X.; Jiang, H.; Zhang, Z. G.; Chopp, M. Sensitization of cerebral tissue in nude mice with photodynamic therapy induces ADAM17/TACE and promotes glioma cell invasion. *Cancer Lett* **2008**, *265* (2), 177-87.

[68] Hynes, R. O. Integrins: Bidirectional, Allosteric Signaling Machines. *Cell* **2002**, *110* (6), 673-687.

[69] (a) Gladson, C. L.; Wilcox, J. N.; Sanders, L.; Gillespie, G. Y.; Cheresh, D. A. Cerebral microenvironment influences expression of the vitronectin gene in astrocytic tumors. *Journal of Cell Science* **1995**, *108* (3), 947-956; (b) Friedlander, D. R.; Zagzag, D.; Shiff, B.; Cohen, H.; Allen, J. C.; Kelly, P. J.; Grumet, M. Migration of Brain Tumor Cells on Extracellular Matrix Proteins *in Vitro* Correlates with Tumor Type and Grade and Involves αv and β1 Integrins. *Cancer Research* **1996**, *56* (8), 1939-1947; (c) Wild-Bode, C.; Weller,

M.; Rimner, A.; Dichgans, J.; Wick, W. Sublethal Irradiation Promotes Migration and Invasiveness of Glioma Cells. *Cancer Research* **2001**, *61* (6), 2744-2750.

[70] (a) Chen, H.-C.; Guan, J.-L. Association of Focal Adhesion Kinase with its Potential Substrate Phosphatidylinositol 3-Kinase. *Proc Natl Acad Sci U S A* **1994**, *91* (21), 10148-10152; (b) Cobb, B. S.; Schaller, M. D.; Leu, T. H.; Parsons, J. T. Stable association of pp60src and pp59fyn with the focal adhesion-associated protein tyrosine kinase, pp125FAK. *Molecular and Cellular Biology* **1994**, *14* (1), 147-155; (c) Schaller, M. D.; Thomas Parsons, J. Focal adhesion kinase and associated proteins. *Current Opinion in Cell Biology* **1994**, *6* (5), 705-710; (d) Zhang, X.; Chattopadhyay, A.; Ji, Q.-s.; Owen, J. D.; Ruest, P. J.; Carpenter, G.; Hanks, S. K. Focal adhesion kinase promotes phospholipase C-γ1 activity. *Proc Natl Acad Sci U S A* **1999**, *96* (16), 9021-9026.

[71] Avraham, H.; Park, S.-Y.; Schinkmann, K.; Avraham, S. RAFTK/Pyk2-mediated cellular signalling. *Cellular Signalling* **2000**, *12* (3), 123-133.

[72] (a) Obara, S.; Nakata, M.; Takeshima, H.; Kuratsu, J.-i.; Maruyama, I.; Kitajima, I. Inhibition of migration of human glioblastoma cells by cerivastatin in association with focal adhesion kinase (FAK). *Cancer Letters* **2002**, *185* (2), 153-161; (b) Zagzag, D.; Nomura, M.; David, R. F.; Blanco, C. Y.; Gagner, J.-P.; Nomura, N.; Newcomb, E. W. Geldanamycin inhibits migration of glioma cells *in vitro*: A potential role for hypoxia-inducible factor (HIF-1alpha) in glioma cell invasion. *Journal of Cellular Physiology* **2003**, *196* (2), 394-402; (c) Ling, J.; Liu, Z.; Wang, D.; Gladson, C. L. Malignant astrocytoma cell attachment and migration to various matrix proteins is differentially sensitive to phosphoinositide 3-OH kinase inhibitors. *Journal of Cellular Biochemistry* **1999**, *73* (4), 533-544.

[73] Varga, I.; Hutoczki, G.; Petras, M.; Scholtz, B.; Miko, E.; Kenyeres, A.; Toth, J.; Zahuczky, G.; Bognar, L.; Hanzely, Z.; Klekner, A. Expression of Invasion-Related Extracellular Matrix Molecules in Human Glioblastoma *Versus* Intracerebral Lung Adenocarcinoma Metastasis. *Cen Eur Neurosurg* **2010**.

[74] Ulrich, T. A.; de Juan Pardo, E. M.; Kumar, S. The Mechanical Rigidity of the Extracellular Matrix Regulates the Structure, Motility, and Proliferation of Glioma Cells. *Cancer Research* **2009**, *69* (10), 4167-4174.

[75] Sarkar, S.; Nuttall, R. K.; Liu, S.; Edwards, D. R.; Yong, V. W. Tenascin-C Stimulates Glioma Cell Invasion through Matrix Metalloproteinase-12. *Cancer Research* **2006**, *66* (24), 11771-11780.

[76] Ziu, M.; Schmidt, N. O.; Cargioli, T. G.; Aboody, K. S.; Black, P. M.; Carroll, R. S. Glioma-produced extracellular matrix influences brain tumor tropism of human neural stem cells. *Journal of Neuro-Oncology* **2006**, *79* (2), 125-133.

[77] Hu, B.; Jarzynka, M. J.; Guo, P.; Imanishi, Y.; Schlaepfer, D. D.; Cheng, S. Y. Angiopoietin 2 induces glioma cell invasion by stimulating matrix metalloprotease 2 expression through the alphavbeta1 integrin and focal adhesion kinase signaling pathway. *Cancer Res* **2006**, *66* (2), 775-83.

[78] Xie, D.; Yin, D.; Tong, X.; O'Kelly, J.; Mori, A.; Miller, C.; Black, K.; Gui, D.; Said, J. W.; Koeffler, H. P. Cyr61 Is Overexpressed in Gliomas and Involved in Integrin-Linked Kinase-Mediated Akt and β-Catenin-TCF/Lef Signaling Pathways. *Cancer Research* **2004**, *64* (6), 1987-1996.

[79] Fortin, S.; Mercier, M. L.; Camby, I.; Spiegl-Kreinecker, S.; Berger, W.; Lefranc, F.; Kiss, R. Galectin-1 Is Implicated in the Protein Kinase C ε/Vimentin-Controlled Trafficking of Integrin-β1 in Glioblastoma Cells. *Brain Pathol* **2010**, *20* (1), 39-49.

[80] Thomas, S. L.; Alam, R.; Lemke, N.; Schultz, L. R.; Gutierrez, J. A.; Rempel, S. A. PTEN augments SPARC suppression of proliferation and inhibits SPARC-induced migration by suppressing SHC-RAF-ERK and AKT signaling. *Neuro-Oncology* **2010**, *Advance Access*, noq048.

[81] (a) Okamoto, I.; Kawano, Y.; Tsuiki, H.; Sasaki, J.-i.; Nakao, M.; Matsumoto, M.; Suga, M.; Ando, M.; Nakajima, M.; Saya, H. CD44 cleavage induced by a membrane-associated metalloprotease plays a critical role in tumor cell migration. *Oncogene* **1999**, *18* (7), 1435-1446; (b) Kajita, M.; Itoh, Y.; Chiba, T.; Mori, H.; Okada, A.; Kinoh, H.; Seiki, M. Membrane-Type 1 Matrix Metalloproteinase Cleaves Cd44 and Promotes Cell Migration. *The Journal of Cell Biology* **2001**, *153* (5), 893-904.

[82] Yu, Q.; Stamenkovic, I. Localization of matrix metalloproteinase 9 to the cell surface provides a mechanism for CD44-mediated tumor invasion. *Genes & Development* **1999**, *13* (1), 35-48.

[83] Murai, T.; Miyazaki, Y.; Nishinakamura, H.; Sugahara, K. N.; Miyauchi, T.; Sako, Y.; Yanagida, T.; Miyasaka, M. Engagement of CD44 Promotes Rac Activation and CD44 Cleavage during Tumor Cell Migration. *Journal of Biological Chemistry* **2004**, *279* (6), 4541-4550.

[84] Mendelsohn, C. L.; Wimmer, E.; Racaniello, V. R. Cellular receptor for poliovirus: Molecular cloning, nucleotide sequence, and expression of a new member of the immunoglobulin superfamily. *Cell* **1989**, *56* (5), 855-865.

[85] Sloan, K.; Eustace, B.; Stewart, J.; Zehetmeier, C.; Torella, C.; Simeone, M.; Roy, J.; Unger, C.; Louis, D.; Ilag, L.; Jay, D. CD155/PVR plays a key role in cell motility during tumor cell invasion and migration. *BMC Cancer* **2004**, *4* (1), 73.

[86] Sloan, K. E.; Stewart, J. K.; Treloar, A. F.; Matthews, R. T.; Jay, D. G. CD155/PVR enhances glioma cell dispersal by regulating adhesion signaling and focal adhesion dynamics. *Cancer Res* **2005**, *65* (23), 10930-7.

[87] Sloan, K. E.; Stewart, J. K.; Treloar, A. F.; Matthews, R. T.; Jay, D. G. CD155/PVR Enhances Glioma Cell Dispersal by Regulating Adhesion Signaling and Focal Adhesion Dynamics. *Cancer Research* **2005**, *65* (23), 10930-10937.

[88] Barbero, S.; Bonavia, R.; Bajetto, A.; Porcile, C.; Pirani, P.; Ravetti, J. L.; Zona, G. L.; Spaziante, R.; Florio, T.; Schettini, G. Stromal Cell-derived Factor 1α Stimulates Human Glioblastoma Cell Growth through the Activation of Both Extracellular Signal-regulated Kinases 1/2 and Akt. *Cancer Research* **2003**, *63* (8), 1969-1974.

[89] Wu, M.; Chen, Q.; Li, D.; Li, X.; Li, X.; Huang, C.; Tang, Y.; Zhou, Y.; Wang, D.; Tang, K.; Cao, L.; Shen, S.; Li, G. LRRC4 inhibits human glioblastoma cells proliferation, invasion, and proMMP-2 activation by reducing SDF-1alpha/CXCR4-mediated ERK1/2 and Akt signaling pathways. *Journal of Cellular Biochemistry* **2008**, *103* (1), 245-255.

[90] Zhang, J.; Sarkar, S.; Yong, V. W. The chemokine stromal cell derived factor-1 (CXCL12) promotes glioma invasiveness through MT2-matrix metalloproteinase. *Carcinogenesis* **2005**, *26* (12), 2069-2077.

[91] Sciaccaluga, M.; Fioretti, B.; Catacuzzeno, L.; Pagani, F.; Bertollini, C.; Rosito, M.; Catalano, M.; D'Alessandro, G.; Santoro, A.; Cantore, G.; Ragozzino, D.; Castigli, E.; Franciolini, F.; Limatola, C. CXCL12-induced glioblastoma cell migration requires

intermediate conductance Ca2+-activated K+ channel activity. *American journal of physiology. Cell physiology* **2010**, *299* (1), C175-84.

[92] Hoelzinger, D. B.; Nakada, M.; Demuth, T.; Rosensteel, T.; Reavie, L. B.; Berens, M. E. Autotaxin: a secreted autocrine/paracrine factor that promotes glioma invasion. *J Neurooncol* **2008**, *86* (3), 297-309.

[93] Malchinkhuu, E.; Sato, K.; Horiuchi, Y.; Mogi, C.; Ohwada, S.; Ishiuchi, S.; Saito, N.; Kurose, H.; Tomura, H.; Okajima, F. Role of p38 mitogen-activated kinase and c-Jun terminal kinase in migration response to lysophosphatidic acid and sphingosine-1-phosphate in glioma cells. *Oncogene* **2005**, *24* (44), 6676-6688.

[94] Shashidhar, S.; Lorente, G.; Nagavarapu, U.; Nelson, A.; Kuo, J.; Cummins, J.; Nikolich, K.; Urfer, R.; Foehr, E. D. GPR56 is a GPCR that is overexpressed in gliomas and functions in tumor cell adhesion. *Oncogene* **2005**, *24* (10), 1673-82.

[95] Shashidhar, S.; Lorente, G.; Nagavarapu, U.; Nelson, A.; Kuo, J.; Cummins, J.; Nikolich, K.; Urfer, R.; Foehr, E. D. GPR56 is a GPCR that is overexpressed in gliomas and functions in tumor cell adhesion. *Oncogene* **2005**, *24* (10), 1673-1682.

[96] (a) Esteve, P.-O.; Tremblay, P.; Houde, M.; St-Pierre, Y.; Mandeville, R. *In vitro* expression of MMP-2 and MMP-9 in glioma cells following exposure to inflammatory mediators. *Biochimica et Biophysica Acta (BBA) - Molecular Cell Research* **1998**, *1403* (1), 85-96; (b) Esteve, P. O.; Chicoine, E.; Robledo, O.; Aoudjit, F.; Descoteaux, A.; Potworowski, E. F.; St-Pierre, Y. Protein Kinase C-ζ Regulates Transcription of the Matrix Metalloproteinase-9 Gene Induced by IL-1 and TNF-α in Glioma Cells *via* NF-κB. *Journal of Biological Chemistry* **2002**, *277* (38), 35150-35155.

[97] Krammer, P. H. CD95's deadly mission in the immune system. *Nature* **2000**, *407* (6805), 789-795.

[98] Suda, T.; Takahashi, T.; Golstein, P.; Nagata, S. Molecular cloning and expression of the fas ligand, a novel member of the tumor necrosis factor family. *Cell* **1993**, *75* (6), 1169-1178.

[99] Barnhart, B. C.; Legembre, P.; Pietras, E.; Bubici, C.; Franzoso, G.; Peter, M. E. CD95 ligand induces motility and invasiveness of apoptosis-resistant tumor cells. *The EMBO journal* **2004**, *23* (15), 3175-85.

[100] Kumar, M.; Makonchuk, D. Y.; Li, H.; Mittal, A.; Kumar, A. TNF-Like Weak Inducer of Apoptosis (TWEAK) Activates Proinflammatory Signaling Pathways and Gene Expression through the Activation of TGF-{beta}-Activated Kinase 1. *The Journal of Immunology* **2009**, *182* (4), 2439-2448.

[101] Panner, A.; Crane, C. A.; Weng, C.; Feletti, A.; Fang, S.; Parsa, A. T.; Pieper, R. O. Ubiquitin-specific protease 8 links the PTEN-Akt-AIP4 pathway to the control of FLIPS stability and TRAIL sensitivity in glioblastoma multiforme. *Cancer Research* **2010**, *70* (12), 5046-53.

[102] Wang, J.; Yao, L.; Zhao, S.; Zhang, X.; Yin, J.; Zhang, Y.; Chen, X.; Gao, M.; Ling, E. A.; Hao, A.; Li, G. Granulocyte-colony stimulating factor promotes proliferation, migration and invasion in glioma cells. *Cancer biology & therapy* **2012**, *13* (6).

[103] Bettinger, I.; Thanos, S.; Paulus, W. Microglia promote glioma migration. *Acta Neuropathologica* **2002**, *103* (4), 351-355.

[104] Wagner, S.; Czub, S.; Greif, M.; Vince, G. H.; Suss, N.; Kerkau, S.; Rieckmann, P.; Roggendorf, W.; Roosen, K.; Tonn, J. C. Microglial/macrophage expression of interleukin 10 in human glioblastomas. *Int J Cancer* **1999**, *82* (1), 12-6.

[105] Webb, T. R.; Slavish, J.; George, R. E.; Look, A. T.; Xue, L.; Jiang, Q.; Cui, X.; Rentrop, W. B.; Morris, S. W. Anaplastic lymphoma kinase: role in cancer pathogenesis and small-molecule inhibitor development for therapy. *Expert Rev Anticancer Ther* **2009**, *9* (3), 331-56.

[106] Lu, K. V.; Jong, K. A.; Kim, G. Y.; Singh, J.; Dia, E. Q.; Yoshimoto, K.; Wang, M. Y.; Cloughesy, T. F.; Nelson, S. F.; Mischel, P. S. Differential Induction of Glioblastoma Migration and Growth by Two Forms of Pleiotrophin. *Journal of Biological Chemistry* **2005**, *280* (29), 26953-26964.

[107] (a) Baker, B. J.; Park, K. W.; Qin, H.; Ma, X.; Benveniste, E. N. IL-27 inhibits OSM-mediated TNF-alpha and iNOS gene expression in microglia. *Glia* **2010**, *58* (9), 1082-1093; (b) Krona, A.; Aman, P.; Orndal, C.; Josefsson, A. Oncostatin M-induced genes in human astrocytomas. *International journal of oncology* **2007**, *31* (6), 1457-63.

[108] Raidoo, D. M.; Sawant, S.; Mahabeer, R.; Bhoola, K. D. Kinin receptors are expressed in human astrocytic tumour cells. *Immunopharmacology* **1999**, *43* (2-3), 255-63.

[109] Montana, V.; Sontheimer, H. Bradykinin promotes the chemotactic invasion of primary brain tumors. *The Journal of neuroscience : the official journal of the Society for Neuroscience* **2011**, *31* (13), 4858-67.

[110] Kikuchi, A.; Yamamoto, H. Tumor formation due to abnormalities in the beta-catenin-independent pathway of Wnt signaling. *Cancer science* **2008**, *99* (2), 202-8.

[111] Kamino, M.; Kishida, M.; Kibe, T.; Ikoma, K.; Iijima, M.; Hirano, H.; Tokudome, M.; Chen, L.; Koriyama, C.; Yamada, K.; Arita, K.; Kishida, S. Wnt-5a signaling is correlated with infiltrative activity in human glioma by inducing cellular migration and MMP-2. *Cancer science* **2011**, *102* (3), 540-8.

[112] (a) Kanu, O.; B Hughes; Di, C.; Lin, N.; Fu, J.; Bigner, D.; Yan, H.; Adamson, D. Glioblastoma multiforme oncogenomics and signaling pathways. *Clin Med Oncol* **2009**, *3*, 39-52; (b) Singh, S. K.; Clarke, I. D.; Terasaki, M.; Bonn, V. E.; Hawkins, C.; Squire, J.; Dirks, P. B. Identification of a cancer stem cell in human brain tumors. *Cancer Res* **2003**, *63* (18), 5821-8.

[113] Wakimoto, H.; Kesari, S.; Farrell, C. J.; Curry, W. T.; Zaupa, C.; Aghi, M.; Kuroda, T.; Stemmer-Rachamimov, A.; Shah, K.; Liu, T.-C.; Jeyaretna, D. S.; Debasitis, J.; Pruszak, J.; Martuza, R. L.; Rabkin, S. D. Human Glioblastoma,ÄìDerived Cancer Stem Cells: Establishment of Invasive Glioma Models and Treatment with Oncolytic Herpes Simplex Virus Vectors. *Cancer Research* **2009**, *69* (8), 3472-3481.

[114] Lathia, J. D.; Gallagher, J.; Heddleston, J. M.; Wang, J.; Eyler, C. E.; MacSwords, J.; Wu, Q.; Vasanji, A.; McLendon, R. E.; Hjelmeland, A. B.; Rich, J. N. Integrin Alpha 6 Regulates Glioblastoma Stem Cells. *Cell Stem Cell* **2010**, *6* (5), 421-432.

[115] Mendez, O.; Zavadil, J.; Esencay, M.; Lukyanov, Y.; Santovasi, D.; Wang, S.-C.; Newcomb, E. W.; Zagzag, D. Knock down of HIF-1alpha in glioma cells reduces migration *in vitro* and invasion *in vivo* and impairs their ability to form tumor spheres. *Molecular Cancer* **2010**, *9*, 133.

[116] Fu, Y.; Zheng, Y.; Li, K.; Huang, R.; Zheng, S.; An, N.; Liang, A. Mutations in isocitrate dehydrogenase 2 accelerate glioma cell migration *via* matrix metalloproteinase-2 and 9. *Biotechnology letters* **2012**, *34* (3), 441-6.

[117] Hsieh, D.; Hsieh, A.; Stea, B.; Ellsworth, R. IGFBP2 promotes glioma tumor stem cell expansion and survival. *Biochemical and Biophysical Research Communications* **2010**, *397* (2), 367-72.

[118] Hjelmeland, A. B.; Wu, Q.; Wickman, S.; Eyler, C.; Heddleston, J.; Shi, Q.; Lathia, J. D.; MacSwords, J.; Lee, J.; McLendon, R. E.; Rich, J. N. Targeting A20 Decreases Glioma Stem Cell Survival and Tumor Growth. *PLoS Biol* **2010**, *8* (2), e1000319.

[119] Song, L.; Liu, L.; Wu, Z.; Lin, C.; Dai, T.; Yu, C.; Wang, X.; Wu, J.; Li, M.; Li, J. Knockdown of stomatin-like protein 2 (STOML2) reduces the invasive ability of glioma cells through inhibition of the NF-kappaB/MMP-9 pathway. *The Journal of pathology* **2012**, *226* (3), 534-43.

[120] Ziv-Av, A.; Taller, D.; Attia, M.; Xiang, C.; Lee, H. K.; Cazacu, S.; Finniss, S.; Kazimirsky, G.; Sarid, R.; Brodie, C. RTVP-1 expression is regulated by SRF downstream of protein kinase C and contributes to the effect of SRF on glioma cell migration. *Cell Signal* **2011**, *23* (12), 1936-43.

[121] Edwards, L. A.; Woolard, K.; Son, M. J.; Li, A.; Lee, J.; Ene, C.; Mantey, S. A.; Maric, D.; Song, H.; Belova, G.; Jensen, R. T.; Zhang, W.; Fine, H. A. Effect of brain- and tumor-derived connective tissue growth factor on glioma invasion. *J Natl Cancer Inst* **2011**, *103* (15), 1162-78.

[122] Ding, T.; Ma, Y.; Li, W.; Liu, X.; Ying, G.; Fu, L.; Gu, F. Role of aquaporin-4 in the regulation of migration and invasion of human glioma cells. *International journal of oncology* **2011**, *38* (6), 1521-31.

[123] Delic, S.; Lottmann, N.; Jetschke, K.; Reifenberger, G.; Riemenschneider, M. J. Identification and functional validation of CDH11, PCSK6 and SH3GL3 as novel glioma invasion-associated candidate genes. *Neuropathology and applied neurobiology* **2012**, *38* (2), 201-12.

[124] Mei, P. J.; Bai, J.; Liu, H.; Li, C.; Wu, Y. P.; Yu, Z. Q.; Zheng, J. N. RUNX3 expression is lost in glioma and its restoration causes drastic suppression of tumor invasion and migration. *Journal of cancer research and clinical oncology* **2011**, *137* (12), 1823-30.

[125] Cavalla, P.; Piva, R.; Bortolotto, S.; Grosso, R.; Cancelli, I.; Chio, A.; Schiffer, D. p27/kip1 expression in oligodendrogliomas and its possible prognostic role. *Acta Neuropathol* **1999**, *98* (6), 629-34.

[126] See, W. L.; Miller, J. P.; Squatrito, M.; Holland, E.; Resh, M. D.; Koff, A. Defective DNA double-strand break repair underlies enhanced tumorigenesis and chromosomal instability in p27-deficient mice with growth factor-induced oligodendrogliomas. *Oncogene* **2010**, *29* (12), 1720-31.

[127] See, W. L.; Heinberg, A. R.; Holland, E. C.; Resh, M. D. p27 deficiency is associated with migration defects in PDGF-expressing gliomas *in vivo*. *Cell Cycle* **2010**, *9* (8), 1562-7.

[128] Concha, C.; Besson, A. p27Kip1 is needed...for glioma invasion. *Cell Cycle* **2010**, *9* (8), 1457.

[129] Yang, J.; Liao, D.; Wang, Z.; Liu, F.; Wu, G. Mammalian target of rapamycin signaling pathway contributes to glioma progression and patients' prognosis. *The Journal of surgical research* **2011**, *168* (1), 97-102.

[130] White, P. S.; Thompson, P. M.; Gotoh, T.; Okawa, E. R.; Igarashi, J.; Kok, M.; Winter, C.; Gregory, S. G.; Hogarty, M. D.; Maris, J. M.; Brodeur, G. M. Definition and characterization of a region of 1p36.3 consistently deleted in neuroblastoma. *Oncogene* **2005**, *24* (16), 2684-94.

[131] Dong, Z.; Pang, J. S.; Ng, M. H.; Poon, W. S.; Zhou, L.; Ng, H. K. Identification of two contiguous minimally deleted regions on chromosome 1p36.31-p36.32 in oligodendroglial tumours. *Br J Cancer* **2004**, *91* (6), 1105-11.

[132] Bharti, S.; Handrow-Metzmacher, H.; Zickenheiner, S.; Zeitvogel, A.; Baumann, R.; Starzinski-Powitz, A. Novel membrane protein shrew-1 targets to cadherin-mediated junctions in polarized epithelial cells. *Mol Biol Cell* **2004**, *15* (1), 397-406.

[133] Schreiner, A.; Ruonala, M.; Jakob, V.; Suthaus, J.; Boles, E.; Wouters, F.; Starzinski-Powitz, A. Junction Protein Shrew-1 Influences Cell Invasion and Interacts with Invasion-promoting Protein CD147. *Mol Biol Cell* **2007**, *18* (4), 1272-1281.

[134] (a) Schwechheimer, K.; Zhou, L.; Birchmeier, W. E-Cadherin in human brain tumours: loss of immunoreactivity in malignant meningiomas. *Virchows Arch* **1998**, *432* (2), 163-7; (b) Utsuki, S.; Sato, Y.; Oka, H.; Tsuchiya, B.; Suzuki, S.; Fujii, K. Relationship between the expression of E-, N-cadherins and beta-catenin and tumor grade in astrocytomas. *J Neurooncol* **2002**, *57* (3), 187-92.

[135] Utsuki, S.; Oka, H.; Sato, Y.; Kawano, N.; Tsuchiya, B.; Kobayashi, I.; Fujii, K. Invasive meningioma is associated with a low expression of E-cadherin and beta-catenin. *Clin Neuropathol* **2005**, *24* (1), 8-12.

[136] McDonald, J. M.; Dunlap, S.; Cogdell, D.; Dunmire, V.; Wei, Q.; Starzinski-Powitz, A.; Sawaya, R.; Bruner, J.; Fuller, G. N.; Aldape, K.; Zhang, W. The SHREW1 gene, frequently deleted in oligodendrogliomas, functions to inhibit cell adhesion and migration. *Cancer biology & therapy* **2006**, *5* (3), 300-4.

[137] Grzmil, M.; Hemmings, B. A. Deregulated signalling networks in human brain tumours. *Biochimica et Biophysica Acta (BBA) - Proteins & Proteomics* **2010**, *1804* (3), 476-483.

[138] (a) Rusciano, D.; Lorenzoni, P.; Burger, M. M. Constitutive Activation of c-Met in Liver Metastatic B16 Melanoma Cells Depends on Both Substrate Adhesion and Cell Density and Is Regulated by a Cytosolic Tyrosine Phosphatase Activity. *Journal of Biological Chemistry* **1996**, *271* (34), 20763-20769; (b) Sundberg, C.; Rubin, K. Stimulation of beta1 integrins on fibroblasts induces PDGF independent tyrosine phosphorylation of PDGF beta-receptors. *The Journal of Cell Biology* **1996**, *132* (4), 741-752; (c) Moro, L.; Venturino, M.; Bozzo, C.; Silengo, L.; Altruda, F.; Beguinot, L.; Tarone, G.; Defilippi, P. Integrins induce activation of EGF receptor: role in MAP kinase induction and adhesion-dependent cell survival. *Embo J* **1998**, *17* (22), 6622-6632; (d) Wang, R.; Kobayashi, R.; Bishop, J. M. Cellular adherence elicits ligand-independent activation of the Met cell-surface receptor. *Proc Natl Acad Sci U S A* **1996**, *93* (16), 8425-8430.

[139] Van Brocklyn, J. R. Sphingolipid Signaling Pathways as Potential Therapeutic Targets in Gliomas. *Mini Reviews in Medicinal Chemistry* **2007**, *7*, 984-990.

CHAPTER 10

Tyrosyl-DNA Phosphodiesterase 1 as a Target for Anticancer Therapy

Thomas S. Dexheimer[1], Shar-yin N. Huang[2], Smitha Antony[2], Christophe Marchand[2] and Yves Pommier[*,2]

[1]NIH Chemical Genomics Center, National Center for Advancing Translational Sciences, National Institutes of Health, 9800 Medical Center Dr., Rockville, MD 20850, USA; [2]Laboratory of Molecular Pharmacology, Center for Cancer Research, National Cancer Institute, National Institutes of Health, 37 Convent Dr., Building 37, Room 5068, Bethesda, Maryland, MD 20892-4255, USA

Abstract: Tyrosyl-DNA phosphodiesterase 1 (*Tdp1*) was initially discovered as an enzyme that catalyzes the hydrolysis of 3'-phosphotyrosyl bonds. Such linkages are transiently introduced *in vivo* by the DNA processing activity of topoisomerase I (Top1). For this reason, *Tdp1* has been implicated in the repair of irreversible Top1-DNA covalent complexes (Top1cc), which can be generated by either exogenous or endogenous factors. *Tdp1* has been regarded as a potential therapeutic co-target of Top1 in that it seemingly counteracts the effects of Top1 inhibitors, such as camptothecin and its clinically used derivatives. Thus, by reducing the repair of Top1-DNA lesions, *Tdp1* inhibitors have the potential to augment the anticancer activity of Top1-targeting drugs. *Tdp1* inhibitors may also selectively target cancer cells with defects in alternative repair pathways for Top1cc, *e.g.* DNA checkpoint and repair pathways. Human *Tdp1* can also hydrolyze other 3'-end DNA alterations including 3'-phosphoglycolates and 3'-abasic sites indicating it may function as a general 3'-end processing repair enzyme. The importance of *Tdp1* in humans is highlighted by the observation that a recessive mutation in the human *Tdp1* gene is responsible for the inherited disorder, spinocerebellar ataxia with axonal neuropathy (SCAN1). This review provides a summary of the biochemical and cellular processes performed by *Tdp1* as well as the rationale behind the development of *Tdp1* inhibitors for anticancer therapy.

Keywords: Tyrosyl-DNA phosphodiesterase, topoisomerase, DNA repair, PARP, proteasome, PNK, camptothecin, indenoisoquinoline.

***Address correspondence to Yves Pommier:** Laboratory of Molecular Pharmacology, Center for Cancer Research, National Cancer Institute, NIH, Building 37, Rm. 5068, Bethesda, MD 20892-4255, USA; Tel: 301-496-5944; Fax: 301-402-0752; E-mail: pommier@nih.gov

Michelle Prudhomme (Ed)

1. INTRODUCTION

Cancer is commonly characterized by the presence of endogenous DNA damage. However, while DNA damage underlies carcinogenesis, it has also been exploited as a means to treat cancer. For example, the cytotoxic effects of the two main therapeutic modalities that are clinically used to treat malignances (*i.e.* chemotherapy or radiation) are directly related to their propensity to generate DNA damage. Moreover, DNA damage is also responsible for many of the side effects of these therapies, including bone marrow suppression, gastrointestinal toxicities, and hair loss. The sensitivity of cancer cells to DNA damaging agents is probably related to intrinsic deficiencies in DNA repair and checkpoint mechanisms. However, the capacity of cancer cells to recognize DNA damage and initiate DNA repair is a key mechanism for therapeutic resistance to chemotherapy. Therefore, targeting DNA repair enzymes can serve as a strategy to potentiate the cytotoxicity of the currently available DNA damaging agents toward cancer cells and to take advantage of known cancer-related deficiencies in DNA repair pathways. In this review we will summarize the enzymatic activities, the biological and cellular functions of tyrosyl-DNA phosphodiesterase 1 (*Tdp1*), as well as discuss the rationale for targeting *Tdp1* for cancer therapy.

2. TOPOISOMERASE I

2.1. Biological Functions and Catalytic Mechanism

DNA topoisomerase IB (Top1) is a ubiquitous enzyme that regulates DNA topology by relaxing positive and negative supercoiling in the DNA. These changes in the DNA topological state permit efficient processing of the genetic material during fundamental cellular events such as replication, transcription, and chromatin remodeling [1-4]. More importantly, Top1 has emerged as an important therapeutic target in cancer chemotherapy following the discovery that camptothecin (CPT) is a specific Top1 inhibitor [5]. FDA has since approved two additional CPT derivatives, topotecan and irinotecan, for clinical use [7].

The catalytic mechanism of Top1 involves a reversible transesterification reaction, as shown in Fig. (**1A**). Following DNA binding, the Top1 catalytic cycle is initiated by the nucleophilic attack of the phenolic hydroxyl group of the active site tyrosine (Tyr723 for human Top1) on the scissile phosphate, which generates a covalent complex between the protein and the 3'-phosphate of the DNA *via* a phosphotyrosyl bond. This transient DNA single-strand break (*i.e.* cleavage complex) subsequently allows controlled rotation of the cleaved DNA strand around its intact complement, effectively removing any local helical tension. Once the DNA is relaxed, the covalent intermediate is reversed *via* a second transesterification reaction, wherein the free DNA 5'-hydroxyl acts as a nucleophile to attack the 3'-phosphotyrosyl linkage; thus restoring the continuity of the original DNA duplex. For more extensive reviews covering the biochemistry and biology of DNA topoisomerase I, see references [1-4][1].

2.2. The Formation of Irreversible Top1 Cleavage Complexes

Under normal circumstances, the rate of religation is much faster than the rate of cleavage, which allows the Top1-DNA cleavage complexes (Top1cc) to be a transitory intermediate of the Top1 catalytic cycle [1]. However, a variety of conditions (schematized in Fig. **1B**), have been shown to increase the frequency of Top1cc by slowing the religation reaction rate (for reviews see [7, 8]). For example, Top1 inhibitors, such as camptothecin (CPT) and its clinically used derivatives, as well as several non-CPT Top1 inhibitors including the indenoisoquinolines and the indolocarbazoles, selectively and reversibly bind to the Top1-DNA interface [6, 9] and slow the rate of Top1-mediated DNA religation. This is especially the case when Top1 relaxes positive supercoiling [10]. Failure to reseal this normally transient break in the DNA results in a Top1-linked DNA single-strand break that can be transformed into a persistent double-stranded break following collision of replication forks with the drug-stabilized cleavage complex [11-14]. In a similar manner, a number of naturally occurring DNA lesions, such as strand breaks [15], abasic sites, base mismatches, and certain oxidized or modified bases [16] are capable of physically blocking the Top1 religation reaction *in vitro*, due to misalignment of the 5'-hydroxyl with the tyrosyl-DNA phosphodiester backbone. Both UV irradiation- [17] and

[1]Pommier, Y. Drugging topoisomerases: lessons and challenges. *ACS Chemical Biology*, **2013**, *8*, 82-95.

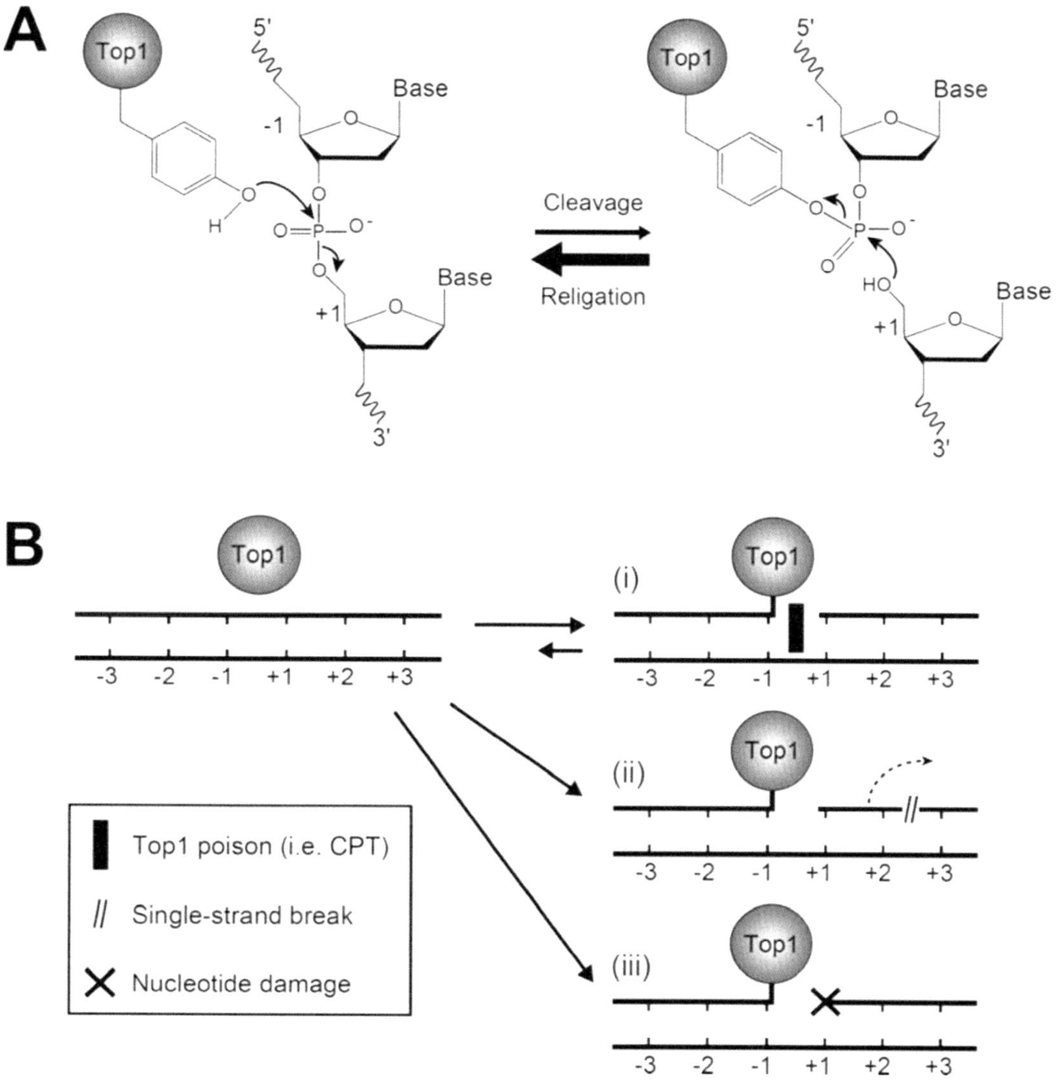

Fig. (1). **A**) Human Top1-mediated DNA cleavage and religation mechanisms. Tyr723 is the active site tyrosine involved in the transesterification reaction. The bases flanking the Top1 cleavage site are referred to as -1 and +1 for the bases at the 3' and 5' DNA termini, respectively. **B**) Representative circumstances resulting in the formation of trapped Top1 cleavage complexes [*i.e.* (i) Top1 inhibitors or preexisting DNA lesions, such as (ii) DNA strand breaks or (iii) nucleotide damage].

hydrogen peroxide-induced [18] DNA damage have also been shown to trap Top1cc in cells. Repair of these irreversible Top1-DNA cleavage complexes is an important part of DNA metabolism given that mutants defective in specific DNA repair pathways demonstrate increased sensitivity to Top1 inhibitors. However,

All repair pathways require DNA termini consisting of a 5'-phosphate and 3'-hydroxyl for appropriate processing by DNA ligase. Thus, Top1-DNA lesions present a unique challenge for the DNA repair machinery given that the DNA strand breakis encumbered with a protein adduct, which must be removed before the DNA can be ligated.

3. TYROSYL-DNA PHOSPHODIESTERASE

3.1. Discovery and Physiological Function of *Tdp1*

In 1996, Nash and coworkers discovered an enzymatic activity in yeast *S. cerevisiae* that specifically hydrolyzes the covalent bond between a tyrosine residue and a DNA 3'-phosphate [19]. Because Top1 is the only known enzyme to generate 3'-phosphotyrosine linkages *in vivo*, the observed enzymatic activity was proposed to be associated with the repair of DNA lesions that develop from abortive Top1-DNA catalytical cycle [19, 20]. The yeast gene encoding this activity was subsequently cloned and named tyrosyl-DNA phosphodiesterase 1 (*Tdp1*) [20]. In addition, *Tdp1*-defective yeast strains demonstrate hypersensitivity to conditions that increase Top1cc, suggesting involvement of *Tdp1* in repair [20, 21].

All eukaryotic species examined to date contain a well-conserved *Tdp1* ortholog. Recently, *Tdp1* genes have also been identified in the kinetoplastid parasite *Leishmaniadonovani* [22] and in plants (*i.e. Medicago truncatula* [23] and *Arabidopsis thaliana* [24]). The human genome encodes a single copy of *Tdp1* [14q32.11] consisting of 17 exons: two 5' non-coding exons and 15 coding exons. Human *Tdp1* has been shown to possess a similar 3'-phosphotyrosyl-processing activity as the yeast enzyme [25], despite sharing minimal sequence identity (~15%) [26]. The greatest sequence variance resides in the N-terminal domain of *Tdp1* orthologs, which is poorly conserved or absent in lower eukaryotes. The N-terminus (aa 1-148) of human *Tdp1* is dispensable for enzymatic activity [25], yet seems to have evolved to play a regulatory function. For example, a serine residue in the N-terminal domain of human *Tdp1* (S81) has been shown to undergo post-translational modification by phosphorylation, subsequently mediating specific protein-protein interactions (*i.e.* XRCC1 and DNA ligase III) [27, 28]. A recent report also identified SUMOylation at a lysine residue in the N-terminal domain (K111), which appears to promote accumulation of *Tdp1* at sites of DNA damage [29]. In addition, the *Arabidopsis thaliana Tdp1* protein contains a distinct SMAD/FHA (forkhead-associated) domain in the N-terminal region that is necessary for targeting the enzyme to the nucleus [24]. An *in silico* search of the human *Tdp1* protein sequence also reveals two putative nuclear localization signals (NLSs) in the N-terminal domain, one of which is located in the nonessential region (Fig. **2A**). This is in agreement with studies using fluorescence microscopy demonstrating most intense localization of *Tdp1* to the nucleus in human cells [30]. However, recent studies have demonstrated that *Tdp1* is also present in mitochondria where it functions to repair oxidative damage of mitochondrial DNA [31].

Tdp1 is physiologically important in humans given that a homozygous mutation in the *Tdp1* gene (A1478G), where in an active site histidine is mutated to arginine (H493R, shown in italics in Fig. **2A**). This mutation is responsible for the rare autosomal recessive neurodegenerative disease, spinocerebellar ataxia with axonal neuropathy (SCAN1) [32, 33]. To date, SCAN1 has been limited to nine patients from a single Saudi Arabian family, three of which have been clinically evaluated. The disease phenotype is characterized by early onset ataxia (~15 years), cerebellum atrophy, and peripheral neuropathy [32, 33]. In addition, individuals harboring the SCAN1 mutation display mild hypercholesterolemia and hypoalbuminemia [32]. In contrast to other diseases associated with defects in DNA repair proteins, the SCAN1 patients have not been noted to have an increase in cancer susceptibility. Initially, it was thought that the mutation disrupted the *Tdp1* active site symmetry leading to a loss-of-function [32, 34, 35]. Indeed, the H493R mutation decreases catalytic activity 20- to 40-fold [36]. However, additional studies have shown that the residual *Tdp1* activity of the H493R mutant results in trapping of *Tdp1*-DNA intermediates, which might be responsible for the DNA damage leading to the SCAN1 phenotype (see Fig. **3**, legend) [36]. Thus, both quantitative and qualitative changes in *Tdp1* may contribute to the SCAN1 phenotype.

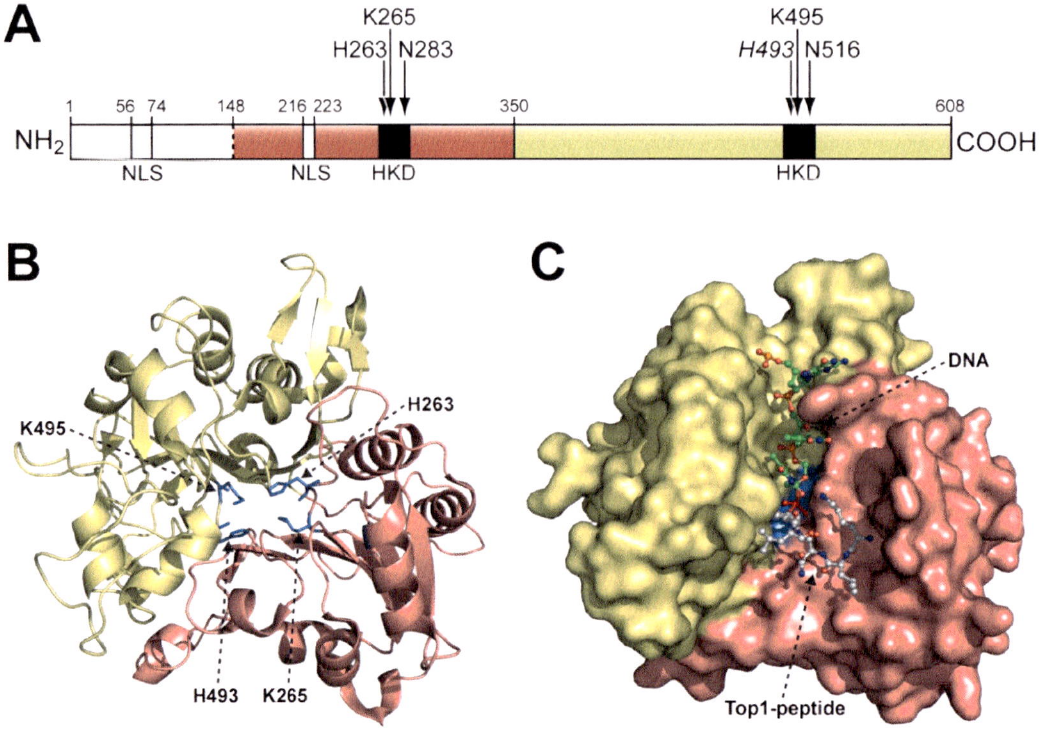

Fig. (2). A) Schematic representation of the human *Tdp1* domain structure. The N-terminal and C-terminal domains correspond to residues 1-350 and 351-608, respectively. Positions of the "HKN" motifs and NLS (nuclear localization signals) motifs are shown in black and white, respectively. Arrows indicate active site residues. **B**) Ribbon diagram of *Tdp1* structure (Δ148). Domain colors correspond to those shown in (**A**). The active site residues (H263, K265, H493, and K495) are shown as stick structures in blue (figure modified from [48]). **C**) Structure of the *Tdp1*-vanadate-peptide-DNA complex (1NOP). The orientation and domain colors of *Tdp1* are identical as in (**B**). *Tdp1* is shown as a molecular surface and the vanadate-peptide-DNA substrate mimic is shown as ball-and-stick structures with the DNA colored in green, the vanadate colored in red, and the Top1-derived peptide colored in white (figure modified from [49]).

3.2. Structure and Catalytic Mechanism of *Tdp1*

Tdp1 is a member of the phospholipase D superfamily [25], which encompasses a diverse group of enzymes that catalyze phosphodiester bond cleavage on substrates ranging from phospholipids to DNA, or in the case of *Tdp1*, protein-DNA complexes. The sequence identity between *Tdp1* and the members of the PLD family is mostly restricted to two copies of a signature motif H(X)K(X_4)D (HKD motif) that has been implicated in the catalytic mechanism of these enzymes [37-39]. Two such motifs are present in the N- and C-terminal domains of human *Tdp1*, both of which contain the conserved histidine and lysine residues (^{263}HTK^{265} and ^{495}HIK^{497}) but lack the aspartate residues that exist in other HKD motifs (Fig. **2A**). Alternatively, two highly conserved asparagine residues cluster near the active site (N283 and N516). Thus, *Tdp1* has been suggested to represent a distinct subclass of the PLD superfamily based on its unique "HKN" motifs. The importance of the two signature HKN motifs for *Tdp1* enzymatic activity has been further established by site-directed mutagenesis. Indeed, mutation of H263 produces a catalytically inactive enzyme, whereas mutating H495, K265, or K497 results in impaired enzymatic activity [25, 40]. These results are consistent with studies performed on other members of the PLD family [41-45].

The affiliation of *Tdp1* with the PLD superfamily has been further established through comparative analysis of the three-dimensional structure of the N-terminal truncated human *Tdp1* (Δ1-148) (Fig. **2A**) [46] with the crystal structures of two members of the PLD superfamily, a PLD from *Streptomyces* [37] and a bacterial nuclease from *Salmonella tryphimurium* [47]. Despite their low sequence identity, these three enzymes share a strikingly similar tertiary structure. In addition, the superimposition of their active sites suggests that all three enzymes employ analogous reaction chemistry. The crystallographic studies of human *Tdp1* reveals a monomeric structure comprised of two topologically similar α-β-α domains. Each domain contributes a histidine and lysine residue to form the active site, which is centrally located at the pseudo-two-fold axis of symmetry between the two domains (Fig. **2B**). The *Tdp1* crystal structure also positions four additional conserved residues: N283, Q294, N516, and E538, near the active site [46].

In order to gain further insight into the substrate binding properties and catalytic mechanism of *Tdp1*, co-crystal structures were solved of human *Tdp1* bound to vanadate [48, 49], an oxyanion form of pentavalent vanadium. Unlike the phosphate ion, vanadate can form five-coordinate species allowing it to serve as a transition state analogue while eliminating enzyme turnover. The molecular assembly of vanadate, *Tdp1*, a Top1-derived peptide containing the active site tyrosine, and a single-stranded DNA oligonucleotide into a quaternary structure is shown in Fig. (**2C**). Initial examination of the quaternary structure revealed an asymmetrical substrate-binding channel that extended in opposite directions from

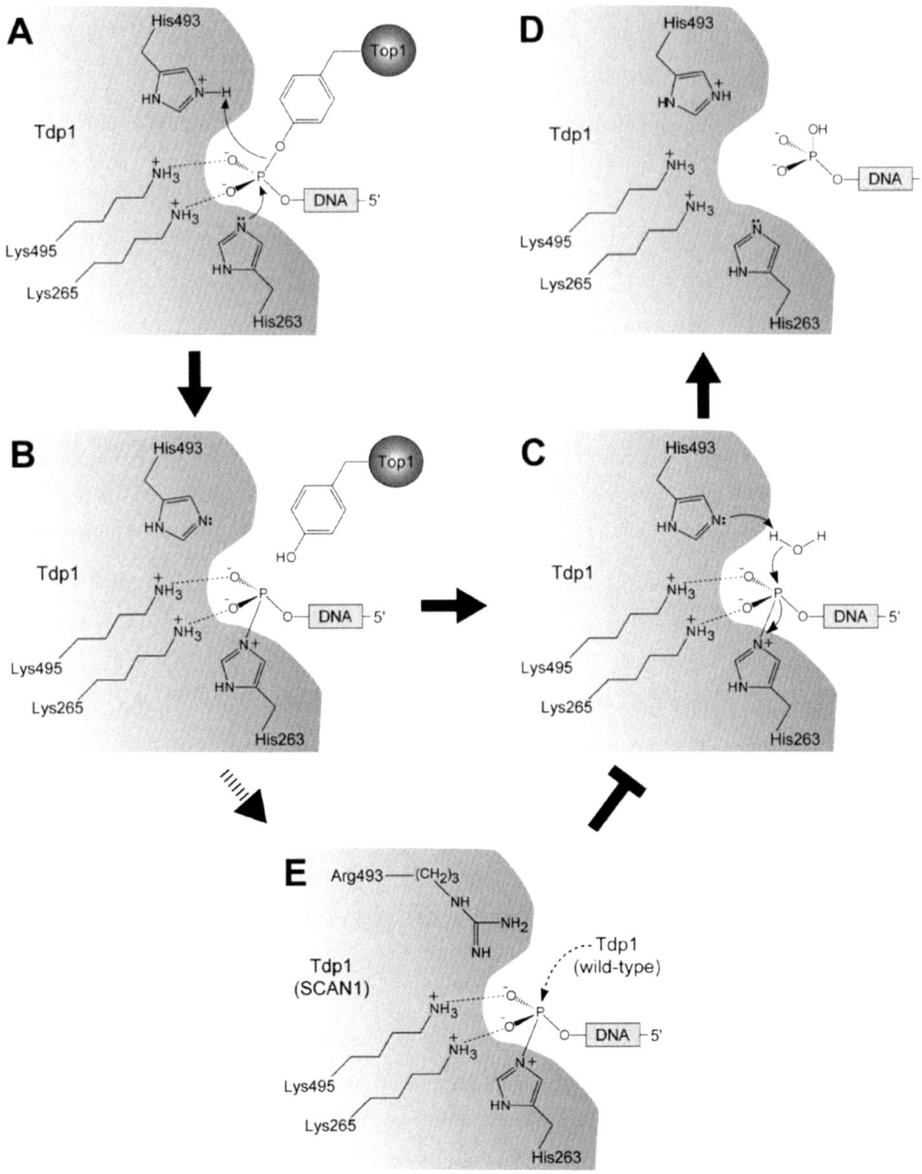

Fig. (3). Proposed reaction mechanism for human *Tdp1*. **A**) The first step of the reaction involves the nucleophilic attack of the phosphodiester-containing substrate by the imidazole Nε2 atom of H263. H493 donates a proton to the tyrosyl moiety of the leaving group. The phosphohistidine intermediate is shown in (**B**). Interactions between the non-bridging oxygens and the active site lysine residues (K265 and K495) serve to stabilize the transition intermediate. **C**) The next step of the reaction involves a second nucleophilic attack by a water molecule activated by H493, generating final 3'-phosphate product and free *Tdp1* (**D**) (A-D modified from [48]). (**E**) The SCAN1 mutation (H493R) leads to an accumulation of the *Tdp1*-DNA intermediate and a defect in *Tdp1* turnover rate.

the active site across the entire surface of *Tdp1*. The DNA moiety bound to one side of the active site in a relatively narrow, positively charged cleft (Fig. **2C**, shown behind the DNA (green)). The peptide moiety bound to the other side of the active site in a larger and more open cleft that contains a mixed charge distribution (Fig. **2C**, shown behind the peptide (white)) [46, 48, 49]. Interestingly, the DNA-binding groove is highly conserved among *Tdp1* orthologs, while the peptide-binding pocket shows much less sequence conservation between different species [49, 50].

A closer look into the active site of the quaternary structure [48, 49] shows that the vanadate ion exhibits trigonal bipyramidal geometry, which is consistent with a transition state of an S_N2 nucleophilic attack on phosphate. The apical coordination to the vanadate molecule is occupied by the imidazole Nε2 atom of the *Tdp1* active site H263 residue and the oxygen atom of the tyrosine side chain of the Top1-derived peptide, whereas the 3'-hydroxyl of the DNA oligonucleotide occupies one of the three equatorial positions. The remaining two equatorial oxygens, which represent the non-bridging oxygens of the phosphodiester substrate, form hydrogen bonds with the amino groups of K265 and K495. Because the incoming and outgoing groups in an S_N2 reaction occupy the two axial positions of a trigonal bipyramid [51], the *Tdp1*-vanadate structure indicates that the first step in the *Tdp1* catalytic mechanism involves the nucleophilic attack of the phosphotyrosyl bond by the H263 residue from the N-terminal HKN motif. Additionally, the H493 residue from the C-terminal HKN motif acts as a general acid and donates a proton to the apical tyrosine-containing peptide-leaving group (Fig. **3A**). This results in the formation of a transient covalent phosphoamide bond between the Nε2 atom of H263 and the 3'-phosphate of the DNA (Fig. **3B**). Hydrolysis of this covalent intermediate is presumably carried out by a water molecule that is activated by the H493 residue acting as a general base (Fig. **3C**) [48]. The second S_N2 reaction step in the *Tdp1* catalytic mechanism is supported by *in vitro* biochemical studies with the SCAN1 H493R mutant, which leads to an accumulation of *Tdp1*-DNA covalent intermediate [36]. Overall, the final product released after *Tdp1* catalysis is a DNA molecule with a 3'-phosphate end (Fig. **3D**).

3.3. *Tdp1* Substrates

A stalled Top1-DNA complex is an unmanageable substrate for *Tdp1* because of the limited access of the scissile phosphotyrosyl bond, which is internally located within the Top1-DNA complex [52]. Indeed, the processing of full-length human Top1 covalently linked to a DNA oligonucleotide by *Tdp1* is poor [19, 53, 54]. Thus, the Top1cc is likely to undergo modification, presumably unfolding or proteolysis, prior to *Tdp1* processing [19]. Recently, Interthal and Champoux demonstrated that *Tdp1* can cleave a substrate with as many as 108 amino acids attached to the 3'-end of DNA [55]. They also showed that the *Tdp1* processing efficiency decreases as the length of the polypeptide extends [55], consistent with a previous report by Debethune *et al.* [53]. Several studies have shown that Top1 is degraded following CPT treatment, suggesting that enhanced proteolysis of Top1 could contribute to CPT resistance [56-59]. Conversely, prevention of Top1 degradation by the proteasome inhibitors, MG132 [57] or the clinically used drug bertozomide (Velcade®; PS-341) [60], results in increased sensitivity to CPT. Proteasome inhibitors also prevent formation of covalent *Tdp1*-DNA complex normally present in the CPT-treated SCAN1 cells [55]. Combined, these studies imply that Top1 degradation *via* an ubiquitin-proteasome pathway prepares Top1cc for processing *via* by a *Tdp1*-dependent repair pathway.

In addition to a Top1-derived peptide and a single tyrosine residue, a variety of other moieties that block DNA 3'-ends from being substrates for DNA polymerases or ligases are hydrolyzed by *Tdp1* (Fig. **4B**, **C**), although less effectively than a 3'-phosphotyrosyl end [19]. The broad substrate specificity of *Tdp1* is consistent with analysis of the human *Tdp1* structure bound to a Top1-derived peptide, which demonstrates that there are no specific contacts between the tyrosine and the *Tdp1* polypeptide [49]. One physiologically relevant *Tdp1* substrate is the 3'-phosphoglycolate (Fig. **4B**), which is generated by oxidative DNA damage [61]. In addition, wild-type *Tdp1* has been shown to hydrolyze the covalent phosphoamide intermediate proposed to form in SCAN1 cells between H493R mutant *Tdp1* and DNA (Fig. **3E**) [54]. Other naturally occurring substrates for *Tdp1* include 3'-nucleosides, 3'-ribonucleosides, 3'-α,β-unsaturated aldehyde (3'-dRP), and 3'-abasic sites (Fig. **4B**) [54, 62]. *Tdp1* is only able to remove a single terminal 3'-mononucleoside and is incapable of further processing the resulting 3'-phosphate ends [54, 63]. However, the concerted action of *Tdp1* and the 3'-phosphatase activity of polynucleotide kinase phosphatase (PNKP) may act as a 3'-exonuclease. A recent report also suggests that *Tdp1* processes internal abasic sites, raising the possibility that *Tdp1* possesses an AP lyase activity and potentially plays a role in an APE-independent base excision repair (BER) pathway [64].

Yeast *Tdp1* was reported to process topoisomerase II cleavage complexes (Top2cc) (*i.e.* 5'-phosphotyrosyl bonds) [65] prior to the discovery of tyrosyl-DNA phosphodiesterase 2 (Tdp2), which specifically processes Top2cc [66]. Recently, it was demonstrated that human *Tdp1* is capable of processing 5'-phosphotyrosyl bonds, albeit at low efficiency [62]. The same study also showed that *Tdp1*-deficient chicken cells are hypersensitive to Top2 inhibitors, while the effects of Top2 inhibitors on *Tdp1*-deficient yeast cells are less clear [21, 65, 67]. Finally, overexpression of *Tdp1* in mammalian cells has been shown to significantly reduce the DNA damage caused by Top2 inhibitors, indicating a role for *Tdp1* in repairing Top2 cleavage complexes [30].

Besides the physiological substrates, numerous synthetic *Tdp1* substrates have been identified (Fig. **4C**). Specifically, phosphotyrosine analogues, such as 3'-(4-nitro)phenol and 3'-(4-methyl)phenol, have been used in kinetic analysis of the *Tdp1* catalytic mechanism [40]. Other artificial substrates include a 3'-linker-biotin [54], a fluorescent 3'-4-methylumbelliferone [68], and a 3'-linker-fluorescein [63], which could potentially be employed in high-throughput screens for *Tdp1* inhibitors, similar to how the 3'-BV tag has been used [69]. It is also interesting to note that a phosphorothioate linkage at the scissile phosphate position prevents hydrolysis by *Tdp1* and thus could also be exploited for high-throughput screening purposes [63].

Tdp1 activity is also influenced by the substrate DNA attached to Top1. Indeed, it has been shown that the efficiency of *Tdp1* to hydrolyze peptide-DNA substrates decreases when the length of the oligonucleotide is shortened from 13 to 4 nucleotides [53]. These findings have been corroborated recently by Interthal and Champoux [55]. Several structural variations of the Top1cc which mimic substrates that *Tdp1* may encounter *in vivo* have also been examined, such as

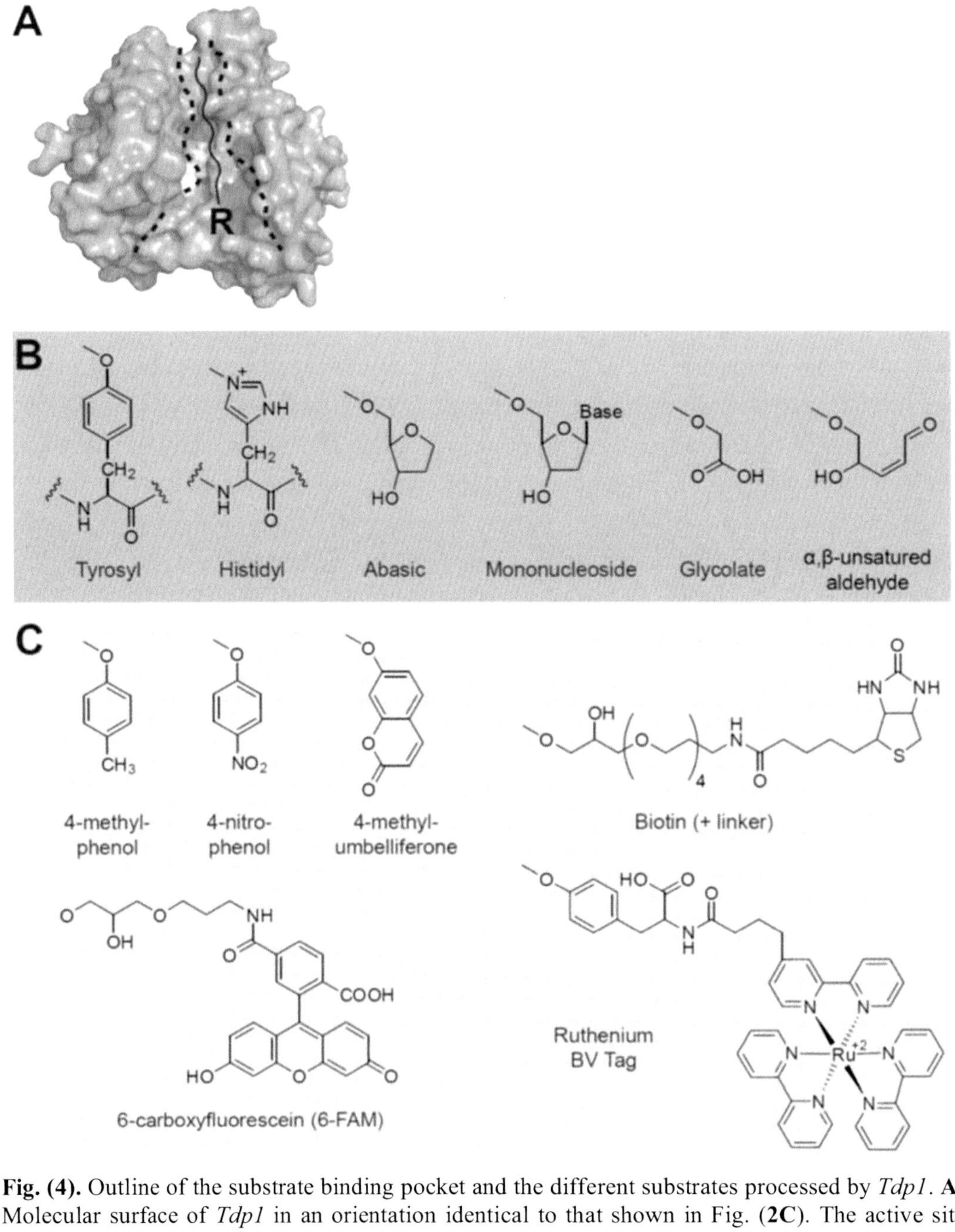

Fig. (4). Outline of the substrate binding pocket and the different substrates processed by *Tdp1*. **A**) Molecular surface of *Tdp1* in an orientation identical to that shown in Fig. (**2C**). The active site region is shown in white. The black dotted lines define the substrate binding pocket (figure modified from [48]). The R-group refers to the structures shown in (**B**) and (**C**). **B**) and **C**) illustrate the physiological and non-physiological substrates of *Tdp1* (Figure modified and updated from [76]).

single-strand, tailed duplex, gapped duplex, and nicked duplex. *Tdp1* is able to cleave all the substrates listed with varying degrees of efficiency [19, 21, 70]. In general, the structure of the DNA segment as well as the size and identity of lesion determines the biochemical activity of *Tdp1*. For example, *Tdp1* processing of 5'-phosphotyrosyl linkages is dependent on DNA structure. Specifically, the 5'-phosphotyrosine is removed most efficiently from 5'-overhang substrates, which mimics Top2cc, but not from blunt-ended substrates [62].

3.4. *Tdp1*-Dependent Repair Pathway

The 3'-phosphate-end generated by *Tdp1* must be hydrolyzed to a 3'-hydroxyl for further DNA repair. PNKP, a bifunctional enzyme with 5'-kinase and 3'-phosphatase activities, is the most plausible candidate in human cells for the repair of these 3'-phosphate lesions. *In vitro* studies have shown that T4 kinase, the bacteriophage equivalent of PNKP, can hydrolyze the resulting 3'-phosphate produced by *Tdp1* [19]. It has also been shown that human A549 cells that are defective in PNKP accrue similar levels of CPT-induced strand breaks in comparison to SCAN1 cells [34], suggesting that *Tdp1* and PNKP function in the same repair pathway in human cells. Furthermore, PNKP is known to interact with the XRCC1 protein, which together with the other BER proteins, such as DNA polymerase β, DNA ligase III, and poly (ADP-ribose)polymerase 1 (PARP1) forms a multiprotein DNA repair complex [71]. *Tdp1* participates in the BER repair complex through its interactions with DNA ligase III [34] and XRCC1 [72]. These protein-protein interactions are promoted by ATM- and/or DNA-PK-mediated phosphorylation of *Tdp1* on S81 following DNA damage [27]. Accordingly, XRCC1-deficient cells are hypersensitive to CPT and defective in *Tdp1* activity, which is in agreement with a direct role of *Tdp1* in association with the BER complex for the removal and repair of Top1-mediated DNA damage [72]. In addition, the interaction of XRCC1 with PNKP has been shown to stimulate both the 5'-kinase and 3'-phosphatase activities of this enzyme [71]. Similarly, XRCC1 interacts with DNA ligase III and increases the intracellular stability of the ligase [73, 74]. The association of PARP1 with the XRCC1 complex has also been observed. PARP1 is a nuclear enzyme often termed a molecular nick sensor, which recognizes and binds to DNA single- or double-strand breaks [75]. Indeed, the hypersensitivity of PARP1-deficient cells to CPT has been shown to be directly related to a functional defect in *Tdp1* [76]. Moreover, it has recently been shown that PARP1 inhibition fails to enhance the cytotoxicity of CPT in *Tdp1*$^{-/-}$ cells, indicating that PARP functions together with *Tdp1* in a common repair pathway [77]. Finally, SUMOylation at K111 has recently been reported to promote *Tdp1* accumulation at DNA damage sites [29], thus promoting DNA repair by *Tdp1*. Cells expressing SUMOylation-deficient mutant *Tdp1* (K111R) accumulate more CPT-induced Top1cc than cells expressing wild type *Tdp1* [29].

Based on these observations and several others, a scheme for the role of BER in the repair of Top1-mediated DNA lesions is outlined in Fig. (**5**) [8]. Following degradation or unfolding of Top1 to expose the phosphotyrosyl linkage, *Tdp1* hydrolyzes the Top1-DNA bond. Next, PNKP hydrolyzes the resulting 3'-phosphate end and catalyzes the phosphorylation of the 5'-end of the DNA. Lastly, DNA polymerase β replaces the missing DNA segment and DNA ligase III reseals the DNA.

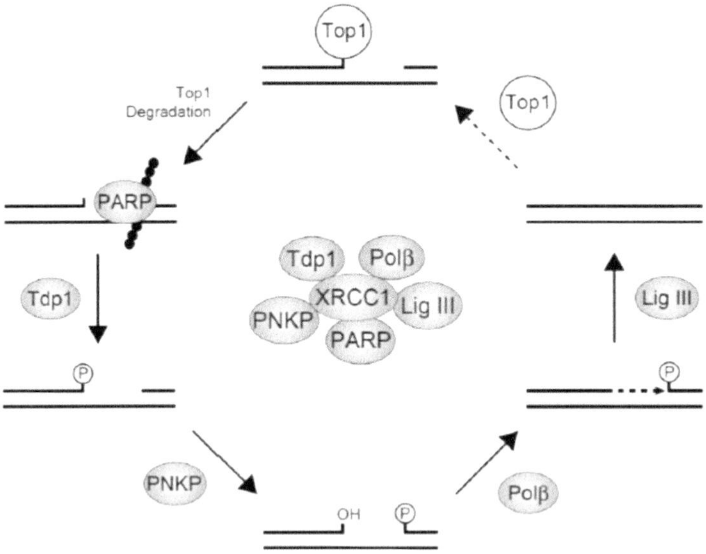

Fig. (5). Repair of Top1 cleavage complexes by the XRCC-1-dependent pathway. The XRCC1 complex including the associated repair enzymes is shown in the center of the figure. *Tdp1* hydrolyzes the Top1 phosphotyrosyl bond. PNKP hydrolyzes the resulting 3'-phosphate and phosphorylates the 5'-hydroxyl. DNA polymerase β fills the gap and DNA ligase III reseals the DNA. PARP-1 may play a role in the initial recognition of the Top1-mediated DNA damage (Figure modified from [8, 19, 99]).

3.5. *Tdp1*-Independent Repair Pathways

The initial understanding of the role of *Tdp1* in DNA repair and the rationale for targeting *Tdp1* for anticancer therapy in combination with CPT came from the wealth of information provided by yeast genetics. Indeed, a number of genetic alterations in yeast have been shown to confer hypersensitivity to Top1-mediated damage [76]. The yeast *Tdp1* knockout has been shown to be viable and insensitive to CPT [20]. It is only when secondary mutations in other DNA repair or checkpoint genes are present that sensitivity of *Tdp1*-defective yeast to CPT can be observed. For instance, significant sensitization to CPT is observed when *Tdp1* and the checkpoint gene *Rad9* are simultaneously inactivated [21]. It is still unclear whether inactivation of the homologous recombination pathways sensitize *Tdp1*-deficient yeast cells to CPT [78]. Recently, we found that CtIP inactivation further sensitizes to CPT in *Tdp1* knockout DT40 cells [62]. CPT sensitivity in *Tdp1*-defective yeast is also conditional upon mutations in three structure-specific endonucleases, which demonstrates the relevance of 3'-endonuclease redundant pathways to remove Top1cc. One such endonuclease is *Rad1-Rad10* (*XPF-ERCC1*), which also functions in the nucleotide excision repair pathway and cleaves on the 5'-side of the repair bubble formed around bulky DNA lesions [79-81]. Recently, XPF-ERCC1 has been shown to be involved not only in the repair of replication-associated DNA damage, but also in the repair of replication-independent DNA damage generated by Top1 in human cells [77]. *Mus81-Mms4* (*Mus81-Eme1*) and *Mre11-Rad50-Xrs2* (*Mre11-Rad50-Nbs1* or *MRN* complex), which cleave 3'-flap structures upstream of DNA branch points [82, 83], also function independently from the *Tdp1* pathway (Fig. **6A**) [84, 85]. There are specific human homologs for each of the genes mentioned above (shown in parentheses), with the exception of *Rad9*.

In humans, there is no single *Rad9* ortholog readily identifiable, but rather a family of tandem BRCT domain-containing proteins that act in the checkpoint response. Some of the *Rad9* human orthologs include BRCA1, CtIP, 53BP1, and MDC1, which are commonly referred to as checkpoint mediators [86]. Recently, these findings in yeast were recapitulated in human cells, in which improved sensitivity to the CPT analog gimatecan was demonstrated following dual siRNA knockdown of *Tdp1* and BRCA1 [87]. Taken together, these studies suggest two redundant pathways for the repair of Top1-mediated DNA damage in humans (Fig. **6A**) [77]. The first is a *Tdp1*-dependent pathway involving the previously mentioned XRCC1 and PARP complex. The second is a *Tdp1*-independent-dependent 3'-endonuclease-dependent pathway. The redundancy in the removal and repair of Top1cc provides a rationale for the development of *Tdp1* inhibitors as deficiencies in checkpoint and DNA repair mechanisms are a common feature in cancer cells [88]. For example, if cancers are defective in checkpoint inactivation or the 3'-endonuclease pathway, then *Tdp1* becomes the principle source for the removal of Top1cc (Fig. **6B**).

3.6. Rationale for Targeting *Tdp1* for Cancer Therapy

Despite their clinical effectiveness, inherent resistance has been reported for Top1 inhibitors. Given that the cytotoxic effect of most Top1 inhibitors is dependent on the persistent stabilization of the Top1-DNA complex, it is reasonable to predict that reduction (*i.e.* repair) of such complexes may play a role in the acquired resistance. Indeed, increased repair of Top1-DNA lesions has been reported in CPT-resistant cell lines [89, 90]. Consequently, a viable therapeutic approach to modulate the sensitivity of Top1 inhibitors is to inactivate DNA repair enzymes, such as *Tdp1*. Initial studies performed in human cells harboring the physiologically relevant SCAN1 *Tdp1* mutant established the first line of evidence for the development of *Tdp1* inhibitors in combination with Top1-targeting drugs in anticancer therapy. Specifically, homozygous mutant SCAN1 cells have been shown to accumulate more total DNA strand breaks than normal lymphoblastoid cells after treatment with CPT [34, 91]. SCAN1 cells have also demonstrated enhanced sensitivity to CPT [36, 91]. Moreover, *Tdp1* knockout mice as well as human cells deficient in *Tdp1* show increased sensitivity to CPT [27, 92-94], while overexpression of *Tdp1* results in reduction of CPT-induced DNA damage [30, 87, 95]. Taken together, these data demonstrate that a single defect in *Tdp1* activity is sufficient for enhancing sensitivity to Top1 inhibitors, which is in contrast to the conditional mutations required in *Tdp1*-deficient yeast cells. Thus, inhibition of *Tdp1* should potentiate or synergize with the cytotoxic effects of the clinically used Top1 inhibitors. *Tdp1* inhibitors might also enhance the selectivity of bleomycin, Top2 inhibitors, and alkylating agents in cells with preexisting DNA repair and cell cycle checkpoint deficiencies.

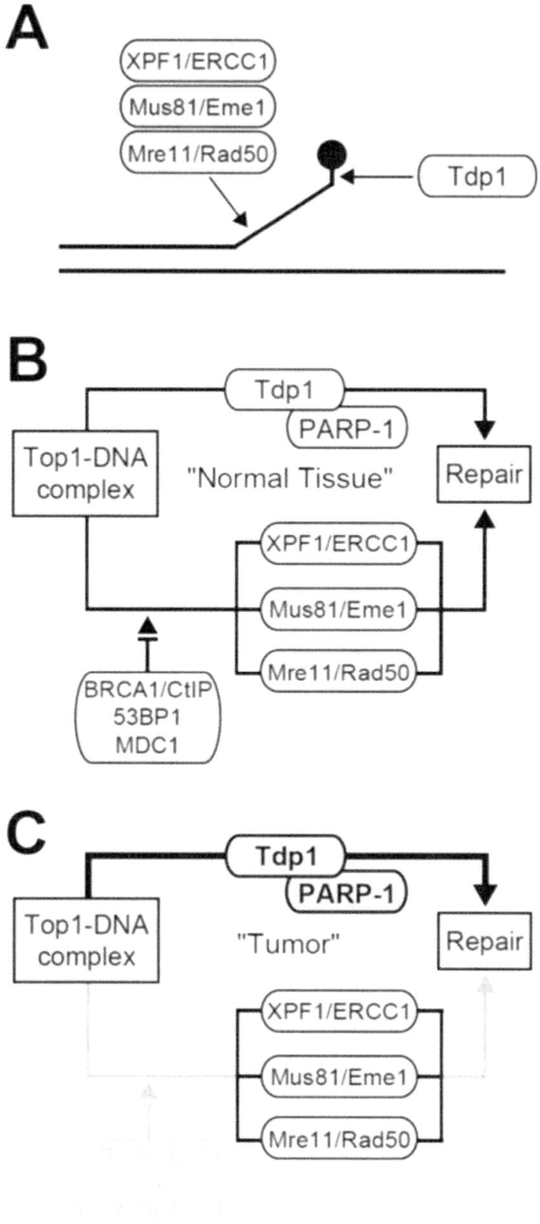

Fig. (6). Redundant pathways involved in the repair of Top1cc in mammalian cells. **A**) The processing of Top1cc by *Tdp1* and three different structure-specific 3'-endonucleases. **B**) Schematic representation of the *Tdp1*-dependent pathway and checkpoint-dependent 3'-endonuclease pathway, which together are implicated in the repair of Top1cc. **C**) DNA repair and checkpoint deficiencies often seen in cancer cells, results in greater dependency on the *Tdp1*-dependent pathway for repair of Top1cc.

3.7. *Tdp1* Inhibitors

Both vanadate and tungstate inhibit *Tdp1* at millimolar concentrations because of their ability to mimic the transition state of *Tdp1* substrate (Fig. **7**) [48]. Vanadate and tungstate have been useful in co-crystallization studies, such as in the case of *Tdp1* [48, 49], but their pharmacological use is limited due to their lack of selectivity. The aminoglycoside antibiotic neomycin is also a millimolar inhibitor of *Tdp1* (IC_{50}, 8 mM) (Fig. **7**) [96], which was originally tested based on its reported ability to inhibit PLD [97].

Furamidine (NSC 305831), a compound in Phase III clinical trials against the human African trypanosomiasis (Fig. **7**), was identified as a micromolar inhibitor of *Tdp1* by an electrochemiluminescent-based assay used to screen the NCI Developmental Therapeutics Program plated set repository [69]. Furamidine was shown to interact with *Tdp1* and its single stranded DNA substrate therefore its mechanism of action is distinct from the known double-stranded DNA binding properties of furamidine. Furamidine is well known to bind selectively the DNA minor groove at AT-rich sites and to intercalate between GC base pairs in double-stranded DNA.

A steroid derative (NSC 88915) was also identified by the same screening assay [69, 98]. This compound bears an aromatic sulfonyl ester group that mimics the Top1 catalytic phosphotyrosine (Fig. **7**), demonstrating that *Tdp1* can be inhibited by phosphotyrosine mimetics. Methyl-3,4-dephostatin is another phosphotyrosine mimetic identified by a high-throughput Alpha Screen 1536-plate-based assay used to screen the NIH Molecular Libraries [69, 98]. This aromatic amine contains a hydroxyl-substituted benzyl ring, which simulates a phosphotyrosine group and inhibits *Tdp1* at sub-micromolar concentrations. Interestingly, dephostatin with a hydroxyl-substituted benzyl ring at different position is completely inactive [69, 98]. Recently, a natural product from an anamorphic fungus with cytotoxic properties has been reported to inhibit *Tdp1* in the micromolar range [100]. This tetracyclic compound offers some similarities with the ring system geometry of the steroid derivative NSC 88915 (Fig. **7**).

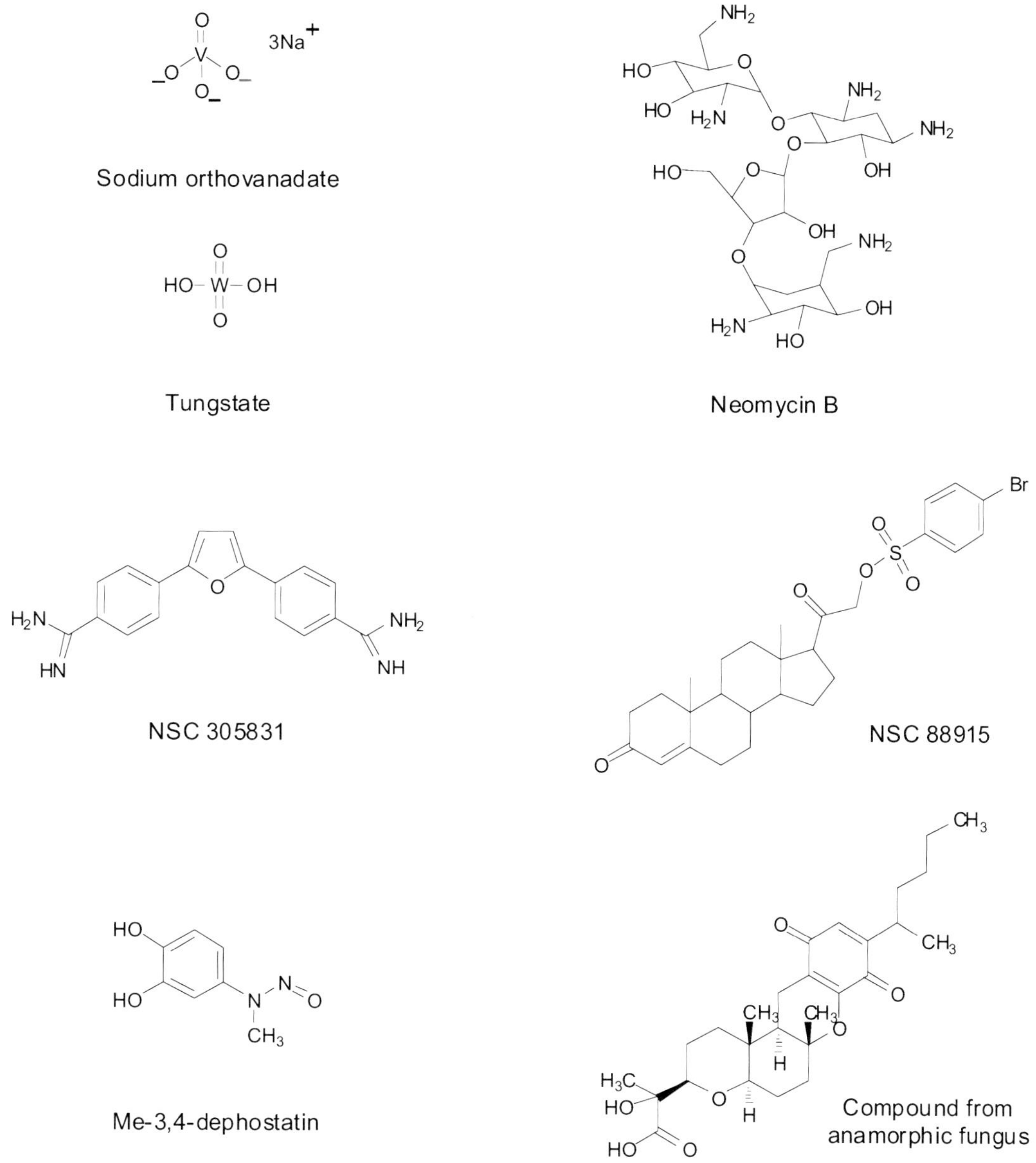

Fig. (7). Chemical structures of *Tdp1* inhibitors reported to date.

Unfortunately, none of these inhibitors inhibit *Tdp1* in cellular systems; therefore, continued search for novel *Tdp1* inhibitors synergyzing with Top1 inhibitors in such systems is warranted.

4. SUMMARY AND PERSPECTIVES

The discovery of novel *Tdp1* inhibitors is now possible as *Tdp1* can be expressed as a biological active recombinant protein and high throughput assays are relatively easy to set up. In addition to biochemical screening, *Tdp1* crystal structures could provide a means for *in silico* screening of chemical libraries. Lead optimization also will benefit from existing crystal structures and from the generation of new co-crystal structures with *Tdp1* inhibitors. Recently, we have generated *Tdp1* knockout DT40 cells complemented with human *Tdp1*. *Tdp1* inhibitors should enhance the cytotoxicity of camptothecins and delay the removal of Top1cc in cell culture, thereby providing a cellular system for compound selection. The overall therapeutic goal is the development of new drugs that would selectively enhance the activity of Top1 inhibitors in tumors with preexisting DNA repair and cell cycle checkpoint deficiencies.

CONFLICT OF INTEREST

The authors declare that there is no conflict of interest.

ACKNOWLEDGEMENTS

Declared none.

DISCLOSURE

This e-Book chapter is an updated version of the review article entitled "Tyrosyl-DNA phosphodiesterase as a target for anticancer therapy" published in *Anti-Cancer Agents in Medicinal Chemistry*, **2008**, *8*, 381-389.

REFERENCES

[1] Champoux, J. J. (2001) DNA topoisomerases: structure, function, and mechanism, *Annual review of biochemistry 70*, 369-413.

[2] Keck, J. L., and Berger, J. M. (1999) Enzymes that push DNA around, *Nature structural biology6*, 900-902.

[3] Pommier, Y., Pourquier, P., Fan, Y., and Strumberg, D. (1998) Mechanism of action of eukaryotic DNA topoisomerase I and drugs targeted to the enzyme, *Biochimica et biophysica acta1400*, 83-105.

[4] Wang, J. C. (2002) Cellular roles of DNA topoisomerases: a molecular perspective, *Nature reviews3*, 430-440.

[5] Hsiang, Y. H., Hertzberg, R., Hecht, S., and Liu, L. F. (1985) Camptothecin induces protein-linked DNA breaks *via* mammalian DNA topoisomerase I, *The Journal of biological chemistry260*, 14873-14878.

[6] Pommier, Y. (2006) Topoisomerase I inhibitors: camptothecins and beyond, *Nat Rev Cancer6*, 789-802.

[7] Pourquier, P., and Pommier, Y. (2001) Topoisomerase I-mediated DNA damage, *Advances in cancer research80*, 189-216.

[8] Pommier, Y., Redon, C., Rao, V. A., Seiler, J. A., Sordet, O., Takemura, H., Antony, S., Meng, L., Liao, Z., Kohlhagen, G., Zhang, H., and Kohn, K. W. (2003) Repair of and checkpoint response to topoisomerase I-mediated DNA damage, *Mutation research532*, 173-203.

[9] Marchand, C., Antony, S., Kohn, K. W., Cushman, M., Ioanoviciu, A., Staker, B. L., Burgin, A. B., Stewart, L., and Pommier, Y. (2006) A novel norindenoisoquinoline structure reveals a common interfacial inhibitor paradigm for ternary trapping of the topoisomerase I-DNA covalent complex, *Molecular cancer therapeutics5*, 287-295.

[10] McClendon, A. K., and Osheroff, N. (2006) The geometry of DNA supercoils modulates topoisomerase-mediated DNA cleavage and enzyme response to anticancer drugs, *Biochemistry45*, 3040-3050.

[11] Chen, A. Y., and Liu, L. F. (1994) DNA topoisomerases: essential enzymes and lethal targets, *Annual review of pharmacology and toxicology34*, 191-218.

[12] Pommier, Y., Pourquier, P., Urasaki, Y., Wu, J., and Laco, G. S. (1999) Topoisomerase I inhibitors: selectivity and cellular resistance, *Drug Resist Updat2*, 307-318.

[13] Strumberg, D., Pilon, A. A., Smith, M., Hickey, R., Malkas, L., and Pommier, Y. (2000) Conversion of topoisomerase I cleavage complexes on the leading strand of ribosomal DNA into 5'-phosphorylated DNA double-strand breaks by replication runoff, *Molecular and cellular biology20*, 3977-3987.

[14] Furuta, T., Takemura, H., Liao, Z. Y., Aune, G. J., Redon, C., Sedelnikova, O. A., Pilch, D. R., Rogakou, E. P., Celeste, A., Chen, H. T., Nussenzweig, A., Aladjem, M. I., Bonner, W. M., and Pommier, Y. (2003) Phosphorylation of histone H2AX and activation of Mre11, Rad50, and Nbs1 in response to replication-dependent DNA-double-strand breaks induced by mammalian DNA topoisomerase I cleavage complexes, *The Journal of biological chemistry278*, 20303-20312.

[15] Pourquier, P., Pilon, A. A., Kohlhagen, G., Mazumder, A., Sharma, A., and Pommier, Y. (1997) Trapping of mammalian topoisomerase I and recombinations induced by damaged DNA containing nicks or gaps. Importance of DNA end phosphorylation and camptothecin effects, *The Journal of biological chemistry272*, 26441-26447.

[16] Pourquier, P., Ueng, L. M., Kohlhagen, G., Mazumder, A., Gupta, M., Kohn, K. W., and Pommier, Y. (1997) Effects of uracil incorporation, DNA mismatches, and abasic sites on cleavage and religation activities of mammalian topoisomerase I, *The Journal of biological chemistry272*, 7792-7796.

[17] Lanza, A., Tornaletti, S., Rodolfo, C., Scanavini, M. C., and Pedrini, A. M. (1996) Human DNA topoisomerase I-mediated cleavages stimulated by ultraviolet light-induced DNA damage, *The Journal of biological chemistry271*, 6978-6986.

[18] Daroui, P., Desai, S. D., Li, T. K., Liu, A. A., and Liu, L. F. (2004) Hydrogen peroxide induces topoisomerase I-mediated DNA damage and cell death, *The Journal of biological chemistry279*, 14587-14594.

[19] Yang, S. W., Burgin, A. B., Jr., Huizenga, B. N., Robertson, C. A., Yao, K. C., and Nash, H. A. (1996) A eukaryotic enzyme that can disjoin dead-end covalent complexes between DNA and type I topoisomerases, *Proceedings of the National Academy of Sciences of the United States of America93*, 11534-11539.

[20] Pouliot, J. J., Yao, K. C., Robertson, C. A., and Nash, H. A. (1999) Yeast gene for a Tyr-DNA phosphodiesterase that repairs topoisomerase I complexes, *Science286*, 552-555.

[21] Pouliot, J. J., Robertson, C. A., and Nash, H. A. (2001) Pathways for repair of topoisomerase I covalent complexes in Saccharomyces cerevisiae, *Genes Cells6*, 677-687.

[22] Banerjee, B., Roy, A., Sen, N., and Majumder, H. K. (2010) A tyrosyl DNA phosphodiesterase 1 from kinetoplastid parasite Leishmania donovani (Ld*Tdp1*) capable of removing topo I-DNA covalent complexes, *Mol Microbiol78*, 119-137.

[23] Macovei, A., Balestrazzi, A., Confalonieri, M., and Carbonera, D. (2010) The tyrosyl-DNA phosphodiesterase gene family in Medicago truncatula Gaertn.: bioinformatic investigation and expression profiles in response to copper- and PEG-mediated stress, *Planta232*, 393-407.

[24] Lee, S. Y., Kim, H., Hwang, H. J., Jeong, Y. M., Na, S. H., Woo, J. C., and Kim, S. G. (2010) Identification of tyrosyl-DNA phosphodiesterase as a novel DNA damage repair enzyme in Arabidopsis, *Plant Physiol154*, 1460-1469.

[25] Interthal, H., Pouliot, J. J., and Champoux, J. J. (2001) The tyrosyl-DNA phosphodiesterase *Tdp1* is a member of the phospholipase D superfamily, *Proceedings of the National Academy of Sciences of the United States of America98*, 12009-12014.

[26] Cheng, T. J., Rey, P. G., Poon, T., and Kan, C. C. (2002) Kinetic studies of human tyrosyl-DNA phosphodiesterase, an enzyme in the topoisomerase I DNA repair pathway, *European journal of biochemistry / FEBS269*, 3697-3704.

[27] Das, B. B., Antony, S., Gupta, S., Dexheimer, T. S., Redon, C. E., Garfield, S., Shiloh, Y., and Pommier, Y. (2009) Optimal function of the DNA repair enzyme *TDP1* requires its phosphorylation by ATM and/or DNA-PK, *EMBO J28*, 3667-3680.

[28] Chiang, S. C., Carroll, J., and El-Khamisy, S. F. (2010) *TDP1* serine 81 promotes interaction with DNA ligase IIIalpha and facilitates cell survival following DNA damage, *Cell Cycle9*, 588-595.

[29] Hudson, J. J., Chiang, S. C., Wells, O. S., Rookyard, C., and El-Khamisy, S. F. (2012) SUMO modification of the neuroprotective protein *TDP1* facilitates chromosomal single-strand break repair, *Nat Commun3*, 733.

[30] Barthelmes, H. U., Habermeyer, M., Christensen, M. O., Mielke, C., Interthal, H., Pouliot, J. J., Boege, F., and Marko, D. (2004) *TDP1* overexpression in human cells counteracts DNA damage mediated by topoisomerases I and II, *The Journal of biological chemistry279*, 55618-55625.

[31] Das, B. B., Dexheimer, T. S., Maddali, K., and Pommier, Y. (2010) Role of tyrosyl-DNA phosphodiesterase (*TDP1*) in mitochondria, *Proceedings of the National Academy of Sciences of the United States of America107*, 19790-19795.

[32] Takashima, H., Boerkoel, C. F., John, J., Saifi, G. M., Salih, M. A., Armstrong, D., Mao, Y., Quiocho, F. A., Roa, B. B., Nakagawa, M., Stockton, D. W., and Lupski, J. R. (2002)

Mutation of *TDP1*, encoding a topoisomerase I-dependent DNA damage repair enzyme, in spinocerebellar ataxia with axonal neuropathy, *Nature genetics32*, 267-272.

[33] Walton, C., Interthal, H., Hirano, R., Salih, M. A., Takashima, H., and Boerkoel, C. F. (2010) Spinocerebellar ataxia with axonal neuropathy, *Adv Exp Med Biol685*, 75-83.

[34] El-Khamisy, S. F., Saifi, G. M., Weinfeld, M., Johansson, F., Helleday, T., Lupski, J. R., and Caldecott, K. W. (2005) Defective DNA single-strand break repair in spinocerebellar ataxia with axonal neuropathy-1, *Nature434*, 108-113.

[35] Zhou, T., Lee, J. W., Tatavarthi, H., Lupski, J. R., Valerie, K., and Povirk, L. F. (2005) Deficiency in 3'-phosphoglycolate processing in human cells with a hereditary mutation in tyrosyl-DNA phosphodiesterase (*TDP1*), *Nucleic acids research33*, 289-297.

[36] Interthal, H., Chen, H. J., Kehl-Fie, T. E., Zotzmann, J., Leppard, J. B., and Champoux, J. J. (2005) SCAN1 mutant *Tdp1* accumulates the enzyme--DNA intermediate and causes camptothecin hypersensitivity, *EMBO J24*, 2224-2233.

[37] Stuckey, J. A., and Dixon, J. E. (1999) Crystal structure of a phospholipase D family member, *Nature structural biology6*, 278-284.

[38] Ponting, C. P., and Kerr, I. D. (1996) A novel family of phospholipase D homologues that includes phospholipid synthases and putative endonucleases: identification of duplicated repeats and potential active site residues, *Protein Sci5*, 914-922.

[39] Waite, M. (1999) The PLD superfamily: insights into catalysis, *Biochimica et biophysica acta1439*, 187-197.

[40] Raymond, A. C., Rideout, M. C., Staker, B., Hjerrild, K., and Burgin, A. B., Jr. (2004) Analysis of human tyrosyl-DNA phosphodiesterase I catalytic residues, *Journal of molecular biology338*, 895-906.

[41] Gottlin, E. B., Rudolph, A. E., Zhao, Y., Matthews, H. R., and Dixon, J. E. (1998) Catalytic mechanism of the phospholipase D superfamily proceeds *via* a covalent phosphohistidine intermediate, *Proceedings of the National Academy of Sciences of the United States of America95*, 9202-9207.

[42] Iwasaki, Y., Horiike, S., Matsushima, K., and Yamane, T. (1999) Location of the catalytic nucleophile of phospholipase D of Streptomyces antibioticus in the C-terminal half domain, *European journal of biochemistry / FEBS264*, 577-581.

[43] Rudolph, A. E., Stuckey, J. A., Zhao, Y., Matthews, H. R., Patton, W. A., Moss, J., and Dixon, J. E. (1999) Expression, characterization, and mutagenesis of the Yersinia pestis murine toxin, a phospholipase D superfamily member, *The Journal of biological chemistry274*, 11824-11831.

[44] Sung, T. C., Roper, R. L., Zhang, Y., Rudge, S. A., Temel, R., Hammond, S. M., Morris, A. J., Moss, B., Engebrecht, J., and Frohman, M. A. (1997) Mutagenesis of phospholipase D defines a superfamily including a *trans*-Golgi viral protein required for poxvirus pathogenicity, *Embo J16*, 4519-4530.

[45] Xie, Z., Ho, W. T., and Exton, J. H. (2000) Association of the N- and C-terminal domains of phospholipase D. Contribution of the conserved HKD motifs to the interaction and the requirement of the association for Ser/Thr phosphorylation of the enzyme, *The Journal of biological chemistry275*, 24962-24969.

[46] Davies, D. R., Interthal, H., Champoux, J. J., and Hol, W. G. (2002) The crystal structure of human tyrosyl-DNA phosphodiesterase, *Tdp1*, *Structure10*, 237-248.

[47] Leiros, I., Secundo, F., Zambonelli, C., Servi, S., and Hough, E. (2000) The first crystal structure of a phospholipase D, *Structure8*, 655-667.

[48] Davies, D. R., Interthal, H., Champoux, J. J., and Hol, W. G. (2002) Insights into substrate binding and catalytic mechanism of human tyrosyl-DNA phosphodiesterase (*Tdp1*) from vanadate and tungstate-inhibited structures, *Journal of molecular biology324*, 917-932.

[49] Davies, D. R., Interthal, H., Champoux, J. J., and Hol, W. G. (2003) Crystal structure of a transition state mimic for *Tdp1* assembled from vanadate, DNA, and a topoisomerase I-derived peptide, *Chemistry & biology10*, 139-147.

[50] Davies, D. R., Interthal, H., Champoux, J. J., and Hol, W. G. (2004) Explorations of peptide and oligonucleotide binding sites of tyrosyl-DNA phosphodiesterase using vanadate complexes, *Journal of medicinal chemistry47*, 829-837.

[51] Lowe, G., Cullis, P. M., Jarvest, R. L., Potter, B. V., and Sproat, B. S. (1981) Stereochemistry of phosphoryl transfer, *Philosophical transactions of the Royal Society of London293*, 75-92.

[52] Redinbo, M. R., Stewart, L., Kuhn, P., Champoux, J. J., and Hol, W. G. (1998) Crystal structures of human topoisomerase I in covalent and noncovalent complexes with DNA, *Science279*, 1504-1513.

[53] Debethune, L., Kohlhagen, G., Grandas, A., and Pommier, Y. (2002) Processing of nucleopeptides mimicking the topoisomerase I-DNA covalent complex by tyrosyl-DNA phosphodiesterase, *Nucleic acids research30*, 1198-1204.

[54] Interthal, H., Chen, H. J., and Champoux, J. J. (2005) Human *Tdp1* cleaves a broad spectrum of substrates, including phosphoamide linkages, *The Journal of biological chemistry280*, 36518-36528.

[55] Interthal, H., and Champoux, J. J. (2011) Effects of DNA and protein size on substrate cleavage by human tyrosyl-DNA phosphodiesterase 1, *Biochem J436*, 559-566.

[56] Beidler, D. R., and Cheng, Y. C. (1995) Camptothecin induction of a time- and concentration-dependent decrease of topoisomerase I and its implication in camptothecin activity, *Molecular pharmacology47*, 907-914.

[57] Desai, S. D., Li, T. K., Rodriguez-Bauman, A., Rubin, E. H., and Liu, L. F. (2001) Ubiquitin/26S proteasome-mediated degradation of topoisomerase I as a resistance mechanism to camptothecin in tumor cells, *Cancer research61*, 5926-5932.

[58] Desai, S. D., Liu, L. F., Vazquez-Abad, D., and D'Arpa, P. (1997) Ubiquitin-dependent destruction of topoisomerase I is stimulated by the antitumor drug camptothecin, *The Journal of biological chemistry272*, 24159-24164.

[59] Zhang, H. F., Tomida, A., Koshimizu, R., Ogiso, Y., Lei, S., and Tsuruo, T. (2004) Cullin 3 promotes proteasomal degradation of the topoisomerase I-DNA covalent complex, *Cancer research64*, 1114-1121.

[60] Cusack, J. C., Jr., Liu, R., Houston, M., Abendroth, K., Elliott, P. J., Adams, J., and Baldwin, A. S., Jr. (2001) Enhanced chemosensitivity to CPT-11 with proteasome inhibitor PS-341: implications for systemic nuclear factor-kappaB inhibition, *Cancer research61*, 3535-3540.

[61] Inamdar, K. V., Pouliot, J. J., Zhou, T., Lees-Miller, S. P., Rasouli-Nia, A., and Povirk, L. F. (2002) Conversion of phosphoglycolate to phosphate termini on 3' overhangs of DNA double strand breaks by the human tyrosyl-DNA phosphodiesterase h*Tdp1*, *The Journal of biological chemistry277*, 27162-27168.

[62] Murai, J., Huang, S. Y., Das, B. B., Dexheimer, T. S., Takeda, S., and Pommier, Y. (2012) Tyrosyl-DNA phosphodiesterase 1 (*TDP1*) repairs DNA damages induced by

topoisomerases I and II, and base alkylation in vertebrate cells, *The Journal of biological chemistry*.

[63] Dexheimer, T. S., Stephen, A. G., Fivash, M. J., Fisher, R. J., and Pommier, Y. (2010) The DNA binding and 3'-end preferential activity of human tyrosyl-DNA phosphodiesterase, *Nucleic acids research38*, 2444-2452.

[64] Lebedeva, N. A., Rechkunova, N. I., and Lavrik, O. I. (2011) AP-site cleavage activity of tyrosyl-DNA phosphodiesterase 1, *FEBS Lett585*, 683-686.

[65] Nitiss, K. C., Malik, M., He, X., White, S. W., and Nitiss, J. L. (2006) Tyrosyl-DNA phosphodiesterase (*Tdp1*) participates in the repair of Top2-mediated DNA damage, *Proceedings of the National Academy of Sciences of the United States of America103*, 8953-8958.

[66] Cortes Ledesma, F., El Khamisy, S. F., Zuma, M. C., Osborn, K., and Caldecott, K. W. (2009) A human 5'-tyrosyl DNA phosphodiesterase that repairs topoisomerase-mediated DNA damage, *Nature461*, 674-678.

[67] Murai, J., Huang, S.-Y. N., Das, B. B., Dexheimer, T. S., Takeda, S., and Pommier, Y. (2012) Tyrosyl-DNA phosphodiesterase 1 (*TDP1*) repairs DNA damages induced by topoisomerases I and II, and base alkylation in vertebrate cells., *The Journal of biological chemistry*.

[68] Rideout, M. C., Raymond, A. C., and Burgin, A. B., Jr. (2004) Design and synthesis of fluorescent substrates for human tyrosyl-DNA phosphodiesterase I, *Nucleic acids research32*, 4657-4664.

[69] Antony, S., Marchand, C., Stephen, A. G., Thibaut, L., Agama, K. K., Fisher, R. J., and Pommier, Y. (2007) Novel high-throughput electrochemiluminescent assay for identification of human tyrosyl-DNA phosphodiesterase (*Tdp1*) inhibitors and characterization of furamidine (NSC 305831) as an inhibitor of *Tdp1*, *Nucleic acids research35*, 4474-4484.

[70] Raymond, A. C., Staker, B. L., and Burgin, A. B., Jr. (2005) Substrate specificity of tyrosyl-DNA phosphodiesterase I (*Tdp1*), *The Journal of biological chemistry280*, 22029-22035.

[71] Whitehouse, C. J., Taylor, R. M., Thistlethwaite, A., Zhang, H., Karimi-Busheri, F., Lasko, D. D., Weinfeld, M., and Caldecott, K. W. (2001) XRCC1 stimulates human polynucleotide kinase activity at damaged DNA termini and accelerates DNA single-strand break repair, *Cell104*, 107-117.

[72] Plo, I., Liao, Z. Y., Barcelo, J. M., Kohlhagen, G., Caldecott, K. W., Weinfeld, M., and Pommier, Y. (2003) Association of XRCC1 and tyrosyl DNA phosphodiesterase (*Tdp1*) for the repair of topoisomerase I-mediated DNA lesions, *DNA repair2*, 1087-1100.

[73] Caldecott, K. W., Tucker, J. D., Stanker, L. H., and Thompson, L. H. (1995) Characterization of the XRCC1-DNA ligase III complex *in vitro* and its absence from mutant hamster cells, *Nucleic acids research23*, 4836-4843.

[74] Taylor, R. M., Wickstead, B., Cronin, S., and Caldecott, K. W. (1998) Role of a BRCT domain in the interaction of DNA ligase III-alpha with the DNA repair protein XRCC1, *Curr Biol8*, 877-880.

[75] de Murcia, G., and Menissier de Murcia, J. (1994) Poly (ADP-ribose) polymerase: a molecular nick-sensor, *Trends in biochemical sciences19*, 172-176.

[76] Pommier, Y., Barcelo, J. M., Rao, V. A., Sordet, O., Jobson, A. G., Thibaut, L., Miao, Z. H., Seiler, J. A., Zhang, H., Marchand, C., Agama, K., Nitiss, J. L., and Redon, C. (2006)

Repair of topoisomerase I-mediated DNA damage, *Progress in nucleic acid research and molecular biology81*, 179-229.

[77] Zhang, Y. W., Regairaz, M., Seiler, J. A., Agama, K. K., Doroshow, J. H., and Pommier, Y. (2011) Poly (ADP-ribose) polymerase and XPF-ERCC1 participate in distinct pathways for the repair of topoisomerase I-induced DNA damage in mammalian cells, *Nucleic acids research39*, 3607-3620.

[78] Vance, J. R., and Wilson, T. E. (2001) Repair of DNA strand breaks by the overlapping functions of lesion-specific and non-lesion-specific DNA 3' phosphatases, *Mol. Cell. Biol.21*, 7191-7198.

[79] Roberts, J. A., and White, M. F. (2005) DNA end-directed and processive nuclease activities of the archaeal XPF enzyme, *Nucleic acids research33*, 6662-6670.

[80] Vance, J. R., and Wilson, T. E. (2002) Yeast *Tdp1* and Rad1-Rad10 function as redundant pathways for repairing Top1 replicative damage, *Proceedings of the National Academy of Sciences of the United States of America99*, 13669-13674.

[81] Bardwell, A. J., Bardwell, L., Tomkinson, A. E., and Friedberg, E. C. (1994) Specific cleavage of model recombination and repair intermediates by the yeast Rad1-Rad10 DNA endonuclease, *Science265*, 2082-2085.

[82] Bastin-Shanower, S. A., Fricke, W. M., Mullen, J. R., and Brill, S. J. (2003) The mechanism of Mus81-Mms4 cleavage site selection distinguishes it from the homologous endonuclease Rad1-Rad10, *Molecular and cellular biology23*, 3487-3496.

[83] D'Amours, D., and Jackson, S. P. (2002) The Mre11 complex: at the crossroads of dna repair and checkpoint signalling, *Nature reviews3*, 317-327.

[84] Deng, C., Brown, J. A., You, D., and Brown, J. M. (2005) Multiple endonucleases function to repair covalent topoisomerase I complexes in Saccharomyces cerevisiae, *Genetics170*, 591-600.

[85] Liu, C., Pouliot, J. J., and Nash, H. A. (2002) Repair of topoisomerase I covalent complexes in the absence of the tyrosyl-DNA phosphodiesterase *Tdp1*, *Proceedings of the National Academy of Sciences of the United States of America99*, 14970-14975.

[86] Zhou, B. B., and Elledge, S. J. (2000) The DNA damage response: putting checkpoints in perspective, *Nature408*, 433-439.

[87] Perego, P., Cossa, G., Tinelli, S., Corna, E., Carenini, N., Gatti, L., De Cesare, M., Ciusani, E., Zunino, F., Luison, E., Canevari, S., Zaffaroni, N., and Beretta, G. L. (2012) Role of tyrosyl-DNA phosphodiesterase 1 and inter-players in regulation of tumor cell sensitivity to topoisomerase I inhibition, *Biochem Pharmacol83*, 27-36.

[88] Dasika, G. K., Lin, S. C., Zhao, S., Sung, P., Tomkinson, A., and Lee, E. Y. (1999) DNA damage-induced cell cycle checkpoints and DNA strand break repair in development and tumorigenesis, *Oncogene18*, 7883-7899.

[89] Park, S. Y., Lam, W., and Cheng, Y. C. (2002) X-ray repair cross-complementing gene I protein plays an important role in camptothecin resistance, *Cancer research62*, 459-465.

[90] Fujimori, A., Gupta, M., Hoki, Y., and Pommier, Y. (1996) Acquired camptothecin resistance of human breast cancer MCF-7/C4 cells with normal topoisomerase I and elevated DNA repair, *Molecular pharmacology50*, 1472-1478.

[91] Miao, Z. H., Agama, K., Sordet, O., Povirk, L., Kohn, K. W., and Pommier, Y. (2006) Hereditary ataxia SCAN1 cells are defective for the repair of transcription-dependent topoisomerase I cleavage complexes, *DNA repair*.

[92] El-Khamisy, S. F., Katyal, S., Patel, P., Ju, L., McKinnon, P. J., and Caldecott, K. W. (2009) Synergistic decrease of DNA single-strand break repair rates in mouse neural cells lacking both *Tdp1* and aprataxin, *DNA repair8*, 760-766.

[93] Katyal, S., el-Khamisy, S. F., Russell, H. R., Li, Y., Ju, L., Caldecott, K. W., and McKinnon, P. J. (2007) *TDP1* facilitates chromosomal single-strand break repair in neurons and is neuroprotective *in vivo*, *EMBO J26*, 4720-4731.

[94] Hirano, R., Interthal, H., Huang, C., Nakamura, T., Deguchi, K., Choi, K., Bhattacharjee, M. B., Arimura, K., Umehara, F., Izumo, S., Northrop, J. L., Salih, M. A., Inoue, K., Armstrong, D. L., Champoux, J. J., Takashima, H., and Boerkoel, C. F. (2007) Spinocerebellar ataxia with axonal neuropathy: consequence of a *Tdp1* recessive neomorphic mutation?, *EMBO J26*, 4732-4743.

[95] Nivens, M. C., Felder, T., Galloway, A. H., Pena, M. M., Pouliot, J. J., and Spencer, H. T. (2004) Engineered resistance to camptothecin and antifolates by retroviral coexpression of tyrosyl DNA phosphodiesterase-I and thymidylate synthase, *Cancer chemotherapy and pharmacology53*, 107-115.

[96] Liao, Z., Thibaut, L., Jobson, A., and Pommier, Y. (2006) Inhibition of human tyrosyl-DNA phosphodiesterase by aminoglycoside antibiotics and ribosome inhibitors, *Molecular pharmacology70*, 366-372.

[97] Huang, Y., Qureshi, I. A., and Chen, H. (1999) Effects of phosphatidylinositol 4,5-bisphosphate and neomycin on phospholipase D: kinetic studies, *Molecular and cellular biochemistry197*, 195-201.

[98] Dexheimer, T. S., Gediya, L. K., Stephen, A. G., Weidlich, I., Antony, S., Marchand, C., Interthal, H., Nicklaus, M., Fisher, R. J., Njar, V. C., and Pommier, Y. (2009) 4-Pregnen-21-ol-3,20-dione-21-(4-bromobenzenesulfonate) (NSC 88915) and related novel steroid derivatives as tyrosyl-DNA phosphodiesterase (*Tdp1*) inhibitors, *Journal of medicinal chemistry52*, 7122-7131.

[99] Caldecott, K. W. (2003) DNA single-strand break repair and spinocerebellar ataxia, *Cell112*, 7-10.

[100] Takagi M, Ueda JY, Hwang JH, Hashimoto J, Izumikawa M, Murakami H, Sekido Y, and Shin-ya K. (2012) Tyrosyl-DNA phosphodiesterase 1 inhibitor from an anamorphic fungus, 75, 764-767.

INDEX

A

Michelle Prudhomme (Ed)

B

C

D

G

J

K

L

M

N

O

P

R

S

T

U

V

W

X

Made in United States
Orlando, FL
04 November 2026

90205811R00297